Dynamic Pathways to Recovery from Alcohol Use Disorder

Alcohol use disorder is by far the most prevalent substance use disorder in the general population and is a major contributor to disease worldwide. Recovery from the disorder is a dynamic process of change, and individuals take many different routes to resolve their alcohol problems within their search to achieve a life worth living. Total abstention is not the only solution, and robust recovery involves more than changing drinking practices. This volume brings together multidisciplinary research on recovery processes, contexts, and outcomes, as well as new ideas about the multiple pathways involved. Experts chart the individual, social, contextual, community, economic, regulatory, policy, and structural influences that are vital to understanding alcohol use disorder and recovery. The book recommends new approaches to conceptualizing and assessing recovery alongside new avenues for research, community engagement, and policy that constitute a major shift in the practice and policy landscape.

JALIE A. TUCKER is Professor of Health Education and Behavior and Director of the Center for Behavioral Economic Health Research at the University of Florida, USA. Her numerous awards include the Betty Ford Award from the Association for Medical Education and Research in Substance Abuse.

KATIE WITKIEWITZ is Regents' Professor of Psychology at the University of New Mexico, USA, and Director of the Addictive Behaviors and Quantitative Research Laboratory. She has received numerous awards, including a Presidential Citation from the American Psychological Association for early career contributions.

Dynamic Pathways to Recovery from Alcohol Use Disorder

Meaning and Methods

Edited by

Jalie A. Tucker

University of Florida

Katie Witkiewitz

University of New Mexico

CAMBRIDGE
UNIVERSITY PRESS

CAMBRIDGE
UNIVERSITY PRESS

University Printing House, Cambridge CB2 8BS, United Kingdom

One Liberty Plaza, 20th Floor, New York, NY 10006, USA

477 Williamstown Road, Port Melbourne, VIC 3207, Australia

314–321, 3rd Floor, Plot 3, Splendor Forum, Jasola District Centre, New Delhi – 110025, India

103 Penang Road, #05–06/07, Visioncrest Commercial, Singapore 238467

Cambridge University Press is part of the University of Cambridge.

It furthers the University's mission by disseminating knowledge in the pursuit of education, learning, and research at the highest international levels of excellence.

www.cambridge.org
Information on this title: www.cambridge.org/9781108838719
DOI: 10.1017/9781108976213

First published 2022

A catalogue record for this publication is available from the British Library.

Library of Congress Cataloging-in-Publication Data
Names: Tucker, Jalie A. (Jalie Ann), 1954- editor. | Witkiewitz, Katie, editor.
Title: Dynamic pathways to recovery from alcohol use disorder : meaning and methods / edited by Jalie A. Tucker, University of Florida, Katie Witkiewitz, University of New Mexico.
Description: Cambridge, United Kingdom ; New York, NY : Cambridge University Press, 2022. | Includes bibliographical references and index.
Identifiers: LCCN 2021020782 (print) | LCCN 2021020783 (ebook) | ISBN 9781108838719 (hardback) | ISBN 9781108972260 (paperback) | ISBN 9781108976213 (epub)
Subjects: LCSH: Alcoholism–Relapse–Prevention. | Alcoholics–Rehabilitation.
Classification: LCC HV5275 .D93 2022 (print) | LCC HV5275 (ebook) | DDC 362.292/8–dc23
LC record available at https://lccn.loc.gov/2021020782
LC ebook record available at https://lccn.loc.gov/2021020783

ISBN 978-1-108-83871-9 Hardback
ISBN 978-1-108-97226-0 Paperback

To G. Alan Marlatt, our mentor and muse (JAT & KW)
To my son, who found his recovery pathway (JAT)

Contents

PART III Macro Level: Creating Environments, Resources, Incentives, and Policies to Promote Harm Reduction and Recovery

Conclusions and Future Directions

Figures

Tables

Contributors

SAMUEL F. ACUFF, MS, Department of Psychology, University of Memphis, Memphis, Tennessee, United States

ROBERT D. ASHFORD, PhD, MSW, Substance Use Disorders Institute, University of the Sciences in Philadelphia, Philadelphia, Pennsylvania, United States

MARSHA E. BATES, PhD, Department of Kinesiology and Health and Center of Alcohol & Substance Use Studies, Rutgers University – New Brunswick, New Jersey, United States

KARA BENSLEY, PhD, MSc, Department of Public Health, Bastyr University, Seattle, Washington, United States

MEREDITH S. BERRY, PhD, Department of Health Education and Behavior, Department of Psychology, and Center for Behavioral Economic Health Research, University of Florida, Gainesville, Florida, United States

DAVID BEST, PhD, Department of Criminology, University of Derby, Derby, United Kingdom

LOVELLA BLACK BEAR, Downtown Emergency Service Center, Seattle, Washington, United States

THOMAS BRITTON, BA, Center of Alcohol and Substance Use Studies and the Graduate School of Applied and Professional Psychology, Rutgers, The State University of New Jersey, Piscataway, New Jersey, United States

COLIN BOULTER, BA, Center of Alcohol and Substance Use Studies and Graduate School of Applied and Professional Psychology, Rutgers, The State University of New Jersey, Piscataway, New Jersey, United States

ALICE BOWEN, MSc, King's College London, London, United Kingdom

SARAH BOWEN, PhD, School of Professional Psychology, Pacific University, Hillsboro, Oregon, United States

DELISA G. BROWN, PhD, Department of Psychiatry and Behavioral Sciences, Medical University of South Carolina, Charleston, South Carolina, United States

JENNIFER F. BUCKMAN, PhD, Department of Kinesiology and Health and Center of Alcohol & Substance Use Studies, Rutgers University – New Brunswick, New Jersey, United States

JEEWON CHEONG, PhD, Department of Health Education and Behavior and Center for Behavioral Economic Health Research, University of Florida, Gainesville, Florida, United States

SEEMA L. CLIFASEFI, PhD, MSW, Department of Psychiatry and Behavioral Sciences, University of Washington, Seattle, Washington, United States

SUSAN E. COLLINS, PhD, Department of Psychology, Washington State University, Pullman, Washington, United States

ASHLEY A. DENNHARDT, PhD, Department of Psychology, University of Memphis, Memphis, Tennessee, United States

MICHAEL L. DENNIS, PhD, Chestnut Health Systems, Normal, Illinois, United States

NOAH N. EMERY, PhD, Department of Psychology, Colorado State University, Fort Collins, Colorado, United States

EMERY FRICK, BA, Center of Alcohol and Substance Use Studies and Graduate School of Applied and Professional Psychology, Rutgers, The State University of New Jersey, Piscataway, New Jersey, United States

MELANIE GETTY, Aurora Project, London, United Kingdom

KATHRYN S. GEX, MS, Department of Psychology, University of Memphis, Memphis, Tennessee, United States

KEVIN A. HALLGREN, PhD, Behavioral Research in Technology and Engineering Center, Department of Psychiatry and Behavioral Sciences, University of Washington, Seattle, Washington, United States

CHARLOTTE HARGREAVES, PhD, Department of Criminology, University of Derby, Derby, United Kingdom

PHILIP HODGSON, PhD, Department of Criminology, University of Derby, Derby, United Kingdom

CASANDRA HOGAN, Create Recovery, London, United Kingdom

BRADY P. HORN, PhD, Department of Economics and Center for Alcohol, Substance use, And Addictions, University of New Mexico, Albuquerque, New Mexico, United States

AMBER M. JARNECKE, PhD, Department of Psychiatry and Behavioral Sciences, Medical University of South Carolina, Charleston, South Carolina, United States

WILLIAM C. KERR, PhD, Alcohol Research Group, Public Health Institute, Emeryville, California, United States

KAAN KIDEYS, BA, Center of Alcohol and Substance Use Studies and Graduate School of Applied and Professional Psychology, Rutgers, The State University of New Jersey, Piscataway, New Jersey, United States

HEDY KOBER, PhD, Yale University School of Medicine, New Haven, Connecticut, United States

THE LEAP COMMUNITY ADVISORY BOARD, Downtown Emergency Service Center, Seattle, Washington, United States

JUHAN LEE, PhD, Yale University School of Medicine, New Haven, Connecticut, United States

MATTHEW R. LEE, PhD, Center of Alcohol and Substance Use Studies and Graduate School of Applied and Professional Psychology, Rutgers, The State University of New Jersey, Piscataway, New Jersey, United States

PAUL LENNON, Aurora Project, London, United Kingdom

YIMEI LI, MA, Center of Alcohol and Substance Use Studies and Graduate School of Applied and Professional Psychology, Rutgers, The State University of New Jersey, Piscataway, New Jersey, United States

ASHLEY N. LINDEN-CARMICHAEL, PhD, Edna Bennett Pierce Prevention Research Center, Pennsylvania State University, University Park, Pennsylvania, United States

ELLE LONG, Mindwave Ventures, London, United Kingdom

STEPHEN A. MAISTO, PhD, Department of Psychology, Syracuse University, Syracuse, New York, United States

ALEXANDER J. MELKONIAN, PhD, Department of Psychiatry and Behavioral Sciences, Medical University of South Carolina, and the Ralph H. Johnson Veterans Administration Medical Center, Charleston, South Carolina, United States

WILLIAM R. MILLER, PhD, Department of Psychology and Center for Alcohol, Substance use, And Addictions, University of New Mexico, Albuquerque, New Mexico, United States

JAMES G. MURPHY, PhD, Department of Psychology, University of Memphis, Memphis, Tennessee, United States

JOANNE NEALE, PhD, King's College London, London, United Kingdom

DAVID PATTON, PhD, Department of Criminology, University of Derby, Derby, United Kingdom

MATTHEW R. PEARSON, PhD, Center on Alcohol, Substance use, And Addictions, University of New Mexico, Albuquerque, New Mexico, United States

JULIANNE L. PRICE, PhD, Department of Kinesiology and Health and Center of Alcohol & Substance Use Studies, Rutgers University – New Brunswick, New Jersey, United States

COREY R. ROOS, PhD, Yale University School of Medicine, New Haven, Connecticut, United States

JENNA SAVIANO, BA, Center of Alcohol and Substance Use Studies and Graduate School of Applied and Professional Psychology, Rutgers, The State University of New Jersey, Piscataway, New Jersey, United States

LAURA SCHMIDT, PhD, MSW, MPH, Philip R. Lee Institute for Health Policy Studies and Department of Humanities and Social Sciences, School of Medicine, University of California, San Francisco, California, United States

FRANK J. SCHWEBEL, PhD, Center on Alcohol, Substance use, And Addictions, University of New Mexico, Albuquerque, New Mexico, United States

CHRISTY K. SCOTT, PhD, Chestnut Health Systems, Chicago, Illinois, United States

KENNETH J. SHER, PhD, Department of Psychological Sciences, University of Missouri, Columbia, Columbia, Missouri, United States

CLAIRE SNELL-ROOD, PhD, School of Public Health, University of California, Berkeley, Berkeley, California, United States

DOUGLAS STEINLEY, PhD, Department of Psychological Sciences, University of Missouri, Columbia, Columbia, Missouri, United States

SIR JOHN STRANG, MBBS, FRCPsych, FRCP, MD, FMedSci, National Addiction Center, King's College London, London, United Kingdom

SAMUEL W. STULL, MS, Department of Biobehavioral Health, Pennsylvania State University, University Park, Pennsylvania, United States

MEENAKSHI S. SUBBARAMAN, PhD, Alcohol Research Group, Public Health Institute, Emeryville, California, United States

J. SCOTT TONIGAN, PhD, Center on Alcohol, Substance use, And Addictions, University of New Mexico, Albuquerque, New Mexico, United States

JALIE A. TUCKER, PhD, MPH, Department of Health Education and Behavior and Center for Behavioral Economic Health Research, University of Florida, Gainesville, Florida, United States

GROVER "WILL" WILLIAMS, Downtown Emergency Service Center, Seattle, Washington, United States

ADAM D. WILSON, PhD, Department of Psychology and Center on Alcohol, Substance use, And Addictions, University of New Mexico, Albuquerque, New Mexico, United States

KATIE WITKIEWITZ, PhD, Department of Psychology and Center on Alcohol, Substance use, And Addictions, University of New Mexico, Albuquerque, New Mexico, United States

ALI M. YURASEK, PhD, Department of Health Education and Behavior and Center for Behavioral Economic Health Research, University of Florida, Gainesville, Florida, United States

YIHONG ZHAO, PhD, Center of Alcohol and Substance Use Studies and Graduate School of Applied and Professional Psychology, Rutgers, The State University of New Jersey, Piscataway, New Jersey, United States

Foreword

Alcohol use disorder (AUD) abounds around the world, and most people who recover (as most indeed do) never receive help from formal treatment or mutual help groups. For most of those who do seek specialist care, their recovery began long before the first treatment contact and continues long afterward. Understanding recovery requires a wide perspective, and that is exactly what this book offers. It spans international contexts, professional and lived experience, biology and economics, clinical and research expertise, and vistas ranging from micro to macro.

I am personally pleased that our field's purview has broadened from treatment to recovery. Whatever clinical services people may receive comprise a very small amount of time within their lifespan. Neither treatment nor recovery is an event, but rather a process that unfolds over time. Treatment for addiction has so often been thought of as an acute episode after which the case is closed, but recovery is developmental and evolving. Like AUD, recovery is not binary: present or absent. It encompasses physical and mental health, social functioning, well-being, and spirituality. Aristotle observed that one swallow or one day does not make a summer, and a drink does not terminate recovery. It is a moment in a life story.

The addiction field has been more generally plagued by dichotomous thinking, often with a moralistic good/bad overtone. Urine samples (and by implication, people) are "clean" or "dirty." Based on an arbitrary cut-off point on a continuum of severity, people are classified as having or not having a disorder. We talk about "success rates" – a concept seldom used in managing chronic conditions like diabetes or hypertension. The concept of relapse is dishonestly binary as well, implying that there are only two possible outcomes: perfection or disaster. In fact, recovery outcomes vary all along a number of continuous dimensions. In AUD treatment samples, about one in four people abstain for at least a year, a discouraging "failure rate," but among the rest alcohol consumption decreases by 86 percent on average with improved health and functioning. Better to broaden the horizon beyond seeing only day or night to appreciate the richly varied hues of recovery.

This book was completed during the COVID-19 pandemic, affording an apt parallel for conceptualizing both the scope and the resolution of AUD. Those with severe symptoms represented a small minority of all who contracted the virus. Mortality was only about 2 percent on average but with the sheer scope of the pandemic the numbers grew to tragic and almost unimaginable proportions. There were health disparities for people of color. For some, recovery with or without treatment was relatively rapid whereas other survivors suffered long-term complications. Containing the pandemic required a perspective far broader than treating individual cases, and misinformation hobbled prevention.

This volume offers a fresh array of lenses through which to understand recovery. You can try them on much as an optometrist flips through lenses in search of clear resolution. For scientists there is a rich array of methodology for future research. There are interventions and levels of analysis for individuals, families, social contingencies, and communities. It is a suitable menu of perspectives within a public health understanding of AUD. Sample your accustomed areas of interest, and also venture into what are for you less familiar offerings. It's a rich feast.

William R. Miller, Ph.D.
University of New Mexico

Preface

Based on 50 years of research, the alcohol field has shifted from a monolithic abstinence-oriented view of alcohol problems, treatment approaches, and recovery pathways to a pluralistic view that recognizes the heterogeneous, multi-dimensional nature of these central features of alcohol use disorder (AUD). Positive change is a dynamic process that occurs over time and ranges from reduced alcohol use and associated problems to abstinence and improved functioning and well-being. Although extant recovery definitions vary with respect to the emphasis placed on abstinence, consensus has emerged that successful recovery is broader than beneficial reductions in drinking practices and entails improvements in health, functioning, and well-being. Most individuals who develop an AUD or have sub-clinical problems eventually reduce their risky drinking practices and experience AUD symptom reduction, and some will further achieve and maintain "recovery," broadly defined as encompassing improved health, well-being, and life circumstances.

This edited book assembles chapters by leading experts whose work informs the current state of knowledge concerning pathways to recovery from AUD, which are diverse and dynamic in nature. The book gathers together knowledge about AUD recovery offered by multiple disciplines and stakeholder groups, including alcohol researchers, service providers, policy-makers, mutual help groups, and persons with AUD. In line with this expanded view of recovery pathways, the book is organized using a socio-ecological model of influences on health and well-being that range from individual to social and community to regulatory, policy, and structural influences. Chapters present recovery research that ranges from micro to meso to macro approaches to understanding, investigating, and promoting positive behavior change and improved well-being. Historically, the bulk of work on recovery was conducted from an individual, often clinical perspective, with emphasis on promoting abstinence. While these contributions are present in the book, additional chapters cover topics that broaden the domains of potential contextual influence to include social, community, economic, and structural variables. The book also extends the focus of assessment in recovery research to include changes in functioning, life circumstances, and well-being, in addition to drinking practices. Chapters on methodologies that have utility for the different levels of investigation are also included and present illustrative examples from AUD research. Methodology chapters are written for researchers who may consider using the methods and are not necessarily expert methodologists.

Following an introductory chapter that summarizes historical and contemporary views of AUD recovery, the book is divided into three main sections organized around micro, meso, and macro levels of analysis. Each section includes substantive content chapters followed by chapters on methodologies useful for research within each level of analysis.

The micro level chapters share a focus on the individual as change agent, the dominant view of much clinical research and practice. The five content chapters cover individual level research in relevant domains, including biopsychosocial processes of change in AUD recovery (Witkiewitz & Maisto), self-regulation strategies in recovery (Roos, Bowen, & Kober), neuropsychological and biological influences on drinking behavior change (Bates, Price, & Buckman), lifespan developmental perspectives on recovery mechanisms (Lee, Zhao, Britton, Saviano, Kideys, Li, Boulter, Frick, & Sher), and mutual help approaches and mechanisms of change (Tonigan). Two methodology chapters describe quantitative methods useful in micro level research on AUD recovery processes and outcomes, including time-varying effect modeling (Linden-Carmichael, Stull, Scott, & Dennis) and latent variable mixture modeling (Cheong, Wilson, & Lee). Taken together, these chapters contribute to a broader understanding of how individual behaviors and biopsychosocial processes associated with individual behavior change may interact to dynamically influence AUD recovery processes over time.

The meso level chapters share a focus on understanding and promoting individual behavior change within the natural environments in which change occurs across the spectrum of problem severity from mild to moderate to serious. Although the meso level chapters focus on individual change, they move beyond an exclusive focus on the minority of affected persons who seek treatment and consider broader contextual influences on beneficial change in alcohol-related and alcohol-free behavior patterns. The four content chapters variously cover patterns, contexts, and the behavioral economics of natural recovery from AUD, the dominant pathway in the population with problems (Tucker); individual behavioral interventions to incentivize sobriety and enrich the natural environment with appealing alternatives to drinking (Murphy, Dennhardt, & Gex); family and social processes in AUD recovery (Jarnecke, Brown, & Melkonian); and community-based harm reduction approaches for AUD (Collins, Clifasefi, Williams, Black Bear, & The LEAP Community Advisory Board). Three methodology chapters describe assessment tools and quantitative methods useful in meso level research on AUD recovery, including mobile technology to understand and improve recovery (Pearson, Emery, & Schwebel), quantitative methods for measuring and modeling social network data in studies of recovery in social context (Hallgren), and measures assessing substance use contexts and substance-free reinforcement (Yurasek, Acuff, & Berry). Collectively, these chapters contribute to a broader understanding of the economic, social, and other contextual features that promote recovery within the environments in which individuals seek to change.

The macro level chapters move beyond concern with directly influencing individual behavior change and share a focus on understanding and creating environments, resources, incentives, and policies to promote harm reduction and recovery. Four content chapters describe recovery communities, resources, settings, and "recovery capital" (Best, Hargreaves, Hodgson, & Patton); disparities in alcohol treatment access in rural areas and opportunities for change (Snell-Rood, Bensley, & Schmidt); recovery-oriented systems of care and the organized recovery movement (Ashford); and alcohol control policy and regulations to promote AUD recovery (Kerr & Subbaraman). Three methodology chapters variously describe causal inference approaches to studying recovery (Steinley), a community-academic collaboration to design a mobile application ("SURE Recovery") for use by people experiencing alcohol and drug problems (Bowen, Getty, Hogan, Lennon, Long, Strang, & Neale) and economic methods to evaluate AUD recovery programs including outcome domains and policy issues (Horn). Together, these chapters contextualize micro and meso level influences on recovery within broader macro environments spanning community organizations and resources, treatment accessibility, economic factors, and drug-related policies.

The chapter authors comprise a diverse multi-disciplinary group of experts on their chapter topic who range from very senior to rising scholars in the field. Their collective body of work covers established and new knowledge about AUD recovery from multiple perspectives and levels of analysis and will guide the path forward for recovery research and application. In our final concluding chapter (Witkiewitz & Tucker), we revisit chapter material and conceptualizations of recovery, identify and describe key measurement domains, and identify unresolved issues and directions for future research. Based on the latest research and topics discussed throughout the book, our main conclusion is that the field is at a critical turning point for understanding and supporting AUD recovery. After nearly a century focused on abstinence as the only possible path to recovery, the broader research, treatment, community, and policy landscape has started to consider extending definitions of recovery to include alternative pathways and a conceptualization of recovery as outlined in the introductory chapter of the book. Correspondingly, new research, assessment, analysis, and community engagement methods are needed to capture nuanced changes in life-health functioning and the dynamic contextual and multilevel influences that will support heterogeneous recovery pathways.

Consistent with the diverse chapter authors and scope of topics, the book is intended for a similarly broad readership, including addiction scholars and practitioners as well as trainees ranging from advanced undergraduates to graduate students to post-doctoral fellows. Given current emphasis on the delivery of evidence-based AUD services, a volume that compiles established and cutting edge findings on how to understand and promote recovery should be useful for clinical and public health practitioners, health care administrators, policy-makers, legal and drug court personnel, and other professionals who are not addiction scholars and contribute in other vital ways to addressing the societal harm and cost of AUD. However, this book is not directly focused on treatments for AUD and other addictive disorders, about which many books have been written. Far fewer academic texts have been written about recovery, and nearly all of them focus on recovery at the individual level typically in the context of treatment or mutual help group participation. Very few present multi-disciplinary and multi-level scientific approaches to understanding and promoting recovery, and none explicitly cover methodologies important for advancing recovery research.

Overall, the book is intended to advance understanding and empirical work on recovery from an expanded perspective that includes multiple levels of analysis spanning individual to contextual to policy levels and broadens the domains of assessment important for understanding and promoting recovery. The book seeks to represent the best of current scientific work on recovery grounded in the practical realities of reaching persons with AUD for service delivery. In contrast to longstanding views that emphasize the chronic nature of AUD and the essential role of treatment and sustained abstinence in recovery, our hope is to change the narrative to highlight the high likelihood of recovery among both treated and untreated persons with AUD, the importance of achieving improvements in valued areas of living in addition to changing drinking practices, and the overarching importance of helping persons with AUD find a recovery pathway that appeals to and works for them. There are many such pathways, and our recovery-relevant theories, treatments, education, and policies need to be revised accordingly.

Acknowledgments

We share a common scientist-practitioner and clinical scientist heritage and a longstanding interest in understanding the forces that shape the development and resolution of alcohol-related problems. We have had the privilege of learning from pioneering scientist-practitioners in the alcohol field, including Mark and Linda Sobell, G. Alan Marlatt, and William R. Miller, who posed and made great advances in addressing big picture questions of enduring significance and centrality: Who recovers and who relapses, what is the role of treatment in promoting recovery, what individual characteristics and extra-therapeutic factors help or hinder progress, and how do we characterize and serve the heterogeneity of pathways to positive change that span treatment-assisted and natural recovery and involve outcomes other than sustained abstinence from alcohol?

This book builds on their seminal work and is aimed at the heart of the matter: Who recovers, how do they do it, and how do we investigate and promote it? We stepped away from the longstanding pathology-oriented view of alcohol use disorder and addiction that focuses on problem severity, symptom reduction, abstinence, and preventing relapse; and moved towards a strength-based view that expands the definition of recovery to encompass improvements in functioning, health, life circumstances, and well-being. Early behavioral conceptions of alcohol-related problems included the latter focus, but it has received short shrift in the decades since the 1970s. We argue that the field has matured sufficiently to tackle these issues directly and to reframe recovery as a dynamic process that moves people towards a life worth living and involves myriad changes other than stopping drinking.

We are indebted to these pioneers and other basic and applied behavioral and public health scientists who laid the groundwork for this shift. We also thank the National Institute of Alcohol Abuse and Alcoholism for their research support over the years, and the University of Florida for providing J.A.T. with a sabbatical leave in the Fall of 2019 at the University of New Mexico and Center on Alcohol, Substance use, And Addictions. This gave us the gift of time to develop the book prospectus and was an uncommon opportunity for creativity and collaboration in a natural setting that inspires big thinking. The writing itself was done during the first year of the tragic COVID-19 pandemic. Several of our contributors endured losses, and most had significant hardships of one kind or another. But this is a resilient, thoughtful, and caring group of expert contributors, and their chapters collectively offer the field a rich multi-disciplinary roadmap forward to understand and promote the many pathways to recovery from alcohol use disorder.

Introduction

1 Historical and Contemporary Perspectives on Pathways to Recovery from Alcohol Use Disorder

Jalie A. Tucker and Katie Witkiewitz

Historical and Contemporary Perspectives on Pathways to Recovery from Alcohol Use Disorder

Substance use disorders (SUD) are among the most prevalent mental health disorders worldwide. Alcohol is the most commonly used substance and contributes to 5 percent of the global burden of disease (World Health Organization [WHO], 2018). Globally, it has been estimated that over 100.4 million people meet current criteria for an alcohol use disorder (AUD; GBD 2016 Alcohol and Drug Use Collaborators, 2018), and many more persons engage in risky drinking or experience negative consequences related to drinking that fall short of clinical diagnostic criteria. Thus, alcohol use is a major public health problem associated with enormous social and economic costs (US National Institute on Alcohol Abuse & Alcoholism [NIAAA], 2020).

Despite the ubiquity and burden of risky alcohol use and AUD, most individuals who develop an AUD or have subclinical problems will eventually reduce or resolve their problem (Dawson et al., 2005, 2007; Fan et al., 2019; Kelly et al., 2017; Sobell et al., 1996). This contrasts with long-held views of alcohol problems as chronic and intractable and is based on evidence from many sources including epidemiological surveys, prospective observational studies, and randomized clinical trials of patients with AUD (Tucker et al., 2020; Witkiewitz et al., 2020). Many will reduce risky drinking practices and experience AUD symptom reduction, and some will further achieve and maintain "recovery." Although different stakeholders (e.g., researchers, government agencies, service providers, mutual help groups, and persons with AUD) have defined recovery somewhat differently, most definitions emphasize improvements in health, functioning, and well-being. The extent to which definitions focus on reductions in risky drinking practices or require abstinence is more variable.

Scientific work on AUD recovery is maturing and has propelled a shift from a monolithic abstinence-oriented view of alcohol problems, treatment approaches, and recovery pathways to a pluralistic view that recognizes the heterogeneous, multidimensional nature of these central features of AUD. This chapter describes historical and contemporary perspectives and empirical findings concerning the multiple pathways to alcohol problem reduction and AUD recovery, including illustrative research on the epidemiology of recovery and longitudinal studies of drinking behavior change in different populations. The chapter concludes with consideration of the research, practice, and public health implications of revised views of beneficial behavior change across the AUD severity spectrum that are grounded in scientific evidence.

Historical Views and Definitions of Recovery

Concerns with how to enjoy drinking in moderation while guarding against the harms of excessive consumption were core issues in early medical approaches to managing chronic inebriation that continue in contemporary definitions of recovery and approaches to promoting it. In the late 1700s, American physician Benjamin Rush (1785) wrote about potential remedies for "curing the ardent use of spirits on the body and mind." He viewed abstinence from distilled spirits as critical but allowed for consumption of larger quantities of beer or wine as a temporary substitute for liquor. This very early harm reduction approach contrasts with later approaches epitomized by the Temperance Movement during the nineteenth and early twentieth centuries, which focused on eradicating alcohol use through alcohol education and legal prohibition of alcohol sales that failed as an alcohol control strategy.

Founded in the 1930s, Alcoholics Anonymous (AA) offered a mutual help program defined by 12 steps in the recovery process of achieving and maintaining lifelong abstinence that continues to influence many modern concepts of recovery and treatment approaches. However, the "Big Book" of AA (1939) also made clear that abstinence was not sufficient to define recovery and described recovery as a lifelong journey involving transformative changes that lead to improved health, functioning, and well-being. In the mid-twentieth century, Jellinek (1960) formalized the concept of "alcoholism" as a progressive chronic disease with several variants or "species," including "gamma alcoholics" who were unable to limit their drinking and for whom lifelong abstinence was essential. Edwards and Gross (1976) refined the disease concept by developing the "alcohol dependence syndrome," defined as a narrowing of the drinking repertoire, increased salience of the need to drink over competing needs and responsibilities, tolerance and withdrawal symptoms, and reinstatement of dependence after abstinence. Thus, early modern work was heavily influenced by AA, and abstinence achieved through treatment or AA participation was widely considered critical for recovery until the late twentieth century.

In the late 1970s, Pattison, M. B. Sobell, and L. C. Sobell (1977) advanced a reconceptualization of alcohol dependence that remains influential today. They described alcohol dependence as a serious health problem and emphasized a "continuum from non-pathological to severely pathological problem development" that "follows variable patterns over time and does not necessarily proceed inexorably to severe fatal stages." Further, "[r]ecovery ... bears no necessary relation to abstinence, although such a concurrence is frequently the case" (pp. 4–5). This framework influenced behavior therapy research and practice from the 1970s to the present and generated evidence-based AUD treatments in use today, including relapse prevention, motivational interviewing, reinforcement-based treatments, and cognitive-behavioral therapy.

The Sobells also conducted treatment research that showed a subset of inpatients with severe alcohol dependence maintained controlled (i.e., moderate or low-risk) drinking for several years after treatment, a finding that ignited controversy by challenging the view that recovery required lifelong abstinence (1995). Their findings concerning moderation have since been widely replicated and extended (Tucker et al., 2020a). Although criteria for low- versus high-risk drinking vary across studies and countries (Furtwængler & De Visser, 2013), low-risk drinking among persons previously diagnosed with AUD is firmly established as a favorable outcome in addition to abstinence.

Concurrent with the controlled drinking controversy, research emerged on "natural" recovery in the absence of treatment. Vaillant's (1996) pioneering longitudinal study of the "natural history of alcoholism" indicated that some individuals with AUD could recover without treatment. Room (1977) reviewed then segregated research on recovery observed in population surveys and clinical studies and wrote about the "two worlds of alcohol problems." Whereas clinical researchers studied relatively homogeneous samples of treatment seekers with severe AUD, survey researchers studied population rates of alcohol use, AUD, and remission. Surveys revealed the variable nature of problem severity and the substantial remission of risky drinking and AUD, often without treatment, that was largely hidden from clinical researchers. As discussed later, bridging these bodies of work is fundamental to understanding and promoting reduction in alcohol-related problems across clinical and nonclinical populations.

Contemporary Views and Definitions of Recovery

Current literature includes four somewhat overlapping approaches to defining recovery: (1) remission of symptoms included in clinical diagnostic schemes for AUD; (2) cessation of risky drinking, typically defined as sustained abstinence; (3) comprehensive definitions that focus on improved functioning and well-being; and (4) views of recovery among persons with AUD. Research has favored the first two approaches because they provide quantifiable, albeit limited, measures of improvement. The second two approaches are more comprehensive concerning the scope of changes important for recovery, but their measurement is less well developed. A challenge at hand is expanding recovery research beyond drinking and symptom reduction to include a focus on improved well-being.

Clinical Diagnosis of AUD and Remission

The American Psychiatric Association (APA) and the WHO offer clinical diagnostic systems used, respectively, within and outside the United States. The *APA Diagnostic and Statistical Manual*, 5th edition (DSM-5; 2013), defines AUD based on meeting criteria for 2 or more of 11 symptoms in the past 12 months that fall within 4 clusters: physiological correlates of alcohol use ((1) tolerance, (2) craving, (3) symptoms of withdrawal); loss of control over alcohol use ((4) drinking longer or larger amounts than intended, (5) unsuccessful efforts to cut down or control drinking); alcohol taking over other meaningful activities ((6) time spent in activities related to alcohol, (7) other activities given up because of alcohol); and problems resulting from alcohol use ((8) failure to fulfill role obligations, (9) social or interpersonal problems, (10) physical or psychological problems, (11) use in situations that are physically hazardous). "Remission" from AUD is defined based on the length of time that symptoms other than craving are no longer present, including early (>3 months and <12 months) and sustained (>12 months) remission.

The *WHO International Classification of Diseases*, 10th edition (ICD-10; 1992) defines alcohol dependence based on having 2 or more of 6 symptoms in the past 12 months, including (1) tolerance; (2) craving; (3) physiological withdrawal; (4) loss of control over drinking; (5) drinking taking over other activities; and (6) problems resulting from alcohol use. Later supplements and revisions included early and sustained remission codes identical to the DSM-5 or reduced the number of core features defining AUD.

Thus, DSM-5 bases remission on not meeting symptoms of the disorder and is silent about alcohol consumption. The ICD schemes require abstinence for full remission, whereas partial remission requires reductions in drinking and the absence of symptoms.

Cessation of Risky Drinking

The large alcohol treatment outcome literature has relied heavily on drinking practices as an outcome metric, typically using NIAAA (2005, 2020) quantity–frequency criteria considered indicative of higher-risk drinking (any occasions of >14 drinks weekly or >5 drinks daily for men; >7 drinks weekly or >4 drinks daily for women in the past year). However, as discussed in Witkiewitz and Tucker (2020), such consumption-based thresholds lack sensitivity and specificity for predicting problems related to drinking and do not differentiate individuals based on measures of health, functioning, and well-being. Moreover, risk of AUD continues to increase above the 4+/5+ cut-points through approximately 10 drinks for women and 11 drinks for men (Linden-Carmichael et al., 2019). Cut-points also ignore the influence of weight, sex, and health status in determining effects of different levels of drinking (Pearson et al., 2016). They also ignore the temporal patterning and manner of drinking over time that can contribute to risk and recovery; e.g., excessive infrequent drinking has been associated with greater risk than stable levels of heavy alcohol consumption (Grønbaek, 2009).

On balance, risky drinking cut-points may be useful for screening for AUD risk in general and medical populations. But in isolation, they do not offer a useful dimension to characterize AUD severity and are insufficient to characterize risk reduction during a recovery attempt.

Stakeholder Definitions of Recovery

In contrast to this limited focus on drinking practices, recent recovery definitions advanced by key stakeholders emphasize the importance of functioning, health, and well-being in defining recovery. For example, the Betty Ford Consensus Panel (2007) defined recovery as "a voluntarily maintained lifestyle characterized by sobriety, personal health, and citizenship" (p. 222). The US Substance Abuse and Mental Health Administration (SAMHSA, 2011) defined recovery as "a process of change through which individuals improve their health and wellness, live a self-directed life, and strive to reach their full potential." Abstinence is cited as one avenue to achieving improved health. In 2017, a Recovery Science Research Collaborative meeting convened by recovery researchers examined the concept of recovery based on a literature review and ideas generated by group members (Ashford et al., 2019). They concluded that "[r]ecovery is an individualized, intentional, dynamic, and relational process involving sustained efforts to improve wellness" in health, psychosocial, and functional domains (p. 5). The National Institute on Alcohol Abuse and Alcoholism (NIAAA, 2020) defined recovery as maintenance of remission from DSM-5 AUD symptoms and cessation from heavy drinking. They further noted that recovery often encompasses "fulfillment of basic needs, enhancements in social support and spirituality, and improvements in physical and mental health, quality of life, and other dimensions of well-being." Two additional categories defined by more limited improvements were remission from AUD symptoms as defined by DSM-5 criteria (excluding craving) or cessation from heavy drinking.

These stakeholder definitions focus on improved health, well-being, and functioning in areas adversely affected by drinking and do not emphasize or are silent about achieving abstinence. Similar to the Big Book of AA, abstinence, without improvement in functioning or well-being would not be considered recovery. These are similar to recovery definitions for other psychiatric disorders (e.g., schizophrenia, depression) that emphasize recovery of functioning and do not require the absence of symptoms, but differ from recovery definitions for health conditions (e.g., cancer) that require symptom reduction/elimination but do not require improved functioning and well-being.

Views of Recovery among Persons with AUD

Mixed methods research has identified recovery elements from the perspective of persons seeking to resolve AUD. Consistent with recent stakeholder definitions and quantitative research discussed later, elements involving improved well-being were generally endorsed to a greater extent than outcomes focused solely on level of substance use or absence of symptoms.

For example, Kaskutas et al. (2014) had over 9,000 persons self-identified as in recovery rate the extent to which specific elements belonged in their personal definition of recovery. A four-factor solution was found: (1) abstinence, (2) essentials of recovery (e.g., dealing with challenging negative feelings, realistic self-appraisal), (3) enriched recovery (e.g., self-care, inner peace, living a life that contributes to others and society), and (4) spirituality. Using the same data set, Witbrodt and colleagues (2015) identified five latent classes of recovery elements characterized as the following: (1) 12-step traditionalist, (2) 12-step enthusiast, (3) secular, (4) self-reliant, and (5) atypical. Those in the 12-step traditionalist and enthusiast classes were mostly abstinent and engaged in AA or other 12-step programs, whereas those in the secular, self-reliant, and atypical recovery classes were less likely to be abstinent or engaged in 12-step programs. Across all classes, commonly endorsed items were (1) being honest with myself, (2) handling negative feelings without using, (3) being able to enjoy life, and (4) growth and development. Similarly, Neale and colleagues (2016) developed a patient-reported outcome measure of recovery from drug and alcohol dependence, named the Substance Use Recovery Evaluator (SURE). Factor analyses yielded a five-factor solution: (1) substance use, (2) material resources, (3) outlook on life, (4) self-care, and (5) relationships.

Related work has focused on the role of social networks and social capital in recovery (Best et al., 2016; Granfield & Smith, 1999; Humphreys et al., 1999). Granfield and Smith (1999) introduced the concept of "recovery capital" in the context of understanding and promoting natural recovery without treatment. They focused on building and using internal and external resources (e.g., social, physical, cultural, community) needed to initiate and sustain recovery, which is variable across individuals and changeable over time. Best and colleagues (2016) proposed that an individual's social identity shifts during recovery and becomes increasingly defined by the norms and behaviors of people in their lives who do not drink alcohol compared to those who do. This is consistent with research showing that higher rates of AA attendance are associated with greater rates of abstinence and with members reporting having more non-drinking friends (Humphreys et al., 1999).

Finally, it is important to acknowledge the term "recovery" is strongly associated with AA and similar mutual help groups. Although the term is widely used in clinical research and practice, many persons attempting to stop or reduce risky drinking do not identify with being in recovery (Kelly et al., 2017) and reject labels indicative of AUD, especially those attempting to resolve a drinking problem on their own (Sobell et al., 1996). Therefore, caution should be exercised when using the term recovery.

Empirical Research on AUD Recovery Rates, Patterns, and Outcomes

Studies of recovery-relevant patterns, processes, and outcomes include the following: (1) population surveys of large representative samples of drinkers that are cross-sectional or have short-term (e.g., 1 year) follow-ups, and (2) longitudinal studies with longer follow-ups that tend to employ smaller, less representative samples. Both approaches have methodological strengths and limitations. For example, of necessity, surveys typically employ brief measures that cannot assess recovery in the comprehensive manner described earlier, and the cross-sectional designs and brief follow-ups are poorly suited to investigate recovery as a dynamic behavior change process. Longitudinal research provides superior information about change processes and outcomes, but the follow-up intervals rarely exceed 3–5 years, although there are notable exceptions with follow-ups of 8–10 years or more (Brennan et al., 2011; Vaillant et al., 1996). Together, these two bodies of research reveal a coherent, complementary, and optimistic view of the extent, nature, and dynamics of positive drinking behavior change.

Epidemiology of Recovery and Relationships with Help-Seeking and Problem Severity

As reviewed by Tucker et al. (2020a), population surveys have consistently shown that most individuals who develop an AUD or have subclinical alcohol problems will reduce or resolve their problem on their own or with assistance from professional alcohol treatment or mutual help groups (e.g., Dawson et al., 2005, 2007; Fan et al., 2019; Kelly et al., 2017; Sobell et al., 1996). Specific improvement rates vary depending on the intervals over which drinking status was assessed (e.g., lifetime or shorter interval), how improvement or recovery/remission was measured, and participant problem severity, help-seeking, and demographic characteristics. The number of quit attempts before stable change is achieved is also variable; some persons succeed on the first attempt, while others require many tries (Kelly et al., 2019). But improvement over time is a robust finding, regardless of help-seeking status.

In contrast, seeking help for drinking problems is uncommon (SAMHSA, 2019). Most surveys indicate that less than 25 percent of persons in need utilize alcohol-focused helping resources from professional treatment or community and peer resources such as mutual help groups. Within the professional sector, care is dispersed through the mental health, medical, and community services systems, and only a minority receive alcohol-focused services from qualified professionals or programs (Kelly et al., 2017; SAMHSA, 2017). This remains the case even though alcohol services have improved and expanded considerably (SAMHSA, 2017; Tucker & Simpson, 2011) and yield benefits for most recipients. Mutual help groups have likewise expanded in focus and availability. In addition to AA, they include groups such as Self-Management and Recovery Training (SMART) Recovery (www.smartrecovery.org/) and LifeRing Secular Recovery (www.lifering.org/).

Among persons who resolve their drinking problems, the great majority do so without interventions. Surveys indicate that over 70 percent of problem resolutions occur outside the context of treatment, and stable, low-risk drinking is a relatively more common outcome in untreated than treated samples (Fan et al., 2019; Sobell et al., 1996). This is likely due in part to the stigma of alcohol and drug treatment participation, barriers to treatment availability (e.g., cost, accessibility, capacity limitations), and emphasis on abstinence in many treatment programs. As a result, treatment seeking is generally associated with higher problem severity (Fan et al., 2019), and individuals with more severe AUD appear to practice some degree of appropriate self-selection into treatment (Tuithof et al., 2016) and may require more change attempts before achieving stable change (Kelly et al., 2019). Nevertheless, characteristics and outcomes of treated and untreated samples overlap. Recoveries that involve abstinence or low-risk drinking are present in both, and some high-severity treatment seekers achieve recoveries involving low-risk drinking (Witkiewitz et al., 2019).

Fan and colleagues (2019) demonstrated these relationships between help-seeking, problem severity, and drinking-related outcomes using data from the 2012-2013 National Epidemiologic Survey on Alcohol and Related Conditions (NESARC-III; Grant et al., 2015). Respondents who met AUD criteria prior to the past year (n = 7785) were assessed with respect to their current (past year) status based on DSM-5 symptom counts and quantity-frequency criteria indicative of risky drinking. Only 22.8 percent reported any lifetime treatment utilization. Over the one-year timeframe of assessment, 34.2 percent had persistent AUD, whereas most respondents showed some improvement: Abstinence or low-risk drinking without symptoms was achieved by 16.0 percent and 17.9 percent, respectively, and asymptomatic low-risk drinking was more common among never treated (20.4 percent) than treated (9.7 percent) respondents. Also, the majority of treated respondents tended to belong to the persistent AUD (39.2 percent) or abstinent (30.4 percent) outcome groups that are generally associated with higher problem severity.

This illustrative survey, among others, reveals a more optimistic and variable view of recovery pathways and outcomes than suggested by early treatment research. Most affected individuals have less serious problems than the minority who seek treatment, and many improve on their own and maintain abstinence or low-risk drinking without problems.

Recovery across the Lifespan

As discussed in Tucker et al. (2020a), cross-sectional surveys and longitudinal research on age-related trends (Grant et al., 2015; Grucza et al., 2018; SAMHSA, 2019) generally show that alcohol use increases during adolescence and early adulthood and then decreases across the adult lifespan beginning in the mid-20s. Prevalence of past-year binge drinking (45 percent) and AUD (19 percent) are highest in the early 20s (Lee & Sher, 2018) and then decrease continuing well after early adulthood. This nonlinear trajectory, typically termed "maturing out," has been attributed to adult role transitions (e.g., employment, marriage, parenthood) and personal maturation (e.g., decreased impulsivity) common in early adulthood (Lee & Sher, 2018; Lee et al., 2018; Vergés et al., 2013). Treatment participation is uncommon (SAMHSA, 2019).

There are notable exceptions to this general trend. Some young adults who engage in risky alcohol use and develop AUD in early adulthood show persistent or escalating drinking problems in later life, and alcohol use before age 21 predicts persistence and severity of problems throughout the lifespan (Hingson et al., 2006). Nevertheless, reductions in problem drinking in early adulthood occur more often among individuals with the most severe problems at earlier ages (Lee et al., 2018). Development of AUD is less common after age 25, and reductions in problem drinking, including AUD recovery, continue past early adulthood through late middle and old age (60 to over 80 years) (Brennan et al., 2011; Lee et al., 2018). Reductions at older ages are predicted by relatively heavier alcohol use in early old age that prompted complaints from concerned others (Brennan et al., 2011).

Research that separated age-related associations between problem onset, remission, and recurrence rates also qualify this general lifespan trajectory (Lee & Sher, 2018; Lee et al., 2018; Vergés et al., 2013). In the NESARC surveys, rates of persistence of alcohol problems over time were relatively stable across ages 18 to 50 years and older, whereas rates of new problem onset and recurrence or relapse from earlier problems declined with age (Vergés et al., 2013). "Desistance" from moderate to severe AUD occurred among younger age groups (ages 25–29 and 30–34), whereas desistance rates from mild AUD were stable across age groups (Lee et al., 2018). Thus, resolution of severe AUD contributes heavily and distinctively to the prevalence of early adulthood remission. These different contributing processes further suggest that maturing out as young people assume adult roles is not a sufficient account of remission rates across the lifespan (Lee & Sher, 2018), and the variable age-related associations between problem onset, remission, and recurrence rates can guide the timing and targeting of interventions.

Finally, natural recoveries tend to occur in mid-life (Kelly et al., 2019; Sobell et al., 1996; Tucker et al., 2020b), which is also when alcohol treatment entry tends to occur (Dawson et al., 2005), typically a decade or more after problem recognition (Tucker & Simpson, 2011). Recovery in mid-life and later ages is associated with an accumulation of alcohol-related problems coupled with life contexts that support and reinforce reduced drinking and involve post-resolution improvements in functioning and well-being (Moos & Moos, 2007; Tucker et al., 2021). Nevertheless, a few studies observed increased binge drinking among middle-aged and older adults (e.g., Grucza et al., 2018), suggesting there may be dynamic mid-life changes that have not been well researched.

Role of Gender and Race/Ethnicity in Recovery and Help-Seeking

Studies of improvement rates by gender and race/ethnicity suggest that many observed differences involve variations in the timing and extent of reductions in binge drinking and AUD during either young adulthood or older age, even though all groups tend to show overall patterns similar to the population as a whole. For example, using NESARC-III data, Vasilenko et al. (2017) found that while AUD prevalence generally peaked in the 20s and declined steadily with age, prevalence was higher for White persons at younger ages and higher for Black persons at older ages. This cross-over pattern typically occurred around age 60. In mid-life, Black individuals and White individuals had similar prevalence of AUD. Also, White individuals reported higher AUD rates than Hispanic individuals at all ages, and men reported higher AUD rates than women until older age, when women were more likely than men to report AUD in their 70s.

Cohort effects in the age of peak binge drinking prevalence also have been observed. Based on drinking data from 27 cohorts of the annual Monitoring the Future surveys (1976–2004) (Patrick et al., 2019), women in more recent cohorts reported significantly higher binge drinking prevalence than women in earlier cohorts from ages 21 through 30, with risk remaining high throughout the 20s. The shifts toward older age of peak binge drinking prevalence signify extended risks in young adulthood, especially for women.

Sex differences are more apparent in help-seeking than in recovery patterns. Women have lower help-seeking rates than men even after controlling for the higher prevalence of AUD and greater problem severity among men (Gilbert et al., 2019; Zemore et al., 2014). With respect to race/ethnicity, White individuals are proportionately more likely to utilize alcohol services than Black and Hispanic individuals (Gilbert et al., 2019; SAMHSA, 2015; Zemore et al. 2009, 2014). For example, using pooled data from multiple waves of the national probability samples collected in the US National Alcohol Surveys, Zemore et al. (2009) found very low rates of lifetime service utilization among Latinx participants. A later study (Zemore et al., 2014) found lower service utilization among Latinx and Black individuals (vs. Whites) and women (vs. men). Overall, recovery research on race/ethnicity and help-seeking is not extensive, and groups other than White, Black, and Hispanic/Latinx individuals have not been well studied.

Prospective Studies of Recovery Outcomes in Different Populations

Quantitative recovery research ranging from treatment outcome to naturalistic observational studies examined changes in functioning and well-being (in addition to drinking practices) and found that pathways to recovery are heterogeneous and involve improved functioning and life circumstances. For example, using Project MATCH (1997) data, Witkiewitz and colleagues (2019) investigated patterns of longer term treatment outcomes in clinical trials targeting AUD. Three years after treatment, four outcome profiles were identified based on intensity and frequency of alcohol consumption and other indicators of health and well-being: (1) low functioning frequent heavy drinkers, (2) low functioning infrequent heavy drinkers, (3) high functioning occasional heavy drinkers, and (4) high functioning infrequent non-heavy drinkers. High functioning occasional heavy drinkers had lower baseline alcohol dependence severity, abstinence self-efficacy, and AA involvement compared to high functioning infrequent non-heavy drinkers, but did not differ on other measures of functioning. The high functioning occasional heavy drinkers also had significantly higher purpose in life compared to the two poor functioning profiles and had greater satisfaction with life compared to abstainers.

In prospective research that followed a community sample of drinkers for over 20 years, Moos and colleagues found that greater self-efficacy and friendship relationships, more negative events, less depression, and viewing drinking as a significant problem predicted long-term reductions in drinking (2007; Brennan et al., 2011). Any alcohol use did not predict long-term negative outcomes, but persistent average heavy drinking and heavy episodic drinking were each associated with greater problems related to alcohol use (Holahan, 2017).

Natural recovery research also highlights the role of life contexts and non-drinking behaviors on drinking outcomes. In a series of prospective studies guided by behavioral economics, Tucker and colleagues (2020b, 2021) followed individuals with AUD who had recently stopped heavy drinking without treatment for 1–2 years. Many participants maintained abstinence or low-risk drinking without problems throughout the follow-up, and those who maintained low-risk drinking were distinguished from other outcome groups by how they spent their money. Prior to stopping heavy drinking, participants who achieved stable low-risk drinking had more balanced allocations between spending on alcohol versus saving money for the future compared to those who abstained or relapsed and who had higher proportionate alcohol spending. After stopping, low-risk drinkers shifted their spending in unique ways that led to receipt of delayed large rewards (e.g., housing) that offered continuing lifestyle benefits. Those who abstained or relapsed spent less overall and appeared to substitute alcohol with small frequent substance-free rewards like entertainment, gifts, and consumable goods. Thus, problem drinkers who organize their behavioral allocation over longer intervals, even while drinking heavily, appear better able to transition to stable moderation compared to those with shorter allocation time horizons.

Taken together, these studies support a comprehensive definition of recovery that recognizes the heterogeneity of positive outcomes and pathways and focuses on enhanced access to non-drinking rewards and improved functioning in areas adversely affected by drinking.

Conceptualizing Recovery and Directions for Research and Practice

Based on prior definitions and recent empirical work, we conclude that recovery is a dynamic process of behavior change in which improvements in biopsychosocial functioning and life satisfaction are fundamental. This expanded conceptualization is aligned with definitions advanced by stakeholders such as SAMHSA and the Recovery Science Research Collaborative and with findings about recovery elements considered important by people with AUD. Available research, however, questions the validity of definitions of recovery that are limited to achieving abstinence or remission of AUD symptoms and do not include changes in these other domains. Such definitions fail to capture the multidimensional and heterogeneous pathways to recovery that are evident in the general population, among patients who receive alcohol treatment, and among those who attempt to recover on their own. Abstinence is certainly important to start the recovery process for some individuals and can contribute to the reduction of many AUD symptoms. But it is neither a necessary nor a sufficient condition to achieve the improvements in life functioning and well-being that are central to a comprehensive definition of recovery.

This conceptualization involves a shift away from a pathology-based model of AUD recovery towards a strength-based, resilience-building model of change that helps people live their "best" life (Seligman & Csikszentmihalyi, 2000). The approach differs from clinical treatment models and practices that focus on reducing illness and curing disease. Tactics useful in a strength-based model of change include increasing rewards and activities that do not involve alcohol use, building and strengthening social and community ties, and increasing healthy behaviors like physical activity and meditation. Many service providers who use evidence-based treatments and a whole person approach to care already practice to some degree in line with this conceptualization, which recognizes that achieving family and financial stability, housing and food security, and good physical and mental health are vitally important.

Expanded concern with improved functioning is incorporated into many current recovery definitions and is a future research priority. The relevant research base, while growing, lags behind the larger literature focused on changes in AUD symptoms and drinking practices. Moreover, with the notable exception of cognitive-behavioral treatments for AUD, many treatment programs, particularly in the United States, remain focused on the initiation and maintenance of abstinence and offer little to promote improved functioning and well-being. Thus, some progress has been made in shifting away from a pathology-based model toward a strength-based model of AUD recovery, but these developments remain uneven in research and practice.

A caveat in pursuing this shift is that it should not require unrealistic changes or focus too heavily on good citizenship and giving back to the community. Lancaster (2017) noted that such expectations, if excessive, "fail to take into account the differences in the normative and social contexts of people's lives" (p. 758). Some individuals pursuing recovery live in disadvantaged circumstances and experience difficulties and discrimination that cannot be resolved through individual effort and are exacerbated by the stigma of addiction (Vilsaint et al., 2019).

Given that adult alcohol use is legal and consuming alcohol without problems is socially normative, requiring complete abstinence for one subgroup (persons meeting AUD criteria) but not for another much larger subgroup (those not meeting AUD criteria) likely compounds the stigma of AUD. Taking a public health perspective instead suggests that it is critical to focus on reducing risks associated with drinking as a goal for all population members, not just those with AUD. This follows from the documented harmful effects of excessive drinking on health (Grønbaek, 2009; Witkiewitz et al., 2017) and from the well-established prevention paradox (Rose, 2001) – i.e., even small reductions in alcohol misuse among the far greater number of risky drinkers with less serious problems will result in greater improvements in population health and associated costs than by reductions large or small among the minority with severe AUD (Witkiewitz & Tucker, 2020). In addition, presenting information about AUD as lying on a continuum of severity, as compared to a binary disease based on the presence or absence of AUD, may promote early problem recognition and help-seeking (Morris et al., 2020).

A final generalization from available research concerns the limited contribution of alcohol treatment or other alcohol-focused services to increasing recovery prevalence in the population. Low rates of service utilization have persisted despite expanded access and coverage of alcohol services provided, for example, by the US Affordable Care Act and the evidence-based improvements in services over the past several decades (Tucker & Simpson, 2011). Closing the gap between need and service utilization and improving recovery rates will likely require offering interventions outside of the healthcare system to at-risk communities and individuals and utilizing social networks and public health tools for intervention dissemination. Priority should be given to reaching broader segments of the at-risk population of drinkers with less serious problems who contribute most of the harm and cost of alcohol-related problems. Nevertheless, a sizeable subset of individuals with AUD will improve or recover without interventions. Important future research questions are how to distinguish among individuals or risk groups for whom natural recovery is a high probability outcome, and how to segment the market so that treatment services are targeted and available for those in need who are not likely to achieve recovery on their own.

In conclusion, problem reduction (including recovery) is the most common outcome among persons with problem alcohol use, and non-abstinent recovery is possible, even among those with more severe AUD. Changing the narrative to highlight the high likelihood of recovery and the importance of improvements in valued areas of living may help motivate more individuals to attempt problem resolution using a pathway that appeals to and works for them. More research is needed to develop and validate operational definitions of recovery that recognize that positive changes lie along continua and involve multiple domains, and that there are many pathways to stable change. This will depend on interdisciplinary work that dissolves the longstanding silos between epidemiological, clinical, and naturalistic studies of recovery and is fundamental to improving recovery models, methods, and outcomes.

References

American Psychiatric Association (2013). *Diagnostic and statistical manual of mental disorders* (5th ed.). https://doi.org/10.1176/appi.books.9780890425596

Anonymous (1939). *Alcoholics Anonymous: The story of how many thousands of men and women have recovered from alcoholism.* Works Publishing.

Ashford, R. D., Brown, A., & Brown, T. (2019). Defining and operationalizing the phenomena of recovery: A working definition from the recovery science research collaborative. *Addiction Research & Theory, 27*(3), 179–188. https://doi.org/10.1080/16066359.2018.1515352

Best, D., Beckwith, M., Haslam, C., Haslam, S. A., Jetten, J., Mawson, E., & Lubman, D. I. (2016). Overcoming alcohol and other drug addiction as a process of social identity transition: The social identity model of recovery (SIMOR). *Addiction Research & Theory, 24*(2), 111–123. https://doi.org/10.3109/16066359.2015.1075980

Betty Ford Institute Consensus Panel (2007). What is recovery? A working definition from the Betty Ford Institute. *Journal of Substance Abuse Treatment, 33*(3), 221–228. https://doi.org/10.1016/j.jsat.2007.06.001

Brennan, P. L., Schutte, K. K., Moos, B. S., & Moos, R. H. (2011). Twenty-year alcohol-consumption and drinking-problem trajectories of older men and women. *Journal of Studies on Alcohol and Drugs, 72*(2), 308–321. https://doi.org/10.15288/jsad.2011.72.308

Dawson, D. A., Goldstein, R. B., & Grant, B. F. (2007). Rates and correlates of relapse among individuals in remission from DSM-IV alcohol dependence: A 3-year follow-up. *Alcoholism: Clinical and Experimental Research, 31*(12), 2036–2045. https://doi.org/10.1111/j.1530-0277.2007.00536.x

Dawson, D.A., Grant, B. F., Stinson, F. S., Chou, S. P., Huang, B., & Ruan, W. J. (2005). Recovery from DSM-IV alcohol dependence: United States, 2001–2002. *Addiction, 100*(3), 281–292. https://doi.org/10.1111/j.1360-0443.2004.00964.x

Edwards, G., & Gross, M. M. (1976). Alcohol dependence: Provisional description of a clinical syndrome. *Alcohol Health and Research World, 19(1)*, 44–45.

Fan, A. Z., Chou, S. P., Zhang, H., Jung, J., & Grant, B. F. (2019). Prevalence and correlates of past-year recovery from DSM-5 alcohol use disorder: Results from National Epidemiologic Survey on Alcohol and Related Conditions – III. *Alcoholism: Clinical and Experimental Research, 43*(11), 2406–2420. https://doi.org/10.1111/acer.14192

Furtwængler, N. A. F., & De Visser, D. O. (2013). Lack of international consensus in low-risk drinking guidelines. *Drug and Alcohol Review, 32*, 11–18. https://doi.org/10.1111/j.1465-3362.2012.00475.x

Gilbert, P. A., Pro, G., Zemore, S. E., Mulia, N., & Brown, G. (2019). Gender differences in use of alcohol treatment services and reasons for nonuse in a national sample. *Alcoholism: Clinical and Experimental Research, 43*(4), 722–731. https://doi.org/10.1111/acer.13965

GBD 2016 Alcohol and Drug Use Collaborators (2018). The global burden of disease attributable to alcohol and drug use in 195 countries and territories, 1990–2016: A systematic analysis for the Global Burden of Disease Study 2016. *Lancet Psychiatry, 5*, 987–1012. http://dx.doi.org/10.1016/S2215–0366(18)30337-7

Granfield, R., & Smith, W. (1999). *Coming clean: Overcoming addiction without treatment*. New York University Press.

Grant, B. F., Goldstein, R. B., Saha, T. D., Chou, S. P., Jung, J., Zhang, H., Pickering, R. P., Ruan, W. J., Smith, S. M., Huang, B., & Hasin, D. S. (2015). Epidemiology of DSM-5 Alcohol Use Disorder: Results from the National Epidemiologic Survey on Alcohol and Related Conditions III. *JAMA Psychiatry, 72*(8):757–766. https://doi.org/10.1001/jamapsychiatry.2015.0584

Grønbaek, M. (2009). The positive and negative health effects of alcohol – and the public health implications. *Journal of Internal Medicine, 265(4)*, 407–420. https://doi.org/10.1111/j.1365-2796.2009.02082.x

Grucza, R. A., Sher, K. J., Kerr, W. C., Krauss, M. J., Lui, C. K., McDowell, Y. E., Hartz, S., Virdi, G., & Bierut L. J. (2018). Trends in adult alcohol use and binge drinking in the early 21st-century United States: A meta-analysis of 6 national survey series. *Alcoholism: Clinical and Experimental Research, 42*(10), 1939–1950. https://doi.org/10.1111/acer.13859

Hingson, R. W., Hereen, T., & Winter, M. R. (2006). Age at drinking onset and alcohol dependence: Age at onset, duration, and severity. *Archives of Pediatric and Adolescent Medicine, 160*(7), 739–746. https://doi.org/10.1001/archpedi.160.7.739.40

Holahan, C. J., Brennan, P. L., Schutte, K. K., Holahan, C. K., Hixon, J. G., & Moos, R. H. (2017). Late-life drinking problems: The predictive roles of drinking level vs. drinking pattern. *Journal of Studies on Alcohol and Drugs, 78*(3), 435–441. https://doi.org/10.15288/jsad.2017.78.435

Humphreys, K. N., Mankowski, E. S., Moos, R. H., & Finney, W. H. (1999). Do enhanced friendship networks and active coping mediate the effect of self-help groups on substance abuse? *Annals of Behavioral Medicine, 21*(1), 24–60. https://doi.org/10.1007/BF02895034

Jellinek, E. M. (1960). *The disease concept of alcoholism*. Hillhouse Press.

Kaskutas, L. A., Borkman, T. J., Laudet, A., Ritter, L. A., Witbrodt, J. Subbaraman, M. S., Stunz, A., & Bond, J. (2014). Elements that define recovery: The experiential perspective. *Journal of Studies on Alcohol and Drugs, 75*(6), 999–1010. https://doi.org/10.15288/jsad.2014.75.999

Kelly, J. F., Bergman, B., Hoeppner, B. B., Vilsaint, C., & White, W. L. (2017). Prevalence and pathways of recovery from drug and alcohol problems in the United States population: Implications for practice, research, and policy. *Drug and Alcohol Dependence, 81*, 162–169. https://doi.org/10.1016/j.drugalcdep.2017.09.028

Kelly, J. F., Greene, M. C., Bergman, B. G., White, W. L., & Hoeppner, B. B. (2019). How many recovery attempts does it take to successfully resolve an alcohol or drug problem? Estimates and correlates from a national study of recovering US adults. *Alcoholism: Clinical and Experimental Research, 43*(7), 1533–1544. https://doi.org/10.1111/acer.14067

Lancaster, K. (2017). Rethinking recovery. *Addiction, 112*(5), 758–759. https://doi.org/10.1111/add.13552

Lee, M. R., Boness, C. L., McDowell, Y. E., Vergés, A., Steinley, D. L., & Sher, K. J. (2018). Desistance and severity of alcohol use disorder: A lifespan-developmental investigation. *Clinical Psychological Science, 6*(1):90–105. https://doi.org/10.1177/2167702617736852

Lee, M. R., & Sher, K. J. (2018). "Maturing out" of binge and problem drinking. *Alcohol Research: Current Reviews*, *39*(1), 31–42. PMID 30557146.

Linden-Carmichael, A. N., Russell, M. A., & Lanza, S. T. (2019). Flexibly modeling alcohol use disorder risk: How many drinks should we count? *Psychology of Addictive Behaviors, 33*(1), 50–57. https://doi.org/10.1037/adb0000431

Moos, R. H., & Moos, B. S. (2007). Protective resources and long-term recovery from alcohol use disorders. *Drug and Alcohol Dependence, 86*(1), 46–54. https://doi.org/10.1016/j.drugalcdep.2006.04.015

Morris, J., Albery, I. P., Heather, N., & Moss, A. C. (2020). Continuum beliefs are associated with higher problem recognition than binary beliefs among harmful drinkers without addiction experience. *Addictive Behaviors, 105*, 106292. https://doi.org/10.1016/j.addbeh.2020.106292

National Institute on Alcohol Abuse and Alcoholism (2020). *NIAAA recovery research definitions*. www.niaaa.nih.gov/research/niaaa-recovery-from-alcohol-use-disorder/definitions

(2005). *Helping patients who drink too much: A clinician's guide*. https://pubs.niaaa.nih.gov/publications/practitioner/cliniciansguide2005/guide.pdf

(2020). *Alcohol facts and statistics.* www.niaaa.nih.gov/alcohol-facts-and-statistics

Neale, J., Vitoratou, S., Finch, E., Lennon, P., Mitcheson, L., Panebianco, D., Rose, D., Strang, J., Wykes, T., & Marsden, J. (2016). Development and validation of SURE: A patient reported outcome measure for recovery from drug and alcohol dependence. *Drug and Alcohol Dependence, 165*, 159–167. https://doi.org/10.1016/j.drugalcdep.2016.06.006

Patrick, M. E., Terry-McElrath, Y. M., Lanza, S. T., Jager, J., Schulenberg, J. E., O'Malley, P. M. (2019). Shifting age of peak binge drinking prevalence: Historical changes in normative trajectories among young adults aged 18 to

30. *Alcoholism: Clinical and Experimental Research, 43*(2), 287–298. https://doi.org/10.1111/acer.13933

Pattison, E. M., Sobell, M. B., & Sobell, L. C. (Eds.) (1977). *Emerging concepts of alcohol dependence*. Springer.

Pearson, M. R., Kirouac, M., & Witkiewitz, K. (2016). Questioning the validity of the 4+/5+ binge or heavy drinking criterion in college and clinical populations. *Addiction, 111*(10), 1720–1726. https://doi.org/10.1111/add.13210

Project MATCH Research Group (1997). Matching alcoholism treatments to client heterogeneity: Project MATCH posttreatment drinking outcomes. *Journal of Studies on Alcohol, 58(1)*, 7–29. https://doi.org/10.15288/jsa.1997.58.7

Room, R. (1977). Measurement and distribution of drinking patterns and problems in general populations. In G. Edwards, M. S. Gross, M. Keller, J. Moser, & R. Room (Eds.), *Alcohol-related disabilities* (pp. 61–87). World Health Organization.

Rose, G. (2001). Sick individuals and sick populations. *International Journal of Epidemiology, 30*(3), 427–432. https://doi.org/10.1093/ije/30.3.427

Rush, B. (1785). *An inquiry into the effects of ardent spirits upon the human body and mind*. Tract Association of Friends.

Seligman, M. E., & Csikszentmihalyi, M. (2000). Positive psychology. An introduction. *American Psychologist, 55*(1), 5–14. https://doi.org/10.1037/0003-066X.55.1.5

Sobell, L. C., Cunningham, J. A., & Sobell, M. B. (1996). Recovery from alcohol problems with and without treatment: Prevalence in two population studies. *American Journal of Public Health, 86* (7), 966–972. https://doi.org/10.2105/ajph.86.7.966

Sobell, M. B., & Sobell, L. C. (1995). Controlled drinking after 25 years: How important was the great debate? *Addiction, 90*(9), 1149–1153; discussion 1157–1177. www.ncbi.nlm.nih.gov/pubmed/7580815

Substance Abuse and Mental Health Services Administration (2011). *SAMHSA working definition of recovery: 10 guiding principles of recovery*. https://store.samhsa.gov/shin/content//PEP12-RECDEF/PEP12-RECDEF.pdf.

(2015). *Behavioral health trends in the United States: Results from the 2014 National Survey on Drug Use and Health* (HHS Publication No. SMA 15-4927, NSDUH Series H-50). www.samhsa.gov/data/sites/default/files/NSDUH-FRR1-2014/NSDUH-FRR1-2014.htm

(2017). *National Survey of Substance Abuse Treatment Services (N-SSATSA): 2016. Data on substance abuse treatment facilities* (BHSIS Series S-93, HHS Publication No. (SMA) 17-5039). www.samhsa.gov/data/sites/default/files/cbhsq-reports/NSDUHMethodSumm Defs2017/NSDUHMethodSummDefs2017.htm

(2019). *Key substance use and mental health indicators in the United States: Results from the 2018 National Survey on Drug Use and Health* (HHS Publication No. PEP19-5068, NSDUH Series H-54). www.samhsa.gov/data/sites/default/files/cbhsq-reports/NSDUHNationalFindingsReport2018/NSDUHNationalFindings Report2018.pdf

Tucker, J. A., Chandler, S. D., & Witkiewitz, K. (2020a). Epidemiology of recovery from Alcohol Use Disorder. *Alcohol Research: Current Reviews, 40(30).* E-pub 2020 November 12 https://doi.org/10.35946/arcr.v40.3.02

Tucker, J. A., Cheong, J., & Chandler, S. D. (2021). Shifts in behavioral allocation patterns as a natural recovery mechanism: Post-resolution expenditure patterns. *Alcoholism: Clinical and Experimental Research*. https://doi.org/10.1111/acer.14620

Tucker, J. A., Cheong, J., James, T. G., Jung, S., & Chandler, S. D. (2020b). Differentiating pre-resolution drinking problem severity indicators associated with maintaining stable moderation or abstinence using latent profile analysis. *Alcoholism: Clinical and Experimental Research*, *44*(3), 738–745. https://doi.org/10.1111/acer.14287

Tucker, J. A., & Simpson, C. A. (2011). The recovery spectrum: From self-change to seeking treatment. *Alcohol Research & Health*, *33*, 371–379. PMID 23580021

Tuithof, M., ten Have, M., van den Brink, W., Vollebergh, W., & DeGraff, R. (2016). Treatment seeking for alcohol use disorders: Treatment gap or adequate self-selection? *European Addiction Research*, *22*(5), 277–285. https://doi.org/10.1159/000446822

Vaillant, G. E., & Hiller-Sturmhöfel, S. (1996). The natural history of alcoholism. *Alcohol Health & Research World*, *20*(3), 152–161.

Vasilenko, S. A., Evans-Polce, R. J., & Lanza, S. T. (2017). Age trends in rates of substance use disorders across ages 18-90: Differences by gender and race/ethnicity. *Drug and Alcohol Dependence*, *180*, 260–64. https://doi.org/10.1016/j.drugalcdep.2017.08.027

Vergés, A., Haeny, A. M., Jackson, K. M., Bucholz, K. K., Grant, J. D., Trull, T. J., Wood, P. K., & Sher, K. J. (2013). Refining the notion of maturing out: Results from the National Epidemiologic Survey on Alcohol and Related Conditions. *American Journal of Public Health*, *103*(12): e67–73. https://doi.org/10.2105/AJPH.2013.301358

Vilsaint, C. L., Hoffman, L. A., & Kelly, J. F. (2019). Perceived discrimination in addiction recovery: Assessing the prevalence, nature, and correlates using a novel measure in a US national sample. *Drug and Alcohol Dependence*, *206*, 107667. https://doi.org/10.1016/j.drugalcdep.2019.107667

Witbrodt, J., Kaskutas, L. A., & Grella, C. E. (2015). How do recovery definitions distinguish recovering individuals? Five typologies. *Drug and Alcohol Dependence*, *148*, 109–117. https://doi.org/10.1016/j.drugalcdep.2014.12.036

Witkiewitz, K., Hallgren, K. A., Kranzler, H. R., Mann, K. F., Hasin, D. S., Falk, D. E., Litten, R. A., O'Malley, S. S., & Anton, R. F. (2017). Clinical validation of reduced alcohol consumption after treatment for alcohol dependence using the World Health Organization risk drinking levels. *Alcoholism: Clinical and Experimental Research*, *41*(1), 179–186. https://doi.org/10.1111/ACER.13272

Witkiewitz, K., Montes, K., Schwebel, F., & Tucker, J. A. (2020). What is recovery? *Alcohol Research: Current Reviews, 40(3).* E-pub 2020 September 30 www.arcr.niaaa.nih.gov/arcr403/article01.htm

Witkiewitz, K., & Tucker, J. A. (2020). Abstinence not required: Expanding the definition of recovery from alcohol use disorder. *Alcoholism: Clinical and Experimental Research*, *44*(1), 36–40. https://doi.org/10.1111/acer.14235

Witkiewitz, K., Wilson, A. D., Pearson, M. R., Montes, K. S., Kirouac, M., Roos, C., Hallgren, K. A., & Maisto, S. A. (2019). Profiles of recovery from alcohol use disorder at three years following treatment: Can the definition of recovery be extended to include high functioning heavy drinkers? *Addiction, 114*(1), 69–80. https://doi.org/10.1111/add.14403

World Health Organization (1992). *The ICD-10 classification of mental and behavioral disorders: Clinical descriptions and diagnostic guidelines.* www.who.int/classifications/icd/en/bluebook.pdf

(2018). *Global status report on alcohol and health 2018.* https://apps.who.int/iris/handle/10665/274603

Zemore, S. E., Mulia, N., Ye, Y., Borges, G., & Greenfield, T. K. (2009). Gender, acculturation, and other barriers to alcohol treatment utilization among Latinos in three national alcohol surveys. *Journal of Substance Abuse Treatment, 36*(4), 446–456. https://doi.org/10.1016/j.jsat.2008.09.005

Zemore, S. E., Murphy, R. D., Mulia, N., Gilbert, P. A., Martinez, P., Bond, J., & Polcin, D. L. (2014). A moderating role for gender in racial/ethnic disparities in alcohol services utilization: Results from the 2000–2010 National Alcohol Surveys. *Alcoholism: Clinical and Experimental Research, 38*(8), 2286–2296. https://doi.org/10.1111/acer.12500

PART I

Micro Level: The Individual as Change Agent

2 Biopsychosocial Process of Change in Alcohol Use Disorder Recovery

Katie Witkiewitz and Stephen A. Maisto

Biopsychosocial Process of Change in Alcohol Use Disorder Recovery

Recovery from alcohol use disorder (AUD) has been described as "an individualized, intentional, dynamic, and relational process involving sustained efforts to improve wellness" (p. 5) (Ashford et al., 2019) and as a process of behavior change (Witkiewitz, Montes, et al., 2020). The goal of this chapter is to review the latest empirical literature that has examined recovery as a dynamic process of behavior change and explore the biological, psychological, social, and contextual factors that are associated with AUD recovery. We also review models of AUD remission and AUD relapse, and offer some possible extension of these models to our understanding of AUD recovery. Importantly, research on biopsychosocial processes of AUD recovery has been primarily retrospective cross-sectional studies of individuals who identify as being in recovery (Kaskutas et al., 2014; Kelly et al., 2018; Neale et al., 2016), and there are only a few prospective, longitudinal studies examining recovery processes over time (Moos & Moos, 2005; Tucker et al., 2016; Witkiewitz, Pearson, et al., 2020). Thus, in the current chapter we focus on a broad range of research that has examined biopsychosocial predictors and correlates of AUD remission, AUD relapse, and AUD recovery processes in the course of treatment, participation in Alcoholics Anonymous (AA) and other mutual help groups, and in the context of natural recovery.

Definitions of AUD Remission, Relapse, and Recovery

The *Diagnostic and Statistical Manual for Mental Disorders*, 5th edition (DSM-5) (American Psychiatric Association, 2013) defines remission from AUD as the absence of symptoms of AUD, other than craving, which can persist after other symptoms of AUD are no longer present. The *International Classification of Diseases* (ICD), 11th edition (World Health Organization, 2018) defines remission as abstinence from alcohol and no ICD-11 symptoms. True to their being part of a clinical diagnostic system, both the DSM and ICD definitions define both remission and recovery within the boundaries of those systems, that is, according to the absence of symptoms (criteria) that constitute the respective AUD diagnoses. Although the criteria themselves may pertain to disruptions due to drinking in the individual's life and the lives of those associated with them, the narrow focus on the absence of diagnostic criteria in defining remission and recovery is a limitation recognized in many other definitions that define recovery using additional and considerably broader criteria (Ashford et al., 2019; Substance Abuse and Mental Health Services Administration, 2011; Witkiewitz, Montes, et al., 2020). In these broader definitions, remission and recovery are viewed as part of a process of change rather than the endpoint implied by the presence or absence of diagnostic symptoms at a given time point.

For example, the Substance Abuse and Mental Health Services Administration (SAMHSA, 2011) defines recovery as "a process of change through which individuals improve their health and wellness, live a self-directed life, and strive to reach their full potential." The *Betty Ford Consensus Panel* in 2007 defined recovery as "a voluntarily maintained lifestyle characterized by sobriety, personal health, and citizenship" (p. 222) (2007). Current data on recovery definitions from the perspectives of multiple stakeholders (e.g., the person who is in the course of AUD change, treatment providers, family/friends, third party payors) also seem to be consistent with a trend toward a broader definition of recovery. Among a large nationally representative sample of 39,809 individuals who resolved an alcohol or drug problem (Kelly, Greene, et al., 2018), participants recalled nonlinear patterns of improvements in multiple indices of well-being, including increases in happiness, self-esteem, and decreases in distress over the course of the first decade after resolving an alcohol or other drug problem. The majority of individuals who had resolved an alcohol or drug problem did not identify with the term "recovery" (Kelly, Abry, et al., 2018), and those who identified as being "in recovery" were more likely to have participated in mutual help organizations, used recovery support, received formal treatment, and/or were diagnosed with a substance use disorder. Importantly, some individuals viewed the "recovery" label as negative, which reflects the unfortunate stigma associated with AUD and recovery from AUD that still persists in our society.

As described in greater detail in the first chapter of this book and previously (Witkiewitz, Montes, et al., 2020), we have defined recovery as a dynamic process of change characterized by improvements in biopsychosocial functioning and well-being. In contrast to narrower definitions of remission and recovery embodied in diagnostic classification schemes, recovery is not limited to a view of AUD as a medical problem to be resolved (e.g., through detoxification, abstinence, and remission of symptoms). The broader definition of recovery proposed in this book considers AUD as caused and maintained by multilevel and multivariable biological (e.g., genes, neurobiology), psychological (e.g., cognitions, behaviors, emotions), and social/environmental/contextual (e.g., social network, socioeconomics, systemic facilitators and barriers) factors. As such, a broader definition of AUD recovery represents an emphasis on ongoing maintenance of change processes that are multivariable and determined by biological, psychological, and socioenvironmental factors. The proposed biopsychosocial model of AUD recovery proposed herein draws on the larger literature that has examined AUD relapse as a dynamic biopsychosocial process of behavior change and on research that has examined the biological, psychological, social, and contextual factors that are associated with AUD recovery.

Processes of Change from Remission to Relapse to Recovery

The concept that remission, relapse, and recovery are markers of a multifaceted dynamic process of change in substance use has evolved from almost five decades of empirical study of change in substance use and related problems and maintenance of change. In 1971 Hunt and colleagues published a combined analysis of 84 studies that examined "relapse" (defined as any use) curves following "successfully completing" (defined as abstinence) a substance use disorder treatment program, with a specific focus on opioid, alcohol, and nicotine use disorders. Results indicated that the majority of individuals who achieved abstinence during treatment had returned to some level of substance use in the year following treatment (1971). Relapse rates rapidly accelerated during approximately the first three months after treatment and slowed thereafter.

Hunt et al.'s (1971) contribution to understanding AUD clinical course and change was considerable, and it generated a very substantial amount of basic and clinical research on change in substance use and related problems and its maintenance that influenced both clinical practice and research. Over the last half century, the field has moved toward a greater understanding of the dynamic process of change that occurs following alcohol treatment or reductions in drinking that occur outside of the treatment context (Chow et al., 2015; Tucker & Simpson, 2011; Witkiewitz & Marlatt, 2004). This newer body of knowledge has shown consistently that viewing relapse as an end point does not accurately represent AUD clinical course. For example, research since the 1980s has shown that any alcohol use following a period of voluntary abstinence from it does not represent a "fall from the wagon" (Miller, 1996). As Miller (1996) noted, "[s]-uccessful behavior change typically involves successive approximations to goals, and this process is not adequately captured in the value-laden concept of relapse" (p. s26). Empirical findings indicate that most people who reduce their drinking, even short of total abstinence from alcohol, report positive outcomes, such as significant improvements in quality of life and physical health functioning (Witkiewitz et al., 2018), as well as reductions in mental health symptoms (Witkiewitz, Falk, et al., 2019).

The difficult question, then, is how best to model the dynamic process of behavior change, when a binary definition of success versus failure (e.g., drinking versus abstinence) does not adequately capture the experience of individuals who recover from AUD. The methodological chapters in this volume (Linden-Carmichael et al., Chapter 7; Cheong et al., Chapter 8) provide a detailed overview of different approaches to studying recovery processes over time, and we highlight a few examples from our work here. Results from longitudinal mixture analyses conducted by our team indicate that relapse, remission, and recovery are best described as a process of behavior change characterized by numerous transitions in drinking statuses over time (Maisto et al., 2018; Witkiewitz, Wilson, et al., 2019), occasional sudden transitions between drinking and non-drinking states (Chow et al., 2015; Witkiewitz et al., 2007), as well as periods of stable maintenance of improvements in functioning, regardless of the level of drinking (Witkiewitz, Pearson, et al., 2020).

Maisto and colleagues (2018) provided an in-depth analysis of transitions in drinking statuses during the first year following outpatient alcohol treatment in the Project MATCH study (Project MATCH Research Group, 1993) and found that the majority of individuals transitioned between periods of heavy drinking (i.e., "relapse") and remission from heavy drinking at least once in the year following treatment. Importantly, regardless of any one relapse episode, those who were more likely to achieve some level of remission from heavy drinking had the best psychosocial functioning at three years following treatment. These findings were recently replicated in the COMBINE study sample (Anton et al., 2006) and extended to examine longer term outcomes. Results indicated that participants who reduced their occasions of heavy drinking during the first year following treatment continued to report improvements in general health, psychological functioning, and purpose in life in follow-ups that spanned nearly a decade (Maisto et al., 2020). Using the same Project MATCH and COMBINE study datasets examined by Maisto and colleagues (2018, 2020), but using a different set of analyses, we found that recovery can be characterized by improvements in psychosocial functioning and quality of life that are sustained for up to 10 years following AUD treatment (Witkiewitz, Pearson, et al., 2020; Witkiewitz, Wilson, et al., 2020).

These findings highlight the dynamic nature of recovery, as well as the importance of psychosocial functioning and well-being in defining the recovery process. Nevertheless, similar to the work of Hunt and colleagues (1971), the recent work of Maisto, Witkiewitz, and colleagues focused on characterizing the process of changes in drinking (2018) and the changes in drinking and life functioning (Witkiewitz, Pearson, et al., 2020; Witkiewitz, Wilson, et al., 2019) without giving much consideration to predictors of patterns of change over time. As such, this body of work has been largely descriptive of the process of change and has not focused on characterizing predictors that might explain why individuals change in particular ways over time. Prior to examining potential predictors suggested by a biopsychosocial model of recovery, we first consider factors that have been found influential in biopsychosocial models of relapse. We selectively highlight this research next, because it may foreshadow a productive path for future research on recovery.

Biopsychosocial Model of the Relapse Process

As noted earlier, the Hunt et al. (1971) study initiated a large volume of empirical study of AUD relapse that has influenced clinical practice in major ways. We do not view recovery as the absence of relapse or the absence of pathology, thus relapse and recovery are not interchangeable; however, several factors that are important in predicting alcohol relapse processes are also likely to be important in the process of recovery. Marlatt's seminal work on defining and characterizing high-risk situations for relapse (1985) led to a large scale research project funded by the National Institute on Alcohol Abuse and Alcoholism (NIAAA) aimed at replicating and extending Marlatt's relapse taxonomy (Lowman et al., 1996). Several aspects of the original relapse taxonomy were not empirically supported, such as the hierarchical classification and the requirement that only one category be selected for defining relapse situations (Maisto et al., 1996). Nevertheless, many of the contextual factors included in the original taxonomy – including negative emotional states, urges and temptations, and interpersonal stressors – were associated with drinking events in the replication project (Marlatt, 1996). As cautioned by Marlatt (1996), it is important not to be "oblivious of the dynamic interplay of cognitive and behavioral factors in the ongoing process of relapse and recovery" (p. S151), and "there may be fifty ways to leave the wagon . . . [and] fifty corresponding ways to get back on" (p. S152).

The relapse taxonomy replication results and a growing appreciation in the psychological sciences for nonlinear dynamical systems theory led Witkiewitz and Marlatt (2004) to develop a reconceptualized model of relapse that proposed complex interactions between background "distal" (also referred to as "tonic") risk factors and "proximal" (also referred to as "phasic") processes that could dynamically interact to predict drinking events (Witkiewitz & Marlatt, 2004). The theoretical proposition that distal and proximal risk factors might interact in nonlinear ways to predict drinking was also supported in empirical work using a nonlinear dynamical systems model, based on catastrophe theory (Chow et al., 2015; Witkiewitz et al., 2007). Empirical research over the past 15 years continues to provide evidence in support of the dynamic model of relapse and points to a number of biological, psychological, environmental, and social factors that interact in the moment to predict alcohol use (Hendershot et al., 2011; Maisto et al., 2014; Sliedrecht et al., 2019).

For example, negative emotional states were originally proposed in the Marlatt relapse taxonomy, and empirical research over the decades continues to indicate that negative affective states are strongly associated with alcohol use (Swan et al., 2020). Neurobiological models of addiction developed in animal research and tested more recently in human studies also point to negative emotionality and aversive experiences as key processes in the addiction cycle (Koob & Volkow, 2016). Relatedly, chronic stressors, experiences of acute stress, and experiences of physical pain have been shown to be associated with alcohol lapse (any drinking) and relapse (heavy drinking) (Jakubczyk et al., 2016; Sinha, 2011), often mediated by negative affect (Maisto et al., 2017; Witkiewitz et al., 2015). Related to emotionality and affect, experiences of urges (i.e., temptation, craving) to drink have been shown to predict risk for drinking lapses and level of consumption when drinking (Witkiewitz, 2011, 2013). Craving appears to be a multidimensional construct that involves several neural substrates and a variety of affective and cognitive processes.

Cognitive processes are also critical in the relapse process, with numerous studies showing that self-efficacy – the belief in one's ability to engage in or execute a behavior (e.g., abstinence self-efficacy) – in particular is a key predictor of alcohol use and relapse (Maisto et al., 2015; McKay et al., 2005). Outcome expectancies, especially positive outcome expectancies for the desired effects of alcohol, attentional bias, and neuropsychological functioning, have also been shown to be associated with alcohol lapse and relapse, although prior research in this area has been somewhat limited by measurement issues and small samples (Sliedrecht et al., 2019).

Coping skills – defined as engaging in a behavior or set of behaviors (e.g., seeking social support, engaging in positive activities) to deal with situational, interpersonal, or intrapersonal experiences that are stressful, induce negative affect, or disrupt self-regulation capacity – have been described as critical to preventing alcohol use lapses and relapse, and the ability to implement an effective coping response was considered the final juncture in Marlatt's cognitive behavioral model of relapse (Marlatt & Gordon, 1985). Several empirical studies have also found coping to be a strong predictor of alcohol use (Moos & Moos, 2005; Witkiewitz & Masyn, 2008). More recent work has pointed to the importance of coping flexibility and the ability to implement the best coping strategy for a given context in reducing drinks per drinking day, drinking-related problems, and percent of days abstinent (Roos & Witkiewitz, 2017).

Interpersonal relationships, degree and quality of social support, and social network support or social network feedback about drinking have all been shown to serve as either protective or risk factors for alcohol use and relapse (Delucchi & Kaskutas, 2010; George & Tucker, 1996; Maisto et al., 2015). Several other distal risk factors have been shown to elevate risk for alcohol use, including family history of AUD, psychiatric comorbidity, severity of AUD, and spirituality/purpose in life (Sliedrecht et al., 2019).

Biopsychosocial Model of Recovery

By comparison to the literature on alcohol relapse, fewer studies have examined biopsychosocial factors that are associated with the process of recovery from AUD. As described earlier, research in this area has largely focused on individuals who identify as being in recovery (Kaskutas et al., 2014; Kelly et al., 2018; Neale et al., 2016) or individuals who participated in longitudinal studies that measured recovery processes over time (Moos & Moos, 2005; Tucker et al., 2016; Witkiewitz, Pearson, et al., 2020).

Among those who identify as being in recovery, Kaskutas and colleagues (2014) identified 35 elements that were important in recovery, which could be summarized by four factors: (1) level of substance use, (2) essentials of recovery, (3) enriched recovery, and (4) spirituality in recovery. The "essentials of recovery" (e.g., dealing with challenging negative feelings, realistic self-appraisal) was considered distinct from the "enriched recovery" factor that revolved around interpersonal and intrapersonal engagement with life and self-care (e.g., inner peace, living a life that contributes to others and society). The factor "spirituality in recovery" included religiosity, but also included aspects of gratitude, giving back, and helping other people. Similarly, using an iterative mixed-methods approach among individuals in recovery and addiction psychiatrists/staff, Neale and colleagues (2016) identified 21 items that corresponded to recovery, summarized by five factors: (1) substance use, (2) material resources, (3) outlook on life, (4) self-care, and (5) relationships. Both of these mixed methods studies point to aspects of recovery that are biological (e.g., improvements in physical health, sleep, and reductions in level of substance use), psychological (e.g., outlook on life, dealing with negative emotions, inner peace), and social (e.g., importance of relationships, giving back, and helping others). These studies also point to the importance of material resources, including stable housing "that is not overrun with alcohol or drugs" (p. 1004; Kaskutas et al., 2014) and financial resources (e.g., stable income, managing finances).

Related research has examined "recovery capital," defined as "the sum total of one's resources that can be brought to bear on the initiation and maintenance of substance misuse cessation" (p. 1972; Cloud & Granfield, 2008). Using cross-sectional survey designs, three domains of recovery capital were identified, including personal recovery capital (intrapersonal, psychological resources), social recovery capital (interpersonal, social resources), and community recovery capital (material resources, financial and housing stability) (Best et al., 2020). Consistent with the mixed-methods work, this research supports the role of biopsychosocial processes in AUD recovery initiation and maintenance, along with the importance of adequate material resources.

Quantitative studies that variously examined prospective outcomes among individuals treated for AUD (Witkiewitz, Pearson, et al., 2020), individuals who attempted to resolve an alcohol problem outside of the treatment context (Tucker et al., 2009, 2016), and individuals who did or did not seek treatment for AUD (Moos & Moos, 2005) similarly found that both biopsychosocial processes of change and resource allocation are critically important to initiation and maintenance of recovery outcomes. Witkiewitz and colleagues (2020) found that individuals who were defined as recovered at three years following treatment based on level of functioning, regardless of level of drinking, had better self-reported health and fewer hospitalizations at 7–9 years post-treatment, as compared to those with fewer environmental resources or those with poorer psychosocial functioning at three years post-treatment (Witkiewitz, Pearson, et al., 2020). An observational study of persons with a history of alcohol-related problems assessed over 16 years found that most participants showed improvement in alcohol-related functioning, life contexts, and coping, and those with more psychosocial support and more social resources predicted stable recovery outcomes (Moos & Moos, 2005). Tucker and her colleagues pioneered the examination of behavioral economic measures in predicting recovery outcomes (see Chapter 9, this volume) and found that pre-resolution spending patterns were associated with long term outcomes, such that individuals who allocated more money to savings were more likely to achieve stable recoveries, particularly non-abstinent recoveries involving some low-risk drinking (Tucker et al., 2009, 2016).

Together, this series of longitudinal studies point to many of the same factors that were relevant to a biopsychosocial model of relapse, such as negative emotional states, coping, and social support, while also highlighting the importance of material resources and economic factors in supporting recovery outcomes.

Future Directions in Studying Recovery as a Biopsychosocial Process of Change

In this chapter we have shown that the field has made considerable progress in conceptualizing AUD clinical course and AUD recovery as a process of behavior change associated with myriad biological, psychological, social, and contextual factors. The shift from an abstinence-only view of recovery to a biopsychosocial model of recovery that extends beyond drinking practices has influenced clinical research and practice and continues to do so. Moreover, the current state of the science and practice of AUD recovery point to several paths of future investigation and development that will likely further advance the field. These paths concern issues related to defining recovery, theoretical models of recovery, and measurement of recovery. Following discussion of each of these areas in turn, we conclude with implications for clinical practice.

Definition of Recovery

It is reasonable to begin any discussion of AUD recovery by asking whether the construct itself has heuristic value; that is, does it facilitate the generation of research and help to advance knowledge? As noted earlier, one major argument against the term "recovery" is that, despite the amount of attention given to defining it, a widely accepted consensus definition has not been forthcoming from either the practice or research community. In addition, a segment of individuals who have resolved their alcohol problems disavow self-identification as "in recovery," "recovered," or "recovering" and do not regard their drinking problem as severe enough to seek treatment (Kelly et al., 2018; Klingemann & Sobell, 2007).

Nevertheless, there are a few compelling reasons to retain the construct, and, rather than dropping it, address its shortcomings so that it acquires heuristic value. Perhaps the most compelling reason is that the term is entrenched in the addictions treatment field and is part of everyday clinical practice worldwide. For example, the United States Surgeon General's report on addiction (US Department of Health & Human Services, 2016) devotes an entire chapter to recovery. The construct has become mainstream in addictions treatment and is not likely to disappear from usage any time soon.

If the construct of recovery is retained, several questions about and problems with it need to be addressed. On the one hand, there are specific clinical and research contexts in which a narrower definition, such as presence of AUD diagnosis, may be warranted. Examples of such contexts are to aid communication in clinical practice or in studies of the predictive validity of psychiatric diagnostic systems. On the other hand, however, research reviewed in this chapter shows clearly that the trend in the field is toward a broader definition of recovery that encompasses multiple areas of life functioning in addition to a dimension of substance consumption. If a broader definition of recovery is accepted as the working definition, then several lines of inquiry are needed for standardization of an operational definition and easier communication in the field. Suggested lines of inquiry include the following: Which dimensions of life functioning are critical? Is a dimension of abstinence from alcohol or other drug use necessary, or is reduction in use sufficient? Or is no dimension of consumption needed at all, such as in DSM-5? Some available data address the latter question. For instance, Garner et al. (2014) showed that an abstinence dimension did not load strongly on a multi-factored latent recovery variable. Similarly, recent studies have found abstinence is not required for long-term improved life functioning among individuals who received treatment for AUD nearly a decade earlier (Witkiewitz, Pearson, et al., 2020; Witkiewitz, Wilson, et al., 2020).

On balance, despite the empirical literature devoted to defining recovery from substance use disorders (e.g., Dodge et al., 2010; Laudet, 2007), the field has not generated systematic research that empirically compares and contrasts competing multidimensional definitions of recovery that might support or direct the development of a conceptualization that earn consensus status in clinical research and practice.

Theory Development

Once there is increased clarity about what the construct of recovery represents, good theoretical models would give the field a foundation for generating hypotheses that could be evaluated empirically. Given our broader definition of AUD recovery as part of a dynamic change process involving biopsychosocial factors, the basic task of a theory would seem to be to explain how the multiple factors purportedly involved in the recovery process change over long periods of time and how desired changes are maintained. This framing suggests a study in lifespan development, and that any theoretical model of AUD recovery should reflect that perspective. Life course theory is a historical-contextual approach to understanding human behavior (Elder et al., 2003), and it has the potential to offer new insights and approaches to the understanding of AUD recovery. It is interesting to note that much of the published empirical studies of AUD recovery have not emphasized human development in a historical and social context. A notable exception is the work on reliable age-related reductions in risky drinking and AUD during earlier adulthood (e.g., Lee et al., 2018; cf. Chapter 5 this volume).

According to Elder Jr. et al. (2003), there are five principles of life course theory: (1) human development and aging are life-long processes; (2) individuals construct their own life course through the choices and actions they take within the opportunities and constraints of history and social circumstance; (3) an individual's life course is embedded by the historical times and places they experience during their lifetime; (4) the developmental antecedents and consequences of life transitions, events, and behavioral patterns vary according to their timing in a person's life; and (5) lives are lived interdependently, and socio-historical influences are expressed through this network of shared relationships.

From a life course perspective, emphasis is placed on prospective, longitudinal research designs. Although cross-sectional, retrospective studies have played a large part in advancing knowledge about AUD recovery; further advances will likely depend on more prospective research if informative tests of hypotheses about recovery are to be undertaken. A prominent factor in developmental research in the behavioral sciences that has been largely ignored in AUD clinical research is cohort effects. Cohort effects point to a connection between chronological age and historical context in determining human behavior. AUD treatment research rarely has referred to cohort factors and how they may relate to a treatment being evaluated and how participants fare following treatment (remission, recovery, or relapse). Instead, age is generally represented by aggregated categories such as adolescent, emerging adult, or adult. Given the wide age range encompassed by the term "adult" (usually 18 years or older), it is critical for researchers to consider history-related differences in how initiation and maintenance of change in AUD might be perceived and experienced by individuals in different age cohorts. Also critical are possible sub-group differences within cohorts, because the same historical or social events may differentially affect individuals of the same age in the same location defined both broadly (e.g., country of residence) and narrowly (local residence). Finally, a life course theory perspective suggests that recovery researchers include more "macro" variables in what have been called distal determinants of outcomes (see Witkiewitz & Marlatt, 2004), as well as transitions in social roles that may occur over the course of a study of individuals in recovery.

Measurement Development

A number of measures of the broader construct of recovery have been generated (Laudet, 2009; White, 2007), but only a small number of them have sound psychometric properties. Further validation of self-report assessment measures is essential. Developing a consensus definition of recovery also would be useful, and a successful one will almost certainly include multiple functional considerations. For example, the Substance Use Recovery Evaluator (SURE) (Neale et al., 2016) is a patient reported outcome measure designed to measure recovery processes across five domains: (1) substance use, (2) material resources, (3) outlook on life, (4) self-care, and (5) relationships. The SURE has recently been deployed as a mobile application to help people who use alcohol or other drugs, identify as in recovery, or are thinking about recovery (see Neale et al., Chapter 21, this volume, for more information). Similarly, the Brief Assessment of Recovery Capital (Vilsaint et al., 2017) and the Strengths and Barriers Recovery Scale (Best et al., 2020) were designed to assess psychological, physical, social, and environmental resources considered important for achieving and maintaining recovery.

Conclusions and Recommendations

Overall, advances in knowledge about AUD recovery and its application in clinical practice and in the study of natural recovery will depend on addiction scientists' coordinated and systematic efforts to develop explanatory theories of AUD recovery as a biopsychosocial process of change and to incorporate relevant measures, such as the SURE and Brief Assessment of Recovery Capital, to evaluate those theories. The analysis of definitions, conceptualizations, and empirical studies of AUD recovery presented in this chapter focus on recovery as a dynamic biopsychosocial process of change. From this perspective, we encourage a broadening of the research agenda to focus on dynamic interactions between biological, psychological, social, contextual, cultural, and life course developmental factors in predicting the onset and maintenance of recovery processes. Ongoing communication between addiction scientists, treatment providers, individuals in the process of recovery from AUD, and mutual help group communities is essential to increase the dissemination and implementation of public health approaches and clinical interventions that promote the recovery process and support maintenance of change. Longitudinal studies that incorporate theoretical grounding and validated measures will be critical in advancing a scientifically-based understanding of recovery and its determinants.

Acknowledgments

The author's research on the biopsychosocial model as applied to understanding alcohol use disorder recovery was supported, in part, by grants from the National Institute on Alcohol Abuse and Alcoholism (R01 AA022328 and K05AA016928).

References

American Psychiatric Association. (2013). *Diagnostic and statistical manual of mental disorders* (5th ed.). https://doi.org/10.1176/appi.books.9780890425596

Anton, R. F., O'Malley, S. S., Ciraulo, D. A., Cisler, R. A., Couper, D., Donovan, D. M., Gastfriend, D. R., Hosking, J. D., Johnson, B. A., LoCastro, J. S., Longabaugh, R., Mason, B. J., Mattson, M. E., Miller, W. R., Pettinati, H. M., Randall, C. L., Swift, R., Weiss, R. D., Williams, L. D., & Zweben, A. (2006). Combined pharmacotherapies and behavioral interventions for alcohol dependence: the COMBINE study: A randomized controlled trial. *JAMA*, *295*(17), 2003–2017. https://doi.org/10.1001/jama.295.17.2003

Ashford, R. D., Brown, A., Brown, T., Callis, J., Cleveland, H. H., Eisenhart, E., Groover, H., Hayes, N., Johnston, T., Kimball, T., Manteuffel, B., McDaniel, J., Montgomery, L., Phillips, S., Polacek, M., Statman, M., & Whitney, J. (2019). Defining and operationalizing the phenomena of recovery: A working definition from the recovery science research collaborative. *Addiction Research and Theory*, *27*(3), 179–188. https://doi.org/10.1080/16066359.2018.1515352

Best, D., Vanderplasschen, W., & Nisic, M. (2020). Measuring capital in active addiction and recovery: The development of the strengths and barriers recovery scale (SABRS). *Substance Abuse: Treatment, Prevention, and Policy*, *15*(1), 1–8. https://doi.org/10.1186/s13011–020-00281-7

Betty Ford Institute Consensus Panel. (2007). What is recovery? A working definition from the Betty Ford Institute. *Journal of Substance Abuse Treatment*, *33*(3), 221–228. https://doi.org/10.1016/j.jsat.2007.06.001

Chow, S.-M., Witkiewitz, K., Grasman, R. P., & Maisto, S. A. (2015). The cusp catastrophe model as cross-sectional and longitudinal mixture structural equation models. *Psychological Methods*, *20*(1), 142–164. https://doi.org/10.1037/a0038962

Cloud, W., & Granfield, R. (2008). Conceptualizing recovery capital: Expansion of a theoretical construct. *Substance Use & Misuse*, *43*(12–13), 1971–1986. https://doi.org/10.1080/10826080802289762

Delucchi, K. L., & Kaskutas, L. A. (2010). Following problem drinkers over eleven years: Understanding changes in alcohol consumption. *Journal of Studies on Alcohol and Drugs*, *71*(6), 831–836. www.ncbi.nlm.nih.gov/pubmed/20946739

Dodge, K., Krantz, B., & Kenny, P. J. (2010). How can we begin to measure recovery? *Substance Abuse Treatment, Prevention, and Policy*, *5*(1), 31. https://doi.org/10.1186/1747-597X-5-31

Elder, G. H., Johnson, M. K., & Crosnoe, R. (2003). The emergence and development of life course theory. In J. T. Mortimer & M. J. Shanahan (Eds.), *Handbook of the life course* (pp. 3–19). Springer. https://doi.org/10.1007/978-0-306-48247-2_1

Garner, B. R., Scott, C. K., Dennis, M. L., & Funk, R. R. (2014). The relationship between recovery and health-related quality of life. *Journal of Substance Abuse Treatment*, *47*(4), 293–298. https://doi.org/10.1016/j.jsat.2014.05.006

George, A. A., & Tucker, J. A. (1996). Help-seeking for alcohol-related problems: Social contexts surrounding entry into alcoholism treatment or alcoholics anonymous.

Journal of Studies on Alcohol, *57*(4), 449–457. https://doi.org/10.15288/jsa.1996.57.449

Project MATCH Research Group (1993). Project MATCH: Rationale and methods for a multisite clinical trial matching patients to alcoholism treatment. *Alcoholism: Clinical and Experimental Research*, *17*(6), 1130–1145. https://doi.org/10.1111/j.1530-0277.1993.tb05219.x

Hendershot, C. S., Witkiewitz, K., George, W. H., & Marlatt, G. A. (2011). Relapse prevention for addictive behaviors. *Substance Abuse Treatment, Prevention, and Policy*, *6*(1747–597X, 1747–597X), 17. https://doi.org/10.1186/1747-597X-6-17

Hunt, W. A., Barnett, L. W., & Branch, L. G. (1971). Relapse rates in addiction programs. *Journal of Clinical Psychology*, *27*(4), 455–456. www.ncbi.nlm.nih.gov/pubmed/5115648

Jakubczyk, A., Ilgen, M. A., Kopera, M., Krasowska, A., Klimkiewicz, A., Bohnert, A., Blow, F. C., Brower, K. J., & Wojnar, M. (2016). Reductions in physical pain predict lower risk of relapse following alcohol treatment. *Drug and Alcohol Dependence*, *158*, 167–171. https://doi.org/10.1016/j.drugalcdep.2015.11.020

Kaskutas, L. A., Borkman, T. J., Laudet, A., Ritter, L. A., Witbrodt, J., Subbaraman, M. S., Stunz, A., & Bond, J. (2014). Elements that define recovery: The experiential perspective. *Journal of Studies on Alcohol and Drugs*, *75*(6), 999–1010. https://doi.org/10.15288/jsad.2014.75.999

Kelly, J. F., Abry, A. W., Milligan, C. M., Bergman, B. G., & Hoeppner, B. B. (2018). On being “in recovery”: A national study of prevalence and correlates of adopting or not adopting a recovery identity among individuals resolving drug and alcohol problems. *Psychology of Addictive Behaviors*, *32*(6), 595–604. https://doi.org/10.1037/adb0000386

Klingemann, H. K., & Sobell, L. C. (2007). *Promoting self-change from addictive behaviors: Practical implications for policy, prevention, and treatment.* Springer.

Koob, G. F., & Volkow, N. D. (2016). Neurobiology of addiction: A neurocircuitry analysis. *Lancet Psychiatry, 3 (8)*, 760–773. https://doi.org/10.1016/S2215–0366(16)00104-8

Laudet, A. B. (2007). What does recovery mean to you? Lessons from the recovery experience for research and practice. *Journal of Substance Abuse Treatment*, *33* (3), 243–256. https://doi.org/10.1016/j.jsat.2007.04.014

(2009). *Environmental scan of measures of recovery*. Substance Abuse and Mental Health Services Administration.

Lee, M. R., Boness, C. L., McDowell, Y. E., Vergés, A., Steinley, D. L., & Sher, K. J. (2018). Desistance and severity of alcohol use disorder: A lifespan-developmental investigation. *Clinical Psychological Science*, *6*(1), 90–105. https://doi.org/10.1177/2167702617736852

Lowman, C., Allen, J., Stout, R. L., Connors, G., Longabaugh, R., Maisto, S. A., Miller, W. R., Rubin, A., Stour, R. L., Waldron, D., Westerberg, V. S., & Zywiak, W. H. (1996). Replication and extension of Marlatt’s taxonomy of relapse precipitants: Overview of procedures and results. *Addiction*, *91*, S51–S71. https://doi.org/10.1111/j.1360-0443.1996.tb02327.x

Maisto, S. A., Connors, G. J., & Zywiak, W. H. (1996). Construct validation analyses on the Marlatt typology of relapse precipitants. *Addiction, 91*(12s1), 89–98. https://doi.org/10.1046/j.1360-0443.91.12s1.19.x

Maisto, S. A., Hallgren, K. A., Roos, C. R., & Swan, J. E. (2020). Patterns of transitions between relapse to and remission from heavy drinking over the first year after outpatient alcohol treatment and their relation to long-term outcomes. *Journal of Consulting and Clinical Psychology 88* (12), 1119–1132. https://doi.org/10.1037/ccp0000615

Maisto, S. A., Hallgren, K. A., Roos, C. R., & Witkiewitz, K. (2018). Course of remission from and relapse to heavy drinking following outpatient treatment of alcohol use disorder. *Drug and Alcohol Dependence, 187*, 319–326. https://doi.org/10.1016/j.drugalcdep.2018.03.011

Maisto, S. A., Kirouac, M., & Witkiewitz, K. (2014). Alcohol use disorder clinical course research: Informing clinicians' treatment planning now and in the future. *Journal of Studies on Alcohol and Drugs, 75*(5), 799–807. https://doi.org/10.15288/jsad.2014.75.799

Maisto, S. A., Roos, C. R., O'Sickey, A. J., Kirouac, M., Connors, G. J., Tonigan, J. S., & Witkiewitz, K. (2015). The indirect effect of the therapeutic alliance and alcohol abstinence self-efficacy on alcohol use and alcohol-related problems in Project MATCH. *Alcoholism: Clinical and Experimental Research, 39*(3), 504–513. https://doi.org/10.1111/acer.12649

Maisto, S. A., Xie, F. C., Witkiewitz, K., Ewart, C. K., Connors, G. J., Zhu, H., Elder, G., Ditmar, M., & Chow, S.-M. (2017). How chronic self-regulatory stress, poor anger regulation, and momentary affect undermine treatment for alcohol use disorder: Integrating social action theory with the dynamic model of relapse. *Journal of Social and Clinical Psychology, 36*(3), 238–263. https://doi.org/10.1521/jscp.2017.36.3.238

Marlatt, G. A. (1996). Lest taxonomy become taxidermy: A comment on the relapse replication and extension project. *Addiction, 91*(12s1), 147–154. https://doi.org/10.1046/j.1360-0443.91.12s1.5.x

Marlatt, G. A., & Gordon, J. R. (Eds.) (1985). *Relapse prevention: Maintenance strategies in addictive behavior change*. Guilford Press.

McKay, J. R., Lynch, K. G., Shepard, D. S., Morgenstern, J., Forman, R. F., & Pettinati, H. M. (2005). Do patient characteristics and initial progress in treatment moderate the effectiveness of telephone-based continuing care for substance use disorders? *Addiction, 100*(2), 216–226. https://doi.org/10.1111/j.1360-0443.2005.00972.x

Miller, W. R. (1996). What is a relapse? Fifty ways to leave the wagon. *Addiction, 91* (Suppl.), S15–27. https://doi.org/10.1111/j.1360-0443.1996.tb02324.x

Moos, R. H., & Moos, B. S. (2005). Sixteen-year changes and stable remission among treated and untreated individuals with alcohol use disorders. *Drug and Alcohol Dependence, 80*(3), 337–347. https://doi.org/10.1016/j.drugalcdep.2005.05.001

Neale, J., Vitoratou, S., Finch, E., Lennon, P., Mitcheson, L., Panebianco, D., Rose, D., Strang, J., Wykes, T., & Marsden, J. (2016). Development and validation of SURE: A patient reported outcome measure for recovery from drug and alcohol dependence. *Drug and Alcohol Dependence, 165*, 159–167. https://doi.org/10.1016/j.drugalcdep.2016.06.006

Roos, C. R., & Witkiewitz, K. (2017). A contextual model of self-regulation change mechanisms among individuals with addictive disorders. *Clinical Psychology Review*, *57*. https://doi.org/10.1016/j.cpr.2017.08.008

Sinha, R. (2011). Effects of adrenal sensitivity, stress- and cue-induced craving, and anxiety on subsequent alcohol relapse and treatment outcomes. *Archives of General Psychiatry*, *68*(9), 942. https://doi.org/10.1001/archgenpsychiatry.2011.49

Sliedrecht, W., de Waart, R., Witkiewitz, K., & Roozen, H. G. (2019). Alcohol use disorder relapse factors: A systematic review. *Psychiatry Research*, *278*, 97–115. https://doi.org/10.1016/j.psychres.2019.05.038

Substance Abuse and Mental Health Services Administration. (2011). *SAMHSA working definition of recovery: 10 guiding principles of recovery*. Department of Health and Human Services.

Swan, J. E., Votaw, V. R., Stein, E., & Witkiewitz, K. (2020). The role of affect in psychosocial treatments for substance use disorders. *Current Addiction Reports*, *7*, 108–116. https://doi.org/10.1007/s40429-020-00304-0

Tucker, J. A., Cheong, J., Chandler, S. D., Lambert, B. H., Pietrzak, B., Kwok, H., & Davies, S. L. (2016). Prospective analysis of behavioral economic predictors of stable moderation drinking among problem drinkers attempting natural recovery. *Alcoholism: Clinical and Experimental Research*, *40*(12), 2676–2684. https://doi.org/10.1111/acer.13245

Tucker, J. A., Roth, D. L., Vignolo, M. J., & Westfall, A. O. (2009). A behavioral economic reward index predicts drinking resolutions: Moderation revisited and compared with other outcomes. *Journal of Consulting and Clinical Psychology*, *77*(2), 219–228. https://doi.org/10.1037/a0014968

US Department of Health & Human Services. (2016). *Facing addiction in America: The surgeon general's report on alcohol, drugs, and health*. Department of Health & Human Services

Vilsaint, C. L., Kelly, J. F., Bergman, B. G., Groshkova, T., Best, D., & White, W. (2017). Development and validation of a Brief Assessment of Recovery Capital (BARC-10) for alcohol and drug use disorder. *Drug and Alcohol Dependence*, *177*, 71–76. https://doi.org/10.1016/j.drugalcdep.2017.03.022

White, W. L. (2007). Addiction recovery: Its definition and conceptual boundaries. *Journal of Substance Abuse Treatment*, *33*(3), 229–241. https://doi.org/10.1016/j.jsat.2007.04.015

Witkiewitz, K. (2011). Predictors of heavy drinking during and following treatment. *Psychology of Addictive Behaviors*, *25*(3), 426–438. https://doi.org/10.1037/a0022889

(2013). Temptation to drink as a predictor of drinking outcomes following psychosocial treatment for alcohol dependence. *Alcoholism: Clinical and Experimental Research*, *37*(3), 529–537. https://doi.org/10.1111/j.1530-0277.2012.01950.x

Witkiewitz, K., Falk, D. E., Litten, R. Z., Hasin, D. S., Kranzler, H. R., Mann, K. F., O'Malley, S. S., & Anton, R. F. (2019). Maintenance of World Health Organization risk drinking level reductions and posttreatment functioning following a large alcohol use disorder clinical trial. *Alcoholism: Clinical and Experimental Research*, *43*(5), 979–987. https://doi.org/10.1111/acer.14018

Witkiewitz, K., Kranzler, H. R., Hallgren, K. A., O'Malley, S. S., Falk, D. E., Litten, R. Z., Hasin, D. S., Mann, K. F., & Anton, R. F. (2018). Drinking risk level reductions associated with improvements in physical health and quality of life among individuals with alcohol use disorder. *Alcoholism: Clinical and Experimental Research*, *42*(12), 2453–2465. https://doi.org/10.1111/acer.13897

Witkiewitz, K., & Marlatt, G. A. (2004). Relapse prevention for alcohol and drug problems: That was Zen, this is Tao. *American Psychologist*, *59*(4), 224–235. https://doi.org/10.1037/0003-066X.59.4.224

Witkiewitz, K., & Masyn, K. E. (2008). Drinking trajectories following an initial lapse. *Psychology of Addictive Behaviors*, *22*(2), 157–167. https://doi.org/10.1037/0893-164X.22.2.157

Witkiewitz, K., McCallion, E. A., Vowles, K. E., Kirouac, M., Frohe, T., Maisto, S. A., Hodgson, R., & Heather, N. (2015). Association between physical pain and alcohol treatment outcomes: The mediating role of negative affect. *Journal of Consulting and Clinical Psychology*, *83*(6), 1044–1057. https://doi.org/10.1037/ccp0000033

Witkiewitz, K., Montes, K. S., Schwebel, F. J., & Tucker, J. A. (2020). What is recovery? A narrative review of definitions of recovery from alcohol use disorder. *Alcohol Research: Current Reviews*, *40*(3), 1–12. https://doi.org/10.35946/arcr.v40.3.01

Witkiewitz, K., Pearson, M. R., Wilson, A. D., Stein, E. R., Votaw, V. R., Hallgren, K. A., Maisto, S. A., Swan, J. E., Schwebel, F. J., Aldridge, A., Zarkin, G. A., & Tucker, J. A. (2020). Can alcohol use disorder recovery include some heavy drinking? A replication and extension up to nine years following treatment. *Alcoholism: Clinical and Experimental Research, 44,* 1862–1873. https://doi.org/10.1111/acer.14413

Witkiewitz, K., Van Der Maas, H. L. J., Hufford, M. R., & Marlatt, G. A. (2007). Nonnormality and divergence in posttreatment alcohol use: Re-examining the Project MATCH data "another way." *Journal of Abnormal Psychology*, *116*(2), 378–394. https://doi.org/10.1037/0021-843X.116.2.378

Witkiewitz, K., Wilson, A. D., Pearson, M. R., Montes, K. S., Kirouac, M., Roos, C. R., Hallgren, K. A., & Maisto, S. A. (2019). Profiles of recovery from alcohol use disorder at three years following treatment: Can the definition of recovery be extended to include high-functioning heavy drinkers? *Addiction*, *114*(1), 69–80. https://doi.org/10.1111/add.14403

World Health Organization. (2018). *International classification of diseases for mortality and morbidity statistics (11th Revision)*. World Health Organization. https://icd.who.int/browse11/l-m/en

3 The Role of Self-Regulation Strategies in Recovery from Alcohol Use Disorder

Corey R. Roos, Sarah Bowen, and Hedy Kober

The Role of Self-Regulation Strategies in Recovery from Alcohol Use Disorder

As human beings, we continually strive toward short- and long-term future desired outcomes. This goal-directed behavior is commonly termed "self-regulation" (Carver & Scheier, 2001), and self-regulation strategies are overt and covert behaviors executed during goal pursuit. As discussed in this chapter, cognitive reappraisal, problem solving, mindful awareness, and seeking social support are examples of self-regulation strategies that people use to pursue their goals. For individuals with alcohol use disorder (AUD), self-regulation strategies are thought to play a critical role in the process of recovery and are often the target of interventions (Kober, 2014; Marlatt & Donovan, 2005; Roos & Witkiewitz, 2017; Witkiewitz & Marlatt, 2009).

In the context of AUD recovery, one might immediately focus on self-regulation strategies directed toward reducing or stopping drinking. However, in our view – and as described throughout this book – defining AUD recovery strictly based on alcohol use is limited and potentially stigmatizing. Instead, a broadened view of AUD recovery encompasses striving toward and achieving personal well-being in the context of past or ongoing problems related to alcohol use. Thus, in this chapter, we define AUD recovery as "a dynamic process over time, occurring in the context of past or ongoing alcohol-related problems, in which individuals increasingly achieve and maintain personally chosen valued goals in various life domains, such as relationships and social life, occupation, roles and responsibilities, recreation and leisure, physical and mental health, substance-related behaviors, spirituality/religiosity, community involvement, and personal growth." Notably, alcohol use is not central to this definition, but is one among multiple domains within which individuals may pursue personally valued goals. Within this framework, this chapter considers the role of self-regulation strategies in AUD recovery, as defined here. We first examine mechanisms that perpetuate AUD and then discuss how various self-regulation strategies can promote AUD recovery.

Mechanisms That Maintain AUD

Before discussing self-regulation strategies in AUD recovery, it is important to review mechanisms thought to maintain AUD at the individual

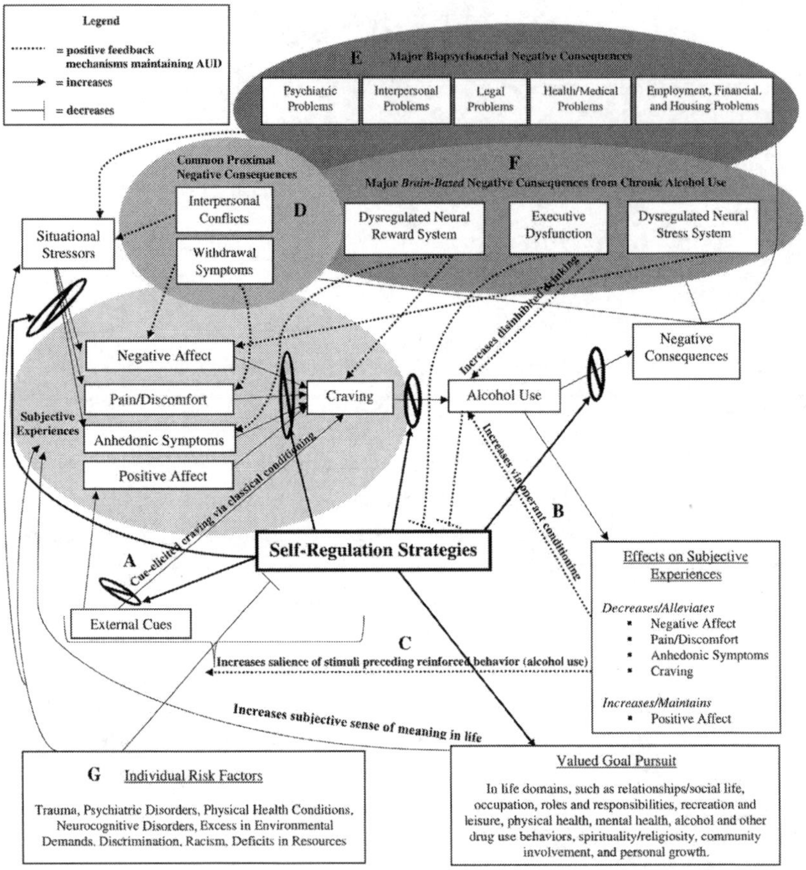

Figure 3.1 *Theorized mechanisms maintaining alcohol use disorder (AUD) and the role of self-regulation strategies.*

level (Cheetham et al., 2010; Everitt & Robbins, 2005; Goldstein & Volkow, 2011; Kober, 2014; Koob & Volkow, 2010, 2016; McHugh & Kneeland, 2019; Skinner & Aubin, 2010; Sliedrecht et al., 2019; Wise & Koob, 2014; Witkiewitz & Marlatt, 2009). For heuristic purposes, Figure 3.1 provides a depiction of multiple mechanisms hypothesized to maintain AUD and relationships among them, as well as the potential role of self-regulation strategies. The figure selectively draws from neuroscience, behavioral, cognitive behavioral, and psychiatric accounts of AUD, and is presented to illustrate the complex set of variables and mechanisms thought to be involved in the self-regulation of alcohol-related behaviors at the individual level.

Starting with Figure 3.1, Parts A and B, classical and operant conditioning are two critical mechanisms demonstrated to maintain AUD (Cheetham et al., 2010; Koob & Volkow, 2010; Skinner & Aubin, 2010). Among individuals who drink alcohol, classical conditioning can occur when neutral stimuli (e.g., walking by a bar, seeing a group of friends, listening to a song) are repeatedly paired with the rewarding effects of alcohol use, thus acquiring the ability to elicit alcohol craving or the subjective state of experiencing a desire to drink alcohol that may contribute to alcohol use (e.g., Schacht et al., 2013; Part A of Figure 3.1). Operant conditioning occurs when the consequence of a behavior increases the likelihood that an individual will repeat that behavior in the future and thus serves as a reinforcer. As shown in Part B of Figure 3.1, the behavior of drinking alcohol often has short-term consequences, such as decreasing/alleviating (1) negative affect (e.g., stress, anxiety, sadness, anger); (2) physical pain and discomfort (e.g., musculoskeletal pain, withdrawal symptoms); (3) anhedonic symptoms (e.g., inability to feel pleasure); (4) alcohol craving; and (5) increasing/maintaining positive affect (e.g., relaxation, excitement, euphoria). These short-term consequences often function as reinforcers, thereby increasing the likelihood of future alcohol use (Wise & Koob, 2014). As part of operant conditioning, the presence of specific stimuli that frequently precede the reinforced behavior of alcohol use – e.g., excitement, social gatherings, anxiety, depressed mood, pain – function as discriminant stimuli that can elicit craving and increase the probability that an individual will drink alcohol because these stimuli have been repeatedly paired with alcohol use (Everitt & Robbins, 2005; Figure 3.1, Part C). In the earlier stages of AUD development, positive reinforcement (via alcohol's ability to increase/maintain positive affect) is hypothesized to play a central role in the progression of AUD (Koob & Volkow, 2016). However, in later and more severe stages of AUD, negative reinforcement (via alcohol's ability to decrease/alleviate challenging subjective experiences) is hypothesized to play a larger role in the progression and maintenance of the disorder (Koob & Volkow, 2016).

Both proximal (Figure 3.1, Part D) and distal (Figure 3.1, Parts E and F) negative consequences from alcohol use (e.g., interpersonal arguments and alcohol-related loss of employment) may variously maintain AUD by increasing distress and concern with loss of future valued rewards and contribute to relapse (e.g., Vuchinich & Tucker, 1996). However, an accumulation of such adverse consequences may also motivate recovery attempts, and improvements in affected areas of functioning after recovery initiation likely reinforce continued engagement in a sober lifestyle (e.g., Tucker et al., 2002).

Additionally, chronic heavy drinking can have negative effects on the brain (Koob & Volkow, 2016), which in turn may maintain AUD (Figure 3.1, Part F). First, chronic heavy drinking can lead to neural changes within reward systems (Koob & Le Moal, 2001), which can increase susceptibility to drug-associated cues and the intensity of cue-elicited craving, as well as disrupt the processing of natural rewards in daily life (e.g., food, social contact). Second, chronic heavy drinking can lead to neural changes in stress systems (Koob et al., 2014), which can increase negative affective reactivity to stressors. Third, chronic heavy drinking can affect the prefrontal cortex and contribute to impairments in executive functioning (Goldstein & Volkow, 2011), which may increase the likelihood of harmful alcohol use.

Finally, several individual risk factors (Figure 3.1, Part G) can play a role in maintaining AUD (Witkiewitz & Marlatt, 2009). Deficits in environmental resources (e.g., education, income, healthcare), excesses in environmental demands (e.g., racism, discrimination, disadvantaged living conditions), and neurocognitive disorders and dispositions (e.g., learning disabilities, attentional deficits, high impulsivity) can impair a person's success in implementing effective self-regulation strategies in daily life (Roos & Witkiewitz, 2017). Moreover, exposure to traumatic events and the presence of comorbid psychiatric disorders (e.g., mood, anxiety, posttraumatic stress, and personality disorders) and physical health conditions (e.g., chronic pain, diabetes) – which all frequently co-occur with AUD – can increase situational stressors and challenging subjective experiences that promote alcohol use (McHugh & Kneeland, 2019).

Self-Regulation as a Mechanism in AUD Recovery

Utilization of adaptive self-regulation strategies is theorized to be a key mechanism in AUD recovery (Kober, 2014; Magill et al., 2020; Roos et al., 2020; Roos & Witkiewitz, 2017). As shown in Figure 3.1, the use of adaptive self-regulation strategies is thought to directly disrupt multiple mechanisms maintaining AUD. Moreover, increased utilization of adaptive self-regulation strategies is thought to increase a person's initial and continued access to a range of valued life goals during the recovery process. In this section, we (1) define specific self-regulation strategies, (2) discuss how each strategy may affect mechanisms that maintain AUD and facilitate AUD recovery, and (3) provide an overview of empirical research on the association between each strategy and recovery outcomes.

As discussed in the following sections, there are two major families of psychosocial interventions that focus on teaching adaptive self-regulation strategies to individuals with substance use disorders including AUD: cognitive behavioral therapies (CBTs; e.g., Carey et al., 2007; Carroll, 1998; Magill et al., 2019; Marlatt & Donovan, 2005; Monti, 2002) and mindfulness- and acceptance-based therapies (MABTs; e.g., Bowen et al., 2011; Cavicchioli et al., 2018; Garland, 2013; Goldberg et al., 2018; Hayes et al., 2011; Linehan, 2015). CBTs and MABTs have several common areas of focus, including teaching self-regulation strategies that can be applied to valued goal pursuit, such as the pursuit of alcohol-specific goals (e.g., reducing alcohol use and related harm). As discussed below, although the supporting evidence is somewhat mixed (Magill et al., 2020; Roos & Witkiewitz, 2017), across the two modalities research has shown that increased utilization of adaptive self-regulation strategies is a statistical mediator of treatment effects on alcohol-related outcomes following CBTs or MABTs for AUD (Garland et al., 2016; Kiluk et al., 2010; Lévesque et al., 2017; Roos et al., 2017, 2020a, 2020b; Witkiewitz et al., 2013, 2018). Some research further suggests that increased utilization of adaptive self-regulation strategies may be a common mechanism of change across multiple psychosocial treatments for AUD (Litt et al., 2018).

Cognitive-Behavioral Self-Regulation Strategies

Cognitive-behavioral self-regulation strategies are focused on directly changing environments (e.g., stimulus control), mental processes (e.g., cognitive reappraisal, distraction, problem solving, goal setting, episodic future thinking), feelings (e.g., arousal reduction, physiological management), and actions (e.g., active communication, seeking social support, positive activity engagement, harm reduction).

Stimulus Control

Stimulus control refers to the operant conditioning process whereby a given response becomes more likely in a particular situation when similar responses in similar situations have previously been reinforced. As applied to behavior change, stimulus control self-regulation strategies involve changing one's environment or modifying one's exposure to stimuli in the environment to promote beneficial behavior patterns (Gross & Thompson, 2007; Marlatt & Donovan, 2005; Monti, 2002). Stimulus control strategies may facilitate AUD recovery by reducing exposure to external cues associated with alcohol consumption, including access to alcohol itself. For example, individuals may intentionally avoid walking by a bar where they used to frequently drink, or they may leave a social gathering when the sight of their favorite alcoholic drink elicits intense craving. Several studies have shown that greater use of stimulus control strategies are associated with reduced alcohol use among individuals with AUD (Dolan et al., 2013; Litt et al., 2003, 2009, 2018; Rohsenow et al., 2001; Roos et al., 2020b; Roos & Witkiewitz, 2016).

Stimulus control strategies may also facilitate valued goal pursuit in many other life domains among individuals on a pathway to AUD recovery. For example, individuals may actively choose to put themselves in situations with new people because they have a goal of finding a romantic partner. Or individuals may walk away from an interpersonal argument to avoid yelling or becoming physically aggressive. There is a lack of research, however, examining the role of stimulus control as a strategy to facilitate goal pursuit (beyond alcohol use) and improve general well-being among individuals with AUD.

Cognitive Reappraisal

Cognitive reappraisal involves changing how one thinks about a situation (Beck, 1979; Gross & Thompson, 2007). Cognitive reappraisal may facilitate AUD recovery by reducing challenging subjective experiences (e.g., negative affect, pain/discomfort, craving) that precede drinking. For example, individuals may replace thoughts about positive consequences of drinking ("drinking would be really fun right now") with thoughts about negative consequences of drinking ("drinking leads to hangovers and causes problems in my marriage"), which may reduce the desire to drink. Numerous studies have demonstrated that greater use of cognitive reappraisal is associated with reduced alcohol use among individuals with AUD (Aase et al., 2018; Chung et al., 2001; Dolan et al., 2013; Dulin & Gonzalez, 2017; Litt et al., 2003, 2009, 2018; Rohsenow et al., 2001; Roos et al., 2020b; Roos & Witkiewitz, 2016). Additionally, two experimental laboratory studies found that the use of cognitive reappraisal during alcohol cue exposure reduced alcohol craving (Naqvi et al., 2015; Suzuki et al., 2020), as well as craving-related neural activity (Suzuki et al., 2020).

Although there is relatively little research on the role of cognitive reappraisal as a strategy to facilitate goal pursuit (beyond reducing alcohol use) and improve general well-being during a recovery attempt, it seems likely that cognitive reappraisal may also facilitate valued goal pursuit in other life domains. For example, individuals in recovery with the goal of keeping a new job may experience frequent anxiety related to the demands of the position. After making a mistake at work and worrying they may get fired, they might use cognitive reappraisal to estimate the actual likelihood of being fired (e.g., "My co-workers have told me they made similar mistakes when they were first starting, and they all still have their jobs"), thus reducing their anxiety and the potential of making a rash decision, such as immediately quitting their job to avoid the anticipated humiliation of being fired.

Distraction

Distraction involves using thoughts or actions to divert attention away from one focus toward a different focus that is more adaptive (Gross & Thompson, 2007; Marlatt & Donovan, 2005; Monti, 2002). Distraction may facilitate AUD recovery by reducing attentional processing of external cues and subjective experiences that precede drinking. For example, individuals may close their eyes and listen to music when seeing a flight attendant begin to serve alcohol to other passengers on an airplane. Substituting non-alcoholic drinks or food for alcohol when experiencing craving can also be viewed as a form of distraction. Several clinical studies have found that use of distraction is associated with reduced alcohol use among individuals with AUD (Dolan et al., 2013; Dulin & Gonzalez, 2017; Litt et al., 2003, 2009, 2018; Roos et al., 2020b; Roos & Witkiewitz, 2016), and one experimental study found that distraction reduced alcohol craving during alcohol cue exposure (Murphy & MacKillop, 2014). Although distraction may reasonably be expected to similarly facilitate valued goal pursuit in other life domains during recovery, there is a lack of research on its use during recovery beyond reducing alcohol use.

Problem Solving

Problem solving involves identifying a specific problem at hand, generating and selecting solutions, and planning and executing steps for addressing the problem

(Nezu et al., 2012). Problem solving may promote AUD recovery by facilitating plans to cope during upcoming high-risk situations or by directly changing situational stressors that precede alcohol use. Several studies have demonstrated that increased use of problem solving is associated with reduced drinking among college student drinkers (Park et al., 2004; Weiss et al., 2017) and individuals receiving treatment for AUD (Chung et al., 2001; Dolan et al., 2013; Litt et al., 2003, 2018; Roos et al., 2020a; Roos & Witkiewitz, 2016). Whether problem solving also improves other life-health functioning during AUD recovery is less well researched.

Goal Setting/Tracking

Goal setting and tracking involves systematically defining one or more specific and measurable target goals and tracking progress towards these goals. Goal setting/tracking in the context of AUD recovery may involve setting a goal to reduce one's drinking frequency over time (e.g., from four days a week to two days a week). One study found that setting a goal to reduce drinking, versus not setting a goal, was associated with reduced alcohol use in heavy drinking college students (Lozano & Stephens, 2010). Research has found that general utilization of goal setting/tracking in life is associated with fewer alcohol-related problems (Carey et al., 2004; Hustad et al., 2009; Pearson et al., 2011).

Beyond alcohol-related goals, goal setting/tracking may facilitate valued goal pursuit in many other life domains during recovery. Goal setting commonly involves identifying smaller and more immediately attainable sub-goals that one can focus on achieving along the way toward pursuing a larger or more distal goal. For example, substance-related interventions guided by behavioral economics seek to help individuals see how discrete acts (e.g., drinking now versus going to an Alcoholics Anonymous meeting) are part of temporally extended behavior patterns that comprise AUD or recovery from AUD (Vuchinich & Tucker, 1996). As discussed in Tucker and Murphy et al. (Chapters 9 and 10, respectively, this volume), recovery is conceptualized as foregoing the immediate rewarding act of drinking – and its attendant longer term negative consequences – in favor of delayed alcohol-free rewards of higher value that in turn reinforce sobriety behaviors. Interventions such as extended daily self-monitoring (Tucker et al., 2012) and the Substance Free Activity Session (SFAS) aimed at increasing substance-free rewards and lengthening time horizons for behavioral allocation (Murphy et al., 2019) have been found to promote the longer view of valued non-drinking goals and contribute to beneficial outcomes among college student heavy drinkers and persons with AUD, respectively.

Episodic Future Thinking

Episodic future thinking similarly involves imagining positive substance-free future events with the aim of motivating behavior that increases their receipt (Mellis et al., 2019; Snider et al., 2016). Episodic future thinking may reduce alcohol use by widening an individual's temporal window during decision making and increasing the value of delayed rewards in the future. For example, vividly imagining the experience of having the job one desires in the future may increase the likelihood that an individual will study for college classes on a Friday night rather than drink heavily with peers. One study found that training individuals with AUD in episodic future thinking increased valuation of future monetary rewards and reduced hypothetical purchasing of alcoholic drinks (Snider et al., 2016). The SFAS, which teaches episodic future thinking (Murphy et al., 2019), has been found to be effective in reducing not only alcohol use, but also depression and anxiety symptoms among heavy drinking college students.

Arousal Reduction

Arousal reduction involves engaging in behaviors to reduce arousal, such as paced breathing and progressive muscle relaxation. Arousal reduction can be used during any experience with high arousal, such as negative affect (e.g., stress, panic, anxiety, anger), positive affect (e.g., excitement), physical pain, or craving. Arousal reduction may facilitate AUD recovery by mitigating the intensity of subjective experiences (see Figure 3.1) preceding drinking that reinforce it. One study found that use of arousal reduction was associated with reduced alcohol use among individuals with AUD (Dolan et al., 2013), and preliminary evidence suggests that training individuals with AUD in biofeedback-enhanced paced breathing may reduce alcohol craving over time (Alayan et al., 2018, 2019). However, as with several other strategies, research is lacking on how arousal reduction may improve functioning and well-being during recovery attempts.

Physiological Management and Self-Care

Physiological management/self-care involves intentional efforts to regulate daily physiological states (energy level, hunger, thirst, etc.) including but not limited to arousal reduction by engaging in health behaviors (nutrition, exercise, sleep, etc.). Physiological management/self-care may facilitate AUD recovery by reducing challenging subjective experiences (e.g., negative affect, craving) that stem from or are exacerbated by physiological dysregulation. One study found that coping by eating healthy food and getting adequate sleep was associated with reduced alcohol use among individuals with AUD (Dolan et al., 2013). A review found that sleep interventions among individuals with AUD improved sleep and reduced depression, but did not appear to affect alcohol abstinence (Miller et al., 2017).

Seeking Social Support

Seeking social support involves seeking out emotional support, validation, and/or information/guidance from other people. Social support may facilitate AUD recovery by reducing the intensity of challenging subjective experiences (e.g., craving, stress) and/or by helping individuals obtain needed guidance and resources when experiencing such challenges. For example, individuals may call their AA sponsor or a supportive family member to prevent themselves from drinking when experiencing a strong craving. Several studies have shown that greater seeking of social support is associated with reduced alcohol use among individuals with AUD (Chung et al., 2001; Dolan et al., 2013; Dulin & Gonzalez, 2017; Litt et al., 2003, 2009, 2018; Roos et al., 2020b; Roos & Witkiewitz, 2016). Additionally, social network support for abstinence is a consistent predictor of reduced alcohol use (Longabaugh et al., 2010; Tucker et al., 2015). Seeking social support may facilitate valued goal pursuit in other life domains among individuals with AUD. For example, one study found that social network support was associated with improved quality of life among individuals in recovery (Best et al., 2012).

Active Communication

Active communication involves communicating one's needs and wishes to other people in a clear and assertive way. Active communication may facilitate AUD recovery by helping to eliminate or reduce drinking opportunities or exposure to external cues, as well as ameliorating interpersonal conflicts that precipitate drinking. For example, individuals may use active communication to refuse drink offers from others (e.g., making direct eye contact, saying "no" clearly, and providing a reason). Several studies have shown that greater use of drink refusal is associated with better alcohol treatment outcomes (Dolan et al., 2013; Litt et al., 2003, 2009, 2018; Roos et al., 2020b; Roos & Witkiewitz, 2016). Further, studies that employed role-play measures to assess the quality with which one implements a drink refusal strategy found that higher quality refusal communications were associated with greater reductions in alcohol use among individuals with AUD (Kadden et al., 1992; Kiluk et al., 2010). Another study found that individuals with AUD who received a drink refusal skills training module versus those who did not had better alcohol treatment outcomes (Witkiewitz et al., 2012). Whether active communication also improves other life-health functioning during AUD recovery is less well researched.

Positive Activity Engagement

Positive activity engagement involves making active efforts to devise, plan, and engage in specific enjoyable activities in one's daily life. Positive activity engagement may facilitate AUD recovery by replacing drinking with other rewarding activities. The SFAS, which involves brief training in substance-free activity engagement, reduced alcohol use and related problems among heavy drinkers, and this effect was mediated by changes in proportional reinforcement from alcohol-free positive activities (Murphy et al., 2019; see Chapter 10 this volume). Other studies have suggested that more frequent engagement in alternative positive activities (other than drinking) is associated with reduced alcohol use among individuals with AUD (Dolan et al., 2013; Litt et al., 2003, 2018;

Roos & Witkiewitz, 2016). Positive activity engagement may also facilitate general well-being among individuals in recovery. For example, the Substance Free Activity Session was effective in reducing depression and anxiety among heavy drinking college students (Murphy et al., 2019).

Harm Reduction

Harm reduction involves intentional efforts to minimize harm while engaging in an activity that potentially poses harm, such as drinking. Harm reduction may facilitate AUD recovery by weakening the link between alcohol use and negative consequences. Examples of harm reduction approaches (often referred to as alcohol-related "protective behavioral strategies") include having a designated driver when drinking, eating before drinking to slow the absorption of alcohol, setting a drink limit for a given occasion, alternating between alcoholic and nonalcoholic drinks, and avoiding drinking games. Harm reduction studies with heavy drinking college students suggest that greater use of such strategies is associated with less alcohol-related problems (Leeman et al., 2016; Pearson, 2013). More broadly, harm reduction is associated with reduced alcohol-related problems among individuals with AUD (Marlatt & Witkiewitz, 2002), and harm reduction strategies can be applied to other domains of life among individuals with AUD, such as sexual activity and other drug use. For example, harm reduction interventions among individuals with AUD and HIV/AIDS are effective in increasing condom use (Scott-Sheldon et al., 2017).

Mindfulness- and Acceptance-Based Therapy (MABT) Self-Regulation Strategies

Mindfulness- and acceptance- based strategies tend to focus less on changing environments, thoughts, feelings, and behaviors, and more on shifting the perspective of and relationship to experiences. This includes increasing awareness of internal and external events, recognition and acceptance of aversive or challenging aspects of life that are outside of one's control, appreciation of naturally reinforcing experiences, and increasing awareness and salience of values that guide personal choices.

Mindful Awareness

Mindful awareness, a component of the two-component model of mindfulness, involves intentional monitoring and recognition of one's experience in the moment (Bishop et al., 2004; Lindsay & Creswell, 2017). Mindful awareness may facilitate AUD recovery by increasing recognition of external and internal antecedents of alcohol use, and by reducing automatic alcohol use. For example, when experiencing a craving to drink, individuals may practice deliberately pausing and observing how the experience of craving feels in their body, instead of automatically acting on the craving. Most studies have examined mindful awareness as a dispositional trait, and have shown that mindful awareness is consistently associated with less alcohol use (Karyadi et al., 2014). Moreover, interventions explicitly targeting mindful awareness via mindfulness meditation training are effective in reducing alcohol use and stress (Li et al., 2017).

Mindful Acceptance

Mindful acceptance, the second component in the two-component model of mindfulness, involves adopting an open, accepting, and nonjudgmental attitude toward momentary experiences, including challenging thoughts, emotions, and sensations. Mindful acceptance may have a positive influence on AUD by reducing cognitive, affective, and physiological reactivity to challenging subjective experiences, and reducing rigid escape- or avoidance-oriented behaviors (including alcohol use). For example, when experiencing negative affect and/or craving, individuals may accept their experience in the moment as it is, instead of judging themselves or trying to change how they feel. Mindful acceptance, as a trait-level disposition, is associated with less alcohol use (Karyadi et al., 2014). Moreover, interventions explicitly targeting mindful acceptance are effective in reducing alcohol use and stress (Li et al., 2017).

Savoring

Savoring involves bringing an attitude of curiosity and appreciation towards one's experience (including sensory experiences and any positive emotions that arise) while engaging in pleasant activities (Garland, 2013). Savoring may facilitate AUD recovery by enhancing the processing of other natural rewards besides alcohol. For example, individuals may practice savoring pleasant activities in daily life, such as drinking coffee, eating, or walking in nature. There is limited research on how savoring is associated with alcohol-related outcomes. Nevertheless, mindfulness-oriented recovery enhancement (MORE), which includes specific training in savoring, has been shown to increase positive affect among individuals with AUD (Garland et al., 2016).

Values Clarification

Values clarification involves identifying, affirming, and committing to living by personal values about what kind of person one aspires to be. Values clarification may facilitate AUD recovery by increasing motivation to engage in the hard work of recovery. For example, individuals may think about their reasons for changing their drinking and about how and why making these changes is personally meaningful to them. Values clarification may also enhance the reinforcement value of alcohol-free valued activities. Values clarification is particularly emphasized in acceptance and commitment therapy (ACT), which has been shown to be effective in reducing alcohol use (Lee et al., 2015). Although there is limited research on how values clarification may also improve other life-health functioning during AUD recovery, this method shares common features with the SFAS, which focuses on bringing current behavior in line with values and goals and has been found efficacious in reducing drinking and improving functioning.

Conclusions and Recommendations

In this chapter, we have described numerous putatively adaptive self-regulation strategies, discussed their demonstrated or likely role in AUD recovery, and provided an overview of research on how use of these strategies may be associated with recovery outcomes. There is some empirical evidence suggesting that each strategy (with the exception of savoring) is associated with reduced alcohol use among individuals with AUD. However, as demonstrated in this chapter, there is considerably less empirical research on how self-regulation strategies are related to AUD recovery outcomes beyond alcohol use. This is an unfortunate gap in the literature, especially for advancing understanding of AUD recovery as a dynamic process over time in which individuals increasingly achieve and maintain personally chosen valued goals in various domains of life functioning. Thus, many important questions regarding the role of self-regulation in AUD recovery remain to be addressed. For example, how can self-regulation strategies improve life satisfaction, social functioning, occupational functioning, meaning in life, and emotional well-being? And which self-regulation strategies may be most important for improving particular recovery outcomes (e.g., meaning in life) or for helping individuals improve their well-being in particular functional domains?

Moreover, our review indicated that there is relatively less research on MABT self-regulation strategies, such as savoring, as compared to CBT self-regulation strategies. This may be because MABTs are newer than CBTs. Hence, further research is needed on how MABT strategies are related to both alcohol-related and broader functional recovery outcomes. Indeed, it is plausible that savoring may be a particularly important strategy for improving well-being in life domains other than alcohol use.

In summary, research on the role of self-regulation strategies in recovery requires expansion to examine relevant functional outcomes beyond alcohol-related outcomes. Such research would be useful for clarifying how self-regulation strategies facilitate a holistic recovery process, not simply changes in alcohol use. Alcohol use and alcohol-related problems are important outcomes to examine, and many individuals with AUD want to reduce their drinking and related problems. However, individuals with AUD often have many other needs and goals in a range of key life domains, not just alcohol use behavior. Their success in addressing these domains of functioning and well-being are likely an important component to achieving and maintaining lasting recovery.

References

Aase, D. M., Gorka, S. M., Greenstein, J. E., Proescher, E., Crane, N. A., Everett, L.-K., Hassan, I., Osborn, A., Schroth, C., & Kennedy-Krage, A. (2018). Cognitive reappraisal moderates the relationship between PTSD symptoms and alcohol use over time in post–9/11 US military veterans. *Drug and Alcohol Dependence*, *191*, 159–164. https://doi.org/10.1016/j.drugalcdep.2018.06.032

Alayan, N., Eddie, D., Eller, L., Bates, M. E., & Carmody, D. P. (2019). Substance craving changes in university students receiving heart rate variability biofeedback: A longitudinal multilevel modeling approach. *Addictive Behaviors*, *97*, 35–41. https://doi.org/10.1016/j.addbeh.2019.05.005

Alayan, N., Eller, L., Bates, M. E., & Carmody, D. P. (2018). Current evidence on heart rate variability biofeedback as a complementary anticraving intervention. *The Journal of Alternative and Complementary Medicine*, *24*(11), 1039–1050. https://doi.org/10.1089/acm.2018.0019

Beck, A. T. (1979). *Cognitive therapy of depression*. Guilford Press.

Best, D., Honor, S., Karpusheff, J., Loudon, L., Hall, R., Groshkova, T., & White, W. (2012). Well-being and recovery functioning among substance users engaged in posttreatment recovery support groups. *Alcoholism Treatment Quarterly*, *30*(4), 397–406. https://doi.org/10.1080/07347324.2012.718956

Bishop, S. R., Lau, M., Shapiro, S., Carlson, L., Anderson, N. D., Carmody, J., Segal, Z. V., Abbey, S., Speca, M., & Velting, D. (2004). Mindfulness: A proposed operational definition. *Clinical Psychology: Science and Practice*, *11*(3), 230–241. https://doi.org/10.1093/clipsy.bph077

Bowen, S., Chawla, N., & Marlatt, G. A. (2011). *Mindfulness-based relapse prevention for addictive behaviors: A clinician's guide*. Guilford Press.

Carey, K. B., Neal, D. J., & Collins, S. E. (2004). A psychometric analysis of the self-regulation questionnaire. *Addictive Behaviors*, *29*(2), 253–260. https://doi.org/10.1016/j.addbeh.2003.08.001

Carey, K. B., Scott-Sheldon, L. A., Carey, M. P., & DeMartini, K. S. (2007). Individual-level interventions to reduce college student drinking: A meta-analytic review. *Addictive Behaviors*, *32*(11), 2469–2494. https://doi.org/10.1016/j.addbeh.2007.05.004

Carroll, K. (1998). *A cognitive-behavioral approach: Treating cocaine addiction* (NIH Publication Number 98-4308). US Department of Health and Human Services. https://archives.drugabuse.gov/sites/default/files/cbt.pdf

Carver, C. S., & Scheier, M. F. (2001). *On the self-regulation of behavior*. Cambridge University Press.

Cavicchioli, M., Movalli, M., & Maffei, C. (2018). The clinical efficacy of mindfulness-based treatments for alcohol and drug use disorders: A meta-analytic review of randomized and nonrandomized controlled trials. *European Addiction Research*, *24*, 137–162. https://doi.org/10.1159/000490762

Cheetham, A., Allen, N. B., Yücel, M., & Lubman, D. I. (2010). The role of affective dysregulation in drug addiction. *Clinical Psychology Review*, *30*(6), 621–634. https://doi.org/10.1016/j.cpr.2010.04.005

Chung, T., Langenbucher, J., Labouvie, E., Pandina, R. J., & Moos, R. H. (2001). Changes in alcoholic patients' coping responses predict 12-month treatment outcomes. *Journal of Consulting and Clinical psychology*, *69*(1), 92–100. https://doi.org/10.1037/0022-006X.69.1.92

Csabonyi, M., & Phillips, L. J. (2020). Meaning in life and substance use. *Journal of Humanistic Psychology*, *60*(1), 3–19. https://doi.org/10.1177/0022167816687674

Dolan, S. L., Rohsenow, D. J., Martin, R. A., & Monti, P. M. (2013). Urge-specific and lifestyle coping strategies of alcoholics: Relationships of specific strategies to treatment outcome. *Drug and Alcohol Dependence*, *128*(1–2), 8–14. https://doi .org/10.1016/j.drugalcdep.2012.07.010

Dulin, P. L., & Gonzalez, V. M. (2017). Smartphone-based, momentary intervention for alcohol cravings amongst individuals with an alcohol use disorder. *Psychology of Addictive Behaviors*, *31*(5), 601–607. https://doi.org/10.1037/adb0000292

Everitt, B. J., & Robbins, T. W. (2005). Neural systems of reinforcement for drug addiction: From actions to habits to compulsion. *Nature Neuroscience*, *8*(11), 1481–1489. https://doi.org/10.1038/nn1579

Garland, E. L. (2013). *Mindfulness-oriented recovery enhancement for addiction, stress, and pain*. National Association of Social Workers Press.

Garland, E. L., Roberts-Lewis, A., Tronnier, C. D., Graves, R., & Kelley, K. (2016). Mindfulness-oriented recovery enhancement versus CBT for co-occurring substance dependence, traumatic stress, and psychiatric disorders: proximal outcomes from a pragmatic randomized trial. *Behavior Research and Therapy*, 77, 7–16. https://doi.org/10.1016/j.brat.2015.11.012

Goldberg, S. B., Tucker, R. P., Greene, P. A., Davidson, R. J., Wampold, B. E., Kearney, D. J., & Simpson, T. L. (2018). Mindfulness-based interventions for psychiatric disorders: A systematic review and meta-analysis. *Clinical Psychology Review*, *59*, 52–60. https://doi.org/10.1016/j.cpr.2017.10.011

Goldstein, R. Z., & Volkow, N. D. (2011). Dysfunction of the prefrontal cortex in addiction: Neuroimaging findings and clinical implications. *Nature Reviews Neuroscience*, *12*(11), 652–669. https://doi.org/10.1038/nrn3119

Gross, J. J., & Thompson, R. A. (2007). Emotion regulation: Conceptual foundations. In J. J. Gross (Ed.), *Handbook of emotion regulation* (pp. 3–24). Guilford Press.

Hayes, S. C., Strosahl, K. D., & Wilson, K. G. (2011). *Acceptance and commitment therapy: The process and practice of mindful change*. Guilford Press.

Hustad, J. T., Carey, K. B., Carey, M. P., & Maisto, S. A. (2009). Self-regulation, alcohol consumption, and consequences in college student heavy drinkers: A simultaneous latent growth analysis. *Journal of Studies on Alcohol and Drugs*, *70*(3), 373–382. https://doi.org/10.15288/jsad.2009.70.373

Jacobson, N. S., Martell, C. R., & Dimidjian, S. (2001). Behavioral activation treatment for depression: Returning to contextual roots. *Clinical Psychology: Science and Practice*, *8*(3), 255–270. https://doi.org/10.1093/clipsy.8.3.255

Kadden, R. M., Litt, M. D., Cooney, N. L., & Busher, D. A. (1992). Relationship between role-play measures of coping skills and alcoholism treatment outcome. *Addictive Behaviors*, *17*(5), 425–437. https://doi.org/10.1016/0306-4603(92) 90003-E

Karyadi, K. A., VanderVeen, J. D., & Cyders, M. A. (2014). A meta-analysis of the relationship between trait mindfulness and substance use behaviors. *Drug and Alcohol Dependence*, *143*, 1–10. https://doi.org/10.1016/j.drugalcdep.2014.07.014

Kiluk, B. D., Nich, C., Babuscio, T., & Carroll, K. M. (2010). Quality versus quantity: Acquisition of coping skills following computerized cognitive–behavioral therapy for substance use disorders. *Addiction*, *105*(12), 2120–2127. https://doi.org/10.1111/j.1360-0443.2010.03076.x

Kober, H. (2014). Emotion regulation in substance use disorders. In J. J. Gross (Ed.), *Handbook of emotion regulation* (pp. 428–446). Guilford Press.

Kober, H., Kross, E. F., Mischel, W., Hart, C. L., & Ochsner, K. N. (2010). Regulation of craving by cognitive strategies in cigarette smokers. *Drug and Alcohol Dependence*, *106*(1), 52–55. https://doi.org/10.1016/j.drugalcdep.2009.07.017

Koob, G. F., Buck, C. L., Cohen, A., Edwards, S., Park, P. E., Schlosburg, J. E., Schmeichel, B., Vendruscolo, L. F., Wade, C. L., & Whitfield Jr, T. W. (2014). Addiction as a stress surfeit disorder. *Neuropharmacology*, *76*, 370–382. https://doi.org/10.1016/j.neuropharm.2013.05.024

Koob, G. F., & Le Moal, M. (2001). Drug addiction, dysregulation of reward, and allostasis. *Neuropsychopharmacology*, *24*(2), 97–129. https://doi.org/10.1016/S0893–133X(00)00195-0

Koob, G. F., & Volkow, N. D. (2010). Neurocircuitry of addiction. *Neuropsychopharmacology*, *35*(1), 217–238. https://doi.org/10.1038/npp.2009.110

(2016). Neurobiology of addiction: A neurocircuitry analysis *The Lancet Psychiatry*, *3*(8), 760–773. https://doi.org/10.1016/s2215–0366(16)00104-8

Lee, E. B., An, W., Levin, M. E., & Twohig, M. P. (2015). An initial meta-analysis of acceptance and commitment therapy for treating substance use disorders. *Drug and Alcohol Dependence*, *155*, 1–7. https://doi.org/10.1016/j.drugalcdep.2015.08.004

Leeman, R. F., DeMartini, K. S., Gueorguieva, R., Nogueira, C., Corbin, W. R., Neighbors, C., & O'Malley, S. S. (2016). Randomized controlled trial of a very brief, multicomponent web-based alcohol intervention for undergraduates with a focus on protective behavioral strategies. *Journal of Consulting and Clinical Psychology*, *84*(11), 1008–1015. https://dx.doi.org/10.1037%2Fccp0000132

Lévesque, A., Campbell, A. N., Pavlicova, M., Hu, M.-C., Walker, R., McClure, E. A., Ghitza, U. E., Bailey, G., Stitzer, M., & Nunes, E. V. (2017). Coping strategies as a mediator of internet-delivered psychosocial treatment: Secondary analysis from a NIDA CTN multisite effectiveness trial. *Addictive Behaviors*, *65*, 74–80. https://doi.org/10.1016/j.addbeh.2016.09.012

Li, W., Howard, M. O., Garland, E. L., McGovern, P., & Lazar, M. (2017). Mindfulness treatment for substance misuse: A systematic review and meta-analysis. *Journal of Substance Abuse Treatment*, *75*, 62–96. https://doi.org/10.1016/j.jsat.2017.01.008

Lindsay, E. K., & Creswell, J. D. (2017). Mechanisms of mindfulness training: Monitor and acceptance theory. *Clinical Psychology Review*, *51*, 48–59. https://dx.doi.org/10.1016%2Fj.cpr.2016.10.011

Linehan, M. (2015). *DBT skills training manual*. Guilford Press.

Litt, M. D., Kadden, R. M., & Kabela-Cormier, E. (2009). Individualized assessment and treatment program for alcohol dependence: Results of an initial study to train coping skills. *Addiction*, *104*(11), 1837–1838. https://dx.doi.org/10.1111%2Fj.1360-0443.2009.02693.x

Litt, M. D., Kadden, R. M., Cooney, N. L., & Kabela, E. (2003). Coping skills and treatment outcomes in cognitive-behavioral and interactional group therapy for alcoholism. *Journal of Consulting and Clinical Psychology*, *71*(1), 118–128. https://doi.org/10.1037//0022-006x.71.1.118

Litt, M. D., Kadden, R. M., & Tennen, H. (2018). Treatment response and non-response in CBT and network support for alcohol disorders: Targeted mechanisms and common factors. *Addiction*, *113*(8), 1407–1417.

Longabaugh, R., Wirtz, P. W., Zywiak, W. H., & O'malley, S. S. (2010). Network support as a prognostic indicator of drinking outcomes: The COMBINE study. *Journal of Studies on Alcohol and Drugs*, *71*(6), 837–846. https://doi.org/10.1111/add.14224

Lozano, B. E., & Stephens, R. S. (2010). Comparison of participatively set and assigned goals in the reduction of alcohol use. *Psychology of Addictive Behaviors*, *24*(4), 581–591. https://psycnet.apa.org/doi/10.1037/a0021444

Magill, M., Ray, L., Kiluk, B., Hoadley, A., Bernstein, M., Tonigan, J. S., & Carroll, K. (2019). A meta-analysis of cognitive-behavioral therapy for alcohol or other drug use disorders: Treatment efficacy by contrast condition. *Journal of Consulting and Clinical Psychology*, *87*(12), 1093–1105. https://doi.org/10.1037/ccp0000447

Magill, M., Tonigan, J. S., Kiluk, B., Ray, L., Walthers, J., & Carroll, K. (2020). The search for mechanisms of cognitive behavioral therapy for alcohol or other drug use disorders: A systematic review. *Behaviour Research and Therapy, 103648*. https://doi.org/10.1016/j.brat.2020.103648

Marlatt, G. A., & Donovan, D. M. (Eds.) (2005). *Relapse prevention: Maintenance strategies in the treatment of addictive behaviors*. Guilford Press.

Marlatt, G. A., & Witkiewitz, K. (2002). Harm reduction approaches to alcohol use: Health promotion, prevention, and treatment. *Addictive Behaviors*, *27*(6), 867–886. https://doi.org/10.1016/s0306–4603(02)00294-0

McGrath, E., Elliott, R., Millar, T., & Armitage, C. J. (2020). The role of neuropsychological mechanisms in implementation intentions to reduce alcohol consumption among heavy drinkers: A randomized trial. *Journal of Behavioral Medicine*, *43*(4), 576–586. https://doi.org/10.1007/s10865–019-00078-5

McHugh, R. K., & Kneeland, E. T. (2019). Affective vulnerability in substance use disorders. *Current Opinion in Psychology*, *30,* 54–58. https://doi.org/10.1016/j.copsyc.2019.01.011

Mellis, A. M., Snider, S. E., Deshpande, H. U., LaConte, S. M., & Bickel, W. K. (2019). Practicing prospection promotes patience: Repeated episodic future thinking cumulatively reduces delay discounting. *Drug and Alcohol Dependence, 204,* 107507. https://doi.org/10.1016/j.drugalcdep.2019.06.010

Monti, P. M. (2002). *Treating alcohol dependence: A coping skills training guide*. Guilford Press.

Murphy, C. M., & MacKillop, J. (2014). Mindfulness as a strategy for coping with cue-elicited cravings for alcohol: An experimental examination. *Alcoholism: Clinical and Experimental Research*, *38*(4), 1134–1142. https://dx.doi.org/10.1111%2Facer.12322

Murphy, J. G., Dennhardt, A. A., Martens, M. P., Borsari, B., Witkiewitz, K., & Meshesha, L. Z. (2019). A randomized clinical trial evaluating the efficacy of a brief alcohol intervention supplemented with a substance-free activity session or relaxation training. *Journal of Consulting and Clinical Psychology*, *87*(7), 657–669. https://doi.org/10.1037/ccp0000412

Naqvi, N. H., Ochsner, K. N., Kober, H., Kuerbis, A., Feng, T., Wall, M., & Morgenstern, J. (2015). Cognitive regulation of craving in alcohol-dependent and social drinkers. *Alcoholism: Clinical and Experimental Research*, *39*(2), 343–349. https://doi.org/10.1111/acer.12637

Nezu, A. M., Nezu, C. M., & D'Zurilla, T. (2012). *Problem-solving therapy: A treatment manual*. Springer.

Park, C. L., Armeli, S., & Tennen, H. (2004). The daily stress and coping process and alcohol use among college students. *Journal of Studies on Alcohol*, *65*(1), 126–135. https://doi.org/10.15288/jsa.2004.65.126

Pearson, M. R. (2013). Use of alcohol protective behavioral strategies among college students: A critical review. *Clinical Psychology Review*, *33*(8), 1025–1040. https://doi.org/10.1016/j.cpr.2013.08.006

Pearson, M. R., D'Lima, G. M., & Kelley, M. L. (2011). Self-regulation as a buffer of the relationship between parental alcohol misuse and alcohol-related outcomes in first-year college students. *Addictive Behaviors*, *36*(12), 1309–1312. https://doi.org/10.1016/j.addbeh.2011.07.009

Rehm, J., Mathers, C., Popova, S., Thavorncharoensap, M., Teerawattananon, Y., & Patra, J. (2009). Global burden of disease and injury and economic cost attributable to alcohol use and alcohol-use disorders. *The Lancet*, *373*(9682), 2223–2233. https://doi.org/10.1016/s0140–6736(09)60746-7

Rodriguez, L. M., Neighbors, C., & Knee, C. R. (2014). Problematic alcohol use and marital distress: An interdependence theory perspective. *Addiction Research & Theory*, *22*(4), 294–312. https://doi.org/10.3109/16066359.2013.841890

Rohsenow, D. J., Monti, P. M., Rubonis, A. V., Gulliver, S. B., Colby, S. M., Binkoff, J. A., & Abrams, D. B. (2001). Cue exposure with coping skills training and communication skills training for alcohol dependence: 6- and 12-month outcomes. *Addiction*, *96*(8), 1161–1174. https://doi.org/10.1046/j.1360-0443.2001.96811619.x

Roos, C., Bowen, S., & Witkiewitz, K. (2020). Approach coping and substance use outcomes following mindfulness-based relapse prevention among individuals with negative affect symptomatology. *Mindfulness, 11,* 2397–2410. https://doi.org/10.1007/s12671–020-01456-w

Roos, C. R., Carroll, K. M., Nich, C., Frankforter, T., & Kiluk, B. D. (2020a). Short-and long-term changes in substance-related coping as mediators of in-person and computerized CBT for alcohol and drug use disorders. *Drug and Alcohol Dependence, 212,*108044. https://doi.org/10.1016/j.drugalcdep.2020.108044

Roos, C. R., Kirouac, M., Pearson, M. R., Fink, B. C., & Witkiewitz, K. (2015). Examining temptation to drink from an existential perspective: Associations among temptation, purpose in life, and drinking outcomes. *Psychology of Addictive Behaviors*, *29*(3), 716–724. https://dx.doi.org/10.1037%2Fadb0000063

Roos, C.R., Kober, H., Trull, T.J., MacLean, R.R., Mun, C.J. (2020b). Intensive longitudinal methods for studying the role of self-regulation strategies in substance use behavior change. *Current Addiction Reports*, *7*, 301–316. https://doi.org/10.1007/s40429–020-00329-5

Roos, C. R., Maisto, S. A., & Witkiewitz, K. (2017). Coping mediates the effects of cognitive–behavioral therapy for alcohol use disorder among out-patient clients in Project MATCH when dependence severity is high. *Addiction, 112*(9), 1547–1557. https://doi.org/10.1111/add.13841

Roos, C. R., & Witkiewitz, K. (2016). Adding tools to the toolbox: The role of coping repertoire in alcohol treatment. *Journal of Consulting and Clinical Psychology, 84*(7), 599–611. https://doi.org/10.1037/ccp0000102

(2017). A contextual model of self-regulation change mechanisms among individuals with addictive disorders. *Clinical Psychology Review, 57*, 117–128. https://doi.org/10.1016/j.cpr.2017.08.008

Schacht, J. P., Anton, R. F., & Myrick, H. (2013). Functional neuroimaging studies of alcohol cue reactivity: A quantitative meta-analysis and systematic review. *Addiction Biology, 18*(1), 121–133. https://doi.org/10.1111/j.1369-1600.2012.00464.x

Scott-Sheldon, L. A., Carey, K. B., Johnson, B. T., Carey, M. P., & Team, M. R. (2017). Behavioral interventions targeting alcohol use among people living with HIV/AIDS: A systematic review and meta-analysis. *AIDS and Behavior, 21*(2), 126–143. https://dx.doi.org/10.1007%2Fs10461–017-1886-3

Skinner, M. D., & Aubin, H.-J. (2010). Craving's place in addiction theory: Contributions of the major models. *Neuroscience and Biobehavioral Reviews, 34*(4), 606–623. https://doi.org/10.1016/j.neubiorev.2009.11.024

Sliedrecht, W., de Waart, R., Witkiewitz, K., & Roozen, H. G. (2019). Alcohol use disorder relapse factors: A systematic review. *Psychiatry Research, 278*, 97–115. https://doi.org/10.1016/j.psychres.2019.05.038

Snider, S. E., LaConte, S. M., & Bickel, W. K. (2016). Episodic future thinking: Expansion of the temporal window in individuals with alcohol dependence. *Alcoholism: Clinical and Experimental Research, 40*(7), 1558–1566. https://doi.org/10.1111/acer.13112

Suzuki, S., Mell, M. M., O'Malley, S. S., Krystal, J. H., Anticevic, A., & Kober, H. (2020). Regulation of craving and negative emotion in alcohol use disorder. *Biological Psychiatry, 5*(2), 239–250. https://dx.doi.org/10.1016%2Fj.bpsc.2019.10.005

Tucker, J. A., Cheong, J., Chandler, S. D., Crawford, S. M., & Simpson, C. A. (2015). Social networks and substance use among at-risk emerging adults living in disadvantaged urban areas in the southern United States: A cross-sectional naturalistic study. *Addiction, 110*(9), 1524–1532. https://doi.org/10.1111/add.13010

Tucker, J. A., Roth, D. L., Huang, J., Crawford, M. S., & Simpson, C. A. (2012). Effects of interactive voice response self-monitoring on natural resolution of drinking problems: Utilization and behavioral economic factors. *Journal of Studies on Alcohol and Drugs, 73*(4), 686–698. https://doi.org/10.15288/jsad.2012.73.686

Tucker, J. A., Vuchinich, R. E., & Rippens, P. D. (2002). Environmental contexts surrounding resolution of drinking problems among problem drinkers with different help-seeking experiences. *Journal of Studies on Alcohol, 63*, 334–341. https://doi.org/10.15288/jsa.2002.63.334

Vuchinich, R. E., & Tucker, J. A. (1996). Life events, alcoholic relapse, and behavioral theories of choice: A prospective analysis. *Experimental and Clinical*

Psychopharmacology, *4*, 19–28. https://psycnet.apa.org/doi/10.1037/1064-1297.4.1.19

Weiss, N. H., Bold, K. W., Sullivan, T. P., Armeli, S., & Tennen, H. (2017). Testing bidirectional associations among emotion regulation strategies and substance use: A daily diary study. *Addiction*, *112*(4), 695–704. https://doi.org/10.1111/add.13698

Wise, R. A., & Koob, G. F. (2014). The development and maintenance of drug addiction. *Neuropsychopharmacology*, *39*(2), 254–262. https://doi.org/10.1038/npp.2013.261

Witkiewitz, K., Bowen, S., Douglas, H., & Hsu, S. H. (2013). Mindfulness-based relapse prevention for substance craving. *Addictive Behaviors*, *38*(2), 1563–1571. https://doi.org/10.1016/j.addbeh.2012.04.001

Witkiewitz, K., Donovan, D. M., & Hartzler, B. (2012). Drink refusal training as part of a combined behavioral intervention: Effectiveness and mechanisms of change. *Journal of Consulting and Clinical Psychology*, *80*(3), 440–449. https://dx.doi.org/10.1037%2Fa0026996

Witkiewitz, K., & Marlatt, G. A. (2009). Relapse prevention for alcohol and drug problems: That was Zen, this is Tao. *American Psychologist*, *59*(4), 224–235. https://doi.org/10.1037/0003-066x.59.4.224

Witkiewitz, K., Roos, C. R., Tofighi, D., & Van Horn, M. L. (2018). Broad coping repertoire mediates the effect of the combined behavioral intervention on alcohol outcomes in the COMBINE study: An application of latent class mediation. *Journal of Studies on Alcohol and Drugs*, *79*(2), 199–207. https://doi.org/10.15288/jsad.2018.79.199

4 Neuropsychological and Biological Influences on Drinking Behavior Change

Marsha E. Bates, Julianne L. Price, and
Jennifer F. Buckman

Neuropsychological and Biological Influences on Drinking Behavior Change

As recently as five years ago, a chapter dedicated to describing the neuropsychological and biological processes underlying drinking behavior change likely would have been organized into two largely distinct sections: one section focused on neuropsychological and cognitive impairments observed in persons with alcohol use disorder (AUD), and one section focused on the biological underpinnings of AUD that persist over time to interrupt recovery trajectories following AUD treatment. Recent efforts to integrate theory and methods across different systems and units of analysis offer newer conceptualizations of changes in drinking behavior and, as a result, have advanced perspectives on recovery from AUD as a nonlinear, multidimensional construct that is best viewed holistically at the individual level (Bates et al., 2019; Buckman et al., 2018).

Multiple conceptual and empirical developments have aligned that foster a holistic, person-centered perspective of AUD and recovery. The National Institute of Mental Health's Research Domain Criteria (RDoC) approach to mental health research seeks to integrate information across different human systems to better understand variation in behavior (Insel et al., 2010). It provides a broad conceptual framework to integrate knowledge across psychological and biological constructs using multiple classes of variables referred to as "units of analysis." The RDoC approach focuses on dimensional concepts that can be used to link heterogeneity in alcohol use and other behaviors to cognitive and biological processes that span normal to abnormal functioning. This aligns with the underlying idea that classifying persons into two groups who do or do not meet diagnostic criteria for a mental disorder, despite its utility in some clinical contexts, may obfuscate understanding of heterogeneity in developmental trajectories of disorders and their recovery, the operation of risk factors, and the outcomes of intervention. Similarly, a sole focus on abstinence from alcohol use as evidence of recovery from AUD has lost favor in many clinical and research arenas due to its oversimplification of the diffusion of drinking behavior change and associated health effects across multiple integrated domains of functioning.

To capture more fully the multidimensional changes that occur across the recovery continuum, we blend the RDoC Arousal/Regulatory Systems and Cognitive Systems Domains with advances put forth in the Alcohol Addiction Research Domain Criteria (AARDoC) (Litten et al., 2015) to consider how drinking behavior change arises from functional improvements in the brain and in peripheral organ systems that together coordinate arousal. This chapter advances physiological arousal as a holistic construct that serves either to support or hinder recovery by linking body state to biology, neurocognition, and overt human behavior. We further consider how the arousal construct may be used to identify more homogeneous subgroups of persons in recovery, such as those who may benefit from arousal-modulation adjuvants to bolster executive cognitive control, affect regulation, and flexible responses to contextual cues.

Behavior Change Depends on Modulation of Arousal to Triggers and Cues

Arousal is defined as a dimension of sensitivity to stimuli to promote interaction with the environment in a contextually-dependent manner. Arousal is elicited by both external and internal stimuli, modulated by both physical and symbolic stimulus characteristics, and regulated by homeostatic factors (Kozak & Cuthbert, 2016). This definition encompasses neural representations of arousal, subjective experiences of arousal state, and physiological arousal evident across the cardiovascular and other organ systems. Many features of drinking behavior change are arousal-dependent, including affective regulation, cue reactivity and craving, and stress modulation. Ample research demonstrates that this arousal dependence is evident across subjective, physiological, and neural domains.

A role for arousal modulation in drinking behavior change is not new; it is interwoven across the domains conceptualized within the AARDoC (Litten et al., 2015), such as affect regulation, executive functions, and incentive salience. It has been studied using RDoC analysis units such as genes, brain circuitry, physiology, behavior, and self-report. A recent human phenotyping study in a sample comprising both healthy adults and persons seeking treatment for AUD found that the domains of executive control, incentive salience, and negative emotionality were intercorrelated, and their severity was associated with genetic, environmental and developmental correlates (Kwako et al., 2019). The results suggested that (1) common processes, as well as domain specific processes, contribute to drinking behavior patterns; and (2) a constellation of personal and environmental factors modulate their expression.

We propose that arousal serves as a common process that supports executive control, negative emotionality, and salience; we further propose that arousal modulation may serve as a holistic intervention target to sustain recovery (Eddie et al., 2020). While challenges certainly remain in how to modify arousal processes that endure over time, the RDoC points to the possibility that multiple units of analysis can be leveraged in this effort. Numerous interventions that modify arousal processes – including but not limited to exercise, mindfulness, meditation, and heart rate variability biofeedback – already exist, but evidence on "dose-response" (i.e., short-term (acute) versus long-term (persisting) effects) and the relative importance of neural, physiological, and subjective system change remain unknown. Interestingly, all of these arousal modification strategies have been linked to cognitive performance, as well as subjective and biological changes.

In addition to arousal as a common process, the holistic influences of arousal underscore the unmet need for person-centered approaches to optimize arousal modification across systems within a person (Buckman et al., 2018). Such approaches are beginning to parse heterogeneous personal and environmental sources of risk into homogeneous clusters (Collins & Varmus, 2015). For example, person-centered approaches have uncovered that characteristics of a person's social support network moderate the impact of their neuropsychological impairment on AUD treatment outcome (Buckman et al., 2007), there are meaningful subtypes of neuropsychological recovery trajectories over one year following AUD treatment (Bates et al., 2013), and men and women differ in their modulation of arousal during alcohol intoxication (Bates et al., 2011).

Arousal Modulation Mechanisms Bridge Brain, Body, and Behavior

In addition to viewing arousal as a "common process" that affects key AARDoC domains (e.g., executive function, negative emotionality, incentive salience), arousal is also a common process across organ systems and one that is experienced subjectively, measurable physiologically, and associated with neural functioning. Here we focus on modulation of arousal through the baroreflex mechanism. The baroreflex is an anatomical body–brain feedback loop that serves to reflexively pair heart and blood vessel activities with blood pressure control. It also influences higher-order behavior by providing an afferent neural pathway that allows visceral feedback from the heart and vessels to become integrated in cognitive and emotional processes mediated by forebrain structures (Bates & Buckman, 2013). The pathway is bidirectional to ensure that efferent neural information is also relayed to the periphery and a coordinated, whole body response to stimuli is generated. This cardiovascular mechanism has been extensively documented in terms of neurophysiology, functional anatomy, and molecular mechanisms in preclinical rodent, primate, and human studies. It supports preparatory functions involving general changes in arousal that make an organism ready for action (e.g., changes in blood pressure and heart rate) and specific changes in arousal needed to initiate a goal-directed behavior (e.g., fleeing from danger, reaching for a drink; Iversen et al., 2000). Moreover, baroreflex dysfunction is observed following acute and chronic alcohol exposure (Bar et al., 2006; Buckman et al., 2015; Fazio et al., 2001).

The RDoC and AARDoC conceptual frameworks emphasize linking subjective self-reports, cognitive assessments, and observations of behavior to neurobiological processes and neural circuits in order to accelerate the translational impact of findings from pre-clinical and human neuroimaging studies. An international initiative (Verdejo-Garcia et al., 2019) similarly proposed the use of a "neuroscience-informed approach" to integrate neurobiological addiction phenomena, human experimental evidence about underlying addiction mechanisms (Ekhtiari et al., 2017), and self-reports of clinically-relevant AUD features to enhance feasibility in AUD treatment contexts (Kwako et al., 2019; Votaw et al., 2020). This initiative primarily has focused on the two behavioral intervention areas of neuromodulation and cognitive training/remediation to improve clinical outcomes. Within these frameworks, neurobiological processes are seen to play a central role in current mental health and addiction models that may inform development of more effective treatments.

Yet, with the exception of the hypothalamic-pituitary-adrenal (HPA) stress axis, body systems are generally absent from neurobiological theories and neuroscience-informed approaches, which may limit their applied value by missing a malleable source of individual variability (Eddie et al., 2020). This gap is not unique to addiction treatment and recovery research. Rather, the intertwined relations between cognition, emotion, multiple health behaviors, and their underlying physiological pathways has been understudied across the lifespan (Jirout et al., 2019). Evidence for the baroreflex mechanism as an accessible extension of the neuroscience-informed approach that directly bridges body–brain communication suggests an integrative target that can begin to address this gap.

The baroreflex can serve as a physiological unit of analysis in the RDoC Arousal/Regulatory System domain to connect self-reports of psychological constructs and performance on neuropsychological tests with biological systems involved in cognitive control, incentive salience, and negative emotionality. There is compelling evidence for three bidirectional information loops between the cardiovascular system and a well-delineated neural circuit often referred to as the "central autonomic network." The baroreflex provides a critical path by which the body continually conveys and receives signals that are components of arousal states and emotional tone to the brain (Critchley, 2005).The bidirectionality of the baroreflex loops indicates that, in addition to the influence of neural inputs at the heart, the cardiovascular system influences the brain via ascending pathways that deliver sensory feedback that becomes embedded in subsequent neural responses (Eddie et al., 2020). Thus, the baroreflex mechanism incorporates neural and cardiovascular biology into the definition of behavior change within the context of cognitive-emotional regulation (Gray et al., 2012).

The baroreflex bridges brain, body, and behavior in several critical ways. First, the baroreflex affects arousal through processes that often operate outside of awareness and contribute to the automaticity of substance use behaviors among individuals with substance use disorders (SUD). Second, neural control of physiological reactivity appears to be predictive as well as reflexive, such that neural prediction errors contribute to exaggerated and blunted cardiovascular stress reactions that undermine adaptive whole-body response to challenge (Gianaros & Jennings, 2018). This is a conceptual departure from predominant psychophysiological theories that have focused on cardiovascular processes as downstream indicators of neural integration, rather than active processes that may enhance or undermine neural regulation. Third, the well-delineated neuroanatomy of the central autonomic network strongly suggests that cardiovascular physiology is not an independent, parallel process of behavior change, but rather an integrated and necessary component of the brain's response to any given challenge. Moreover, the substantial overlap in cardiovascular system and addiction circuitry (Bates & Buckman, 2013; Eddie et al., 2020) suggests the relevance of cardiovascular health and function to understanding heterogeneity in alcohol's acute effects and the development of behavioral rigidity towards alcohol over time (Bates & Buckman, 2013; Buckman et al., 2018; Critchley & Harrison, 2013; Leyro et al., 2019).

While we focus here on the cardiovascular system and its neural substrate in relation to drinking behavior change, we note that arousal modulation can be elaborated in endocrine (Seo & Sinha, 2015) and other biological systems that communicate with one another to control stress reactivity, affective state, cognition, and behavior. The interdependence of cognitive and biological systems is becoming increasingly evident as shown, for example, by the reliable association between psychosocial interventions for diverse mental and physical disorders and improved immune system function (Shields et al., 2020). There is mounting evidence that the baroreflex functions at the crossroads of neurobiology, systems physiology, and human psychology to affect arousal. Behavioral manipulation of cardiovascular system processes directly affects neuroplasticity (i.e., neuromodulation such as altering neural activation to alcohol stimuli [Bates et al., 2019]). Moreover, behavioral interventions developed to directly target cardiovascular functioning have demonstrated efficacy in reducing self-reported stress and anxiety (Goessl et al., 2017) and may reduce craving (Alayan et al., 2018). These findings set the stage for considering a role for physiological arousal in cognitive functioning in parallel to its role in neural and behavioral functioning.

Arousal as "Context" for Cognitive Training: Implications for Intervention and Recovery

Empirically supported behavioral treatments for AUD are often successful in helping persons to stop or greatly reduce drinking. Over time, however, drinking behavior changes instituted during treatment are not sustained in many cases. A central premise of most cognitive behavioral AUD treatments is that strengthening cognitive control will increase an individual's ability to resist impulsive use of alcohol (McCrady & Epstein, 1999). Accordingly, there has been great interest in understanding the extent to which cognitive control processes are impaired in AUD, the time course and extent of such impairments, and whether direct interventions to remediate and restore cognitive function can facilitate and sustain drinking behavior changes.

The effects of alcohol on the neuropsychological underpinnings of effortful cognitive control deficits in person with AUD have been well studied (Goldman, 1995; Nixon & Lewis, 2019). RDoC Cognitive System constructs of attention, declarative and working memory, and cognitive control encompass primary areas of neuropsychological deficits that are related to chronic, excessive alcohol use (Bates et al., 2002). Limitations in attentional capacity, encoding and retrieval of information, the flexible manipulation of information, and modulation of cognitive and emotional processes to accomplish goal-directed behavior have been identified consistently as neurocognitive processes that support conscious intentions to stop or limit drinking (Bates & Buckman, 2013). These same processes, of course, also support a wide spectrum of other health behaviors that contribute to life quality in areas as diverse as employment, interpersonal relationships, and physical health.

Interest in the intersection of cognitive deficits and treatment engagement (e.g., adherence, length of stay, therapeutic alliance) and outcome (e.g., sustained abstinence) initially led to an increased interest in cognitive remediation as an adjunct in the treatment of AUD. The potential of this approach is highlighted by a review of prospective cognitive studies of SUD treatment retention and relapse (defined as consuming alcohol/drugs again after a period of abstinence) suggesting that processing speed and accuracy during attention and reasoning tasks consistently predicted treatment retention, while decision-making tasks predicted relapse (Domínguez-Salas et al., 2016). A subsequent review of substance-specific cognitive predictors found that episodic memory and executive functions predicted future alcohol use (Rolland et al., 2019). Early studies examining whether cognitive remediation adjuncts could be used to improve treatment retention and prevent subsequent substance use modeled lessons learned from studies of other neurological disorders, including stroke and traumatic brain injury (Bates & Buckman, 2013). Goldman and colleagues demonstrated transfer of gains from visuospatial training to enhancement in other cognitive domains (1987). However, the inability to translate gains on cognitive tasks to daily function or treatment outcomes ultimately led to a decade-long quiescence in the field. Nonetheless, research interest remained in exploring the hypothesis that 'experience-dependent' interventions, such as cognitive remediation, could hasten the timeline or augment the extent of neuropsychological recovery during AUD and other drug use disorder treatment, thereby increasing the likelihood of sustaining drinking behavior change.

During the ensuing decades, addiction research added depth to the neurological and cognitive factors that were more susceptible to the effects of chronic alcohol use. The past decade has seen a resurgence in more targeted cognitive remediation. This time, tasks were geared specifically toward inhibitory control and working memory capacity. This was based on evidence that one of the most robust effects of chronic, excessive alcohol use on the brain is to disrupt the function of the prefrontal cortex, which results in substantial impairment of central executive control and inhibitory functions (Abernathy et al., 2010). However, the ability to translate changes in neuropsychological test performance to treatment outcomes and recovery trajectories again has been mixed. Recent detailed reviews further provide evidence for both natural (time-dependent) and experience-dependent (cognitive retraining and rehabilitation) recovery of cognitive functions over time with alcohol abstinence or greatly reduced drinking (Nixon & Lewis, 2019). Yet, evidence remains limited that intervening in such trajectories promotes beneficial changes in drinking behavior. Thus, in-depth reviews of this literature differ in being cautiously optimistic regarding benefits that promote behavior change (Nixon & Lewis, 2019) or emphasizing the failure of working memory task improvements to exhibit much transfer to daily life function or to correlate with substance use behavior change (Verdejo-Garcia et al., 2019). Nonetheless, the idea stands: improvements in neuropsychological functioning and cognitive control should support behavior change. Why has the field not been able to observe this consistently?

As one of several possibilities, we look to the dual process models of neurocognitive function (Bechara, 2005), which propose a conflict between effortful processes that support conscious goals and intentions ("reflective," "executive," "cool," "frontal," or "cortical"), and automatic processes that derive from attention capture by salient cues in the environment and impulsive or habitual modes of affective regulation ("impulsive," "automatic," "hot," or "limbic"). Arousal modulation affects this conflict, operating either to promote impulsive stimulus-driven use, or damping attentional and salience processes to promote cognitive control (Bates et al., 2019). Thus, cognitive retraining/remediation, per se, may have limited impact on unplanned alcohol use behaviors because these behaviors are most often initiated in-the-moment and under conditions of altered (often heightened) arousal (e.g., a negative emotion, the sight of friends drinking). Everyday experiences of stress, negative affect, and salient alcohol cues serve as potent triggers for drinking (Marlatt, 1996) that activate arousal systems and appear to be automatic in the sense that they bypass cognitive plans and conscious intentions not to drink (Tiffany, 1990). A consideration of the internal and environmental precursors that interrupt plans to limit alcohol use (as well as to engage in exercise, get more sleep, and maintain positive interpersonal relations) suggests that the contexts of planned actions are extremely important. Bodily states, both specific (hunger and fatigue) and general (racing heart and sweating), create strong internal contexts. These contexts then influence behavioral regulation both dependent on – and independent of – cognitive strategies set in motion during AUD treatment. Yet, the automatic physiological processes (other than the HPA axis) that dynamically interact with internal affective states and environmental cues to undermine effortful cognitive control rarely have been considered.

Many behavioral interventions for AUD involve operant learning strategies, cognitive and motivational restructuring, and skills building (e.g., drink refusal skills, expectations of self-efficacy to carry out conscious intentions to overcome urges to use alcohol). Yet, the basic human physiology of arousal dictates that automatic visceral processes often outpace and may outcompete cognitive mediation of goal-directed behavior. By definition, these processes mainly occur outside of conscious awareness. If one considers the evidence for cognitive interruptions by automatic arousal processes in parallel to the current state of research on cognitive retraining/remediation, new questions arise as to whether cognitive remediation interventions may need to take into account contextual features related to arousal. First, the potential for cognitive remediation may be limited during states of hyperarousal such as are commonly seen early in recovery. Second, to transfer cognitive gains more fully to "real world" situations, cognitive control training may benefit from embedded contextual features wherein cognitive control can be facilitated during altered arousal states that often serve as triggers for substance use. Third, arousal is a dynamic state; thus, neither neuropsychological functioning nor recovery should be viewed as static, linear processes that happen in isolation. Implementing cognitive remediation in tandem with arousal dampening interventions that can be used on demand could go a long way in allowing cognitive processing to 'keep up' with the often intense automatic, visceral reactions to real life that people in recovery experience.

Adaptive Arousal Modulation as Recovery Capital

Definitions of "recovery" have become increasingly nuanced over the years, both with respect to mental health disorders broadly considered and specifically with respect to AUD and other SUD (National Academies of Sciences Engineering and Medicine, 2016). Singular definitions of recovery as the absence of clinical features in mental health disorders (such as depression) or the absence of drinking/drug taking behaviors in persons with substance use disorders have given way to conceptualizations that acknowledge multiple subjective and objective dimensions of recovery that include the presence of positive life outcomes and skills. For example, the working definition of recovery of the Substance Abuse and Mental Health Services Administration recognizes recovery as "an active process of positive changes in health and wellness that emphasizes self-direction and personal actualization." This perspective is in line with the results of recent re-analyses of data from large AUD treatment outcome studies showing that drinking behaviors can become dissociated from levels of functioning in other life domains following treatment. For example, a subset of individuals who sometimes engaged in heavy drinking also were found to show relatively high levels of psychosocial functioning at 12–15 months after treatment (Wilson et al., 2016) and high levels of psychosocial functioning, employment, life satisfaction, and mental health at three years after treatment (see review by Witkiewitz & Tucker, 2020). Conversely, a subset of alcohol abstainers was identified that reported relatively lower levels of life quality functions. We further observed that women receiving cognitive behavioral therapy for AUD experienced improvements in cardiovascular regulation from pre- to post-treatment, even without stable abstinence (Buckman et al., 2019). Such studies suggest that knowing an individual is abstinent, or alternatively engaging in some level of heavy drinking, provides an incomplete picture of recovery in other dimensions of life functioning.

This nicely dovetails with the AARDoC notion of a continuum of drinking severity ranging from the occasional binge drinker to the chronic relapsing heavy drinker (Litten et al., 2015) and the natural extension of this idea to conceptualizing drinking behavior change during recovery as a continuum ranging from complete abstinence to various levels of low-risk and occasional heavy drinking. It also adds dimension to the definition of recovery by allowing additional behavioral and life quality dimensions to capture more fully the heterogeneity of treatment outcomes (Witkiewitz & Tucker, 2020). Within the context of such biobehavioral changes that actively unfold in persons during recovery, the hypothesis of recovery capital has emerged. Recovery capital refers to the physical and mental resources at a person's avail to negotiate daily stressors and challenges that may interfere with maintaining drinking behavior change (Hennessy, 2017). Baroreflex sensitivity and related cardiovascular arousal modulation processes are often but not always impaired in persons with AUD (Bar et al., 2006), suggesting its potential role as an asset that could be enhanced or as a barrier to be remedied during the recovery process.

Certain characteristics of the recovery process, such as its heterogeneity and nonlinear nature, point to the value of targeting holistic and transbehavioral dimensions of recovery that serve to bolster multiple levels of life functioning (National Academies of Sciences Engineering and Medicine, 2016). Non-linear changes in anxiety, craving, depression, and stress were found over two semesters in a college-attending sample who were in recovery from AUD and other SUD and received an adjunctive heart rate variability biofeedback intervention aimed at reducing craving and negative affect (Alayan et al., 2019; Eddie et al., 2018). Perhaps unsurprisingly, the intervention most benefitted those who entered the study with elevated craving. In some, craving reductions accelerated over time, whereas in others, co-occurring increases in depressive symptoms attenuated biofeedback effects on craving. These observations support that multidimensional, person-level definitions of recovery may be needed to account for the heterogeneous pathways of alcohol use behavior change that have been observed over time.

A systematic review of over 100 behavior change theories identified distinct patterns of explanation for behavior change and behavior change maintenance (Kwasnicka et al., 2016). Self-regulation and resources (psychological and physical) emerged as two of the five themes identified to explain maintenance of behavior change. We consider arousal modulation and cognitive resources as promising targets in the search for routes to sustain AUD recovery. This extends the definition of self-regulation to include self-monitoring of bodily processes as well as the automatic operation of arousal modulation that occurs outside of conscious awareness.

Earlier we highlighted that intentional-cognitive strategies can fail to interrupt drinking behavior when triggers are encountered because automatic-visceral reactions, urges, and craving are not usually subject to cognitive control. In addition, intentional self-control resources, such as self-efficacy and executive control, are not stable across time (Muraven & Baumeister, 2000); rather, they fluctuate within an individual due to ever-changing personal and environmental contexts (Bates et al., 2013; Buckman et al., 2007, 2008). Dealing with triggers like stress and negative mood depletes these resources (Muraven & Baumeister, 2000) and can aggravate arousal states, thereby reducing recovery capital. This suggests that recovery needs to be conceptualized as a time-extended process that may be initiated by behavioral and pharmacological AUD treatments, yet also will require on-demand tools to support active maintenance of drinking behavior change and improvements in quality of life over time.

The idea of arousal modulation as a recovery capital target moves beyond static and trait-like descriptions of behavioral dispositions that may moderate risk for relapse at the level of the group, but cannot predict risk mechanistically at the level of the individual. Long-standing individual differences in arousal modulation prior to the onset of AUD may serve as vulnerability processes (reviewed in Buckman et al., 2018). It is well known that difficulties in effectively modulating emotional arousal are present across the lifespan, observable as infant reactivity to novel stimuli and capacity to be soothed, and the development of externalizing and internalizing problems in childhood and adolescence. Such innate differences between persons in the efficiency of the arousal regulation system may make some more susceptible to developing AUD. Moreover, if not addressed during treatment, difficulties in modulating arousal may increase susceptibility to reinstitute the use of alcohol and other drugs to regulate stress and emotion during recovery. Considerable research has linked reduced basal heart rate variability to reduced health, resiliency, and social competence in childhood and to increased vulnerability to stress, somatic and emotional illnesses, less use of active coping skills, exaggerated pro-inflammatory responses, and cardiovascular and all-cause mortality in adults (as reviewed in Buckman et al., 2018). This suggests that the baroreflex may serve as a viable prevention, intervention, and sustained recovery target that could bolster arousal modulation.

In addition to long-standing and perhaps genetically mediated difficulties in arousal modulation, life experiences can further deplete arousal recovery resources. As stressors are repeatedly encountered and their effects "pile up," a slow resetting of physiological set points in cardiovascular arousal modulation functions also can contribute to reduced arousal modulation. Unlike the abrupt and acute shifts in blood pressure that are initially triggered to mobilize the organism for behavior in the moment, gradual changes in blood pressure induced over time due to chronic stress are not detected by the brain control system (Bates & Buckman, 2013). In addition to cardiovascular conditions such as heart disease and hypertension, which are common in AUD treatment populations, this gradual resetting of cardiovascular set points is in line with McEwen's conceptualization of "allostatic load" (McEwen, 1998). This emphasizes how chronic exposure to stress can instigate a breakdown in the bodily systems (such as the cardiovascular and immune systems) that are needed to manage and control stress. It is possible that the baroreflex may be an important mechanism underlying allostatic load and key to understanding the differential influences of acute versus chronic stressors in recovery from AUD.

Finally, it is important to note that rather than being construed as a return to a prior level of functioning, recovery may well require the development and engagement of *new* processes that either can compensate for persistent changes in functioning due to chronic substance use (Bickel et al., 2019) or make it easier to flexibly align behavior with personal intentions and goals (Eddie et al., 2020). From a practical perspective, consideration of body physiology has the translational advantage of providing an accessible intervention target for persons with long-standing arousal modulation difficulties, as well as those with acute or persistent alcohol-related decrements in baroreflex function. The neurocardiac system can be manipulated using a variety of non-invasive, behavioral techniques to expand the repertoire of available AUD intervention adjuvants and recovery-support boosters. Aerobic exercise, yoga, mindfulness, and other forms of meditation enhance baroreflex function via respiratory features and other mechanisms that may serve to influence the baroreflex. Such strategies that promote physical wellness are becoming increasingly common elements of treatment and recovery plans. Directly targeting baroreflex functioning, such as by heart rate variability biofeedback, has the advantage of having surprisingly few barriers to potential wide-scale dissemination, being easily administered and learned and requiring no expensive laboratory equipment; mobile technology (e.g., iPhone apps and wearables) expands the accessibility of this intervention technique outside the laboratory or clinic. These and other physiology-focused interventions on the horizon hold promise for augmenting current AUD treatments and expanding the available methods by which the expansive influence of arousal on recovery can be studied by researchers and used by persons to support drinking behavior change and improvements in functioning.

Conclusions and Recommendations

At the core of this chapter is neuroplasticity, a concept that is often relegated to cellular and molecular sciences, but also overlaps with the interest of behavioral science in a person's capacity to change to meet the needs imposed by the environment and internal milieu. When a seemingly intractable behavioral repertoire as is seen in SUD demonstrates manageable change as seen in recovery, the behavioral scientist sees behavior change. Beneath this overt change in behavior, however, resides complex biological changes, many of which may serve to lay a foundation for the personal resources and daily-life realignments that are fundamental to recovery. Such biological plasticity is observed throughout the brain as well as across many organ systems; however, the latter has been understudied in persons who differ in drinking behaviors and SUD profiles.

A dynamic systems perspective of neuroplasticity involves consideration of the active processes through which persons adapt to challenge and self-regulate by continuously modifying their behavior based on information about changes in internal states and the environment (Boker, 2001). The inability to generate flexible behavior in response to continually changing life challenges, such as negative affect and salient appetitive cues, is central to the development of AUD and may continue to undermine sustained recovery, even years following treatment (Baker et al., 2004). Prominent models of AUD point to neuroplasticity as a critical phenomenon in drinking behavior change via adaptation and learning processes (Bickel et al., 2018; Koob & Volkow, 2010; Lewis, 2018). This has been supported by preclinical studies (Uhl et al., 2019) and by studies of human risk for AUD (Paulus et al., 2012), the development of drinking behavior trajectories (Squeglia et al., 2015), and AUD diagnosis (Zahr & Pfefferbaum, 2017). Neuroplasticity has further been implicated in recovery pathways that involve body–brain integration (Seo & Sinha, 2015).

We extend these concepts to posit that the ability to adaptively moderate arousal physiologically is a common resource that promotes neuroplasticity. Diminished neurocognitive capacity undermines the effortful regulation of emotional states and contributes to non-adaptive modes of arousal modulation such as the use of alcohol and other drugs. Likewise, decreased autonomic nervous system balance undermines the adaptive regulation of arousal by biasing the system toward sympathetic nervous system control with a resultant loss of inhibitory functions (Berntson & Cacioppo, 2007). While adaptation and self-regulation processes are often cognitively driven and effortful, other critical self-regulation processes are automatic and operate outside of conscious awareness. Cognitive control processes work in tandem with peripheral physiological systems to inhibit and restrain maladaptive behaviors and to promote health and quality of life in human and non-human organisms. Recovery is possible, there are various pathways to recovery, and the recovery process involves multiple systems and is best viewed holistically at the individual level.

References

Abernathy, K., Chandler, L. J., & Woodward, J. J. (2010). Alcohol and the prefrontal cortex. *International Review of Neurobiology*, *91*, 289–320. https://doi.org/10.1016/s0074–7742(10)91009-x

Alayan, N., Eddie, D., Eller, L., Bates, M. E., & Carmody, D. (2019). Substance craving changes in university students receiving heart rate variability biofeedback: A longitudinal multilevel modeling approach. *Addictive Behaviors*, *97*, 35–41. https://doi.org/10.1016/j.addbeh.2019.05.005

Alayan, N., Eller, L., Bates, M. E., & Carmody, D. P. (2018). Current evidence on heart rate variability biofeedback as a complementary anticraving intervention. *Journal of Alternative and Complementary Medicine*, *24*(11), 1039–1050. https://doi.org/10.1089/acm.2018.0019

Baker, T. B., Piper, M. E., McCarthy, D. E., Majeskie, M. R., & Fiore, M. C. (2004). Addiction motivation reformulated: An affective processing model of negative reinforcement. *Psychology Review*, *111*(1), 33–51. https://doi.org/10.1037/0033-295x.111.1.33

Bar, K. J., Boettger, M. K., Boettger, S., Groteluschen, M., Neubauer, R., Jochum, T., Baier, V., Sauer, H., & Voss, A. (2006). Reduced baroreflex sensitivity in acute alcohol withdrawal syndrome and in abstained alcoholics. *Drug and Alcohol Dependence*, *85*(1), 66–74. https://doi.org/10.1016/j.drugalcdep.2006.03.014

Bates, M. E., Bowden, S. C., & Barry, D. (2002). Neurocognitive impairment associated with alcohol use disorders: Implications for treatment. *Experimental and Clinical Psychopharmacology*, *10*(3), 193–212. https://doi.org/10.1037//1064-1297.10.3.193

Bates, M. E., & Buckman, J. F. (2013). Integrating body and brain systems in addiction neuroscience. In P. Miller (Ed.), *Biological research on addiction: Comprehensive addictive behaviors and disorders* (Vol. 2, pp. 187–198). Elsevier.

Bates, M. E., Buckman, J. F., Vaschillo, E. G., Fonoberov, V. A., Fonoberova, M., Vaschillo, B., Mun, E. Y., Mezic, A., & Mezic, I. (2011). The redistribution of power: Neurocardiac signaling, alcohol and gender. *PLoS One*, *6*(12), e28281. https://doi.org/10.1371/journal.pone.0028281

Bates, M. E., Buckman, J. F., Voelbel, G. T., Eddie, D., & Freeman, J. (2013). The mean and the individual: Integrating variable-centered and person-centered analyses of cognitive recovery in patients with substance use disorders. *Frontiers in Psychiatry*, *4*, 177. https://doi.org/10.3389/fpsyt.2013.00177

Bates, M. E., Lesnewich, L. M., Uhouse, S. G., Gohel, S., & Buckman, J. F. (2019). Resonance-paced breathing alters neural response to visual cues: Proof-of-concept for a neuroscience-informed adjunct to addiction treatments. *Frontiers in Psychiatry*, *10*, 624. https://doi.org/10.3389/fpsyt.2019.00624

Bechara, A. (2005). Decision making, impulse control, and loss of willpower to resist drugs: A neurocognitive perspective. *Nature Neuroscience*, *8*(11), 1458–1463. https://doi.org/10.1038/nn1584

Berntson, G. G., & Cacioppo, J. T. (2007). Integrative physiology: Homeostasis, allostasis, and the orchestration of systemic physiology. In J. T. Cacioppo, L. G. Tassinary, &

G. G. Berntson (Eds.), *Handbook of psychophysiology* (pp. 433–452). Cambridge University Press. https://doi.org/10.1017/CBO9780511546396.019.

Bickel, W. K., Crabbe, J. C., & Sher, K. J. (2019). What is addiction? How can animal and human research be used to advance research, diagnosis, and treatment of alcohol and other substance use disorders? *Alcoholism: Clinical and Experimental Research*, *43*(1), 6–21. https://doi.org/10.1111/acer.13912

Bickel, W. K., Mellis, A. M., Snider, S. E., Athamneh, L. N., Stein, J. S., & Pope, D. A. (2018). 21st century neurobehavioral theories of decision making in addiction: Review and evaluation. *Pharmacology, Biochemistry, and Behavior*, *164*, 4–21. https://doi.org/10.1016/j.pbb.2017.09.009

Boker, S. M. (2001). Differential structural equation modeling of intraindividual variability. In L. M. Collins & A. G. Sayer (Eds.), *New methods for the analysis of behavior change* (pp. 5–27). American Psychological Association.

Buckman, J. F., Bates, M. E., & Cisler, R. A. (2007). Social networks and their influence on drinking behaviors: Differences related to cognitive impairment in clients receiving alcoholism treatment. *Journal of Studies on Alcohol and Drugs*, *68* (5), 738–747. https://doi.org/10.15288/jsad.2007.68.738

Buckman, J. F., Bates, M. E., & Morgenstern, J. (2008). Social support and cognitive impairment in clients receiving treatment for alcohol- and drug-use disorders: A replication study. *Journal of Studies on Alcohol and Drugs*, *69*(5), 738–746. https://doi.org/10.15288/jsad.2008.69.738

Buckman, J. F., Eddie, D., Vaschillo, E. G., Vaschillo, B., Garcia, A., & Bates, M. E. (2015). Immediate and complex cardiovascular adaptation to an acute alcohol dose. *Alcoholism: Clinical and Experimental Research*, *39*(12), 2334–2344. https://doi.org/10.1111/acer.12912

Buckman, J. F., Vaschillo, B., Vaschillo, E. G., Epstein, E. E., Nguyen-Louie, T. T., Lesnewich, L. M., Eddie, D., & Bates, M. E. (2019). Improvement in women's cardiovascular functioning during cognitive behavioral therapy for alcohol use disorder. *Psychology of Addictive Behaviors*, *33*(8), 659–668. https://doi.org/10.1037/adb0000524

Buckman, J. F., Vaschillo, E. G., Fonoberova, M., Mezic, I., & Bates, M. E. (2018). The translational value of psychophysiology methods and mechanisms: Multilevel, dynamic, personalized. *Journal of Studies on Alcohol and Drugs*, *79*(2), 229–238. https://doi.org/10.15288/jsad.2018.79.229

Collins, F. S., & Varmus, H. (2015). A new initiative on precision medicine. *New England Journal of Medicine*, *372*(9), 793–795. https://doi.org/10.1056/NEJMp1500523

Critchley, H. D. (2005). Neural mechanisms of autonomic, affective, and cognitive integration. *Journal of Comparative Neurology*, *493*, 154–166. https://doi.org/10.1002/cne.20749

Critchley, H. D., & Harrison, N. A. (2013). Visceral influences on brain and behavior. *Neuron*, *77*(4), 624–638. https://doi.org/10.1016/j.neuron.2013.02.008

Domínguez-Salas, S., Díaz-Batanero, C., Lozano-Rojas, O. M., & Verdejo-García, A. (2016). Impact of general cognition and executive function deficits on addiction treatment outcomes: Systematic review and discussion of neurocognitive pathways. *Neuroscience & Biobehavioral Reviews*, *71*, 772–801. https://doi.org/10.1016/j.neubiorev.2016.09.030

Eddie, D., Bates, M. E., & Buckman, J. F. (2020). Closing the loop between heart and brain: Towards more holistic models of addiction and addiction recovery. *Addiction Biology* e12958. https://doi.org/10.1111/adb.12958

Eddie, D., Conway, F. N., Alayan, N., Buckman, J., & Bates, M. E. (2018). Assessing heart rate variability biofeedback as an adjunct to college recovery housing programs. *Journal of Substance Abuse Treatment*, *92*, 70–76. https://doi.org/10.1016/j.jsat.2018.06.014

Ekhtiari, H., Rezapour, T., Aupperle, R. L., & Paulus, M. P. (2017). Neuroscience-informed psychoeducation for addiction medicine: A neurocognitive perspective. *Progress in Brain Research*, *235*, 239–264. https://doi.org/10.1016/bs.pbr.2017.08.013

Fazio, M., Bardelli, M., Macaluso, L., Fiammengo, F., Mattei, P. L., Bossi, M., Fabris, B., Fischetti, F., Pascazio, L., Candido, R., & Carretta, R. (2001). Mechanics of the carotid artery wall and baroreflex sensitivity after acute ethanol administration in young healthy volunteers. *Clinical Science*, *101*(3), 253–260.

Forsberg, L. K., & Goldman, M. S. (1987). Experience-dependent recovery of cognitive deficits in alcoholics: Extended transfer of training. *Journal of Abnormal Psychology*, *96*(4), 345–353. https://doi.org/10.1037//0021-843x.96.4.345

Gianaros, P. J., & Jennings, J. R. (2018). Host in the machine: A neurobiological perspective on psychological stress and cardiovascular disease. *American Psychologist*, *73*(8), 1031–1044. https://doi.org/10.1037/amp0000232

Goessl, V. C., Curtiss, J. E., & Hofmann, S. G. (2017). The effect of heart rate variability biofeedback training on stress and anxiety: A meta-analysis. *Psychological Medicine*, *47*(15), 2578–2586. https://doi.org/10.1017/s0033291717001003

Goldman, M. S. (1995). Recovery of cognitive functioning in alcoholics – The relationship to treatment. *Alcohol Health and Research World*, *19*(2), 148–154.

Gray, M. A., Beacher, F. D., Minati, L., Nagai, Y., Kemp, A. H., Harrison, N. A., & Critchley, H. D. (2012). Emotional appraisal is influenced by cardiac afferent information. *Emotion*, *12*(1), 180–191. https://doi.org/10.1037/a0025083

Hennessy, E. A. (2017). Recovery capital: A systematic review of the literature. *Addiction Research & Theory*, *25*(5), 349–360. https://doi.org/10.1080/16066359.2017.1297990

Insel, T., Cuthbert, B., Garvey, M., Heinssen, R., Pine, D. S., Quinn, K., Sanislow, C., & Wang, P. (2010). Research domain criteria (RDoC): Toward a new classification framework for research on mental disorders. *American Journal of Psychiatry*, *167*(7), 748–751. https://doi.org/10.1176/appi.ajp.2010.09091379

Iversen, S., Kupfermann, I., & Kandel, E. R. (2000). Emotional states and feelings. In E. R. Kandel, J. H. Schwartz, & T. M. Jessell (Eds.), *Principles of neural science* (4th ed., pp. 982–996). McGraw-Hill.

Jirout, J., LoCasale-Crouch, J., Turnbull, K., Gu, Y., Cubides, M., Garzione, S., Evans, T. M., Weltman, A. L., & Kranz, S. (2019). How lifestyle factors affect cognitive and executive function and the ability to learn in children. *Nutrients*, *11*(8), 1953. https://doi.org/10.3390/nu11081953

Koob, G. F., & Volkow, N. D. (2010). Neurocircuitry of addiction. *Neuropsychopharmacology*, *35*(1), 217–238. https://doi.org/10.1038/npp.2009.110

Kozak, M. J., & Cuthbert, B. N. (2016). The NIMH research domain criteria initiative: Background, issues, and pragmatics. *Psychophysiology*, *53*(3), 286–297. https://doi.org/10.1111/psyp.12518

Kwako, L. E., Schwandt, M. L., Ramchandani, V. A., Diazgranados, N., Koob, G. F., Volkow, N. D., Blanco, C., & Goldman, D. (2019). Neurofunctional domains derived from deep behavioral phenotyping in alcohol use disorder. *American Journal of Psychiatry*, *176*(9), 744–753. https://doi.org/10.1176/appi.ajp.2018.18030357

Kwasnicka, D., Dombrowski, S. U., White, M., & Sniehotta, F. (2016). Theoretical explanations for maintenance of behaviour change: A systematic review of behaviour theories. *Health Psychology Review*, *10*(3), 277–296. https://doi.org/10.1080/17437199.2016.1151372.

Lewis, M. (2018). Brain change in addiction as learning, not disease. *New England Journal of Medicine*, *379*(16), 1551–1560. https://doi.org/10.1056/NEJMra1602872

Leyro, T. M., Buckman, J. F., & Bates, M. E. (2019). Theoretical implications and clinical support for heart rate variability biofeedback for substance use disorders. *Current Opinion in Psychology*, *30*, 92–97. https://doi.org/10.1016/j.copsyc.2019.03.008

Litten, R. Z., Ryan, M. L., Falk, D. E., Reilly, M., Fertig, J. B., & Koob, G. F. (2015). Heterogeneity of alcohol use disorder: Understanding mechanisms to advance personalized treatment. *Alcoholism: Clinical and Experimental Research*, *39*(4), 579–584. https://doi.org/10.1111/acer.12669

Marlatt, G. A. (1996). Taxonomy of high-risk situations for alcohol relapse: evolution and development of a cognitive-behavioral model. *Addiction*, *91*(Suppl.), S37–S49. PMID 8997780

McCrady, B. S., & Epstein, E. (1999). *Addictions: A comprehensive guidebook.* Oxford University Press.

McEwen, B. S. (1998). Stress, adaptation, and disease. Allostasis and allostatic load. *Annals of the New York Academy of Sciences*, *840*, 33–44. https://doi.org/10.1111/j.1749-6632.1998.tb09546.x

Muraven, M., & Baumeister, R. F. (2000). Self-regulation and depletion of limited resources: Does self-control resemble a muscle? *Psychological Bulletin*, *126*(2), 247–259. https://doi.org/10.1037/0033-2909.126.2.247

National Academies of Sciences Engineering and Medicine (2016). *Measuring recovery from substance use or mental disorders: Workshop summary*. The National Academies Press. https://doi.org/10.17226/23589

Nixon, S. J., & Lewis, B. (2019). Cognitive training as a component of treatment of alcohol use disorder: A review. *Neuropsychology*, *33*(6), 822–841. https://doi.org/10.1037/neu0000575

Paulus, M. P., Schuckit, M. A., Tapert, S. F., Tolentino, N. J., Matthews, S. C., Smith, T. L., Trim, R. S., Hall, S. A., & Simmons, A. N. (2012). High versus low level of response to alcohol: Evidence of differential reactivity to emotional stimuli. *Biological Psychiatry*, *72*(10), 848–855. https://doi.org/10.1016/j.biopsych.2012.04.016

Rolland, B., D'Hondt, F., Montègue, S., Brion, M., Peyron, E., D'Aviau de Ternay, J., de Timary, P., Nourredine, M., & Maurage, P. (2019). A patient-tailored evidence-based approach for developing early neuropsychological training programs in addiction settings. *Neuropsychology Review*, *29*(1), 103–115. https://doi.org/10.1007/s11065–018-9395-3

Seo, D., & Sinha, R. (2015). Neuroplasticity and predictors of alcohol recovery. *Alcohol Research, 37*(1), 143–152.

Shields, G. S., Spahr, C. M., & Slavich, G. M. (2020). Psychosocial interventions and immune system function: A systematic review and meta-analysis of randomized clinical trials. *JAMA Psychiatry, 77*(10), 1–13. https://doi.org/10.1001/jamapsychiatry.2020.0431

Squeglia, L. M., Tapert, S. F., Sullivan, E. V., Jacobus, J., Meloy, M. J., Rohlfing, T., & Pfefferbaum, A. (2015). Brain development in heavy-drinking adolescents. *American Journal of Psychiatry, 172*(6), 531–542. https://doi.org/10.1176/appi.ajp.2015.14101249

Tiffany, S. T. (1990). A cognitive model of drug urges and drug-use behavior: Role of automatic and nonautomatic processes. *Psychological Review, 97*(2), 147–168. https://doi.org/10.1037/0033-295x.97.2.147

Uhl, G. R., Koob, G. F., & Cable, J. (2019). The neurobiology of addiction. *Annals of the New York Academy of Science, 1451*(1), 5–28. https://doi.org/10.1111/nyas.13989

Verdejo-Garcia, A., Lorenzetti, V., Manning, V., Piercy, H., Bruno, R., Hester, R., Pennington, D., Tolomeo, S., Arunogiri, S., Bates, M. E., Bowden-Jones, H., Campanella, S., Daughters, S. B., Kouimtsidis, C., Lubman, D. I., Meyerhoff, D. J., Ralph, A., Rezapour, T., Tavakoli, H., Zare-Bidoky, M., Zilverstand, A., Steele, D., Moeller, S. J., Paulus, M., Baldacchino, A., & Ekhtiari, H. (2019). A roadmap for integrating neuroscience into addiction treatment: A consensus of the neuroscience interest group of the international society of addiction medicine. *Frontiers in Psychiatry, 10*, 877. https://doi.org/10.3389/fpsyt.2019.00877

Votaw, V. R., Pearson, M. R., Stein, E., & Witkiewitz, K. (2020). The Addictions Neuroclinical Assessment negative emotionality domain among treatment-seekers with alcohol use disorder: Construct validity and measurement invariance. *Alcoholism: Clinical and Experimental Research, 44*(3), 679–688. https://doi.org/10.1111/acer.14283

Wilson, A. D., Bravo, A. J., Pearson, M. R., & Witkiewitz, K. (2016). Finding success in failure: Using latent profile analysis to examine heterogeneity in psychosocial functioning among heavy drinkers following treatment. *Addiction, 111*(12), 2145–2154. https://doi.org/10.1111/add.13518

Witkiewitz, K., & Tucker, J. A. (2020). Abstinence not required: Expanding the definition of recovery from alcohol use disorder. *Alcoholism: Clinical and Experimental Research, 44*(1), 36–40. https://doi.org/10.1111/acer.14235

Zahr, N. M., & Pfefferbaum, A. (2017). Alcohol's effects on the brain: Neuroimaging results in humans and animal models. *Alcohol Research, 38*(2), 183–206.

5 Lifespan Developmental Perspectives on Natural Mechanisms of Cessation of Risky Alcohol Use and Recovery from Alcohol Use Disorder

Matthew R. Lee, Yihong Zhao, Thomas Britton, Jenna Saviano, Kaan Kideys, Yimei Li, Colin Boulter, Emery Frick, and Kenneth J. Sher

Lifespan Developmental Perspectives on Natural Mechanisms of Cessation of Risky Alcohol Use and Recovery from Alcohol Use Disorder

Given the significance of risky alcohol use and alcohol use disorder (AUD) as public health concerns, understanding natural pathways to drinking reduction and AUD recovery is a key research objective. This chapter is premised on the notion that unique insights can be gleaned from considering pathways to change from a lifespan developmental perspective. We use the term risky alcohol use to refer broadly to a number of interrelated phenomena involving excessive, risky, and consequential drinking, including but not limited to formal diagnostic conditions like AUD (American Psychiatric Association [APA], 2013). This chapter discusses cessation of risky alcohol use and AUD recovery from a lifespan developmental perspective. Topics covered include AUD assessment with an emphasis on lifespan developmental issues, the epidemiology of risky alcohol use with an emphasis on age differences, and influences on risky use, AUD, and recovery in different periods of the lifespan.

Lifespan Developmental Issues in AUD Diagnosis

Chapter 1 of this book reviewed the diagnostic system of the *Diagnostic and Statistical Manual*, 5th edition (DSM-5; 2013) in the context of defining AUD recovery. Here we offer additional related considerations from a lifespan developmental perspective, emphasizing developmental differences across the lifespan related to specific AUD symptoms. One source of such developmental differences pertains to differential symptom validity by age. For instance, Vergés et al.

(2021) summarized reasons to suspect that observed adolescent and early young adult elevations of several AUD symptoms (e.g., tolerance, withdrawal) reflect some false positive endorsements (see also Caetano & Babor, 2006). Further, they noted that such false positive symptom endorsements could spuriously inflate rates of AUD at these ages and thereby inflate rates of subsequent AUD recovery or "desistance" in longitudinal research.

These concerns notwithstanding, there also appear to be valid ways that the meaning of symptoms shifts across the lifespan. For example, Lane et al. (2016) found age reductions in the likelihood that an AUD diagnosis includes endorsement of role impairment symptoms and suggested that this reduced endorsement of role impairment is likely attributable to real developmental increases across early adulthood in the importance of role responsibilities. Another example pertaining to later ages is that older adult AUD diagnoses appear to be less likely to include the symptom of tolerance, perhaps due to countervailing effects of aging related metabolic changes that can increase alcohol sensitivity (the opposite of tolerance; Kuerbis et al., 2017).

A general point pertaining to these examples is that accounting for such age differences could facilitate improved precision in AUD diagnosis (Boness et al., 2019), thereby also supporting improved precision in detecting AUD recovery. More broadly, such age differences can also offer important insights into variability across the lifespan in the ways that AUD manifests.

Epidemiology of Risky Alcohol Use and AUD

In the United States (US), AUD has consistently been more prevalent than all illicit substance use disorders combined (including cannabis), whereas rates of nicotine use disorder are higher than AUD (reviewed by Lee & Sher, 2018). When considering changes in AUD prevalence across recent years, the importance of developmental nuance is highlighted by critically important differences across age groups. The overall US population showed relative stability or modest declines in monthly binge drinking (5+ or 4+ drinks per occasion for males and females, respectively), monthly heavy drinking (5+ binge-drinking days per month), and DSM-IV AUD (abuse or dependence; APA, 1994) from 2002 to 2018 (Substance Abuse and Mental Health Services Administration [SAMHSA], 2019). However, young people have shown more dramatic declines across the same time period, with AUD rates declining from 5.9 percent to 1.6 percent in adolescents and from 17.7 percent to 10.1 percent in young adults over this period (SAMHSA, 2019). In contrast, significant increases have been observed in late midlife and older adulthood; e.g., one meta-analysis of changes from 2002 to 2013 showed heavy drinking increases of 26.8 percent and 38.5 percent for those aged 50–64 and aged 65+, respectively (Gruczca et al., 2018). This trend is concerning given the ongoing aging of the US population and the growing strain this will place on health systems (Ortman, 2014).

Age-Related Changes in Risky Alcohol Use and AUD

Perhaps the most striking demographic feature of risky alcohol use is its robust nonlinear association with age, with increases during adolescence, peaks around ages 18–23, and declines beginning in young adulthood. For example, this can be seen in Figure 5.1 based on our descriptive analyses of baseline data from the National Epidemiologic Survey on Alcohol and Related Conditions (NESARC; Grant et al., 2004).

Of course, caution is warranted in interpreting such cross-sectional age differences, given that what appears to reflect age-related changes could instead reflect confounded cohort or history effects (or various other age-related methodologic confounds). Thus, we also produced the "porcupine figure" shown in Figure 5.2. This figure shows the same cross-sectional age differences in AUD prevalence from Figure 5.1, but it also shows longitudinal age effects from NESARC's baseline data to the three-year follow-up.

In early young adulthood, the longitudinal data do approximately replicate conclusions from the cross-sectional data, showing (1) longitudinal *increases* from ages 18–20 to around ages 21–23 and then (2) longitudinal *decreases* from ages 21–24 to around ages 24–27. However, at later ages, while the cross-sectional data appeared to show continued decline in midlife and older adulthood, the longitudinal data instead appear to show (1) slight escalations during midlife and (2) approximate stability during older adulthood. While these

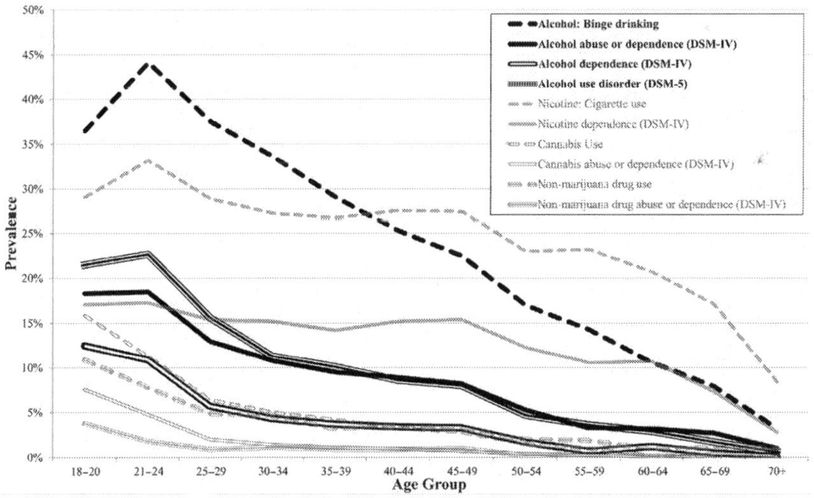

Figure 5.1 *US age-group differences in prevalence rates of past-year risky-drinking indices (other substances included for contrast)*

Note. *Results are from 2001–2002 NESARC data (Grant et al., 2004). Binge drinking was defined as four or more drinks on one occasion for females and five or more drinks on one occasion for males. DSM-5 AUD diagnoses were calculated based on 10 of 11 DSM-5 AUD symptoms because the craving symptom was not assessed in these NESARC data.*

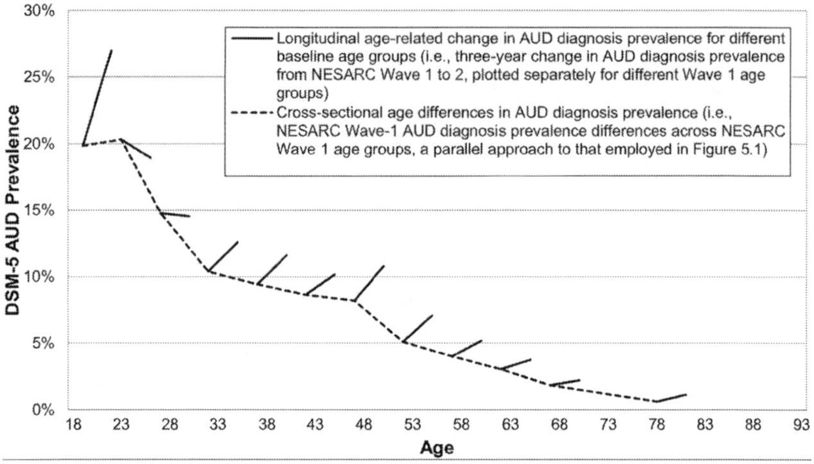

Figure 5.2 *"Porcupine figure" contrasting apparent age-related developmental changes in AUD prevalence from longitudinal versus cross-sectional NESARC data*

Note. *Results are from Wave 1 (2001–2002) and Wave 2 (2004–2005) NESARC data (Grant et al., 2004). Plotted points are DSM-5 AUD prevalence rates, with DSM-5 AUD diagnoses calculated based on 10 of 11 DSM-5 AUD symptoms because the craving symptom was not assessed in the NESARC Wave-1 data.*

analyses are exploratory and far from conclusive, they highlight the need for more empirical attention to drinking in midlife and older adulthood, including addressing questions as fundamental as the shape of normative drinking-related change across these ages.

Age Differences in Transitions In and Out of AUD

In addition to evidence of age-related changes in rates of risky alcohol use and AUD, some research using epidemiologic data has investigated longitudinal AUD-related transitions in a way that pertains more directly to recovery across the lifespan. Vergés et al. (2012) used NESARC data to assess age differences in rates of AUD onset, persistence (i.e., "non-desistance"), and recurrence, thereby characterizing contributions of these three phenomena to overall age-related AUD prevalence reductions. A key conclusion was that the observed age reductions in AUD rates reflected a decreasing propensity for AUD onset as individuals aged. In contrast, Vergés et al. did not find significant age differences in AUD remission, although their plotted results do appear to show a slight young-adulthood peak in remission rates. Perhaps confirming and extending the latter notion, Lee and colleagues (2018) conducted analyses with the same NESARC sample and found that young adult elevations in desistance rates between baseline and follow-up were especially notable for desistance from severe AUD, with desistance rates of 43–50 percent across ages 25–34 versus 22–24 percent across ages 35–55. Thus, the apparent overall young adult elevation in

AUD recovery appears largely attributable to those with severe AUD, a finding that highlights the relevance of the young adult "maturing out" phenomenon to an understanding of recovery.

Cohort Differences in Age-Related Change

Schulenberg et al. (2018) articulated how life course theory guides a multi-level view of developmental psychopathology and highlights historical context as a level of analysis that can moderate developmental change. Recent research has investigated such questions of development-by-history interactions by leveraging the rare US representative, cohort-sequential design of the *Monitoring the Future* (MTF) study (Bachman et al., 2002). This work revealed ways that longitudinal patterns of age-related changes in risky alcohol use and recovery have shifted across cohorts spanning birth years from the late 1970s to the early 2000s (e.g., Patrick et al., 2019). Specifically, for more recent cohorts, initial increases in risky drinking have shifted to begin at later ages of adolescence. However, more recent cohorts have also shown steeper subsequent risky-drinking increases, slightly later ages of peak risky drinking around the early 20s, and less substantial "maturing out" declines in the remainder of the 20s and early 30s.

These shifts in drinking-related age trends over time may reflect historical changes in other social and economic variables. For example, variables associated with young adult maturing out such as age of initial marriage and parenthood have increased during this same time period (Furstenberg, 2010; Settersten & Ray, 2010). However, it should be noted that the MTF study was limited to a focus on heavy drinking, and future research should investigate parallel development-by-history interactions predicting AUD and AUD recovery.

Sociodemographic Differences

Males generally show higher levels of heavy drinking when compared to females, although the differences vary in important ways across age groups. Gender differences in AUD rates have been found to be nonsignificant at the relatively early ages of 12–17, but rates among males surpass females by ages 18–25 (Chung & Jackson, 2019). Similarly, early adolescent alcohol use has been shown to be higher among females than males, but males show more rapid subsequent escalation and surpass females by mid-to-late adolescence (Windle, 2020). These higher rates among males appear to persist throughout the rest of the lifespan, although such gender differences appear to have narrowed in more recent cohorts (Patrick et al., 2019).

More work is needed to understand sociodemographic differences (e.g., by gender and ethnicity), both in the lifespan-developmental course of risky drinking and in risk and protective factors that influence this lifespan-developmental course (Chung & Jackson, 2019). A recent summary of the available evidence concluded that individuals who identify as non-Hispanic and White and American Indian/Alaska Native may initiate alcohol use relatively early, and there is more rapid initial escalation to AUD among those classified as non-Hispanic and White versus those classified as Hispanic or Black/African American. Throughout later parts of the lifespan, alcohol use and risky drinking remains especially high among those who identify as non-Hispanic and White and remains lower among those who identify as Black/African American and Asian (Jackson & Sartor, 2016).

Adolescent Etiology of Risky Alcohol Use

In reviewing etiologic influences on the emergence and escalation of drinking in adolescence, we adopted a framework that emphasizes three interrelated biopsychosocial risk pathways: (1) the "deviance proneness pathway," (2) the "stress/trauma and negative affect pathway," and (3) the "pharmacological effects pathway" (Chassin et al., 2013; Sher & Gotham, 1999). These pathways are viewed as originating from genetic and very early developmental risk factors. In fact, a developmental psychopathology view emphasizes potential "heterotypic continuity" as a parsimonious explanation for associations of earlier risk factors with later risky alcohol use, with such associations viewed as reflecting how the risk underlying a given etiologic pathway can manifest differently across developmental periods (Caspi & Roberts, 1999; Schulenberg et al., 2018).

Deviance Proneness Pathway

Deviance proneness models view risky alcohol use as part of a broader "externalizing spectrum" that includes other problem behaviors (e.g., conduct disorder, other substance-related problems, anti-sociality). These externalizing behaviors are viewed as originating from genetic risk and early impulsivity (i.e., a trait-like tendency to act on impulse without restraint or forethought) that are exacerbated by environmental risks such as family dysfunction (Gottfredson & Hirschi, 1990). Early intrapersonal and environmental risks are viewed as "setting the stage" for academic problems, deviant-peer affiliation, and various other externalizing behaviors including risky alcohol use. Deviance proneness models exemplify the aforementioned notion of heterotypic continuity, as links among problem behaviors across development are thought to reflect ways that deviance proneness manifests differently as development progresses (e.g., as conduct problems in childhood, binge drinking in adolescence, and AUD in adulthood; Schulenberg et al., 2018).

It is important to note instances where strong support has been provided for environmental risk effects, as opposed to the alternative explanation that apparent environmental risk factors may instead be environmental markers that are merely correlated with more causal intrapersonal risk processes. For example, there is evidence for environmental effects of deviant-peer affiliation on risky drinking even when controlling for gene- and impulsivity-related peer selection, and there is evidence for environmental effects of parenting deficits even when controlling for genetic risk and child impulsivity (Chassin et al., 2016). Further, positive environmental influences can offset effects of intrapersonal risk on the development of risky drinking (Chassin et al., 2016). In instances when high-risk individuals are exposed to positive influences, this developmental discontinuity can spark a "turning point" diverting the individual onto a lower-risk trajectory (Schulenberg et al., 2018).

Stress/Trauma and Negative Affect Pathway

Negative affect models have emphasized drinking to alleviate negative emotion, but past research is mixed regarding effects of negative affect on development of risky drinking patterns in adolescents. While this may prompt consideration of alternative explanations for associations between drinking and negative affect (e.g., negative affect as a consequence of heavy drinking), nuanced consideration supports the etiologic relevance of negative affect under certain conditions (Hussong et al., 2019; Schulenberg, 2018). Specifically, effects are more apparent (1) for depression- than anxiety-related negative affect, (2) in later ages of adolescence, and (3) when occurring in conjunction with other risk factors.

Regarding the role of stress and trauma in the negative affect pathway, there is consistent evidence, especially in females, that development of risky drinking patterns is associated with early stress and trauma exposure (e.g., violence, parental abuse/neglect; Cicchetti & Handley, 2019). However, the prediction that early stress and trauma effects are mediated by negative affect has received limited support. It is therefore noteworthy that neurologic effects of stress and trauma appear capable of inducing impulsivity-like deficits via alterations of impulse-control and reward networks in the brain. Thus, it may be more through these mechanisms than through negative affect regulation that early stress and trauma influence risky drinking development (Zucker et al., 2008).

Pharmacological Effects Pathway

Pharmacological effects models focus on individual differences in the effects of alcohol consumption, with these individual differences believed to confer differential risk for problem development. Two competing theories make partially conflicting predictions (Morean & Corbin, 2010). The low level of response model suggests an association between heightened risk for development of risky drinking patterns and overall lower sensitivity to the effects of alcohol. In contrast, the differentiator model suggests an association between heightened drinking risk and lower sensitivity to the sedating and unpleasant effects of alcohol coupled with higher sensitivity to stimulating and rewarding effects. Despite a vast body of past research, inconsistencies between these models remain unresolved (MacKillop & Ray, 2018). Nevertheless, there is evidence that higher drinking-related risks are associated with lower alcohol sensitivity, especially for sedating or unpleasant alcohol effects. Longitudinal research has also characterized mechanisms that appear to mediate the effects of lower alcohol sensitivity on risky drinking development, including (1) heavier drinking to achieve desired effects, (2) selection of heavier drinking peers, and (3) pro-alcohol changes in social norms, alcohol expectancies, and drinking motives (Schuckit et al., 2011).

AUD Recovery across the Adult Lifespan

We next discuss different developmental periods during the adult lifespan, with an emphasis on potential differences in how recovery may occur across these different adult developmental periods.

Late Adolescence and Early Young Adulthood (Approximately Ages 18–23)

The normative peaks in risky alcohol use around ages 18–23 have led to the view that these ages are when risky drinking is especially likely to reflect a "developmental disturbance" (Schulenberg et al., 2018). This term implies temporary elevations in risky drinking among otherwise low-risk individuals, with these temporary elevations driven primarily by environmental risk factors that are specific to this age period (e.g., college-related environmental risks). In contrast, a subset of individuals at these ages have stable intrapersonal risk factors for risky alcohol use (Ashenhurst & Fromme, 2018), which can be viewed as a continuation of an existing high-risk trajectory. For those whose risky alcohol use is best characterized as a developmental disturbance, their subsequent recovery can be conceptualized as a low-risk individual returning to an established low-risk trajectory once they exit a temporary high-risk environment (e.g., upon college graduation). For those whose risky alcohol use is associated with more stable intrapersonal risk factors, their subsequent recovery can be conceptualized as requiring disruption of an established high-risk trajectory, and thus be expected to require a more substantial ameliorative influence than merely exiting a high-risk environment. Such heterogeneity illustrates how conceptualizations of recovery require flexibility to account for a diversity of pathways through which risky drinking patterns develop and subsequent recovery occurs.

Recovery during Young Adulthood

With regard to developmental perspectives on recovery, particular attention has been paid to explaining the normative reductions in risky alcohol use or "maturing out" that occur in young adulthood beginning around the mid-20s, including resolution of AUD symptoms. A common explanation for young adult maturing out is that it is motivated by transitions into adult roles like marriage, parenthood, and full-time employment (Bachman et al., 2002). Young adulthood is marked by widespread adoption of such roles, and developmental theory views these transitions as key young adult developmental tasks (Erikson, 1968). Research has shown that both marriage and parenthood predict young adult reductions in risky drinking (Lee & Sher, 2018) and that either or both can contribute uniquely to these reductions. In contrast, research has often failed to show effects of young adult employment on reductions in risky alcohol use. There is also evidence for the clinical significance of family role related maturing out. This includes findings that the drinking changes following marriage can include AUD desistance (Gotham et al., 2003) and that marriage effects are especially strong among young adults with more severe alcohol-related problems (Lee, Chassin, et al., 2015), thus highlighting a clear relevance of family role-related maturing out to an understanding of recovery. However, research is needed on mediating mechanisms of family role effects to better illuminate more specific components of this pathway to recovery (Lee & Sher, 2018).

Despite a vast literature linking personality to risky drinking patterns (Sher et al., 2018), research has only recently considered how personality may relate to maturing out. A series of studies by Littlefield et al. (2009, 2010a) showed that the drinking reductions that typify young adult maturing out correspond to age-related maturational changes in personality, including increases in conscientiousness and decreases in impulsivity and neuroticism. The associations of impulsivity and neuroticism on maturing out were mediated by reductions in drinking to cope (Littlefield et al. 2010b). Lee, Ellingson et al. (2015) extended this work by examining directionality in associations between personality and changes in drinking and found that lower impulsivity and higher conscientiousness predicted subsequent reductions in risky drinking, and these effects were mediated by family role transitions. For example, young adults with higher conscientiousness at age 21 were more likely to experience a family role entry by age 25, which in turn predicted lower risky drinking at age 29.

Taken together, these findings support a developmental view of recovery as involving maturational improvements in decision making and affectivity, which in turn are associated with taking on new family roles and/or a decreased tendency toward using alcohol to cope. This view is consistent with emerging perspectives on AUD recovery that emphasize broad intrapersonal and interpersonal improvements as central or even definitional components of recovery (Witkiewitz et al., 2020; cf. Chapter 1). Another point of intersection between concepts of young adult development and concepts of recovery pertains to the role of identity. Recovery research has attended to recovery-related shifts in social networks and "social identity" (see Best et al., Chapter 16). Identity formation is also viewed as a key developmental process of adolescence and early young adulthood (Arnett, 2014; Erikson, 1968), and it should therefore receive increased attention as a possible distal influence on young adult maturing out as well as AUD recovery later in life. Recovery research has also incorporated assessments of "choice impulsivity" originating from behavioral economics, and this work has illuminated how the recovery process can involve shifts toward prioritizing longer-term rewards (Tucker et al., 2009; cf. Chapters 9, 10, and 15). Future research should investigate whether such elongation of one's "time horizon" is an additional unique component of personality maturation that contributes to young adult maturing out of risky alcohol use.

Recovery beyond Young Adulthood

This section discusses two topics related to potential differences across the lifespan in the ways that recovery occurs: (1) differences in how recovery has been characterized between the "maturing out" and "natural recovery" literatures, and (2) recovery among older adults and potential links to aging-related health issues.

Maturing Out versus Natural Recovery Models

Predictions regarding lifespan developmental differences in mechanisms of recovery were highlighted in Watson and Sher's (1998) review of conceptual differences between the "maturing out" and "natural recovery" literatures. As discussed earlier, the maturing out literature has focused on young adulthood and has largely viewed desistance of risky drinking as arising from the widespread contextual and intrapersonal changes reflecting maturation toward adulthood during this age period. Importantly, these processes are rarely conceptualized as involving acknowledgement of or concern about one's drinking (Jackson & Sartor, 2016; Watson & Sher, 1998). The natural recovery literature generally rests on a different view of change that primarily occurs in midlife after years of heavy drinking. Informed in part by models of behavior change, this literature views recovery as being motivated by an accumulation of adverse drinking consequences, problem recognition and deliberate reappraisals of one's drinking, and targeted efforts to change one's drinking (Klingemann & Sobell, 2007). It further views the experience of improved functioning, well-being, and life circumstances after initial resolution as being vital to maintaining stable long-term recovery (see Chapter 9).

Thus, maturing out models apply more often to young adulthood and natural recovery models apply more often to midlife and beyond (Lee & Sher, 2018). Recovery in young adulthood may often be understood as one component of the broader maturational change that characterizes this period, which may explain why recovery at these ages can often occur without much direct attention, contemplation, or effort specific to one's drinking. In contrast, recovery in midlife may require relatively more deliberate and alcohol-specific processes of problem recognition and effortful change coupled with positive reinforcement of initial change in valued areas of life-health, particularly those adversely affected by drinking. The latter improvements are a central feature of broadened conceptualizations of recovery discussed throughout this volume. These differences illustrate the potential for lifespan developmental research to help advance a more nuanced understanding of recovery that acknowledges different pathways to recovery are distinctive in different developmental periods over the lifespan.

Recovery in Older Adults

Older adulthood can bring health-related physical and cognitive challenges that may increase in importance as possible mechanisms of recovery in the older adult period of the lifespan. For instance, over 50 percent of older adults in the United States consume alcohol at levels deemed risky in the context of co-occurring medical conditions (Moore et al., 2006). Further, along with aging-related health issues comes increased use of medications that could interact harmfully with alcohol (Gu et al., 2010). The limited literature on older adult drinking indicates that health issues are among the most commonly reported reasons for cessation of drinking and AUD recovery (Schutte et al., 2006). However, studies of prospective associations of health problems with drinking reductions are more equivocal (Moos et al., 2010), perhaps owing to the complex relevance of affect- and coping-related issues in older adult drinking (Schulte & Hser, 2014). For instance, health problems can sometimes promote drinking reductions but can also have the opposite effect for those who drink to cope (Moos et al., 2010).

As noted earlier, there are reasons to view heavy drinking among older adults as an emerging area of particular public health concern in the United States, in part due to the ongoing aging of the "baby boomer" generation, who are projected to increase from under 15 percent of the population in 2012 to over 20 percent in 2030 (Barry & Blow, 2016). Given this generation's increased alcohol involvement relative to the preceding generation (Breslow et al., 2017), the ongoing aging of the baby boomer generation corresponds to ongoing increases in heavy drinking rates among US older adults (Colliver et al., 2006; Gruczca et al., 2018). These trends indicate that there is particular need for empirical and clinical attention to risky drinking and recovery among older adults. We argue for a lifespan developmental framework for such work that identifies components of recovery and role changes that are particularly influential in older adulthood, such as health-related concerns, social isolation, spousal bereavement, retirement, or other financial strain (Kuerbis et al., 2017). Such work may also reveal barriers to recovery and AUD treatment services that are particularly influential in older adulthood (e.g., reduced transportation access, lack of insurance coverage, relative computer illiteracy). Aging-related physiologic increases in alcohol sensitivity is another factor that may have unique relevance to recovery in older adulthood.

Conclusions and Recommendations

This chapter reviewed ways that an understanding of AUD recovery can be informed by a developmental perspective and illuminated the substantial heterogeneity of pathways to recovery, especially across different periods of the adult lifespan. Some of the developmental research on recovery, such as the work characterizing young adult "maturing out" of risky drinking, suggests dynamic pathways to recovery involving complex interplay among multiple interrelated mechanisms such as personality maturation and family role transitions. However, more work is needed to identify and model more components of this apparent rich interplay. Furthermore, additional work is also needed to integrate such findings from developmentally oriented research with pertinent findings from areas that more directly focus on recovery processes and outcomes (e.g., linking developmental and recovery-related views of identity). We argue for a lifespan developmental framework in future recovery research. Such work will likely reveal important differences in how recovery tends to occur across different periods of the adult lifespan, may help to reconcile ostensible discrepancies between different conceptual models of recovery, and show how different conceptual models may be more useful for different developmental periods. Below we discuss in relative detail two objectives that we view as important next steps for lifespan developmental recovery research.

Bridging Developmental Models across the Entire Lifespan

Key questions remain regarding how known etiologic risk factors may influence the likelihood and timing of adult recovery. For instance, among adolescents exhibiting substantial etiologic risk and corresponding risky drinking, to what extent do they mature out in young adulthood as normatively observed in the overall population, and in what ways may this depend on the specific forms of early etiologic risk? Might some, despite substantial early etiologic risk, nonetheless "mature out" in young adulthood if exposed to certain ameliorative influences like the family role transitions of marriage and parenthood? Alternatively, can certain levels or specific forms of early etiologic risk interfere with family role-driven maturing out, either by preventing family role entry or by counteracting the benefits that these roles typically convey?

How early etiologic risk will influence the adulthood course of risky drinking likely depends on the specific nature of the early etiologic risk. For example, research has demonstrated links of early stress and trauma with risky drinking and AUD in adulthood (e.g., Widom et al., 2007), thus supporting the potential relevance of stress and trauma to the adulthood course of risky drinking and recovery. There is also ample reason to predict that early stress and trauma may confer a reduced likelihood of young adult maturing out, in part due to how early stress and trauma may disrupt the key maturing out mechanisms of young adult family role transitions. Another prediction that highlights how attending to early etiology may yield unique insights into AUD course heterogeneity is that early stress and trauma may be especially predictive of a "late-onset" AUD subtype. In Zucker et al.'s (2016) view, this late-onset AUD subtype emerges around late young adulthood or early midlife, is especially related to negative affect, and is more common in women than in men. This is just one example of how one specific early etiologic risk factor may be better understood through a lifespan developmental framework to influence adulthood heterogeneity in the course of risky drinking, AUD, and recovery.

Links to Brain-Based Models of Addiction

Developmental models of the etiology and lifespan course of risky drinking and AUD can be further informed by neurophysiologic research, which has provided clear and consistent evidence of structural and functional alterations in the brain associated with AUD progression (Volkow & Koob, 2015). Certain brain-based models describe three ascending stages through which alcohol addiction can progress (binge/intoxication, withdrawal/negative affect, and preoccupation/anticipation), with each stage being associated with neurobiological alterations in distinct brain systems, and with the changes of each stage interacting with one another and worsening over time. Yet, criticisms of brain-based models have included the minimization of important psychosocial influences on the developmental course of risky drinking and AUD (Volkow & Koob, 2015). Opportunities to address such limitations should increase in the coming years through the availability of large-scale longitudinal datasets such as the National Consortium on Alcohol and Neurodevelopment in Adolescence (NCANDA), the Adolescent Brain Cognitive Development (ABCD) project, and the Enhancing Neuro Imaging Genetics by Meta-Analysis (ENIGMA) project (Luna et al., 2020). Such studies should provide opportunities to investigate brain-based mechanisms in relation to key psychosocial and developmental influences. This research combining psychosocial and developmental influences with brain-based mechanisms has the potential to yield key insights into their combined and interacting influences on the development of risky alcohol use, AUD, and recovery across the lifespan.

Acknowledgments

Writing of this chapter was supported by National Institute on Alcohol Abuse and Alcoholism grants R00-AA024236 to Matthew R. Lee and K05-AA017242 to Kenneth J. Sher. We also wish to thank additional GSAPP students and CAS research trainees who assisted with preparation of this chapter, including Mohammed Ahmed, Yasin Farshchi, Daniel Friedman, Thomas Kwan, Syeda Qasim, and Amy Xu.

References

American Psychiatric Association. (1994). *Diagnostic and statistical manual of mental disorders* (4th ed.).

(2013). *Diagnostic and statistical manual of mental disorders* (5th ed.). https://doi.org/10.1176/appi.books.9780890425596

Arnett, J. (2014). *Emerging adulthood: The winding road from the late teens through the twenties* (2nd ed.). Oxford University Press. https://doi.org/10.1093/oxfordhb/9780199795574.013.9

Ashenhurst, J. R., & Fromme, K. (2018). Alcohol use and consequences across developmental transitions during college and beyond. In H. E. Fitzgerald, & L. I. Puttler (Eds.), *Alcohol use disorders: A developmental science approach to etiology*. Oxford University Press. https://doi.org//oso/9780190676001.003.0015

Bachman, J. G., O'Malley, P. M., Schulenberg, J. E., Johnston, L. D., Bryant, A. L., & Merline, A. C. (2002). *The decline of substance use in young adulthood: Changes in social activities, roles, and beliefs*. Lawrence Erlbaum Associates. https://doi.org/10.4324/9781410606013

Barry, K. L., & Blow, F. C. (2016). Alcohol over the lifespan: Focus on older adults. *Alcohol Research: Current Reviews, 38*(1), 115–120. https://pubmed.ncbi.nlm.nih.gov/27159818/

Boness, C. L., Lane, S. P., & Sher, K. J. (2019). Not all alcohol use disorder criteria are equally severe: Toward severity grading of individual criteria in college drinkers. *Psychology of Addictive Behaviors, 33*(1), 35–49. https://doi.org/10.1037/adb0000443

Breslow, R. L., Castle, I. P., Chen, C. M., & Graubard, B. I. (2017). Trends in alcohol consumption among older Americans: National Health Interview Surveys, 1997–2014. *Alcoholism: Clinical and Experimental Research, 41*(5), 978–986. https://doi.org/10.1111/acer.13365

Caetano, R., & Babor, T. F. (2006). Diagnosis of alcohol dependence in epidemiological surveys: An epidemic of youthful alcohol dependence or a case of measurement error? *Addiction, 101*, 111–114. http://doi.org/10.1111/j.1360-0443.2006.01599.x

Caspi, A., & Roberts, B. W. (1999). Personality change and continuity across the life course. In L. A. Pervin, & O. P. John (Eds.), *Handbook of personality theory and research* (pp. 300–326). Guilford Press.

Chassin, L., Haller, M., Lee, M. R., Handley, E., Bountress, K., & Beltran, I. (2016). Familial factors influencing offspring substance use and dependence. In K. J. Sher (Ed.), *Oxford handbook of substance use and substance use disorders* (pp. 449–482). Oxford University Press. http://doi.org/10.1093/oxfordhb/9780199381678.013.008

Chassin, L., Sher, K. J., Hussong, A., & Curran, P. (2013). The developmental psychopathology of alcohol use and alcohol disorders: Research achievements and future directions. *Development and Psychopathology, 25*(402), 1567. http://doi.org/10.1017/S0954579413000771

Chung, T., & Jackson, K. M. (2019). Adolescent alcohol use. In R. A. Zucker & S. Brown (Eds.) *The Oxford handbook of adolescent substance abuse*. Oxford University Press. http://doi.org/10.1093/oxfordhb/9780199735662.013.007

Cicchetti, D., & Handley, E. D. (2019). Child maltreatment and the development of substance use and disorder. *Neurobiology of Stress, 10*, 100144. https://doi.org/10.1016/j.ynstr.2018.100144

Colliver, J. D., Compton, W. M., Gfroerer, J. C., & Condon, T. (2006). Projecting drug use among aging baby boomers in 2020. *Annals of epidemiology, 16*(4), 257–265.

Erikson, E.H. (1968). *Identity: Youth and crisis*. Norton & Co.

Furstenberg Jr, F. F. (2010). On a new schedule: Transitions to adulthood and family change. *The Future of Children, 20*(1), 67–87.

Gotham, H. J., Sher, K. J., & Wood, P. K. (2003). Alcohol involvement and developmental task completion during young adulthood. *Journal of Studies on Alcohol, 64*(1), 32–42. https://doi.org/10.15288/jsa.2003.64.32

Gottfredson, M., & Hirschi, T. (1990). *A general theory of crime*. Stanford University Press.

Grant, B. F., Stinson, F. S., Dawson, D. A., Chou, S. P., Dufour, M. C., Compton, W., Pickering, R. P., & Kaplan, K. (2004). Prevalence and co-occurrence of substance use disorders and independent mood and anxiety disorders: Results from the National Epidemiologic Survey on Alcohol and Related Conditions. *Archives of General Psychiatry, 61*(8), 807–816. https://doi.org/10.1001/archpsyc.61.8.807

Grucza, R. A., Sher, K. J., Kerr, W. C., Krauss, M. J., Lui, C. K., McDowell, Y. E., Hartz, S., Virdi, G., & Bierut, L. J. (2018). Trends in adult alcohol use and binge drinking in the early twenty-first century United States: A meta-analysis of six national survey series. *Alcoholism: Clinical and Experimental Research, 42* (10), 1939–1950. https://doi.org/10.1111/acer.13859

Gu, Q., Dillon, C. F., & Burt, V. L. (2010). Prescription drug use continues to increase: US prescription drug data for 2007–2008. *NCHS data brief,* (42), 1–8.

Hussong, A. M., Shadur, J., Burns, A. R., Stein, G., Jones, D., Solis, J., & McKee, L. G. (2019). An early emerging internalizing pathway to substance use and disorder. In R. A. Zucker & S. Brown (Eds.), *The Oxford Handbook of adolescent substance abuse* (pp. 319–343). Oxford University Press. https://doi.org/10.1093/oxfordhb/9780199735662.013.015

Jackson, K., & Sartor, C. (2016). The natural course of substance use and dependence. In K. J. Sher (Ed.), *Oxford handbook of substance use and substance use disorders* (pp. 67–131). Oxford University Press. https://doi.org/10.1093/oxfordhb/9780199381678.013.007

Klingemann, H. K., & Sobell, L. C. (2007). *Promoting self-change from addictive behaviors: Practical implications for policy, prevention, and treatment.* Springer. https://doi.org/10.1007/978-0-387-71287-1

Kuerbis, A., Moore, A. A., Sacco, P., & Zanjani, F. (Eds.). (2017). *Alcohol and aging: Clinical and public health perspectives.* Springer. https://doi.org/10.1007/978-3-319-47233-1

Lane, S. P., Steinley, D., & Sher, K. J. (2016). Meta-analysis of DSM alcohol use disorder criteria severities: Structural consistency is only 'skin deep'. *Psychological Medicine, 46*(8), 1769–1784. https://doi.org/10.1017/S0033291716000404

Lee, M. R., Boness, C. L., McDowell, Y. E., Vergés, A., Steinley, D. L., & Sher, K. J. (2018). Desistance and severity of alcohol use disorder: A lifespan-developmental investigation. *Clinical Psychological Science, 6*(1), 90–105. https://doi.org/10.1177/2167702617736852

Lee, M. R., Chassin, L., & MacKinnon, D. (2015). Role transitions and young adult maturing out of heavy drinking: Evidence for larger effects of marriage among more severe pre-marriage problem drinkers. *Alcoholism: Clinical and Experimental Research, 39(6),* 1064–1074. https://doi.org/10.1111/acer.12715

Lee, M. R., Ellingson, J. M., & Sher, K. J. (2015). Integrating social-contextual and intrapersonal mechanisms of "maturing out": Joint influences of familial role transitions and personality maturation on problem drinking reductions. *Alcoholism: Clinical and Experimental Research, 39*(9), 1775–1787. https://doi.org/10.1111/acer.12816

Lee, M. R., & Sher, K. J. (2018). "Maturing out" of binge and problem drinking. *Alcohol Research: Current Reviews, 39*(1), 31–42.

Littlefield, A.K., Sher, K. J., & Wood, P. K. (2009). Is "maturing out" of problematic alcohol involvement related to personality change? *Journal of Abnormal Psychology, 118*(2), 360–374. https://doi.org/10.1037/a0015125

Littlefield, A. K., Sher, K. J., & Wood, P. K. (2010a). A personality-based description of maturing out of alcohol problems: Extension with a five-factor model and robustness to modeling challenges. *Addictive Behaviors, 35*(11), 948–954. https://doi.org/10.1016/j.addbeh.2010.06.008

(2010b). Do changes in drinking motives mediate the relation between personality change and "maturing out" of problem drinking? *Journal of Abnormal Psychology, 119*(1), 93–105. https://doi.org/10.1037/a0017512

Luna, B., Tervo-Clemmens, B., & Calabro, F. J. (2020). Considerations when characterizing adolescent neurocognitive development. *Biological Psychiatry, 89*(2), 96–98. https://doi.org/10.1016/j.biopsych.2020.04.026

MacKillop, J., & Ray, L. A. (2018). The etiology of addiction: A contemporary biopsychosocial approach. In J. MacKillop, G. A. Kenna, L. Leggio, & L. A. Ray (Eds.), *Integrating psychological and pharmacological treatments for addictive disorders: An evidence-based guide* (pp. 32–53). Routledge/Taylor & Francis Group.

Morean, M. E., & Corbin, W. R. (2010). Subjective response to alcohol: A critical review of the literature. *Alcoholism: Clinical and Experimental Research, 34*(3), 385–395. https://doi.org/10.1111/j.1530-0277.2009.01103.x

Moore, A. A., Giuli, L., Gould, R., Hu, P., Zhou, K., Reuben, D., Greendale, G., & Karlamangla, A. (2006). Alcohol use, comorbidity, and mortality. *Journal of the American Geriatrics Society, 54*(5), 757–762. https://doi.org/10.1111/j.1532-5415.2006.00728.x

Moos, R. H., Brennan, P. L., Schutte, K. K., & Moos, B. S. (2010). Older adults' health and late-life drinking patterns: A 20-year perspective. *Aging and Mental Health, 14*(1), 33–43. https://doi.org/10.1080/13607860902918264

Ortman, J. M., Velkoff, V. A., & Hogan, H. (2014). *An aging nation: The older population in the United States.* United States Census Bureau.

Patrick, M. E., Terry-McElrath, Y. M., Lanza, S. T., Jager, J., Schulenberg, J. E., & O'Malley, P. M. (2019). Shifting age of peak binge drinking prevalence: Historical changes in normative trajectories among young adults aged 18 to 30. *Alcoholism: Clinical and Experimental Research, 43*(2), 287–298. https://doi.org/10.1111/acer.13933

Schuckit, M. A., Smith, T. L., Trim, R. S., Allen, R. C., Fukukura, T., Knight, E. E., Cesario, B. A., & Kreikebaum, S. A. (2011). A prospective evaluation of how a low level of response to alcohol predicts later heavy drinking and alcohol problems. *The American Journal of Drug and Alcohol Abuse, 37*(6), 479–486. https://doi.org/10.3109/00952990.2011.598590

Schulenberg, J., Maslowsky, J., & Jager, J. (2018). Substance use and abuse during adolescence and the transition to adulthood are developmental phenomena: Conceptual and empirical considerations. In H. E. Fitzgerald, & L. I. Puttler (Eds.), *Alcohol use disorders: A developmental science approach to etiology.* (pp. 199–222). Oxford University Press. https://doi.org/10.1093/oso/9780190676001.003.0012

Schulte, M. T., & Hser, Y. I. (2014). Substance use and associated health conditions throughout the lifespan. *Public Health Reviews, 35*(2), 1–27. https://doi.org/10.1007/BF03391702

Schutte, K. K., Moos, R. H., & Brennan, P. L. (2006). Predictors of untreated remission from late-life drinking problems. *Journal of Studies on Alcohol*, *67*(3), 354–362. https://doi.org/10.15288/jsa.2006.67.354

Settersten Jr, R. A., & Ray, B. (2010). What's going on with young people today? The long and twisting path to adulthood. *The Future of Children*, *20*(1), 19–41. https://doi.org/10.1353/foc.0.0044

Sher, K. J., & Gotham, H. J. (1999). Pathological alcohol involvement: A developmental disorder of young adulthood. *Development and Psychopathology*, *11*(04), 933–956. https://doi.org/10.1017/s0954579499002394

Sher, K. J., Littlefield, A., & Lee, M. (2018). Personality processes related to the development and resolution of alcohol use disorders. In H. E. Fitzgerald & L. I. Puttler (Eds.), *Alcohol use disorders: A developmental science approach to etiology* (pp. 285–304). Oxford University Press. https://doi.org/10.1093/med-psych/9780190492243.003.0018

Substance Abuse and Mental Health Services Administration. (SAMHSA) (2019). *Key substance use and mental health indicators in the United States: Results from the 2018 National Survey on Drug Use and Health* (HHS Publication No. PEP19–5068, NSDUH Series H-54). Substance Abuse and Mental Health Services Administration.

Tucker, J. A., Roth, D. L., Vignolo, M. J., & Westfall, A. O. (2009). A behavioral economic reward index predicts drinking resolutions: Moderation revisited and compared with other outcomes. *Journal of Consulting and Clinical Psychology*, *77*(2), 219–228. https://doi.org/10.1037/a0014968

Vergés, A., Jackson, K. M., Bucholz, K. K., Grant, J. D., Trull, T. J., Wood, P. K., & Sher, K. J. (2012). Deconstructing the age-prevalence curve of alcohol dependence: Why "maturing out" is only a small piece of the puzzle. *Journal of Abnormal Psychology*, *121*(2), 511–523. https://doi.org/10.1037/a0026027.

Vergés, A., Lee, M. R., Martin, C. S., Trull, T. J., Martens, M. P., Wood, P. K., & Sher, K. J. (2021). Not all symptoms of alcohol dependence are developmentally equivalent: Implications for the false-positives problem. *Psychology of Addictive Behaviors*, *35*(4), 444–457. https://doi.org/10.1037/adb0000723

Volkow, N. D., & Koob, G. (2015). Brain disease model of addiction: Why is it so controversial? *The Lancet Psychiatry*, *2*(8), 677–679. https://doi.org/10.1016/S2215–0366(15)00236-9

Votaw, V. R., Pearson, M. R., Stein, E., & Witkiewitz, K. (2020). The addictions neuroclinical assessment negative emotionality domain among treatment-seekers with alcohol use disorder: Construct validity and measurement invariance. *Alcoholism: Clinical and Experimental Research*, *44*(3), 679–688. https://doi.org/10.1111/acer.14283

Watson, A. L., & Sher, K. J. (1998). Resolution of alcohol problems without treatment: Methodological issues and future directions of natural recovery research. *Clinical Psychology: Science and Practice*, *5*(1), 1–18. https://doi.org/10.1111/j.1468-2850.1998.tb00131.x

White, H. R., Labouvie, E. W., & Papadaratsakis, V. (2005). Changes in substance use during the transition to adulthood: A comparison of college students and their noncollege age peers. *Journal of Drug Issues*, *35*(2), 281–306. https://doi.org/10.1177/002204260503500204

Widom, C. S., White, H. R., Czaja, S. J., & Marmorstein, N. R. (2007). Long-term effects of child abuse and neglect on alcohol use and excessive drinking in middle adulthood. *Journal of Studies on Alcohol and Drugs*, *68*(3), 317–326. https://doi.org/10.15288/jsad.2007.68.317

Windle, M. (2020). Sex differences in substance use from adolescence to young adulthood: Tests of increases in emergent adulthood and maturing out in later young adulthood. *Drug and Alcohol Dependence*, *207*, 107813. https://doi.org/10.1016/j.drugalcdep.2019.107813

Witkiewitz, K., Montes, K. S., Schwebel, F. J., & Tucker, J. A. (2020). What is recovery? *Alcohol Research: Current Reviews*, *40*(3), 1–12. https://doi.org/10.35946/arcr.v40.3.01

Zucker, R. A., Donovan, J. E., Masten, A. S., Mattson, M. E., & Moss, H. B. (2008). Early developmental processes and the continuity of risk for underage drinking and problem drinking. *Pediatrics, 121*(Suppl. 4), S252–S272. https://doi.org/10.1542/peds.2007-2243B

Zucker, R. A., Hicks, B. M., & Heitzeg, M. M. (2016). Alcohol use and the alcohol use disorders over the life course: A cross-level developmental review. In D. Cicchetti (Ed.), *Developmental psychopathology: Maladaptation and psychopathology* (pp. 793–832). John Wiley & Sons, Inc. https://doi.org/10.1002/9781119125556.devpsy318

6 Mutual Help Approaches and Mechanisms of Change

J. Scott Tonigan

Mutual Help Approaches and Mechanisms of Change

Mutual help programs are a popular resource for individuals suffering from alcohol use disorder (AUD), and evidence suggests that a higher proportion of people seek help for their drinking problems from mutual help programs than from formal treatment (e.g., Zemore et al., 2017). Today, there are at least four established mutual help programs in the United States (US), each of which has a literature and prescribed program to alleviate AUD: Alcoholics Anonymous (AA), Women for Sobriety (WFS), LifeRing, and SMART Recovery. While these four mutual help programs have commonalities, there is a sharp distinction in how they view the locus of control to change harmful alcohol use. On one hand, AA considers an affected individual to be *powerless* over alcohol and regards personal change to be dependent upon spiritual growth, with sobriety being contingent upon a relationship with a *higher power*. In contrast, the remaining three mutual help programs emphasize the importance of *empowering* individuals to initiate and sustain changes in their drinking and lifestyles, often incorporating coping skill strategies developed in cognitive behavior therapy. This chapter describes what is currently known about the efficacy of mutual help programs, prescribed practices that are associated with changes in alcohol use, and underlying mechanisms that may explain why, for some individuals, mutual help programs are useful. Given the preponderance of research on AA relative to SMART, LifeRing, and WFS, this discussion will necessarily focus on AA, highlighting where possible what is known about alternative mutual help programs.

AA and Other Mutual Help Programs

AA is the most popular mutual help program for people with AUD trying to achieve alcohol abstinence, and a majority of treatment providers in the United States encourage AA attendance during and after treatment (Alcoholics Anonymous, 2020). AA is a community-based organization that is strictly non-professional, is free to attend, and is widely available. Succinctly stated in the AA preamble, “Alcoholics Anonymous is a fellowship of men and women who share their experience, strength, and hope with each other that they may solve their common problem and help others to recover from alcoholism. The only requirement for membership is a desire to stop drinking" (Alcoholics Anonymous, 1939). According to AA, in 2019 world-wide membership was about 2,077,374, and there were roughly 125,557 meeting locations across 180 countries (Alcoholics Anonymous, 2020). By comparison, Zemore and colleagues (2017) reported that there were about 1,240 meetings when *summing* the number of meetings for the WFS, LifeRing, and SMART Recovery mutual help programs.

The core text of AA, *Alcoholics Anonymous: The Story of How Many Thousands of Men and Women Have Recovered from Alcoholism* (i.e., the "Big Book"; Alcoholics Anonymous, 1939), has sold over 30 million copies to date. Several excellent works have described the history, underlying tenets and assumptions, and implications of AA prescribed practices in the core AA literature (Kurtz, 1979; White & Kurtz, 2008), and a detailed discussion goes beyond the scope of this chapter. Briefly, the *program* of AA is expressed in the 12 Steps, and members are encouraged, with the aid of an AA sponsor, to sequentially work through the steps. Working each of the steps is claimed to confer benefit that ultimately culminates in a fundamental spiritual transformation with the completion of Step 12.

The AA program is strictly abstinence-based. While there is general agreement between *Diagnostic and Statistical Manual*, 5th edition (DSM-5) criteria (American Psychiatric Association, 2013) for the diagnosis of AUD and AA's definition of the "real alcoholic," there is ambiguity within and outside of AA about the distinctions between abstinence, sobriety, and recovery. In AA, alcohol abstinence is considered a necessary prerequisite for sobriety and recovery, a hierarchy that is consistent with the results of a national survey of individuals who had resolved their alcohol problems (96 percent through treatment and/or mutual support groups) and who identified themselves to be in recovery (Kaskutas et al., 2014). The distinction in AA between abstinence and sobriety is nuanced, and sobriety is regarded to be the higher objective. Most aptly described in the 12 promises of AA associated with Step 8 (Alcoholics Anonymous, 1939, pp. 83-84), sobriety is defined as enhanced well-being, awareness of serenity, an absence of economic insecurity, and a positive change in attitude and outlook on life.

The conundrum is, what is meant by recovery in AA, where is it to be placed in this hierarchy of abstinence and sobriety, and how can AA members who are abstinent or who have achieved sobriety both legitimately claim they are in recovery? The answer is deceptively simple. As considered by AA members, recovery is a *verb* and not a *noun*. To be in recovery implies that one is actively engaged in activities that promote abstinence and, directly or indirectly, also move one toward or sustain sobriety. In short, recovery is a means to achieve sobriety, with the acknowledgment in AA that sobriety itself is ephemeral and frequently waxes and wanes contingent upon one's spiritual condition. In this light, efforts to define full remission from AUD as it is conceptualized in AA should focus on the development of operational definitions and measures of sobriety as defined in the AA promises (e.g., Kelly & Greene, 2013).

The origin and practice of alternative mutual help programs may be viewed as reactions to perceived omissions and/or commissions in AA. LifeRing, for example, has a secular orientation and endorses cognitive behavior coping strategies in its core literature and prescriptions (e.g., Nicolaus, 2009). In contrast, WFS is grounded in the belief that the path to recovery for women with AUD is grounded in enhancing self-esteem and positive thinking of women, most aptly seen in the program's Thirteen Statement Program (e.g., Kirkpatrick, 1977). Both LifeRing and WFS are abstinence-based and share with AA the practice of peer-led meetings. Unlike these programs, the SMART Recovery Program (Hardin, 2013) endorses educational and mental health models and meetings are led by trained facilitators. In SMART abstinence is encouraged, but is not the sine qua non in defining success or recovery. Here, the elimination of harmful drinking is considered an acceptable goal for SMART members.

Mutual Help Affiliation Profiles

Mutual help programs differ on key dimensions, including beliefs about the etiology of AUD, the ability and role of an individual to reduce harmful drinking, the task demands placed upon members, and the expected longevity of membership. With this in mind, the study of AA affiliation profiles has a long history, and one of the most robust findings is that alcohol problem severity is the single strongest predictor of AA affiliation, with problem severity encompassing such constructs as loss of control when drinking, alcohol-related problems, and quantity and frequency of alcohol consumption (Emrick et al., 1993; Harris et al., 2003). Not surprisingly given the spiritual focus of AA, studies have also demonstrated that self-declared atheists are significantly less likely to affiliate with AA, relative to agnostic, spiritual, and religious individuals (Tonigan et al., 2002). In general, demographic variables such as ethnicity, age, gender, and SES have demonstrated weak or no association with AA affiliation.

Zemore and colleagues (2017) provided a rare comparison of mutual help affiliation profiles of AA, WFS, SMART, and LifeRing members, divided according to clinical and demographic variables. In general, they found no mean differences in past-year alcohol symptom count and problems between members in the four mutual help groups. Demographically, however, substantial differences emerged in member characteristics. Specifically, members of AA alternatives reported more education and higher income, and members of WFS and LifeRing tended to be married and older relative to AA members. Predictably, more AA members self-identified as religious or spiritual relative to members of the AA alternatives. Zemore and colleagues also reported that "recovery goal" differed significantly between members of the four mutual help programs. AA members reported, on average, higher endorsement of "quit forever" relative to SMART and LifeRing members and, alternatively, SMART and LifeRing members endorsed goals of "abstinent now, may drink in the future" and "use alcohol in a controlled manner/occasionally" relative to AA and WFS members.

Mutual Support and Alcohol Abstinence Outcomes

The body of peer-reviewed research on AA is vast and growing. Between 1950 and 2000 there were over 300 peer-reviewed papers on AA processes and outcomes. Since then, the number of such publications further increased by at least 123 percent (374 peer-reviewed publications) with a majority of these studies including prospective hypothesis testing, longitudinal designs, use of outcome measures with strong psychometric properties, and high follow-up rates. Thus, the application of meta-analytic procedures is an ideal approach to summarize the rapidly expanding AA-focused literature.

Evidence is, at best, circumstantial about the efficacy of WFS, SMART, and LifeRing. In a systematic review of the SMART program, for example, Beck et al., (2017) reported that 8 of the 12 studies investigating alcohol-related outcomes and SMART used a cross-sectional design. Further, only a handful of studies have investigated WFS (e.g., Kaskutas, 1994), and none of these used a longitudinal design that included measures of alcohol use. To date, Zemore and colleagues (2018) have provided the clearest longitudinal picture of the relative efficacy of AA and other alternatives. Based on a national sample they reported relative parity in abstinence outcomes at 6- and 12-month follow-ups between members in AA, SMART, LifeRing, and WFS. It should be noted that a majority of these participants were in relatively stable recovery prior to enrolling in this study, and the findings await replication with individuals during early efforts to reduce their alcohol use.

With this background, there is sufficient consistency in findings across meta-analytic reviews to assert that frequency of AA meeting attendance is associated with subsequent increases in alcohol abstinence, with significant and positive effect size estimates of this relationship ranging from a weighted correlation of $r_w = .21$ to $r_w = .31$ (Emrick et al., 1993; Humphreys et al., 2014; Kelly et al., 2020; Tonigan, 2001; Tonigan et al., 1996, 2018).

It is noteworthy that meta-analytic reviews have arrived at similar conclusions regardless of whether they combined studies targeting special populations such as dually diagnosed AA affiliates (e.g., Tonigan et al., 2018), general population AA samples (e.g., Emrick et al., 1993), or randomized clinical trials that examined AA in combination with 12 Step facilitation treatment (Kelly et al., 2020). The salutary association between AA participation and drinking reductions does not appear to arise from self-selection bias; e.g., individuals who choose to attend AA may be systematically more motivated to change drinking behavior relative to individuals who do not attend AA (e.g., Humphrey et al., 1996; Magura et al., 2012; although see Steinley, Chapter 20 for a critique of propensity score methods used in these prior studies). Collectively, then, when abstinence is the goal, the weight of evidence indicates that AA attendance alone or in combination with professional treatment is an evidence-based practice for the treatment of AUD.

AA Active Ingredients

Meeting Characteristics

A guiding principle in selecting AA active ingredients for discussion is that they have demonstrated an association with increased abstinence. Recent work indicates that fine grained aspects of the AA meeting experience can be reliably measured, and that they, too, are associated with increased abstinence. For example, in a large study of treatment-seeking adults, Zemore and colleagues (2013) reported that having a "declared" AA home group that one frequently attends at 6-month follow-up was significantly associated with increased abstinence at nine months, even after controlling for AA attendance and sponsorship. Likewise, different types of activities associated with AA meetings are associated with increased abstinence, including activities such as whether one "shared" or not in a meeting, helped prepare the room for a meeting, and read the AA preamble *How it Works* at the beginning of a meeting (Rynes & Tonigan, 2013; Zemore et al., 2013). Collectively, these finer grained measures may be important indices of commitment to AA and, consequently, may be influential catalysts for mobilizing change mechanisms.

AA Sponsors

There is strong evidence that getting an AA sponsor is associated with increased abstinence. The primary role of an AA sponsor is to guide a junior member through the 12 Steps of AA, or the "program of AA" (Alcoholics Anonymous, 1939). Secondary roles of sponsors include encouraging AA meeting attendance, offering abstinence-based support, and encouraging service work (Whelan et al., 2009), which reflect AA fellowship activities. These overlapping functions suggest that AA sponsorship may be one of the most potent yet least understood of the active ingredients in AA. Prevalence estimates of AA members with a sponsor vary widely and tend to be time-dependent in the course of recovery (Witbrodt et al., 2012), with the highest rates occurring during the first six months of AA affiliation. The 2007 Triennial AA survey reports that 73 percent of new AA members get an AA sponsor within the first 90 days of AA affiliation. There is some evidence that this estimate may be overly optimistic. Specifically, in a community-based sample of early AA members ($N = 253$) at baseline, 44.3 percent ($n = 112$) of the participants had a sponsor, and this percentage remained relatively constant across the 3-, 6-, and 12-month follow-ups at 44.1 percent, 44.2 percent, and 42.9 percent, respectively (Tonigan & Rice, 2010)

At least 22 longitudinal studies have investigated the association between having an AA sponsor and later increases in abstinence. Meta-analytically combining these studies (as reported in Magill et al., 2015), the overall association between having an AA sponsor and later abstinence was $r_w = .26$ (95 percent CI = .24–.28). Standard research practice for determining whether a participant had a sponsor was accomplished with a binary response to the question, "Do you have a sponsor (yes/no)?" This practice has been criticized and, quite recently, a number of studies have evaluated how to better capture the structure and functions of the sponsor-sponsee relationship (Stevens et al., 2015).

AA Step Work

Fifteen studies have directly investigated whether progress in AA step work was associated with increased abstinence. With few exceptions, step work was assessed by asking respondents to indicate which steps they had "completed." The overall weighted correlation between number of steps completed and abstinence for these 15 studies was $r_w = .23$ (CI: .21–.26; Magill et al., 2015). Work by Greenfield and Tonigan (2013) indicated that directly asking early AA members about the steps they have completed is a poor indicator of their endorsement and practice of the beliefs and practices embedded in the steps. Specifically, they found that participants' endorsement of steps completed was consistently lower than the endorsement of the beliefs and practice abstracted from each of the steps, as measured by the General Alcoholics Anonymous Tools of Recovery (GAATOR; Montgomery et al., 1995), an unobtrusive self-report measure of step progress. It appears, then, that the endorsement of "completing" a step had a higher threshold among participants than the endorsement of practicing specific elements within a step.

Mutual Support Mechanisms of Behavior Change (MOBC)

To date, investigation of the change mechanisms in mutual help programs has been limited to understanding the salutary effects of AA. While there is reason to suspect that many of these same mechanisms may operate in WFS, LifeRing, and SMART, such generalizations should be made cautiously. Conceptually, AA change mechanisms studied thus far may be classified as belonging to one of two categories. In the first class, change mechanisms may be regarded as *common* and *protective* in nature and are present in AA as well as in formal treatment. Here, a presumed mechanism is mobilized to increase in strength by virtue of the action of an AA active ingredient and, in turn, once increased the mechanism should account for increased abstinence (positive a and b paths, respectively, in statistical mediation models). Falling into this class of presumed mechanisms are AA prescribed spiritual practices, abstinence social support, and abstinence self-efficacy. In contrast, a second class of change mechanisms in AA requires the blunting of a pre-existing cognitive, psychological, and/or emotional attribute. In this case, an AA active ingredient is presumed to mobilize reductions in a mechanism because the attribute is thought to predict later alcohol relapse (negative a and b paths, respectively, in mediation models). Examples of this class of MOBC include depression, anger, and selfishness. Of historical interest, this class of mechanisms was later identified and incorporated as common relapse triggers in various relapse prevention models (Marlatt & Donovan, 2005).

Class One: Common and Protective MOBC

In this class, 26 (74 percent) of the 35 studies were funded by the National Institutes of Health (n = 19) or Veterans Administration (n = 7), indicating that these research protocols had undergone peer review. In addition, a majority (68 percent) of these MOBC studies temporally ordered variables of interest, and most studies used psychometrically sound assessments. To illustrate, 67 percent of the studies investigating changes in spiritual practices used the Religious Background and Behaviors measure (RBB; Connors et al., 1996), and 73 percent of the studies investigating self-efficacy used either the Alcohol Abstinence Self-Efficacy Scale (AASE; DiClemente et al., 1994), a modified version of the AASE (Brown et al., 2002), or the Situational Confidence Questionnaire (Annis & Graham, 1988). More variation in measurement tools between studies was found for social support. The most frequently used measure was the Life Stressors and Social Resources Inventory (Moos et al., 1988), followed by the Important People and Activities (IPA; Clifford & Longabaugh, 1991). Thus, it seems unlikely that these effect sizes were inflated because of a disproportionate number of cross-sectional designs or attenuated because of psychometrically weak self-report measures. With this background, the evidence on spiritual change, abstinence-based social support, and self-efficacy as common change mechanisms in AA is summarized next.

Spiritual Practices

Central to AA ideology is the proposition that spiritual growth or awakening is pivotal for AA members to achieve in order to sustain alcohol abstinence. In fact, the core literature states that a time will inevitably come when the AA member is defenseless against the first drink and that such a defense must come from a "Higher power." Spiritual growth is assured in AA doctrine through working the 12 Steps and by actively practicing prayer and meditation. Anecdotally, it is claimed that these prescriptions are heeded by AA newcomers, and converging evidence supports this claim. Young (2013), for example, reported that 73 percent of sponsored AA members prayed daily. Two complementary explanations have been offered to explain the salutary effects of AA prayer. First, Galanter and colleagues (2017), for example, found that reading of AA prayers produced lower reports of craving when presented with alcohol cues (relative to neutral readings) and higher activation of neural mechanisms responsible for attention and emotion control. Second, Kelly et al. (2011) and Tonigan et al. (2013) suggested that prayer serves as a coping mechanism during times of high affective arousal when relapse risk may be highest. Nine studies (5,058 participants) were identified that examined spiritual practices as an explanatory factor accounting for increased abstinence among AA members. Using meta-analytic techniques (as reported in Magill et al., 2015), frequency of AA attendance was found to be significantly and positively associated with later increases in spiritual practices and, in turn, spiritual practices were positively and significantly associated with later increases in alcohol abstinence. Collectively, then, there is circumstantial support that spiritual practices are a change mechanism in AA.

Abstinence Social Support

The AA social network is one of the most plausible change agents in AA, and it is most readily expressed in AA meeting attendance, working with an AA sponsor and newcomers, and social interactions with AA friends. Put simply, the AA social network or AA fellowship is the *practice* of the AA program. Demonstrating the importance of the AA fellowship in AA ideology, the very first tradition in AA states, "Our common welfare should come first; personal recovery depends on AA unity" (Alcoholics Anonymous, 1939). Strong emphasis is voiced for AA newcomers to partake of the AA fellowship. Telephone numbers are readily shared with newcomers to contact a more senior AA member when drinking may occur or at times of personal difficulty. Likewise, AA slogans warn against straying from the AA fellowship (e.g., "The straggler of the herd is the one that is picked off") and encourage disengagement with drinking social networks (e.g., "You need to change your playpens and playmates").

Reviewed by Groh et al. (2008), the nature and influence of AA social network support on outcomes have been investigated from numerous perspectives including type of social support (AA versus non-AA) and social network structure, function, and size. The robustness in positive mediational findings across widely different operational definitions of this construct indicates that it is an important mediator accounting for AA-related benefit. To illustrate, several investigations reported that engagement in AA was associated with significant reductions in the size of pro-drinking social networks and increased size in social support for abstinence, both of which accounted for later increases in alcohol abstinence (Kaskustas et al., 2002; Kelly et al., 2011). Notably, Kaskutas and colleagues also found that abstinence-based social support from AA members was significantly more influential in accounting for 30-day and 90-day alcohol abstinence among new AA members relative to similar support offered by non-AA individuals. Fifteen studies (15,482 participants) were meta-analytically combined to summarize the association between frequency of AA meeting attendance and the AA social network, defined in several ways along numerous dimensions (see meta-analysis results reported by Tonigan in Magill et al, 2015). Overall, AA attendance was associated with significant increases in positive abstinence support and concomitant declines in pro-drinking social networks. These changes in social networks were positively and significantly associated with alcohol abstinence.

Abstinence Self-efficacy

Most directly articulated in the first step of AA ("We admitted we were powerless over alcohol – that our lives had become unmanageable," p. 59, Alcoholics Anonymous, 1939), the core AA literature stresses that loss of control when drinking is a signature feature of AUD along with the belief that willpower is insufficient to avoid the first drink and that "the first drink is too much and a thousand drinks are not enough." In this context, abstinence self-efficacy or one's confidence to abstain in a variety of situations, including situations that are high-risk for drinking, seems an unlikely change mechanism in AA. This view discounts the content and influence of storytelling in AA meetings, however. Specifically, sharing at AA meetings often entails stories of near lapses and relapses due to tragic circumstances, encountering unforeseen and risky situations laden with drinking cues, and voluntary admissions about craving alcohol. Most often, the story ends with an account of how the person avoided alcohol – frequently by employing an AA-specific strategy (e.g., calling a sponsor for help). Bandura (1986) identified vicarious experience by observing others succeed at a task as an important source of self-efficacy, especially so when the observed and observer share much in common. Considered in this light, storytelling in AA meetings may be a potent catalyst for change in AA member abstinence self-efficacy, in spite of the official AA position of powerlessness over alcohol. More parsimoniously, abstinence self-efficacy may simply increase because yesterday's abstinent behavior reinforces the belief that one can be abstinent the next day.

Nine studies (3,739 participants) have investigated if changes in abstinence self-efficacy explained, in part, the association between AA attendance and abstinence (reported in Magill et al., 2015). Overall, the weighted correlation between frequency of AA attendance and abstinence self-efficacy was positive and significant ($r_w = .21$), although it should be noted that the magnitude of changes in self-efficacy was not uniform across studies (r_w range = .11–.31). Likewise, the association between self-efficacy and later abstinence was positive and significant ($r_w = .33$), but the magnitude of this association also was not homogeneous (r_w range = .06–.46). Collectively, the findings indicate that changes in abstinence self-efficacy during early AA attendance accounts, in part, for the positive association between frequency of AA attendance and increased abstinence.

Class Two: Reductions in MOBC

The core AA literature stresses that persons with active AUD are laden with negative affect in the form of selfishness, anger, resentment, and depression. The core AA literature also emphasizes that negative affect is a primary cause for alcohol relapse and, as such, negative affect must be reduced or blunted to achieve and sustain abstinence. A meta-analytic summary of findings in this class is not yet feasible given the limited number of studies, which are discussed below.

Depression

Three prospective and rigorous studies have investigated how changes in depression among participants in AA may mediate AA-related benefit. One study was a large multisite clinical trial including outpatient and aftercare participants (Project MATCH, $N = 1726$; Kelly et al., 2010), the second was a controlled trial contrasting 12 Step facilitation with integrated cognitive behavioral therapy (with pharmacotherapy as a treatment adjunct) with 209 veterans with a major depression diagnosis (MDD; $N = 209$; Worley et al., 2012), and the third was a community-based observational study of early AA members without extensive AA histories ($N = 253$; Wilcox & Tonigan, 2018). All studies employed lagged analyses, two studies measured depression using the Beck Depression Inventory, and one study used the Hamilton Depression rating scale, and all controlled for concurrent drinking (during follow-up) because depressive symptoms often decline simply by virtue of increased abstinence. During the 1-year period after treatment in the Project MATCH sample, Kelly and colleagues (2010) found that frequency of AA attendance did not account for reductions in depression after controlling for concurrent drinking and that, under the same conditions, reductions in depression did not account for increased abstinence and reductions in drinking intensity. In contrast, Worley et al. (2012) reported that within six months of active outpatient treatment for MDD, frequency of AA meeting attendance was significantly associated with lower depression controlling for concurrent drinking, and such reductions in depression were associated with percent days drinking during the three months after treatment. Finally, Wilcox and Tonigan (2018) conducted an observational study that recruited adults very early in their AA experience from the community. Assessments were conducted at baseline and 3, 6, 9, 12, 18, and 24 months after enrollment, and mediational tests were conducted in two stages, early (baseline to 12 months) and late (18–24 months) follow-up. At early follow-up, mediation results were in agreement with Kelly et al.'s (2010) non-significant findings for the outcome measure, percent days abstinent. In contrast, when controlling for concurrent drinking intensity, frequency of AA attendance was associated with later reductions in depression. These reductions, in turn, were associated with reductions in subsequent drinking intensity. Associations were not significant at the later follow-ups.

Reconciling these findings is not straightforward. On one hand, depressive symptom severity was significantly higher in the Worley et al. and Wilcox and Tonigan samples relative to Kelly et al.'s Project MATCH outpatient and aftercare samples. Specifically, the Wilcox and Tonigan sample, on average, reported almost twice the number of BDI symptoms relative to the Project MATCH participants (Wilcox and Tonigan BDI mean = 19.79; Kelly et al. BDI mean = 10.16), and the Worley et al. sample, on average, reported Hamilton Depression scores above the cut off for moderate depression (mean = 28.55). At first glance, it would appear that depressive severity moderates the associations between AA attendance and drinking up to 12 months, controlling for concurrent drinking. On the other hand, however, Wilcox and Tonigan tested this possibility and reported no moderation effect when BDI scores were categorized as either minimal to mild versus moderate to severe.

Anger

In a companion study using the Project MATCH sample, Kelly et al. (2010) questioned whether changes in anger mediated the direct effect of AA on increased abstinence and reductions in drinking intensity, with anger measured by the Spielberger Anger Scale. Across the board, all findings were non-significant in both the aftercare and outpatient arms of the study. Specifically, in lagged analyses, frequency of AA attendance was not associated with later changes in participant anger, and changes in anger were not associated with changes in later percent days abstinent and drinking intensity.

Selfishness

Tonigan and colleagues (2013) examined whether changes in selfishness defined as the total score on the Narcissistic Personality Inventory (NPI; Raskin & Terry, 1988) accounted for the direct effect of frequency of AA attendance on later abstinence and drinking intensity. Participants (N = 130) were recruited from community-based AA groups or as they presented for outpatient treatment (and reported AA attendance in the prior 90 days) in a number of locations in a Southwestern city. In this observational study, participants were interviewed at baseline, three, six, and nine months. Lagged analyses indicated that frequency of AA attendance was unrelated to NPI scores, which were elevated at baseline and remained elevated across the course of the study. Likewise, lagged analyses indicated that NPI scores were not associated with later changes in percent abstinent days and drinking intensity.

Future Directions for Mutual Support Research

This section considers several areas for future AA research and recommendations for promoting research on non-AA mutual help programs. A theme is a call for more ecologically valid depictions of the mutual help experience, including the need for (1) expanding the types of AA active ingredients in research, (2) modeling AA meeting heterogeneity, (3) identifying linkages between life functioning and MOBC, (4) expanding timeframes and methods in AA research, and (5) extending lessons learned from AA research to the investigation of AA alternatives.

Expanding the Types of AA Active Ingredients in MOBC Research

Virtually all AA MOBC studies have used some permutation of frequency of AA attendance as the sole active ingredient in AA that mobilizes presumed change mechanisms. In the early research on AA MOBC, the use of this simple "dose-response" measure had advantages. Measurement of frequency of AA meeting attendance was easily and reliably collected, and the focus on a single active ingredient facilitated aggregating findings across studies. Unfortunately, frequency of AA meeting attendance lacks clinical utility, perhaps most aptly illustrated by the only recommendation that can now be made by AA researchers to clinicians to "encourage AA attendance."

Several classes of AA prescribed behaviors and practices that predict later reductions in alcohol use have been identified in this chapter. It makes sense, then, to drill down and assess the relative importance of these finer grained measures in mobilizing MOBC, as well as to identify potentially new MOBC in AA. Such information would prove useful in guiding clinical recommendations about *how* clients ought to initially engage in AA and/or how to sustain AA participation. Significant measurement challenges will need to be addressed to achieve this objective. As noted earlier, AA sponsorship is a potentially potent active ingredient but, with rare exception (Kelly et al., 2016), the norm in AA research is to use a binary measure of whether an AA member has a sponsor. In addition to the obvious limitations of a binary measure capturing the multidimensional nature of AA sponsorship, a binary measure also lacks utility in longitudinal analyses of AA participation. To illustrate, a study participant may indicate that they have a sponsor at each follow-up in a study. What is not known, however, is whether the study participant has the *same* sponsor throughout the follow-ups. As is well known, the longevity of sponsor-sponsee relationships varies widely, with some dyads lasting only weeks or months and others lasting many years, and there is reason to suspect that the quality and effectiveness of sponsors varies greatly. Therefore, modeling potential shifts in the potency and quality of AA sponsorship is a high priority.

Substantial work is also recommended in refining the measurement of 12-step work and how such work may mobilize change mechanisms and/or predict outcomes. The standard practice of asking study participants which of the 12 Steps they have completed probably results in false negatives, especially when recognizing that each step embodies several precepts. Importantly, the core AA literature identifies proximal outcomes associated with working each step. As examples, progress through Step 2 is felt to instill hope, and Step 9 seeks to repair social relationships damaged by harmful drinking. Assessment of these proximal outcomes and whether they are associated with change mechanisms and outcomes are worthy of investigation.

Modeling AA Meeting Heterogeneity

Evidence suggests that the social dynamics of AA meetings vary. A series of studies that administered the Group Environment Scale (Moos, 1986) reported that AA meetings differed in perceived cohesiveness, expressiveness, aggressiveness, and encouragement to adopt spiritual practices. These perceptions were linked with later increases in AA attendance, greater 12 Step discussion in AA meetings, and later abstinence, even after controlling for concurrent frequency of AA meeting attendance (e.g., Kuerbis & Tonigan, 2018; Tonigan et al., 1995). Modeling perceptions of AA meeting social dynamics may be one of the most vexing challenges for future research. These challenges include the (1) subjectivity of such impressions and whether they correspond with an *objective* observational coding measure of AA meeting social dynamics, (2) perceived and objective stability of AA group social dynamics over time, and (3) taking into account AA member migration to different AA meetings over time. Innovative strategies such as GPS tracking devices, ecological momentary assessment, and mixed method approaches will be necessary to address these challenges in this neglected area of research on AA change processes.

Identifying Linkages between Improvements in Life Functioning and MOBC

Substantial work has shown that AA participation, generally defined as frequency of AA meeting attendance, is associated with improvement in multiple domains of life functioning and reductions in health care utilization (Humphreys et al., 1996; Kelly et al., 2020; Moos & Moos, 2004). The pressing question is what accounts for these psychosocial improvements? There is reason to suggest that the same MOBC that are associated with abstinence in AA also may mobilize improvements in non-alcohol domains, especially so for increases in self-efficacy and spiritual practices. Mapping of these linkages is critical. Understanding which, if any, of the three MOBC contribute to these secondary benefits, coupled with a clearer understanding of the specific AA behaviors that mobilize each of the three MOBCs, will help clinicians know which AA behaviors to encourage in treatment to derive optimal long-term client outcomes.

Expanding Timeframes and Methods for AA Research

Most prospective AA MOBC studies have used a longitudinal design with fixed follow-up points, generally in three month increments. This design has the utility of discerning at relatively low cost the probability that a given MOBC accounts for AA benefits during early AA affiliation. Serious limitations of this approach, however, include requiring a study participant to "average" the daily shifts in state-based MOBC variables and lack of assessment of the finer grained trajectories of multiple mobilized MOBCs during early AA affiliation. Taken together, the standard longitudinal design generates correlation-based findings that are not well suited for testing established criteria to determine causality (Kazdin, 2007).

Mobile technology and daily ecological momentary assessment (EMA) offer significant advancements in how AA-related MOBC can be investigated (see Pearson et al., Chapter 13 for detailed discussion of EMA). To illustrate, we offer an example of how real-time daily assessment can be applied to examine the linkages between AA practices, changes in an MOBC, and drinking. This example considers AA attendance as the active ingredient, spiritual practices as the MOBC, and drinking as the outcome. First, one would test the micro day-by-day dynamic changes in the magnitude of associations between AA attendance and spiritual practices, as well as between spiritual practices and drinking. Here, event-level data represent a significant improvement for making causal inferences about the temporal linkages between variables of interest. One could also test for dose-response linkages between frequency of AA attendance and changes in spiritual practices and, in turn, gradient effects between changes in an MOBC and abstinence. This could be achieved by grouping AA attendance as absent, low, medium, and high and using a similar grouping strategy for spiritual practices. Next, one could investigate the specificity of the linkages of interest. Here, one may choose to control for AA sponsorship status to assess the association between AA meeting attendance and spiritual practices, and control for AA step work when examining the association between spiritual practices and drinking. Finally, because EMA-based data can be easily aggregated in many ways including, but not limited to, daily, weekly, and monthly values, one can seek to replicate the findings reported in fixed longitudinal studies.

Investigating Other Mutual Help Groups

There is a dire need for rigorous prospective longitudinal investigations of the direct and indirect effects of WFS, SMART, and LifeRing, and virtually all of the above recommendations can be applied to this work. Outstanding questions for the AA alternatives include: (1) enhanced understanding of how, if at all, affiliation profiles differ between AA and SMART, WFS, and LifeRing; (2) documentation of a direct and positive linkage between WFS, SMART, and LifeRing attendance and later drinking reductions, especially during early change efforts; (3) identification of the linkages between prescribed activities in these mutual help programs and outcomes; (4) development and testing of the underlying process model depicting *why* individuals will achieve drinking reductions in WFS, SMART, and LifeRing; and (5) identification of subpopulations that may find affiliation with AA alternatives especially advantageous (or not). AA-related findings discussed in this chapter have spanned decades of research. Fortunately, this past work provides a staged-strategy that, if adopted, may accelerate future understanding of WFS, SMART, and LifeRing mutual help programs.

The study of the WFS, SMART, and LifeRing programs poses many unique challenges, and innovative strategies will be required to meaningfully address research questions. Perhaps most critical will be the choice of sampling procedures and how such procedures potentially may bias study findings. Recall, for example, that WFS, SMART, and LifeRing combined offer less than 1 percent of the meetings offered by AA. Zemore et al (2017, 2018) provided one online strategy for accessing WFS and SMART participants and limiting attrition, with a rigorous protocol for assessing the veracity of self-report. Future work may benefit from building upon Zemore and colleague's methodology. Regarding the testing of indirect effects, the SMART program seeks to increase self-reliance as a means to achieve self-identified drinking goals. In testing this indirect effect one must determine if the measurement of self-reliance is defined broadly or targets alcohol/substance use. Similar measurement choices have to be made in testing the indirect effects of purported changes in self-empowerment, which is common to all three AA alternative mutual help programs. Finally, with the exception of spiritual practices, there is good reason to assess whether presumed and established mechanisms in AA generalize to SMART, WFS, and LifeRing, the philosophical and practical differences in mutual help programs notwithstanding.

Conclusions and Recommendations

Mutual help programs are an important resource for addressing AUD, either alone or in combination with formal treatment. While AA remains the most popular program in the United States, the past few decades have witnessed substantial growth in alternative programs such as WFS, SMART, and LifeRing. Preliminary evidence on affiliation profiles suggests that the emergence of these alternatives to AA is, in part, the result of a lack of appetite for the AA focus on spiritual practices and its staunch position on the need for complete and lifelong alcohol abstinence. A large body of correlational research indicates that affiliation with AA is associated with increased abstinence, and confidence in these findings is bolstered by recent high quality prospective lagged studies. Likewise, there is growing evidence that the salutary effects of AA are explained, in part, by increased social support, abstinence self-efficacy, and spiritual practices. Application of innovative assessment strategies such as EMA should help support the conclusion that AA referral is an evidence-based practice and increase understanding of why AA is beneficial for many, but not all, AA affiliates. Emphasized throughout this chapter is the need to extend research initiatives to include the study of AA alternatives such as WFS, SMART, and LifeRing. Such initiatives can build upon the strategies, research questions, and methods developed in the lengthy study of AA and will also require some unique and innovative approaches.

References

Alcoholics Anonymous (1939). *Alcoholics Anonymous: The story of how many thousands of men and women recovered from alcoholism.* The Works Publishing Company.

(2020). General Service Office, New York: A.A. World Services. www.aa.org/assets/en_US/smf-132_en.pdf

American Psychiatric Association (2013). *Diagnostic and statistical manual of mental disorders* (5th ed.). https://doi.org/10.1176/appi.books.9780890425596

Annis, H. & Graham, J. M. (1988). *Situational confidence questionnaire (SCQ): User's guide*. Addiction Research Foundation.

Bandura, A. (1986). The explanatory and predictive scope of self-efficacy theory, *Journal of Social and Clinical Psychology,4*, 359–373. https://doi.org/10.1521/jscp.1986.4.3.359

Beck, A. K., Forbes, E., Baker, A. L., Kelly, P. J., Peter, J., Deane, F. P., Shakeshaft, A., Hunt, D., & Kelly, J. F. (2017). Systematic review of SMART recovery: Outcomes, process variables, and implications for research, *Psychology of Addictive Behaviors, 31* (1), 1–20. https://doi.org/10.1037/adb0000237

Brown, T. G., Seraganian, P., Tremblay, J., & Annis, H. (2002). Process and outcome changes with relapse prevention versus 12 Step aftercare programs for alcohol and other drug abusers. *Addiction, 97,* 677–689. https://doi.org/10.1046/j.1360-0443.2002.00101.x

Clifford, P. R., & Longabaugh, R. (1991). *Manual for the administration of the Important People and Activities Instrument. Adapted for use by Project MATCH for the National Institute on Alcohol Abuse and Alcoholism.* National Institutes of Health/National Institute on Alcohol Abuse and Alcoholism. https://pubs.niaaa.nih.gov/publications/AssessingAlcohol/InstrumentPDFs/39_IPA.pdf

Connors, G., Tonigan, J. S., & Miller, W. R. (1996). Measure of religious background and behavior for use in behavior change research. *Psychology of Addictive Behaviors, 10*(2), 90–96. https://doi.org/10.1037/0893-164X.10.2.90

DiClemente, C. C., Carbonari, J. P., Montgomery, R. P., & Hughes, S. O. (1994). The alcohol abstinence self-efficacy scale. *Journal of Studies on Alcohol, 55*(2), 141–148. https://doi.org/10.15288/jsa.1994.55.141

Emrick, C. D., Tonigan, J. S., Montgomery, H., & Little, L. (1993). *Alcoholics Anonymous: What is currently known?* In B. S. McCrady & W. R. Miller (Eds.), *Research on Alcoholics Anonymous: Opportunities and alternatives* (pp. 41–76). Rutgers Center of Alcohol Studies.

Galanter, M., Josipovic, Z., Dermatis, H., Weber, J., & Millard, M. A., (2017). An initial fMRI study on neural correlates of prayer in members of Alcoholics Anonymous. *The American Journal of Drug and Alcohol Abuse, 43*(1), 44–54. https://doi.org/10.3109/00952990.2016.1141912

Greenfield, B. L., & Tonigan, J. S. (2013). The general Alcoholics Anonymous tools of recovery: The adoption of 12 Step practices and beliefs. *Psychology of Addictive Behaviors, 27*(3), 553–561. https://doi.org/10.1037/a0029268

Groh, D. R., Jason, L. A., & Keys, C. B. (2008). Social network variables in alcoholics anonymous: A literature review. *Clinical Psychology Review, 28* (3), 430–450. https://doi.org/10.1016/j.cpr.2007.07.014

Hardin, R. (2013). *SMART Recovery handbook* (3rd ed.). Alcohol & Drug Abuse Self-Help Network, Inc. dba SMART Recovery.

Harris, J., Best, D., Gossop, M., Marshall, J., Man, L. O., Manning, V., & Strang, J. (2003). Prior Alcoholics Anonymous (AA) affiliation and the acceptability of the 12 Steps to patients entering UK statutory addiction treatment. *Journal of Studies on Alcohol and Drugs, 64*(2), 257–261. https://doi.org/10.15288/jsa.2003.64.257

Humphreys, K., Blodgett, J. C., & Wagner, T. H. (2014). Estimating the efficacy of Alcoholics Anonymous without self-selection bias: An instrumental variables re-analysis of randomized clinical trials. *Alcoholism: Clinical and Experimental Research, 38*(11), 2688–2699. https://doi.org/10.1111/acer.12557

Humphreys, K. & Moos, R. H. (1996). Reduced substance-abuse-related health care costs among voluntary participants in Alcoholics Anonymous. *Psychiatric Services, 47* (7), 709–713. https://doi.org/10.1176/ps.47.7.709

Humphreys, K., Phibbs, C. S., & Moos, R. H. (1996). Addressing self-selection effects in evaluations of mutual help groups and professional mental health services: An introduction to two-stage sample selection models. *Evaluation and Program Planning, 19*(4), 301–308. https://doi.org/10.1016/S0149-7189(96)00028-6

Kaskutas, L. A., (1994). What do women get out of self-help? Their reasons for attending Women for Sobriety and Alcoholics Anonymous. *Journal of Substance Abuse Treatment, 11* (3) 185–195. https://doi.org/10.1016/0740-5472(94)90075-2

Kaskutas, L. A., Bond, J., & Humphreys, K. (2002). Social networks as mediators of the effect of Alcoholics Anonymous. *Addiction, 97*(7), 891–900. https://doi.org/10.1046/j.1360-0443.2002.00118.x

Kaskutas, L. A., Borkman, T. J., Laudet, A., Ritter, L. A., Witbrodt, J., Subbaraman, M. S., Stunz, A., & Bond, J. (2014). Elements that define recovery: The experiential perspective. *Journal of Studies on Alcohol and Drugs, 75* (6), 999–1010. https://doi.org/10.15288/jsad.2014.75.999

Kazdin, A. E. (2007). Mediators and mechanisms of change in psychotherapy research. *Annual Review of Clinical Psychology, 3*, 1–27. https://doi.org/10.1146/annurev.clinpsy.3.022806.091432

Kelly, J. F., Abry, A., Ferri, M., & Humphreys, K. (2020). Alcoholics Anonymous and 12 Step facilitation treatments for alcohol use disorder: A distillation of a 2020 Cochrane Review for clinicians and policy makers. *Alcohol and Alcoholism, 55* (6), 641–651. https://doi.org/10.1093/alcalc/agaa050

Kelly J. F. & Greene, M. C. (2013). The twelve promises of Alcoholics Anonymous: Psychometric measure validation and mediational testing as a 12 Step specific mechanism of behavior change. *Drug and Alcohol Dependence, 133*(2), 633–640. https://doi.org/10.1016/j.drugalcdep.2013.08.006

Kelly, J. F., Greene, M. C., & Bergman, B. G. (2016). Recovery benefits of the "therapeutic alliance" among 12 Step mutual help organization attendees and their sponsors. *Drug and Alcohol Dependence, 162*, 64–71. https://dx.doi.org/10.1016%2Fj.drugalcdep.2016.02.028

Kelly, J. F., Stout, R. L., Magill, M., & Tonigan, J. S. (2011). The role of Alcoholics Anonymous in mobilizing adaptive social network changes: A prospective lagged mediational analysis. *Drug and Alcohol Dependence, 114*, 119–126. https://doi.org/10.1016/j.drugalcdep.2010.09.009

Kelly, J. F., Stout, R. L., Magill, M., Tonigan, J. S., & Pagano, M. E. (2011). Spirituality in recovery: A lagged meditational analysis of Alcoholics Anonymous' principal theoretical mechanism of behavior change. *Alcoholism: Clinical and Experimental Research, 35*(3), 454–463. https://doi.org/10.1111/j.1530-0277.2010.01362.x

Kelly, J. F., Stout, R. L., Tonigan, J. S., Magill, M., & Pagano, M. E. (2010). Negative affect, relapse, and Alcoholics Anonymous (AA): Does AA work by reducing anger? *Journal of Studies on Alcohol and Drugs, 71*(3), 434–444. https://doi.org/10.15288/jsad.2010.71.434

(2010). Mechanisms of behavior change in Alcoholics Anonymous: Does Alcoholics Anonymous lead to better alcohol use outcomes by reducing depression symptoms? *Addiction, 105*(4), 626–636. https://doi.org/10.1111/j.1360-0443.2009.02820.x

Kirkpatrick, J., (1977). *Turnabout: New help for the woman alcoholic*. Women for Sobriety, Inc.

Kurtz, E. (1979). *Not God: A history of Alcoholics Anonymous*. Hazelden Publishing.

Kuerbis, A., & Tonigan, J. S. (2018). More than taking a chair: The perceived group social dynamics of Alcoholics Anonymous related to changes in spiritual practices. *Alcoholism Treatment Quarterly, 36*(3), 314–329. https://doi.org/10.1080/07347324.2017.1420437

Magill, M., Kiluk, B. D. McCrady, B. S., Tonigan, J. S., & Longabaugh, R. (2015). Active ingredients of treatment and client mechanisms of change in behavioral treatments for alcohol use disorders: Progress 10 years later. *Alcoholism: Clinical and Experimental Research, 39* (10), 1852–1862. https://doi.org/10.1111/acer.12848

Magura, S., McKean J., Kosten, S., & Tonigan, J. S. (2012). A novel application of propensity score matching to estimate Alcoholics Anonymous' effect on drinking outcomes. *Drug and Alcohol Dependence, 129* (1-2), 54–59. https://doi.org/10.1016/j.drugalcdep.2012.09.011

Marlatt, G. A., & Donovan, D. M. (Eds.) (2005). *Relapse prevention: Maintenance strategies in the treatment of addictive behaviors*. Guilford Press.

Montgomery, H. A., Miller, W. R., & Tonigan, J. S. (1995). Does Alcoholics Anonymous involvement predict treatment outcome? *Journal of Substance Abuse Treatment, 12*(4), 241–246. https://doi.org/10.1016/0740-5472(95)00018-z

Moos, R. H. (1986). *Group Environment Scale manual*. Consulting Psychologists Press.

Moos, R. H., Fenn, C. B., & Billings, A. G. (1988). Life stressors and social resources: An integrated assessment approach. *Social Science & Medicine, 27* (9), 999–1002. https://doi.org/10.1016/0277-9536(88)90291-2

Moos, R. H., & Moos, B. S. (2004). Long-term influence of duration and frequency of participation in Alcoholics Anonymous on individuals with alcohol use disorders. *Journal of Consulting and Clinical Psychology 72*(1), 81–90. https://doi.org/10.1037/0022-006x.72.1.81

Nicolaus, M. (2009). *Empowering your sober self* (2nd ed.). LifeRing Bookstore.

Raskin, R., & Terry, H. (1988). A principal-components analysis of the Narcissistic personality inventory and further evidence of its construct validity. *Journal of Personality and Social Psychology, 54* (5), 890–902. https://doi.org/10.1037//0022-3514.54.5.890

Rynes, K. N., Tonigan, J. S., & Rice, S. (2013). Interpersonal climate of 12 Step groups predicts reductions in alcohol use. *Alcohol Treatment Quarterly, 31* (2), 167–185. https://doi.org/10.1080/07347324.2013.771983

Stevens, E. B., & Jason, L. A. (2015). Evaluating Alcoholics Anonymous sponsor attributes using conjoint analysis. *Addictive Behaviors, 51,* 12–17. https://doi.org/10.1016/j.addbeh.2015.06.043

Tonigan, J. S. (2001). Benefits of Alcoholics Anonymous attendance: Replication of findings between clinical research sites in Project MATCH. *Alcoholism Treatment Quarterly, 19*(1), 67–77. https://doi.org/10.1300/J020v19n01_05

Tonigan, J. S., Ashcroft, F., & Miller, W. R. (1995). AA group dynamics and 12 Step activity. *Journal of Studies on Alcohol, 54,* 616–621. https://doi.org/10.15288/jsa.1995.56.616

Tonigan, J. S., Miller, W. R., & Schermer, C. (2002). Atheist, agnostics, and Alcoholics Anonymous. *Journal of Studies on Alcohol and Drugs, 63*(5), 534–541. https://doi.org/10.15288/jsa.2002.63.534

Tonigan, J. S., Pearson, M. R., Magill, M., & Hagler, K. J. (2018). AA attendance and abstinence for dually diagnosed patients: A meta-analytic review. *Addiction, 113*(11), 1970–1981. https://doi.org/10.1111/add.14268

Tonigan, J. S., & Rice, S. L. (2010). Is it beneficial to have an Alcoholics Anonymous sponsor? *Psychology of Addictive Behaviors, 24*(3), 397–403. https://doi.org/10.1037/a0019013

Tonigan, J. S., Rynes, K., & McCrady, B. S. (2013) Spirituality as a change mechanism in 12 Step programs: A replication, refinement and extension. *Substance Use and Misuse, 48* (12) 1161–1173. https://doi.org/10.3109/10826084.2013.808540

Tonigan, J. S., Rynes, K., Toscova, R., & Hagler, K. (2013). Do changes in selfishness explain 12 Step benefit? *A prospective lagged analysis.* Substance Abuse, *34* (1), 13–19. https://doi.org/10.1080/08897077.2012.691453

Tonigan, J. S., Toscova, R., & Miller, W. R. (1996). Meta-analysis of the literature on Alcoholics Anonymous: Sample and study characteristics moderate findings. *Journal of Studies on Alcohol, 57*(1), 65–72. https://doi.org/10.15288/jsa.1996.57.65

Whelan, P. J. P., Marshall, E. J., Ball, D. M., & Humphreys, K. (2009). The role of AA sponsors: A pilot study. *Alcohol and Alcoholism, 44*(4) 416–422. https://doi.org/10.1093/alcalc/agp014

White, W., & Kurtz, E. (2008). Twelve defining moments in the history of Alcoholics Anonymous. In M. Galanter & L. A. Kaskutas (Eds.) *Recent developments in alcoholism* (pp. 37–57). Plenum Publishing Corporation.

Wilcox, C., & Tonigan, J. S. (2018). Changes in depression mediate the effects of AA attendance on alcohol use outcomes. *The American Journal of Drug and Alcohol Abuse, 44*(1), 103–112. https://doi.org/10.1080/00952990.2016.1249283

Witbrodt, J., Kaskutas, L., Bond, J., & Delucchi, K. (2012). Does sponsorship improve outcomes above Alcoholics Anonymous attendance? A latent class growth curve analysis. *Addiction, 107*(2), 301–311. https://doi.org/10.1111/j.1360-0443.2011.03570.x

Worley, M. J., Tate, S. R., & Brown, S. A. (2012). Mediational relations between 12 Step attendance, depression, and substance use in patients with comorbid substance dependence and major depression. *Addiction, 107*(11), 1974–1983. https://doi.org/10.1111/j.1360-0443.2012.03943.x

Zemore, S. E., Kaskutas, L. A., Mericle, A., & Hemberg, J. (2017). Comparison of 12 Step groups to mutual help alternatives for AUD in a large, national study: Differences in membership characteristics and group participation, cohesion, and satisfaction. *Journal Substance Abuse Treatment, 73,* 16–26. https://doi.org/10.1016/j.jsat.2016.10.004

Zemore, S. E., Lui, C., Mericle, A., Hemberg, J., & Kaskutas, L. A. (2018). A longitudinal study of the comparative efficacy of Women for Sobriety, LifeRing, SMART Recovery, and 12 Step groups for those with AUD. *Journal of Substance Abuse Treatment, 88,* 18–26. https://doi.org/10.1016/j.jsat.2018.02.004

Zemore, S. E., Subbaraman, M., & Tonigan, J. S., (2013). Involvement in 12 Step activities and treatment outcomes. *Substance Abuse, 34*(1), 60–69. https://doi.org/10.1080/08897077.2012.691452

7 Time-Varying Effect Modeling to Examine Recovery Outcomes across Four Years

Ashley N. Linden-Carmichael, Samuel W. Stull, Christy K. Scott, and Michael L. Dennis

Time-Varying Effect Modeling to Examine Recovery Outcomes across Four Years

Substance use recovery is a dynamic process with widespread effects on multiple domains of life-functioning (Ashford et al., 2019; White, 2007; Witkiewitz & Tucker, 2020). This conceptualization embraces the heterogeneous nature of recovery pathways, while recognizing that different elements of recovery may be more meaningful, relevant, and achievable for different people. The varied pathways of recovery make capturing these phenomena equal parts fascinating and complex, and a concerted effort is needed to quantify all aspects of the recovery process, including the notion that recovery is dynamic, enduring, and has diverse effects on functioning. The goals of this chapter are to outline the substantive elements of recovery; present an empirical demonstration of the effect of an intervention, Recovery Management Check-ups (Scott & Dennis, 2003), on recovery outcomes over four years; and provide a demonstration of time-varying effect modeling (TVEM; Lanza & Linden-Carmichael, 2021; Tan et al., 2012), a nuanced statistical method for studying change over time.

Global Influences on Functioning in Recovery

Abstinence or reductions in substance use have long served as the defining metric of successful recovery from substance use disorder (SUD). Operational definitions include dichotomous outcomes such as abstinence versus substance use or less than weekly substance use versus more than weekly substance use, and continuous outcomes such as duration of abstinence or frequency of use (Donovan et al., 2012; Finney et al., 2003). However, in recent years, the field has shifted to incorporating a larger array of recovery outcomes, a movement that has been primarily geared toward treating alcohol use disorder (Kiluk et al., 2018; Wilson et al., 2016; Witkiewitz et al., 2020; Witkiewitz & Tucker, 2020) and one that is beginning to include other types of SUD as well (Bray et al., 2017; Garner et al., 2014; National Academies of Sciences, Engineering, and Medicine, 2016; Stull et al., 2019). Important outcomes include positive changes in physical, social, and cognitive functioning; improvements in well-being and life satisfaction; and better fulfillment of family, work, and social responsibilities. Although a movement toward broad adoption of positive recovery outcomes is occurring in the field, studies that measure positive changes in recovery are still comparatively uncommon, with abstinence-based or substance use indices remaining as the prevailing mode of measuring and defining recovery (Bjornestad et al., 2020). Positive change indices are key for improving understanding of recovery processes, which unfold over days, months, and years of ongoing recovery.

Recovery as an Ongoing Process

To understand recovery, it is not only important to consider multiple indices of recovery outcomes, but to recognize that fostering these positive changes requires ongoing environmental and social support. Traditionally, interventions for SUD have taken an acute, pathology-oriented focus, but in the last few decades there has been a broader recognition of recovery as a process that requires a continuum of ongoing support (McKay, 2001; McLellan et al., 2005; Scott et al., 2005). Put simply, recovery is rarely quick or sudden, and initial problem recognition to the first help-seeking episode can take about a decade; further, the median time from first treatment episode to a year of abstinence is estimated to be nine years, with three or more treatment episodes occurring in between (Dennis et al., 2005; Simpson & Tucker, 2002). Rather than characterizing a return to substance use as a failure on the path of recovery, it may instead be viewed as a natural part of the recovery process. However, the path to recovery is often slowed by a range of barriers that make it difficult to access treatment.

In the past two decades, a critical solution to this problem has been developed and demonstrated to be efficacious: Recovery Management Check-ups (RMCs). RMCs involve continued tracking after post-treatment discharge, frequent assessment for substance use symptomology, linkage back to treatment if needed, strategies to increase treatment engagement, and continued support to maximize treatment retention (Scott & Dennis, 2009). RMC reduces time to treatment, substance use, and substance use-related problems and has helped spark recognition of SUD as a chronic health condition (Dennis & Scott, 2012). Insights have also been leveraged towards understanding for whom RMC works best; for example, those with greater substance use severity and poor life functioning at baseline receive the most benefit from RMC (Dennis & Scott, 2012). This finding is consistent with the general pattern that those with greater problem severity (e.g., more substance use-related and/or psychological problems) tend to benefit most from treatment and ongoing support, while those with less severity may require less intensive care or may simply recover without treatment (Simpson et al., 2002; Stull et al., 2019; Witkiewitz et al., 2017; Tucker, Chapter 9 & Murphy et al., Chapter 10 this volume). This bifurcation is reflected in treatment- versus population-based studies of recovery, wherein people with greater symptom severity need and benefit most from treatment while those with lower severity may resolve symptoms without treatment (i.e., natural recovery; cf. Tucker, Chapter 9). Thus, distinguishing individuals by their severity level may help determine the type or intensity of appropriate intervention. Another critical piece, yet to be clarified, entails distinguishing the time-varying nature of these recovery outcomes based on pre-treatment severity levels. These issues may help target the appropriate timing of an intervention for specific subgroups of people.

Examining Recovery as a Dynamic Process via Time-Varying Effect Modeling

Recovery unfolds in a dynamic and often nonlinear fashion as relevant personal and environmental factors coalesce and change across days, weeks, and even years to influence positive changes. Intermittent setbacks in positive recovery steps are not a divergence from the path of recovery, but instead, are part of the dynamic process of growth, learning, and continual effort – this underlies the very definition of recovery. The reality is, however, that capturing these dynamic recovery processes is complex from a statistical standpoint, and the research field is only beginning to characterize the nuances of recovery. Prior empirical studies of recovery have often only assessed study outcomes across a few brief timepoints, with less consideration given to how improvements unfold at multiple timepoints across a longer temporal interval. Such time-limited “dipstick” assessments may under- or over-state the benefits of an intervention and may preclude inferences about how an intervention episode may have increasing or diminishing benefits across time. For example, large improvements in coping skills may occur early in treatment, but these skills may diminish over time (Dennis et al., 2007; Moos & Moos, 2007), or perhaps certain positive changes, such as improvements in self-esteem or happiness, may get worse before they get better (Kelly et al., 2018). Collectively, the functional form of these recovery trajectories is often nonlinear and requires statistical methods suited to capture such change.

Time-varying effect modeling (TVEM), introduced in the statistical literature more than two decades ago (Hastie & Tibshirani, 1993; Hoover et al., 1998), and more recently implemented and disseminated in applied research (e.g., Lanza et al., 2016; Linden-Carmichael et al., 2017; Tan et al., 2012), is a statistical method for studying change over time. TVEM is a non-parametric approach that captures the association between a predictor and outcome across continuous time (e.g., see Figure 7.1) without assumptions regarding the nature of the relationship (e.g., linear, quadratic). Specifically, TVEM uses *splines*, or smooth functions comprised of line segments, which permit high flexibility when estimating non-linear shapes. Splines are connected at inflection points or *knots*. Using TVEM, the analyst can specify the number of knots to determine the level of complexity of the curve (for specifics on different types of spline bases, see Li et al., 2017).

This circumvents assumptions about a functional form of an association, which is particularly important when the true nature of the relationship is unknown; it also allows greater precision in capturing fine-grained changes in associations across time. Further, TVEM offers the flexibility of handling binary, continuous, and count outcomes. As in the standard regression framework, TVEM allows the effects of predictors and their interactions on outcomes to be examined and interpreted as the effect of a variable on an outcome at each timepoint. Analyses can include time-varying covariates, and they can be specified to have a time-varying or time-invariant effect.

TVEM may be very useful for understanding aspects pertinent to SUD recovery. First, its non-parametric and flexible properties make TVEM ideally suited for characterizing dynamic changes in substance use and other positive change outcomes naturally observed in the recovery process. TVEM can demonstrate the naturally occurring ebbs and flows of recovery outcomes such as estimating the mean level of alcohol use since the start of treatment. Second, effects of predictors and their interaction on recovery outcomes can be tested in TVEM, such as modeling the effect of an intervention on recovery outcomes across time to identify timepoints at which the intervention is most effective or when intervention boosters are needed, and for whom the intervention is most effective. TVEM can also estimate the effects of time-invariant demographic factors (e.g., sex, age) or relevant time-varying predictors (e.g., readiness to change). Third, TVEM can accommodate recovery outcomes that are assessed dichotomously (e.g., abstinence vs. any drinking), continuously (e.g., level of life satisfaction), or as a standard or zero-inflated count outcome (e.g., number of drinks consumed). Although TVEM has been used in studies of alcohol use disorder (e.g., Evans-Polce & Schuler, 2016; Linden-Carmichael et al., 2018) and symptoms of psychosis, depression and anxiety disorders), limited work has applied TVEM to study SUD recovery processes.

TVEM Example Application: RMC Intervention as a Time-Varying Predictor of Substance Use and Other Recovery Changes across Four Years

In the remainder of this chapter, we present an empirical example to demonstrate the use of TVEM as a statistical tool for capturing dynamic changes over multiple years of the SUD recovery pathway. The data come from the Early Re-Intervention (ERI-2) experiment (Dennis & Scott, 2012) of 446 adults recruited from a large addiction treatment agency in Illinois (including all levels of care across residential and outpatient services) who reported any substance use in the past 90 days and any past-year SUD symptoms. Participants were randomly assigned to RMC ($n = 223$) or an assessment control ($n = 223$, quarterly monitoring-only) group and were assessed quarterly for four years. Using these data, TVEM was used to address key features of the ongoing process of recovery that depend on measuring setbacks in positive recovery steps and capturing changes over several years during an RMC intervention. Specifically, the example demonstrates how the effect of receiving RMC – relative to the quarterly monitoring-only control condition – was associated with commonly measured substance use outcomes (odds of less than weekly alcohol/drug use, number of days without alcohol/drug use, odds of abstinence for all 90 days) and other positive change outcomes (general life satisfaction, cognitive avoidance, self-efficacy) across four years. The presence of multimorbidity (three or more conditions) is a common phenomenon in community and clinical settings (Diederichs et al., 2011; Nicholson, Almirall, & Fortin, 2019) and is often related to substance use and treatment outcomes (Griffith et al., 2018; Wu et al., 2018). Thus, the example also demonstrates moderation effects using TVEM by examining whether the RMC intervention had a differential effect on recovery outcomes depending on individuals' baseline problem severity (i.e., whether they experienced three or more substance-related or psychological problems).

Early Re-Intervention (ERI-2) Method

Approximately half (46 percent) of participants were female, 80 percent were African American, and 87 percent were between 30–49 years old (mean age = 38). Participants reported weekly (or more frequent) use of alcohol (45 percent), cannabis (16 percent), cocaine (53 percent), opioids (22 percent), and other drugs (2 percent); and nearly every participant met lifetime criteria for substance dependence per DSM IV (98 percent), including for alcohol (24 percent), cannabis (5 percent), cocaine (61 percent), opioids (25 percent), or another drug (2 percent). More than half of participants reported one or more internalizing disorders (53 percent), and approximately a third reported one or more externalizing or impulse control disorders (30 percent).

Both groups were followed at three month intervals for four years. At each quarterly assessment, the control group received an assessment only, and the experimental group received an assessment plus a quarterly RMC intervention. The RMC protocol involved locating the individual for a follow-up interview, determining eligibility for intervention and need for treatment, and, if in need of treatment, transferring the participant to a Linkage Manager, who were two masters' level women with 5+ years of experience in the field and were trained and supervised by the third author. The Linkage Manager used motivational interviewing to provide feedback on participants' current substance use and problems, discuss managing their addiction as a chronic condition, discuss treatment barriers and solutions, assess and discuss their motivation for treatment, schedule treatment appointments, and accompany participants to treatment intake. Additional details describing the sample and study procedures can be found in the parent study (Dennis & Scott, 2012).

Baseline Severity Assessment

At baseline, participants were interviewed using the Global Appraisal of Individual Needs (GAIN; Dennis et al., 2003b). The number of problems they reported experiencing in the past year was based on the number of SUD symptoms related to alcohol, cannabis, cocaine, opioids, or other drug use; mood disorder, generalized anxiety disorder, traumatic stress symptoms, suicidal thoughts or ideation, and conduct disorder, and any ADHD, victimization, physical violence, or illegal activity. Consistent with prior definitions of multimorbidity, participants who reported two or fewer of these problems at baseline were coded as *lower risk* (0), and participants who reported three or more problems ("multimorbidity") were coded as *higher risk* (1).

Substance Use Recovery Outcomes

Each quarter, participants reported during the GAIN interview the number of days they had used alcohol, cannabis, cocaine, opioids, or other drugs during the past 90 days. This information yielded three variables regarding participants' past 90-day "positive" behavior, including: (1) whether they used alcohol or other drugs on less than 13 out of 90 days (about 13 weeks) as an indicator of *less than weekly alcohol/drug use* (coded as 0 = used alcohol or other drugs 13 or more days in the past 90 days and 1 = used alcohol or drugs fewer than 13 days in the past 90 days), (2) the *number of days without using alcohol or other drugs*, and (3) whether they were *abstinent* from alcohol or other drugs on all days (coded as 0 = not abstinent/used one or more days, 1 = abstinent all 90 days).

Other Positive Change Recovery Outcomes

Each quarter, participants completed questionnaires that assessed various dimensions of recovery including physical health, mental health, quality of life, and daily functioning. For present purposes, recovery outcomes included general satisfaction with their personal environment and relationships, cognitive avoidance, and self-efficacy. *General satisfaction* was assessed using the General Satisfaction Index (Dennis et al., 2003b), which is a sum of six yes/no questions indicating their satisfaction with their living situation, family relationships, sexual/marital relationships, school/work environment, how they spend their free time, and the degree to which they were coping with or receiving help with their problems. Higher scores represent greater general satisfaction. *Cognitive avoidance* was assessed using an adapted version of the Coping Responses Inventory (Moos, 1993); this six-item scale measured the degree to which participants attempted to avoid thinking realistically about their substance use (presumed likely to lead to continued use). Lower scores represent less cognitive avoidance (a positive outcome). *Self-efficacy* was assessed using the Self-Efficacy Scale, a five-item measure of one's ability to avoid thinking about or using substances in different settings. For this modified Global Appraisal of Individual Needs

(GAIN; Dennis et al., 2003a, 2003b) scale, higher scores indicate greater perceived self-efficacy to resist substance use.

Additional Covariates

The number of times participants attended treatment was recorded for each quarter. Based on findings suggesting it was a key threshold variable (Scott & Dennis, 2009), a covariate was created representing whether they had *attended treatment 10 or more times* in each quarter (coded as 0 = attended <10 times, 1 = attended 10+ times). *Self-help involvement* was measured using the Self-Help Involvement Scale (SHIS; Conrad et al., 2015), a 21-item scale assessing the number of self-help meetings attended and other self-help engagement. Higher scores represent more self-help involvement.

TVEM and Analytic Plan

TVEM examined the effect of the intervention condition on quarterly-assessed substance use outcomes and other positive changes, and the interaction of intervention condition and baseline severity on all outcome variables as a continuous function of time. Because TVEM estimates coefficients and odds ratios (OR) as a function of continuous time, all results were plotted as figures that included the time-varying effect estimate and its associated lower-bound and upper-bound 95 percent confidence intervals (CI). Points at which CIs do not include 1.0 (for binary outcomes or count outcomes) or 0.0 (for normally distributed outcomes) are considered statistically significant. Time, measured along the x-axis in Figures 7.1–7.3, represents the number of months since enrolling in the clinical trial ranging from 0 to 48 months.

All analyses were conducted using the %TVEM macro in SAS version 9.3 (Li et al., 2017). User guides for the %TVEM macro (and its %WeightedTVEM counterpart for analyses involving survey weights; Dziak et al., 2017) provide details on installing and running the macro. The %TVEM macro requires the user to specify a number of arguments; some are required, and some are optional. The %TVEM macro statements used in this chapter include **data**, **ID**, **time**, **dv**, **dist**, **tvary_effect**, **method**, and **knots**. **Data** is the name of the analysis dataset (named "recov" here). **ID** (named "rxpid" here) is the individual participant identification record. **Time** (named "xobs" here) included a maximum of 17 time-points per participant, representing the quarterly assessment period (0, 3, 6, … 48 months). **DV** is the name of the dependent (i.e., outcome) variable. **Dist** is the specification of the outcome variable distribution, with the options of normal, binary, or count (using a Poisson distribution)[1]. **Tvary_effect** are the variables specified to have a time-varying effect. The user can choose to include covariates in their model as having either a time-varying effect (and list them under

[1] A separate macro, %TVEM_ZIP, is also available for fitting zero-inflated Poisson models (Li et al., 2015).

tvary_effect) or a time-invariant effect (and list each variable under an optional **invar_effect** argument). To examine the effect of the intervention condition – relative to the control condition – at each quarterly assessment, the intervention was specified to have a time-varying effect in all analyses. **Method** is the estimation method. As detailed in Li et al. (2017), the user has the option of specifying one of two estimation methods: "P-spline" (where the macro automatically selects the number of knots, as discussed above) or "B-spline" (where the analyst manually conducts model selection to determine the optimal number of knots). For present purposes, P-spline was used in all analyses. Ten **knots** were specified for each time-varying effect (the maximum number of knots for the macro to consider). See Li et al. (2017) for more information on using the % TVEM macro and a full list of the required and optional arguments.

RMC Intervention Effect on Substance Use Outcomes across Time

First, three separate TVEMs were conducted to examine the time-varying effect of the intervention on less than weekly alcohol/drug use, number of days without alcohol/drugs, and abstinence. The intercept (named "x0" in the syntax, a created variable specified to equal one) and the main effect of the intervention were specified as time-varying predictors of each outcome. Less than weekly alcohol/drug use and abstinence are dichotomous outcomes and thus were specified to have a binary distribution. Number of days without alcohol/drug use, a count outcome, was specified to have a Poisson distribution. To facilitate interpretation of the Poisson outcome, coefficients were exponentiated to represent incident rate ratios (IRR). Whether the participant attended 10+ treatment sessions at each timepoint and their self-help involvement at each timepoint were also controlled for by including both variables as time-varying covariates.

RMC Intervention Effect on Other Positive Recovery Outcomes across Time

Second, three separate TVEMs were conducted to examine the time-varying effect of the intervention on self-reported general life satisfaction, cognitive avoidance, and self-efficacy. All of these outcomes are continuous measures and were thus specified as having a normal distribution. In addition to controlling for whether the participant received 10+ treatment sessions and their self-help involvement at each timepoint, all analyses also controlled for the number of days without alcohol or drug use at each timepoint.

Interaction between RMC Intervention and Baseline Severity on Outcomes across Time

Finally, an interaction term was created by multiplying the intervention condition by baseline severity, as measured by the GAIN. Similar to a standard regression model, the intercept, main effect of the intervention condition, main effect of baseline severity, and interaction term were included as time-varying predictors of each outcome in separate analyses. Each model identified time points of significance for the interaction term across time. When the interaction term was significant for at least one time point, simple slopes were examined by testing the main effect of the intervention condition at each level of the moderator (i.e., a binary indicator representing low versus high baseline severity). This required creating separate datasets by baseline severity and examining the time-varying effect of the intervention condition on each outcome for both baseline severity groups. Syntax corresponding to each model shown in the figures is provided in the Appendix.

TVEM Results

RMC Intervention Effect on Substance Use Outcomes across Time

TVEMs were used to examine the effect of the intervention on substance use outcomes across time. An example equation for examining the outcome of odds of less than weekly alcohol/drug use is shown below:

$$ln\left(\frac{P(Less\ than\ Weekly\ Use_i)}{1+P(Less\ than\ Weekly\ Use_i)}\right)$$
$$=\beta_0(t)+\beta_1(t)RMC_i+\beta_2(t)Tx10_i+\beta_3(t)Self\ help_i$$

Here, $Less\ than\ Weekly\ Use_i$ represents whether individual i reported less than weekly use at time t. $\beta_0(t)$ is the intercept function and $\beta_1(t)RMC_i$ is the coefficient function representing the main effect of being in the intervention condition across months. $\beta_2(t)T\times 10_i$ and $\beta_3(t)Self\ help_i$ are the coefficient functions representing whether the individual reported 10+ days of treatment and their self-help involvement across months, respectively.

Figure 7.1a shows the time-varying effect of the RMC intervention condition (relative to the monitoring-only control condition) on odds of less than weekly alcohol/drug use across months 0–48. The solid black line represents the effect of the intervention, controlling for additional days of treatment and self-help involvement. The dashed line represents the associated 95 percent CIs. Individuals in the intervention condition relative to the control condition were at significantly higher odds of less than weekly alcohol/drug use from months 6 to 24. Further, it appears that the effect of the intervention gradually strengthened across months, peaking at month 14 (OR = 1.50) and decreasing until around month 38 (OR = 1.14). The effect of the intervention slightly increased from months 38 to 48.

As shown in Figure 7.1b, a similar time trend was observed for number of days without alcohol/drug use such that the intervention effect gradually increased over months 0–18 (peak IRR = 1.10 at month 18). The effect decreased from months 18 to 38 and slightly increased from months 38 to 48. The intervention was associated with significantly more days without alcohol/drug use from months 10 (IRR = 1.07, CI = 1.01 – 1.14) to 27 (IRR = 1.08, CI = 1.01 – 1.16) A key difference between Figure 7.1a using a dichotomous

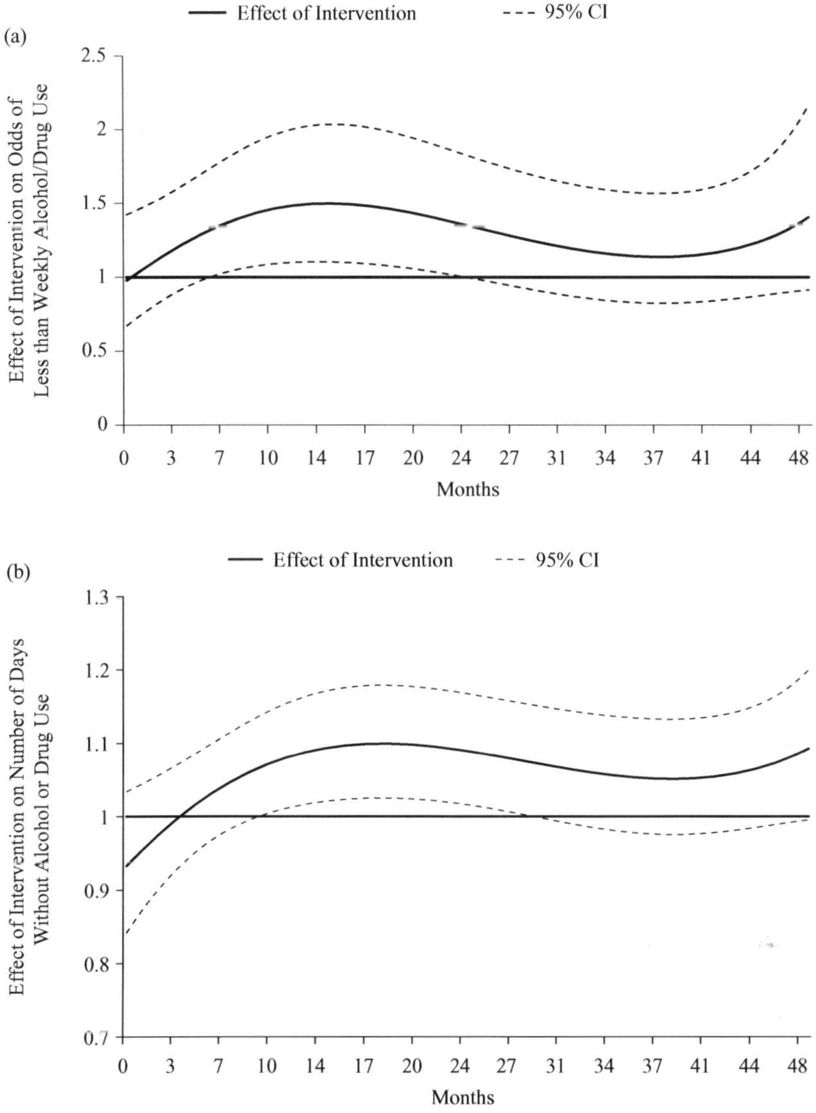

Figure 7.1 *Effect of intervention condition on alcohol/drug use across months since entering treatment (0–48)*

Note. *Figure 7.1a shows the odds of less than weekly alcohol/drug use, and Figure 7.1b shows the number of days without alcohol/drug use across months since entering treatment.*

outcome measure and Figure 7.1b using a count outcome measure was that the 95 percent CIs were narrower for the latter, which reflects greater precision of the estimate.

The effect of the intervention on whether individuals were abstinent all 90 days was non-significant at all time points (not shown).

RMC Intervention Effect on Other Positive Recovery Outcomes across Time

The effect of the intervention on the continuous measures of general life satisfaction, cognitive avoidance, and self-efficacy are presented in Figure 7.2a, 7.2b, and 7.2c, respectively. An example model with the outcome of general life satisfaction is specified as:

$$LifeSat_i = \beta_0(t) + \beta_1(t)RMC_i + \beta_2(t)T \times 10_i + \beta_3(t)Self\,help_i + \beta_4(t)NumDays\,of\,Use_i$$

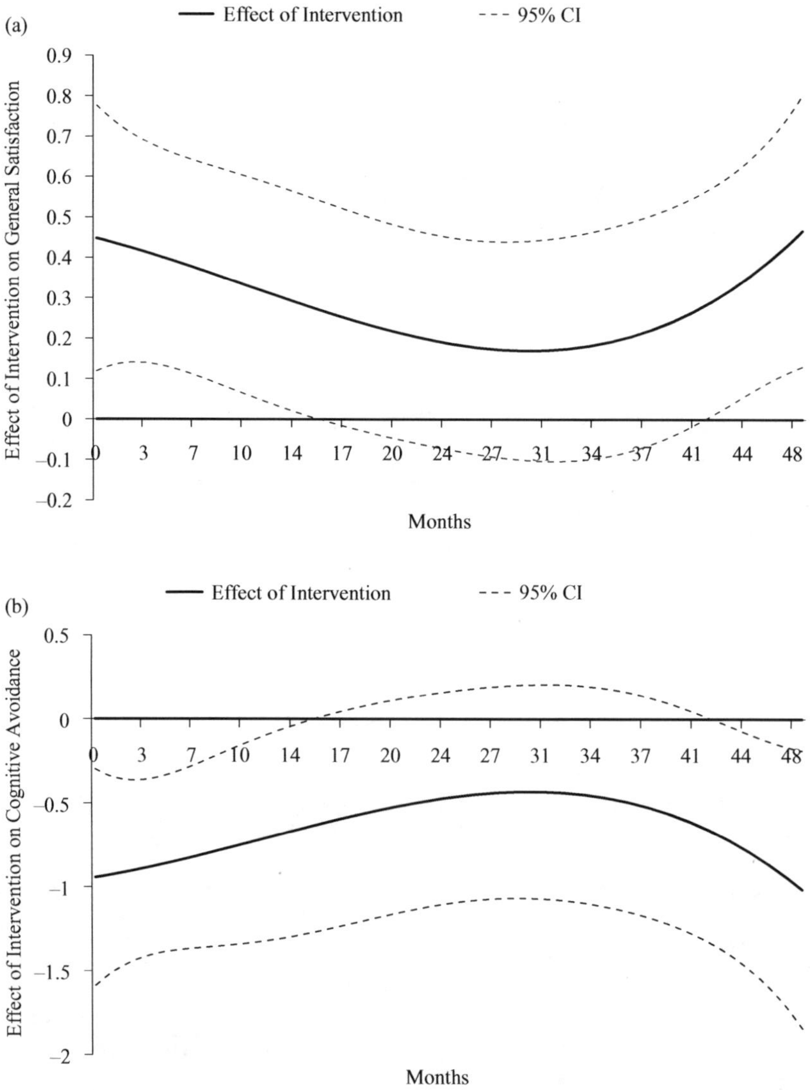

Figure 7.2 *The effect of the intervention condition on general satisfaction, cognitive avoidance, and self-efficacy across months since entering treatment (0–48)*
Note. *Figure 7.2a shows the outcome of general satisfaction, Figure 7.2b shows cognitive avoidance, and Figure 7.2c shows self-efficacy.*

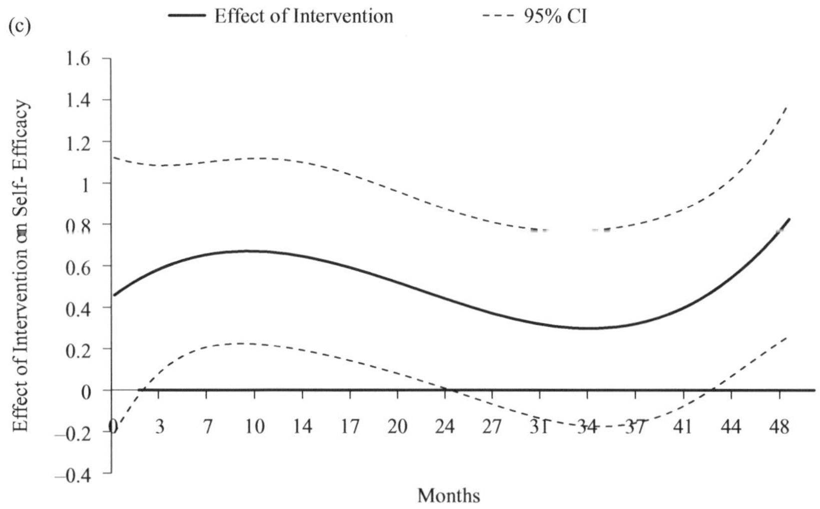

Figure 7.2 *(cont.)*

where life satisfaction ($Life\ Sat_i$) indicates individual *i*'s self-reported life satisfaction score, RMC_i represents individual *i*'s intervention condition, $T \times 10_i$ represents whether individual *i* attended treatment 10+ times, $Self\ help_i$ indicates individual *i*'s self-help involvement, and $NumDays\ of\ Use_i$ represents the number of days individual *i* reported not using alcohol or drugs.

Overall, similar patterns were observed across each positive recovery outcome. Relative to the monitoring-only control condition, RMC recipients reported higher general life satisfaction from months 0 to 15 and from months 42 to 48. The effect tended to weaken from month 0 to month 30 and then gradually increased, peaking at month 48 ($B = 0.47$, $SE = 0.17$, CI = 0.13–0.80). Level of cognitive avoidance was significantly lower for individuals in the intervention relative to control condition from months 0 to 15 and from months 42 to 48. This effect gradually became more positive from month 0 to month 30 ($B = -0.43$, $SE = 0.32$) and then gradually declined. The strongest effect of the intervention on cognitive avoidance was observed at month 48 ($B = -1.01$, $SE = 0.42$). Reported self-efficacy was significantly higher for individuals in the intervention condition from months 2 to 24 and from months 43 to 48. The effect was fairly stable across time, peaking at month 48 ($B = 0.83$, $SE = 0.29$).

Notably, the effect of the RMC intervention, as compared to the control condition, was associated with significantly higher general satisfaction, lower cognitive avoidance, and higher self-efficacy at various timepoints after controlling for additional treatment, self-help involvement, and number of days without alcohol/drug use. Thus, individuals in the RMC intervention condition reported greater positive outcomes at specific quarterly assessments regardless of the number of days abstinent.

Interaction between RMC Intervention and Baseline Severity on Outcomes across Time

Finally, moderation of the intervention effect by baseline severity was tested for all outcomes. The interaction was statistically significant at some timepoints for the outcomes of less than weekly alcohol/drug use, number of days without alcohol/drug use, and odds of abstaining for all 90 days. The interaction was non-significant for general life satisfaction, cognitive avoidance, and self-efficacy. For demonstration purposes, the interaction of intervention condition by baseline severity and associated simple slopes is presented here. The model specified for this outcome is:

$$In\left(\frac{P(Less\ than\ Weekly\ Use_i)}{1 + P(Less\ than\ Weekly\ Use_i)}\right)$$
$$= \beta_0(t) + \beta_1(t)RMC_i + \beta_2(t)Severity_i + \beta_3(t)RMC \times Severity_i$$
$$+ \beta_4(t)T \times 10_i + \beta_5(t)Self\ help_i$$

with main effects of intervention condition (RMC_i) and severity $(Severity_i)$, and their interaction $(RMC \times Severity_i)$.

Figure 7.3a shows the interaction effect for less than weekly alcohol/drug use. Although this outcome is binary (odds of less than weekly alcohol/drug use), similar to standard regression models, when modeling interaction terms, the *B* coefficient curve should be used (instead of the odds ratio curve) for ease of interpretation. The interaction was significant from months 4 to 48, suggesting that the effects of RMC were *not* the same for those with low versus high

(a)

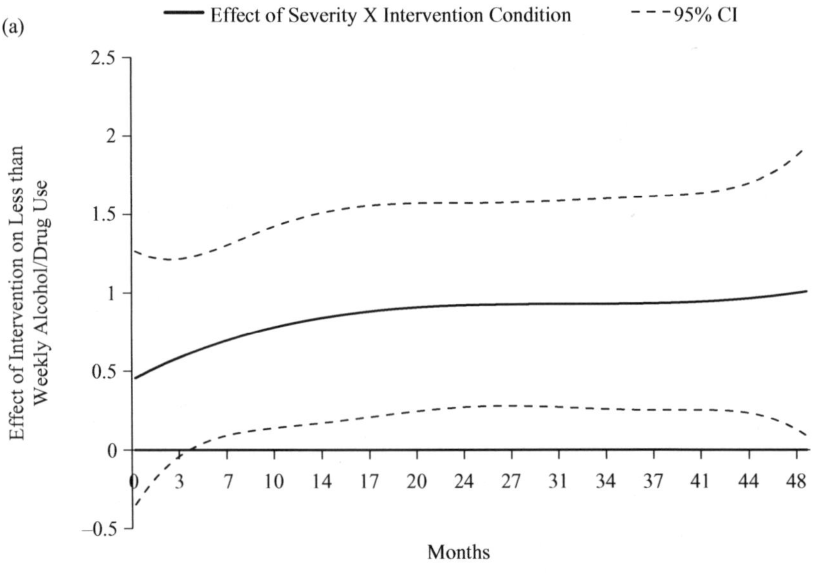

Figure 7.3 *Problem severity and intervention condition interaction effects across months since entering treatment*

Note. *Figure 7.3a shows the interaction for less than weekly alcohol/drug use. Figure 7.3b shows the effect of the intervention for odds of less than weekly alcohol/drug use for individuals with lower problem severity. Figure 7.3c shows the effect of the intervention for odds of less than weekly alcohol/drug use for individuals with higher problem severity.*

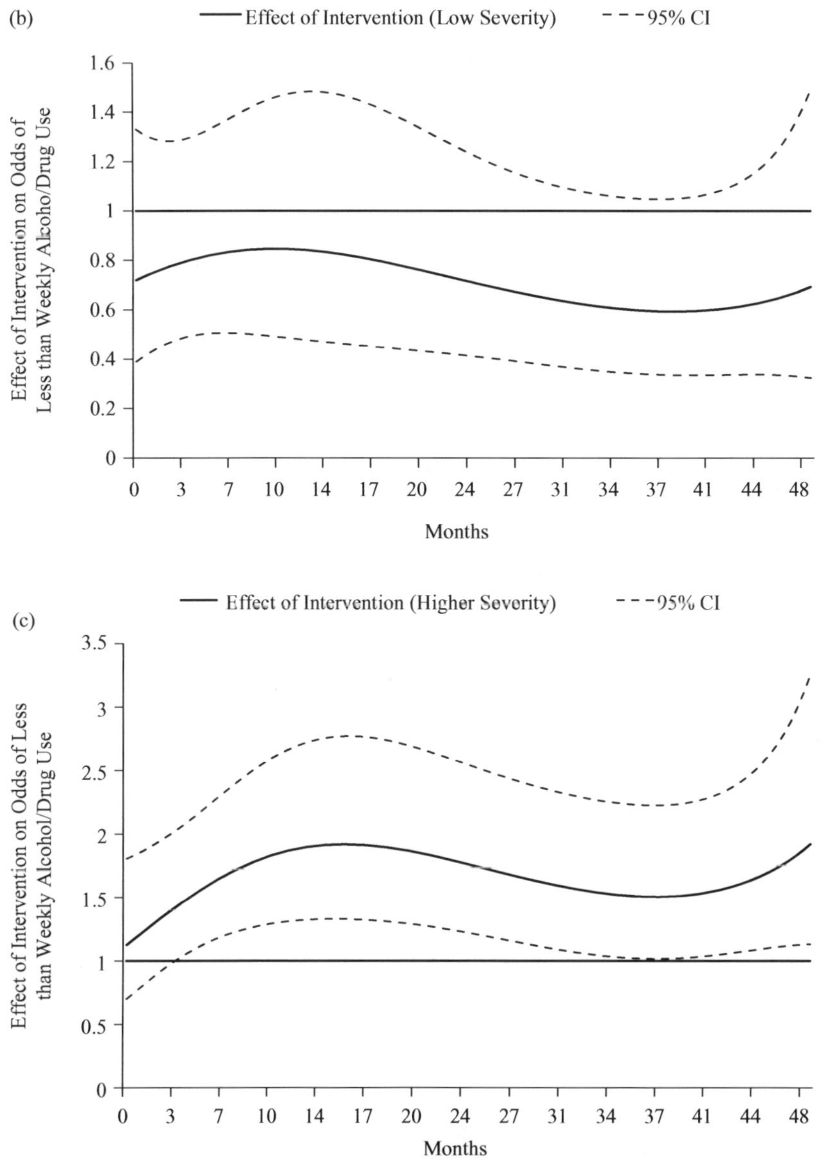

Figure 7.3 (*cont.*)

severity. To probe the interaction effect, we examined the effect of the intervention on odds of less than weekly alcohol/drug use for individuals with lower (Figure 7.3b) and higher (Figure 7.3c) baseline severity. For individuals with lower severity, the intervention condition was not significantly associated with odds of less than weekly alcohol/drug use. For individuals with higher baseline severity, the RMC intervention, as compared to the control condition, was associated with higher odds of less than weekly alcohol/drug use across months 4–48, with odds ratios peaking at month 48 (OR = 1.92).

Conclusions and Recommendations

The RMC intervention had a positive impact by reducing substance use and improving other positive recovery outcomes, including higher general life satisfaction, lower cognitive avoidance, and higher self-efficacy. The TVEM analyses further showed that the intervention generally had a time-varying effect on the assessed outcomes. Specifically, those in the RMC intervention group were more likely to report less than weekly alcohol/drug use and fewer days of alcohol/drug use after approximately two to three quarters of receiving RMC, although this effect dissipated starting around two years of having received RMC. The effect of receiving RMCs on positive change outcomes of satisfaction, cognitive avoidance, and self-efficacy was apparent for approximately the first year after the intervention, waned for years two and three, and then increased during the last few quarters of monitoring.

Given the time-varying nature of these effects and the differential patterns observed by type of recovery outcome, TVEM may be a viable option in lieu of or in addition to using common metrics of "treatment success." For example, a common approach is to determine the effect of an intervention by comparing substance use frequency at baseline and follow-up, with little consideration given to changes between baseline and follow-up. Employing such a traditional method may be a lost opportunity to gain insights into the timepoints for *when* the intervention is most and least effective and – as observed in our interaction analyses – *for whom* the intervention is most and least effective.

Several important findings emerged from these analyses. First, although abstinence from alcohol and/or drugs is a common metric of treatment success, the odds of complete abstinence for all 90 days was not significantly different between the RMC intervention and control condition. Less than weekly use of alcohol or other drugs and/or days of abstinence were more sensitive to change. Moreover, a number of other significant substance use and positive life changes were observed throughout the intervention trial. In concert with recent calls for expanding the definition of recovery from SUD beyond abstinence (National Academies of Sciences, Engineering, and Medicine, 2016; Witkiewitz & Tucker, 2020), it is highly recommended that researchers consider adding alternative measures of treatment success beyond days of abstinence.

Relatedly, positive changes in life satisfaction, cognitive avoidance of alcohol or drug problems, and self-efficacy to resist substance use were observed for approximately the first year of the intervention trial, even after controlling for the number of days without alcohol or drug use. Participants' quality of life and other behavioral outcomes appeared to improve independent of their frequency of substance use and thus are important recovery outcomes to assess.

Finally, simple slope analyses revealed that individuals with lower baseline severity on measures of symptoms of SUD, mental health disorders, physical violence, or illegal activity did not show benefits from the RMC intervention relative to the monitoring-only control condition. In contrast, for those with higher baseline severity, the RMC intervention was associated with significantly better substance use outcomes relative to the control condition. This suggests that investment in RMC applications makes more sense for persons with multiple serious problems who may need more support in navigating treatment and their recovery pathway.

RMC was explicitly designed to shift the traditional acute care model of substance use treatment towards a chronic disease model of care (Scott & Dennis, 2010). While it incorporates several evidence-based practices like motivational interviewing and relapse prevention, a key component is the ongoing monitoring that occurs at least quarterly over several years and early-intervention when problems may escalate (Dennis & Scott, 2012; Scott et al., 2005). This empirical demonstration of TVEM helps establish the value of this longer-term approach to improve outcomes by showing additive effects in the early quarters. However, it also shows a diminishing return of simply continuing to do the same thing indefinitely. RMC and other longer-term interventions will likely require modifications over time to maintain the positive impact.

The empirical example presented here illustrates the utility of using TVEM to examine dynamic changes that occur across time. TVEM has several strengths including its ability to flexibly estimate recovery change (broadly defined) over time without making assumptions about the nature of the association. TVEM can also identify points in time for which the intervention is most effective and for whom the intervention is most effective. Statistical methods presented here might serve generally as a framework for future studies of recovery that aim to assess dynamic processes as they unfold across time. Also, although not discussed in this chapter, researchers considering the use of TVEM in their work may creatively conceptualize "time" in a variety of ways. For example, substance use and other behavioral outcomes can be modeled as a function of cross-sectional or developmental age, in the moment or each day via intensive longitudinal data, historically, or time since an event. TVEM can also accommodate complex features such as sample weights, link functions, and multiple covariates. Examples illustrating these various considerations of time can be found at https://aimlab.psu.edu/tvem/.

It should also be noted that TVEM has limitations, and the analyst should carefully consider whether TVEM is the best fit for their research questions and data. TVEM requires substantial coverage of data points across time to appropriately estimate and capture relevant change processes. To collect such data requires intensive time and study resources, which is often a major barrier for researchers. As with any linear regression framework, causality cannot be inferred, and findings should be interpreted as such. Also, many other methods for analyzing longitudinal data are available and may be better suited depending on the research question(s); these methods include structural equation modeling, multilevel modeling, or linear growth curve modeling. Although TVEM can more flexibly estimate changes in outcomes across time, it is less flexible in modeling individual growth trajectories. TVEM software is also rapidly evolving. The current empirical example used SAS software (from which the macro was originally developed). Work on developing an R package to fit TVEM models is underway, and dynamic structural equation modeling, which combines multilevel modeling, time-series modeling, structural equation modeling, and TVEM, can also be estimated in Mplus software (Asparouhov et al., 2018). Despite the limitations of TVEM, as this empirical demonstration showed, TVEM is a flexible longitudinal analysis method that can be used to answer important research questions about dynamic change during the recovery process.

APPENDIX: SYNTAX FOR MODELS SHOWN

Syntax for Panel Figure 7.1

Figure 7.1a Time-varying effect of intervention (XRA) on whether reported <13 days of alcohol or other drug use in the past 90 days (WKYDR2), controlling for whether reported 10+ days of treatment (TX10) and self-help involvement (SHIS)

```
%TVEM(data = recov,
id = rxpid,
time = xobs,
dv = wkydr2,
dist = binary,
tvary_effect = x0 xra tx10 shis,
method = p-spline,
knots = 10 10 10 10
);
*Exporting data file to Excel;
data XRAonWKYDR2; set tvem_plot_data_or; run;
PROC EXPORT
DATA= XRAonWKYDR2
DBMS=xlsx
OUTFILE="C:\FolderName\XRAonWKYDR2.xlsx";
run;
```

Figure 7.1b Time-varying effect of intervention (XRA) on number of days without alcohol/drugs in the past 90 days (S2S1AR), controlling for controlling for whether reported 10+ days of treatment (TX10) and self-help involvement (SHIS)

```
%TVEM(data = recov,
id = rxpid,
time = xobs,
dv = S2S1AR,
```

```
dist = poisson,
tvary_effect = x0 xra tx10 shis,
method = p-spline,
knots = 10 10 10 10
);
```

Example Syntax for Panel Figure 7.2

Figure 7.2a Time-varying effect of intervention (XRA) on general satisfaction (GSI), controlling for whether reported 10+ days of treatment (TX10), self-help involvement (SHIS), and number of days without using alcohol or drugs (S2S1AR)

```
%TVEM(data = recov,
id = rxpid,
time = xobs,
dv = qsi,
dist = normal,
tvary_effect = x0 xra tx10 shis S2S1AR,
method = p-spline,
knots = 10 10 10 10 10
);
```

Note. Outcomes of cognitive avoidance (Figure 7.2b) and self-efficacy (Figure 7.2c) are also normally distributed and thus have similar syntax.

Syntax for Panel Figure 7.3

Figure 7.3a The time-varying effect interaction (PROBXGRP) of intervention condition (XRA) by baseline severity (PROBCNTB) on whether reported <13 days of alcohol or other drug use in the past 90 days (WKYDR), controlling for whether reported 10+ days of treatment (TX10) and self-help involvement (SHIS)

```
%TVEM(data = recov,
id = rxpid,
time = xobs,
dv = wkydr2,
dist=binary,
tvary_effect = x0 tx10 shis xra probcntB probXgrp,
method = p-spline,
knots = 10 10 10 10 10 10
);
```

Figure 7.3b The time-varying effect of the intervention condition (XRA) on whether reported <13 days of alcohol or other drug use in the past 90 days (WKYDR), among those reporting two or fewer problems at baseline (PROBCNTB = 0), controlling for whether reported 10+ days of treatment (TX10) and self-help involvement (SHIS)

```
*Creating a dataset among only those with 0 to 2 prob-
lems at baseline (PROBCNTB = 0);
data recovLO;
set recov;
where probcntB=0;
run;
%TVEM(data = recovLO,
id = rxpid,
time = xobs,
dv = wkydr2,
dist=binary,
tvary_effect = x0 tx10 shis xra,
method = p-spline,
knots = 10 10 10 10
);
```

Figure 7.3c The time-varying effect of the intervention condition (XRA) on whether reported <13 days of alcohol or other drug use in the past 90 days (WKYDR), among those reporting three or more problems at baseline (PROBCNTB = 1), controlling for whether reported 10+ days of treatment (TX10) and self-help involvement (SHIS)

```
*Creating a dataset among only those with 3+ problems
at baseline (PROBCNTB = 1);
data recovHI;
set recov;
where probcntB=1;
run;
%TVEM(data = recovHI,
id = rxpid,
time = xobs,
dv = wkydr2,
dist=binary,
tvary_effect = x0 tx10 shis xra,
method = p-spline,
knots = 10 10 10 10
);
```

References

Ashford, R. D., Brown, A., Brown, T., Callis, J., Cleveland, H. H., Eisenhart, E., Groover, H., Hayes, N., Johnston, T., Kimball, T., Manteuffel, B., McDaniel, J., Montgomery, L., Phillips, S., Polacek, M., Statman, M. Whitney, J. (2019). Defining and operationalizing the phenomena of recovery: A working definition from the recovery science research collaborative. *Addiction Research & Theory, 27*, 179–188. https://doi.org/10.1080/16066359.2018.1515352

Asparouhov, T., Hamaker, E. L., & Muthén, B. (2018). Dynamic structural equation models. *Structural Equation Modeling: A Multidisciplinary Journal, 25*, 359–388. https://doi.org/10.1080/10705511.2017.1406803

Bray, J. W., Aden, B., Eggman, A. A., Hellerstein, L., Wittenberg, E., Nosyk, B., Stribling, J. C., & Schackman, B. R. (2017). Quality of life as an outcome of opioid use disorder treatment: A systematic review. *Journal of Substance Abuse Treatment, 76*, 88–93. https://doi.org/10.1016/j.jsat.2017.01.019

Conrad, K. M., Conrad, K. J., Passetti, L. L., Funk, R. R., & Dennis, M. L. (2015). Validation of the full and short-form self-help involvement scale against the Rasch measurement model. *Evaluation Review, 39*, 395–427. https://doi.org/10.1177/0193841x15599645

Dennis, M., Scott, C. K., & Funk, R. (2003a). An experimental evaluation of recovery management check-ups (RMC) for people with chronic substance use disorders. *Evaluation and Program Planning, 26*, 339–352. https://doi.org/10.1016/S0149-7189(03)00037-5

Dennis, M. L., Foss, M. A., & Scott, C. K. (2007). An eight-year perspective on the relationship between the duration of abstinence and other aspects of recovery. *Evaluation Review, 31*, 585–612. https://doi.org/10.1177/0193841X07307771

Dennis, M. L., & Scott, C. K. (2012). Four-year outcomes from the early re-intervention (ERI) experiment using recovery management check-ups (RMCs). *Drug and Alcohol Dependence, 121*, 10–17. https://doi.org/10.1016/j.drugalcdep.2011.07.026

Dennis, M. L., Scott, C. K., Funk, R., & Foss, M. A. (2005). The duration and correlates of addiction and treatment careers. *Journal of Substance Abuse Treatment, 28 Suppl 1*, S51–S62. https://doi.org/10.1016/j.jsat.2004.10.013

Dennis, M. L., Titus, J. C., White, M. K., & Unsicker, J. I. (2003b). *Global appraisal of individual needs: Administration guide for the GAIN and related measures. Chestnut Health Systems*. www.gaincc.org/instruments

Diederichs, C., Berger, K., & Bartels, D. B. (2011). The measurement of multiple chronic diseases—A systematic review on existing multimorbidity indices. *The Journals of Gerontology: Series A, 66A*, 301–311. https://academic.oup.com/biomedgerontology/article-abstract/66A/3/301/600233

Donovan, D. M., Bigelow, G. E., Brigham, G. S., Carroll, K. M., Cohen, A. J., Gardin, J. G., Hamilton, J. A., Huestis, M. A., Hughes, J. R., Lindblad, R., Marlatt, G. A., Preston, K. L., Selzer, J. A., Somoza, E. C., Wakim, P. G., Wells, E. A. (2012). Primary outcome indices in illicit drug dependence treatment research: Systematic approach to selection and measurement of drug use end-points in clinical trials. *Addiction, 107*, 694–708. https://doi.org/10.1111/j.1360-0443.2011.03473.x

Dziak, J. J., Li, R., & Wagner, A. T. (2017). *WeightedTVEM SAS macro users' guide* (Version 2.6). [Computer software] https://aimlab.psu.edu/tvem/weighted-tvem-sas-macro/

Evans-Polce, R., & Schuler, M. S. (2016). Rates of past-year alcohol treatment across two time metrics and differences by alcohol use disorder severity and mental health comorbidities. *Drug and Alcohol Dependence, 166*, 194–201. https://doi.org/10.1016/j.drugalcdep.2016.07.010

Finney, J. W., Moyer, A., & Swearingen, C. E. (2003). Outcome variables and their assessment in alcohol treatment studies: 1968–1998. *Alcoholism: Clinical and Experimental Research, 27*, 1671–1679. https://doi.org/10.1097/01.Alc.0000091236.14003.E1

Garner, B. R., Scott, C. K., Dennis, M. L., & Funk, R. R. (2014). The relationship between recovery and health-related quality of life. *Journal of Substance Abuse Treatment, 47*, 293–298. https://doi.org/10.1016/j.jsat.2014.05.006

Griffith, L. E., Gruneir, A., Fisher, K. A., Nicholson, K., Panjwani, D., Patterson, C., Markle-Reid, M., Ploeg, J., Bierman, A. S., Hogan, D. B., & Upshur, R. (2018). Key factors to consider when measuring multimorbidity: Results from an expert panel and online survey. *Journal of Comorbidity, 8*, 2235042X18795306. http://dx.doi.org/10.1177/2235042X18795306

Hastie, T., & Tibshirani, R. (1993). Varying-coefficient models. *Journal of the Royal Statistical Society Series B (Methodological), 55*, 757–796. https://doi.org/10.1111/j.2517-6161.1993.tb01939.x

Hoover, D. R., Rice, J. A., Wu, C. O., & Yang, L.-P. (1998). Nonparametric smoothing estimates of time-varying coefficient models with longitudinal data. *Biometrika, 85*, 809–822. https://doi.org/10.1093/biomet/85.4.809

Kelly, J. F., Greene, M. C., & Bergman, B. G. (2018). Beyond abstinence: Changes in indices of quality of life with time in recovery in a nationally representative sample of US adults. *Alcoholism: Clinical and Experimental Research, 42*, 770–780. https://doi.org/10.1111/acer.13604

Kiluk, B. D., Frankforter, T. L., Cusumano, M., Nich, C., & Carroll, K. M. (2018). Change in DSM-5 alcohol use disorder criteria count and severity level as a treatment outcome indicator: Results from a randomized trial. *Alcoholism: Clinical and Experimental Research, 42*, 1556–1563. https://doi.org/10.1111/acer.13807

Lanza, S. T., & Linden-Carmichael, A. N. (2021). *Time-varying effect modeling for the behavioral, social, and health sciences*. Springer. doi: 10.1007/978-3-030-70944-0

Lanza, S. T., Vasilenko, S. A., & Russell, M. A. (2016). Time-varying effect modeling to address new questions in behavioral research: Examples in marijuana use. *Psychology of Addictive Behaviors, 30*, 939–954. https://doi.org/10.1037/adb0000208

Leadbeater, B. J., Ames, M. E., & Linden-Carmichael, A. N. (2019). Age-varying effects of cannabis use frequency and disorder on symptoms of psychosis, depression and anxiety in adolescents and adults. *Addiction, 114*, 278–293. https://doi.org/10.1111/add.14459

Li, R., Dziak, J. J., Tan, X., Huang, L., Wagner, A. T., & Yang, J. (2017). *TVEM SAS macro users' guide* (Version 3.1.1). [Computer software] https://aimlab.psu.edu/tvem/tvem-sas-macro/

Li, R., Tan, X., Huang, L., Wagner, A. T., & Yang, J. (2015). *%TVEM_zip (time-varying effect model) SAS macro users' guide* (Version 2.1.1). [Computer software] The Methodology Center, Penn State. http://methodology.psu.edu

Linden-Carmichael, A. N., Dziak, J. J., & Lanza, S. T. (2018). Dynamic features of problematic drinking: Alcohol use disorder latent classes across ages 18–64. *Alcohol and Alcoholism, 54*, 97–103. https://doi.org/10.1093/alcalc/agy074

Linden-Carmichael, A. N., Vasilenko, S. A., Lanza, S. T., & Maggs, J. L. (2017). High-intensity drinking versus heavy episodic drinking: Prevalence rates and relative odds of alcohol use disorder across adulthood. *Alcoholism: Clinical and Experimental Research, 41*, 1754–1759. https://doi.org/10.1111/acer.13475

McKay, J. R. (2001). Effectiveness of continuing care interventions for substance abusers: Implications for the study of long-term treatment effects. *Evaluation Review, 25*, 211–232. https://doi.org/10.1177/0193841x0102500205

McLellan, A. T., McKay, J. R., Forman, R., Cacciola, J., & Kemp, J. (2005). Reconsidering the evaluation of addiction treatment: From retrospective follow-up to concurrent recovery monitoring. *Addiction, 100*, 447–458. https://doi.org/10.1111/j.1360-0443.2005.01012.x

Moos, R. H. (1993). *Coping Responses Inventory Youth form: Professional manual.* Psychological Assessment Resources.

Moos, R. H., & Moos, B. S. (2007). Protective resources and long-term recovery from alcohol use disorders. *Drug and Alcohol Dependence, 86*, 46–54. https://doi.org/10.1016/j.drugalcdep.2006.04.015

National Academies of Sciences, Engineering, and Medicine (2016). *Measuring recovery from substance use or mental disorders: Workshop summary.* The National Academies Press. https://doi.org/10.17226/23589

Nicholson, K., Almirall, J., & Fortin, M. (2019). The measurement of multimorbidity. *Health Psychology, 38*(9), 783–790. https://doi.org/10.1037/hea0000739

Scott, C. K., & Dennis, M. L. (2003). *Recovery Management Check-ups: An early re-intervention model.* Chestnut Health Systems.

(2009). Results from two randomized clinical trials evaluating the impact of quarterly recovery management check-ups with adult chronic substance users. *Addiction, 104*, 959–971. https://doi.org/10.1111/j.1360-0443.2009.02525.x

(2010). Recovery management check-ups with adult chronic substance users. In J. F. Kelly & W. L. White (Eds.), *Current clinical psychiatry. Addiction recovery management: Theory, research, and practice* (pp. 87–101). Humana Press.

Scott, C. K., Dennis, M. L., & Foss, M. A. (2005). Utilizing Recovery Management Check-ups to shorten the cycle of relapse, treatment re-entry, and recovery. *Drug and Alcohol Dependence, 78*, 325–338. https://doi.org/10.1016/j.drugalcdep.2004.12.005

Simpson, C. A., & Tucker, J. A. (2002). Temporal sequencing of alcohol-related problems, problem recognition, and help-seeking episodes. *Addictive Behaviors, 27*, 659–674. https://doi.org/10.1016/s0306-4603(01)00200-3

Simpson, D. D., Joe, G. W., & Broome, K. M. (2002). A national 5-year follow-up of treatment outcomes for cocaine dependence. *Archives of General Psychiatry, 59*, 538–544. https://doi.org/10.1001/archpsyc.59.6.538

Stull, S. W., Panlilio, L. V., Moran, L. M., Schroeder, J. R., Bertz, J. W., Epstein, D. H., Preston, K. L., Phillips, K. A. (2019). The chippers, the quitters, and the highly symptomatic: A 12-month longitudinal study of DSM-5 opioid- and cocaine-use problems in a community sample. *Addictive Behaviors, 96*, 183–191. https://doi.org/10.1016/j.addbeh.2019.04.030

Tan, X., Shiyko, M. P., Li, R., Li, Y., & Dierker, L. (2012). A time-varying effect model for intensive longitudinal data. *Psychological Methods, 17*, 61–77. https://doi.org/10.1037/a0025814

White, W. L. (2007). Addiction recovery: Its definition and conceptual boundaries. *Journal of Substance Abuse Treatment, 33*, 229–241. https://doi.org/10.1016/j.jsat.2007.04.015

Wilson, A. D., Bravo, A. J., Pearson, M. R., & Witkiewitz, K. (2016). Finding success in failure: Using latent profile analysis to examine heterogeneity in psychosocial functioning among heavy drinkers following treatment. *Addiction, 111*, 2145–2154. https://doi.org/10.1111/add.13518

Witkiewitz, K., Heather, N., Falk, D. E., Litten, R. Z., Hasin, D. S., Kranzler, H. R., Mann, K. F., O'Malley, S. S., & Anton, R. F. (2020). World Health Organization risk drinking level reductions are associated with improved functioning and are sustained among patients with mild, moderate, and severe alcohol dependence in clinical trials in the United States and United Kingdom. *Addiction, 115*(9), 1668–1680. https://doi.org/10.1111/add.15011

Witkiewitz, K., Pearson, M. R., Hallgren, K. A., Maisto, S. A., Roos, C. R., Kirouac, M., Wilson, A. D., Montes, K. S., & Heather, N. (2017). Who achieves low-risk drinking during alcohol treatment? An analysis of patients in three alcohol clinical trials. *Addiction, 112*(12), 2112–2121. https://doi.org/10.1111/add.13870.

Witkiewitz, K., & Tucker, J. A. (2020). Abstinence not required: Expanding the definition of recovery from alcohol use disorder. *Alcoholism: Clinical and Experimental Research, 44*, 36–40. https://doi.org/10.1111/acer.14235

Wu, L. T., Zhu, H., & Ghitza, U. E. (2018). Multicomorbidity of chronic diseases and substance use disorders and their association with hospitalization: Results from electronic health records data. *Drug and Alcohol Dependence, 192*, 316–323. https://doi.org/10.1016/j.drugalcdep.2018.08.013

8 Latent Variable Mixture Modeling Approaches to Investigating Longitudinal Recovery Processes

JeeWon Cheong, Adam D. Wilson, and Juhan Lee

Latent Variable Mixture Modeling Approaches to Investigating Longitudinal Recovery Processes

The investigation of continuity and change is a central focus in social and behavioral sciences. Many research questions center around patterns of developmental courses that unfold over time, individual differences in those patterns, and possible predictors or outcomes of such individual differences. For example, a researcher might want to know how drinking practices change before and after receiving treatment, whether individuals are different in the magnitude of changes, and what patient characteristics predict greater changes. To address these research questions, longitudinal data are required, assessing the same individuals over multiple measurement occasions (Rogosa, 1988; Willet, 1989).

This chapter is concerned with latent variable modeling approaches that are suitable for person-centered analyses on data collected in panel design studies, where individuals are repeatedly measured for a limited number of occasions (Collins, 2006). For a discussion of longitudinal data with many measurement occasions, we refer interested readers to the chapter on time-varying effect modeling (Linden-Carmichael et al., Chapter 7 this volume). To aid foundational understanding of mixture modeling, we start with a discussion of finite mixture models applied to cross-sectional data (i.e., latent class analysis and latent profile analysis), where subgroups are identified based on the individual patterns of responses to multiple indicators measured concurrently. Then, conventional latent growth curve models and growth mixture models are discussed, where individual patterns of change over time are modeled. We also touch on mediation analysis conducted in a mixture modeling framework.

Important Features of Longitudinal Data for Modeling Changes

Singer and Willett (2003) argued that longitudinal studies need certain features to model changes more accurately. First, data should be collected across three or more occasions. With only two waves of data, change is narrowly conceptualized as linear, i.e., increment/decrement between pre- and post-scores. The difference score between pre- and post-assessments provides an estimate of the total change over the time elapsed (e.g., a year), and the rate of change per time interval (e.g., per month) may be estimated by dividing the difference score by the number of intervals (e.g., 12). With two waves of data, assuming a constant rate of change can be misleading, if the rate of change varies across different time intervals, and it is only possible to model the shape of an individual's trajectory as linear, because necessary information is lacking between the two measurements (Willet, 1989). In addition, with only two waves of data, it is difficult to parse out measurement errors from true change (Rogosa, 1988).

The second feature that is required in the analysis of change is a sensible time metric. Because change is modeled as a function of time, the time unit should be meaningful in relation to the changes in the variable of interest. For example, changes in drinking practices among adult drinkers after treatment, which tend to be highly variable, would be more sensibly captured with weekly or monthly assessments than yearly assessments. For young adolescents who have fewer opportunities and are less likely to drink, yearly assessments of alcohol use might make more sense to capture changes over time. Choosing sensible time metrics can, however, be challenging. In many cases, clear hypotheses are lacking about the timing of when change occurs. Even if such hypotheses exist, the optimal number and spacing of assessments may be limited by cost or feasibility.

Finally, the repeated measures should be equatable, equally valid, and reliable over time (Singer & Willet, 2003). An item is equatable when a given value on that item at one wave equates to the same value at other waves, rendering the interpretation of the magnitude of change meaningful and constant over time. Thus, for example, a problem severity scale value of 3 should represent the same degree of problem severity at age 21 and at age 30. In addition, the instrument tool should be equally valid across time, so the meaning of the item remains the same across time. For example, childhood antisocial behavior indicators may not be valid if applied to individuals in later adolescence. Furthermore, measurement errors should not differ across time if the variable is to be assessed with the same level of precision.

Within-Individual vs. Between-Individual Change

Having multiple waves of data allows characterization of an individual's pattern of change over time and growth trajectory. The change captured by the growth trajectory is *within-individual change* pertinent to the unit of time (e.g., increase occurring per year). The capacity to estimate within-individual change is a strength of longitudinal studies, as the individuals' previous response serves as his/her own control level, rendering the estimated change closer to the true level of change. With cross-sectional data, the change has to be estimated based on differences among individuals. For example, when age is used to predict drinking practices, the coefficient of age is the expected change in drinking by a one year change in age. However, the change in age is based on individuals with different ages, and it could be confounded by other unmeasured individual characteristics.

Between-individual change in the study of change is the question about individual differences in the change rates. Different individuals show different patterns of within-individual change. For example, some people may show greater changes, while others may show no changes or smaller changes, resulting in heterogeneous within-individual changes. Once significant variation is detected, identifying what predicts these individual differences is of interest. The capability to detect and assess predictors of heterogeneity of within-individual changes is important because the predictors of within-individual changes can be quite different from the predictors of between-person differences in cross-sectional data. For example, the predictors of why some people show a greater decrease in drinking than others could be quite different from the predictors explaining why a certain individual drinks more at given times.

Variable-Centered vs. Person-Centered Approaches

Variable-centered approaches focus on the associations among variables. The goal of a variable centered approach is to describe whether and how variables, observed or unobserved (i.e., latent), are related to each other. Variable-centered approaches are based on the assumption that the population is homogeneous with respect to the relations among the variables (Laursen & Hoff, 2006). That is, the association between two variables is assumed to hold for all individuals in the population. Statistical methods used to describe the relative importance of predictor variables in predicting outcomes, such as multiple regression analysis and structural equation modeling, take variable-centered approaches.

On the other hand, *person-centered approaches* focus on relations among individuals. The assumption is that the population is heterogeneous in terms of how individuals respond to the variables. Individuals are probabilistically grouped into categories based on the similarities and differences in the patterns of responses to a set of variables (Magnusson, 2003; Muthén, 2001). Each category contains individuals who are similar to each other and different from those in other categories in terms of their pattern of responses. This categorization is achieved by minimizing the within-category differences and maximizing the between-category differences. The analytic basis of person-centered approaches is finite mixture models, which assume that there are a finite number of subpopulations within the overall population (McLachlan & Peel, 2000; Titterington et al., 1985). In mixture models, the subpopulation group membership is unobserved or latent, and, thus, the probabilistic group membership is estimated. This nature of unobserved or latent group membership allows the integration of person-centered mixture modeling into a general latent variable modeling framework. While latent variables in general latent structural equation modeling are continuous, latent variables in mixture modeling are categorical, representing distinctive categories of latent classes, i.e., subgroups of individuals

(Muthén & Muthén, 2000). Statistical methods such as latent class analysis, cluster analysis, and growth mixture modeling take person-centered approaches.

It should be noted that variable-centered and person-centered approaches are complementary rather than competing approaches (Laursen & Hoff, 2006; Masyn, 2013). The choice between the two approaches should depend on the research questions. When research questions are concerned with the cause-and-effect relations between variables over time, variable-centered approaches are appropriate. Researchers are interested in the relative strengths of predictors and the replications of such strengths across populations. When research questions focus on types or categories of individuals based on different patterns of responses to a set of variables, person-centered approaches are chosen. It is desirable to have a priori hypotheses regarding different patterns of responses that may differentiate persons; however, it is rare. Most empirical studies taking person-centered approaches tend to be exploratory and descriptive, and the replications of the categories of individuals across similar populations are important (Laursen & Hoff, 2006). Although variable-centered and person-centered approaches provide different types of information, it is common that both approaches are employed within a study (Masyn, 2013; Muthén & Muthén, 2000). Taking a person-centered approach, researchers identify subgroups of individuals and then examine predictors or outcomes of group membership by using a variable-centered analysis.

Latent Class Analysis and Latent Profile Analysis

This section provides an overview of latent class analysis (LCA) and latent profile analysis (LPA). Although LCA and LPA are mixture analyses conducted on cross-sectional data and do not involve the analysis of change (Lanza & Cooper, 2016), we discuss these methods to provide the basics of mixture modeling, as these methods can serve as an introductory framework for mixture modeling and can be easily expanded to longitudinal data analysis (e.g., latent class membership predicting an outcome measured later, or LCA of repeated measures). More detailed overview of LCA and applications can be found in Clogg (1995) and Collins and Lanza (2009).

Latent Class Analysis

LCA identifies subgroups or latent classes of individuals based on their response patterns on multiple categorical indicators (Collins & Lanza, 2009). For example, a set of diagnostic symptoms of alcohol use disorder (AUD) have been used in LCA to identify subgroups of college drinkers showing different patterns of presence or absence of various symptoms (e.g., Beseler et al., 2012; Rinker & Neighbors, 2015). The goal is to identify the smallest number of subgroups that can describe the patterns of responses on the observed categorical variables. Each individual's probability of belonging to each class, referred to as posterior class probability, is estimated for all individuals for all classes, and the final class membership (i.e., most likely membership) is determined by the individual's highest probability to be in a specific class. This part of the analysis relating the observed categorical indicators to the categorical latent class variable is analogous to establishing the measurement model in structural equation modeling (Masyn, 2013).

Model Specification

In model specification stage of LCA, researchers decide how many classes will be investigated. However, the number of classes is not known in most cases, even when one can assume that the population is heterogenous. Thus, the model building process starts with a smaller number of classes and adds classes until the model fits the data well and interpretable latent classes are obtained. This process is probably the most challenging part of mixture modeling, as it involves comparison of multiple models with a varying number of classes using various fit indices as well as considering substantive interpretability. In addition, there is no established method that is widely accepted for comparing these models (Masyn, 2013; Nylund et al., 2007).

Commonly, *relative fit indices* are used to compare models in mixture modeling. One set of such fit indices are information criteria (IC)-based fit indices, such as Bayesian Information Criteria (BIC; Schwartz, 1978), Akaike Information Criteria (AIC; Akaike, 1987), and Adjusted BIC (Sclove, 1987). In these criteria, adding parameters improves the model fit but is penalized against model parsimony. A model with lower values on these fit indices is considered a better model. Another set of relative fit indices include Maximum Likelihood-based likelihood ratio tests, such as Lo-Mendell-Rubin test (LMR; Lo et al., 2001) and the Bootstrap Likelihood Ratio Test (BLRT; McLachlan & Peel, 2000). These fit indices are used for comparing nested models, i.e., a model with k classes against a model with $k - 1$ classes. If the test result is significant, a model with one more class is considered better. Among these relative fit indices, BIC (or sample-size adjusted BIC) and BLRT are generally preferred (Nylund et al., 2007).

Inspecting *classification diagnostics* can help model comparisons by informing the precision of latent class assignment for individuals in a candidate model. These diagnostics are based on posterior class probabilities. As the goal of mixture modeling is to extract well-separated classes by maximizing within-class homogeneity and between-class heterogeneity in the response patterns, it is desired that each individual has a very high posterior probability for a specific class. Suppose we estimate a three-class LCA model. Individual 1's posterior probabilities are 0.90, 0.05, and 0.05 for Class 1, 2, and 3, respectively. Individual 2's posterior probabilities are 0.40, 0.25, and 0.35. The most likely class for Individual 1 is clearly Class 1, because the probability of being in Class 1 is much higher than the probabilities of being in other classes. However, Individual 2's posterior probabilities are not quite differentiable. Based on the highest probability, both individuals are assigned to Class 1; but the assignment for Individual 2 may not be accurate. If there are many cases like Individual 1, the overall classification accuracy would be high; if there are many cases like Individual 2, the overall classification accuracy would be low. Entropy is a statistic that assesses the overall accuracy of classification, ranging from zero to one, with higher scores indicating greater accuracy. Entropy, however, should not be used alone for model selection, because it may be high for models with more classes simply by chance (Masyn, 2013). Another index for classification accuracy is average posterior class probability, which is calculated by averaging posterior probabilities across all individuals for each class, ranging from zero to one. While entropy provides an overall classification accuracy, the average posterior probability assesses classification accuracy for a specific class, with a higher value indicating greater accuracy. When the average posterior probabilities are greater than 0.70 for all classes, the classification accuracy is considered adequate (Nagin, 2005).

Additionally, the size of the smallest class (i.e., the class with the fewest individuals most likely classified in that class) should be considered in determining a model because small classes have lower power and lower classification precision than larger classes (Lubke & Neale, 2006). Although model fit would improve as classes are added, if the size of the added class is small (as a rule of thumb, less than 1.0 percent of the entire sample or fewer than 25 individuals), researchers should evaluate the results and justify what is gained by adding the small class (Berlin, Williams et al., 2014).

Assumption of Local Independence

One important assumption in the measurement models of LCA is *local independence* (also termed conditional independence). When the local independence assumption is met, the observed indicators are independent of each other within classes. It implies that the associations between the observed class indicators are fully accounted for by latent class membership. However, this assumption is often violated, as some indicators are related to or dependent on each other (e.g., “passing out as a result of drinking” and “forgetting what happened as a result of drinking”). If local independence is forced in the presence of dependency, the number of latent classes are incorrectly estimated. This occurs because model fit indices are poor if the dependence is not accounted for, leading researchers to incorrectly increase the number of classes in the model building process (Reboussin et al., 2008). Although such solutions improve the fit statistics and may achieve local independence, the extra latent classes may not reflect true subgroups.

Another possible consequence of forcing local independence is biased estimates in the LCA models, even if the number of latent classes is correctly estimated based on a priori hypotheses (Torrance-Rynard & Walter, 1997; Vacek, 1985). The local independence assumption can be evaluated and may be relaxed (see Reboussin et al., 2008). However, it should be noted that local independence in LCA models can only be partially relaxed for model identification for models with more than one class. LCA measurement models will not be identified if all the items are allowed to covary with all other items within class, unless other parameter are constrained (Masyn, 2013).

Latent Profile Analysis

LPA is basically LCA with continuous indicators. LPA has been used in alcohol studies to investigate subgroups of college drinkers showing different profiles of drinking practices (e.g., Lau-Barraco et al., 2017) and to characterize risk profiles using various problem indicators (e.g., Tucker et al., 2020; Yeater et al., 2018). For example, Tucker et al. (2020) assessed distinctive risk profiles in a natural recovery sample, based on pre-resolution drinking days, levels of alcohol dependence (measured on Alcohol Dependence Scale [Skinner and Horn, 1984] and Drinking Problems Scale [Cahalan, 1970]), and a behavioral economic measure assessing relative strength of preference for alcohol compared to savings (Alcohol-Savings Discretionary Expenditure index; Tucker et al., 2006), and examined the relation between problem severity profiles and recovery outcomes.

Analysis procedures described in LCA can be applied to LPA models. The difference lies in the parameters estimated in LCA and LPA. Because the indicators are continuous variables, additional parameters are estimated in LPA models, such as class specific means, variances, and covariances of the indicators. Typically, means of the indicators are allowed to vary across classes, as the goal is to extract latent classes that show different response patterns (mean levels in this case) across indicators. Model specifications on the indicator variances and covariances are quite flexible: they can be constrained to be invariant or variant within-class and also between classes. In addition, unlike LCA, local (conditional) independence can be fully relaxed without causing model identification problems (Masyn, 2013).

The increased flexibility of model specification in LPA, however, could add more complexity in the model specification process and could make the interpretation quite intensive. Masyn (2013) described this issue very well (pp. 586–587), showing that a two-class model with correlated indicators could yield adequate fit statistics comparable to a three-class model with uncorrelated indicators. In such a case, the substantive interpretations of the two LPA models are quite different, and yet choosing one model over the other based on fit statistics is not possible. Thus, the role of theory becomes quite important in specifying and interpreting the LPA models.

Latent Class Regression

While identifying latent classes is an intensive and critical part of mixture modeling, it is the first step in the analyses. Researchers are often interested in relations between the latent class membership and certain background covariates that may be differentially distributed across classes or how class membership predicts outcomes, which are often referred to as distal outcomes (Bandeen-roche et al., 1997; Berlin, Williams et al., 2014). Therefore, once latent classes are identified, predictors and/or outcomes of the latent class membership are introduced in the model.

In this stage of analysis, two methods are typically used: one-step and three-step methods. In the *one-step method,* covariates and/or outcomes, as well as latent class indicators, are included simultaneously in a comprehensive model. When the covariates and/or outcomes are added to the model, they would affect the extraction of the latent classes, as they "become" like the additional class indicators (Asparouhov & Muthén, 2014). Thus, each time covariates and/or outcome are changed, it is necessary to estimate the model again, and quite different solutions of latent classes may be obtained, especially when the classification uncertainty is high (Asparouhov & Muthén, 2014; Bakk, Tekle et al., 2013; Vermunt, 2010). If there are many individuals whose posterior probabilities are rather similar across the classes, such as Individual 2 in the earlier example, class identification in the first step is unstable, and such uncertainty could contribute to different class solutions when adding covariates or outcome variables.

The *three-step method* was developed to overcome the shortcomings of the one-step method (Asparouhov & Muthén, 2014; Bolck et al., 2004; Vermunt, 2010). In the three-step method, classification of individuals into latent classes and estimation of the associations between covariates and/or outcomes and latent class membership are carried out in separate steps, and covariates and/or outcomes are treated as "auxiliary" variables. In the first step, the latent class measurement model is estimated without using the covariates and/or outcome. In the second step, bias-correction for misclassification is made. For example, in the method developed by Bolck et al. (2004) and modified by Vermunt (2010), also known as the Bolck, Croon, and Hagenaars (BCH) method, a class membership variable is created by using the posterior probabilities obtained in the first step and by incorporating the uncertainty of classification to correct the misclassification bias. In the final step, the bias-corrected most likely class is modeled as the outcome of the covariates or as a predictor of a distal outcome. More details of these three-step methods can be found elsewhere (Bolck et al., 2004; Lanza et al., 2013; Vermunt, 2010).

According to simulation studies, the BCH three-step method generally performs as well as or better than the one-step method or other alternative three-step methods (e.g., Lanza et al., 2013) when the entropy is relatively high (entropy $\geq$ 0.6) for both small (100 or 200) and large ($\geq$ 500) samples (Asparouhov & Muthén, 2014; Bakk, Oberski et al., 2016; Bakk et al., 2013; No & Hong, 2018). The one-step method can be used, but extra caution should be taken when the latent class solution changes with and without the predictors or outcomes (Asparouhov & Muthén, 2014). The development of methods for estimating latent class regression models is an active area of research, and methods are continuously being developed and modified. Currently, the BCH method and Lanza et al.'s (2013) method are both implemented in Mplus (Muthén & Muthén, 2014).

Longitudinal Latent Variable Mixture Models

This section focuses on mixture modeling applied to longitudinal data. The goal of longitudinal mixture modeling is to categorize individuals into subgroups characterized by different patterns of changes based on their responses to the same measure assessed over time (i.e., repeated measures). Conventional latent growth modeling (LGM) is discussed first followed by discussion of growth mixture modeling (GMM) because LGM introduces the foundations for modeling trajectories and is considered a special case of GMM.

Latent Growth Curve Modeling

LGM is essentially a confirmatory factor analysis with mean structure. Observed variables assessed repeatedly over time are the indicators of latent variables, referred to as growth factors. These growth factors are the parameters of individual trajectories. A path diagram of a linear growth curve model is shown in Figure 8.1, where the observed variable Y (i.e., $Y_1 - Y_5$) is measured across five time points.

The factor loadings relating the repeated measures and latent factors determine the trajectory shapes. In any functional trajectory form, the factor loadings on the intercept factor (denoted as Intercept in Figure 8.1) are all set to be 1. Specification of the loadings on the slope factor (denoted as Slope in Figure 8.1) is determined by the time scale and hypothesized trajectory shape.

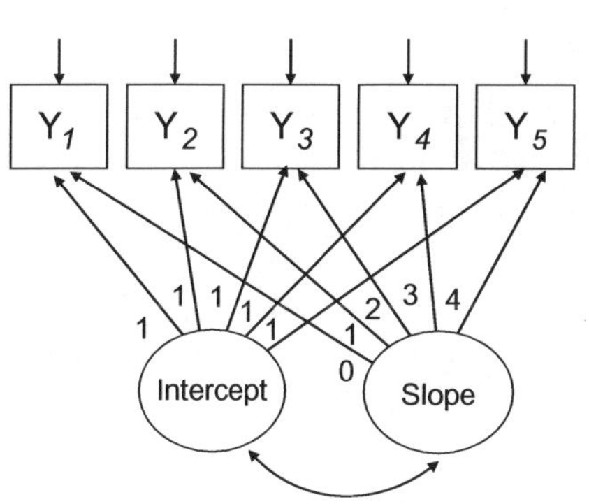

Figure 8.1 *Path diagram for a latent growth curve model specifying a linear trajectory on the variable Y assessed across five time points (Y_1–Y_5). Intercept: Intercept factor; Slope: Slope factor.*

In Figure 8.1, a linear growth curve is modeled by specifying the factor loadings on the slope factor at values increasing linearly, i.e., [0 1 2 3 4]. The value of 0 in the slope factor loading defines the meaning of the intercept factor. In the above example, the slope factor loading of Y_1 is fixed to 0, modeling the intercept factor to capture the mean and the variance of Y at the first assessment (Y_1). This specification also reflects assessments with equal intervals. If the interval between the first and second assessments is half of the other intervals (e.g., baseline, 6-month, 18-month, 30-month, 42-month), the time scale is specified as [0 1 3 5 7], indicating that the interval between Time 1 and Time 2 is half the length of intervals between later waves.

In LGM, the means and the variances of the latent factors have special meaning. The mean of the intercept factor estimates the level of Y at the time point specified as 0 in the slope factor loading, and the variance estimates individual differences in the level at that time point. The mean of the slope factor captures the change rate per time unit. If the time interval is one year, it indicates the increase/decrease expected per year. In our example with unequal intervals, i.e., [0 1 3 5 7], the mean of the slope indicates the change rate per six months. The variance of the slope factor estimates individual differences in the change rate: Some individuals may show greater changes, while other individuals may show no changes or relatively small changes. The covariance between the growth factors reflects how an individual's response level estimated by the intercept factor is related to his/her rate of change. When the variances of the growth factors are significant, predictors can be introduced to explain the individual differences in the intercept and the slope factors.

Modeling trajectory shapes in LGM is quite flexible. If the trajectory is expected to take a quadratic form, a second growth factor is added to the model, and the factor loadings are specified as the squared values of the time scaling of the linear factor. For the model in Figure 8.1, the loadings on the added quadratic factor would be specified as [0 1 4 9 16]. Other types of nonlinear growth curved can be also modeled (Grimm et al., 2011). For example, latent basis growth models (McArdle & Epstein, 1987; Meredith & Tisak, 1990) are a type of growth curve models that provide flexible ways to determine the optimal growth trajectory, linear or non-linear. In these models, the first (Time 1) and the last (Time t) loadings of the slope factor are fixed to 0 and 1, respectively, while other loadings (Time 2 to Time $t-1$) are freely estimated. The mean of the slope factor estimates the total amount of change from Time 1 to Time t, and the estimated loadings indicate the amount of change up to a specific time point proportional to the total amount of change. Estimated factor loadings would suggest the trajectory shape that best describes the observed data. Much more details on LGM are available in several books (e.g., Bollen & Curran, 2005; Singer & Willet, 2003).

In the context of mixture modeling, LGM can be viewed as a GMM with one class, where the trajectories of all individuals take the same functional form. Different individuals may have different levels at baseline and different change

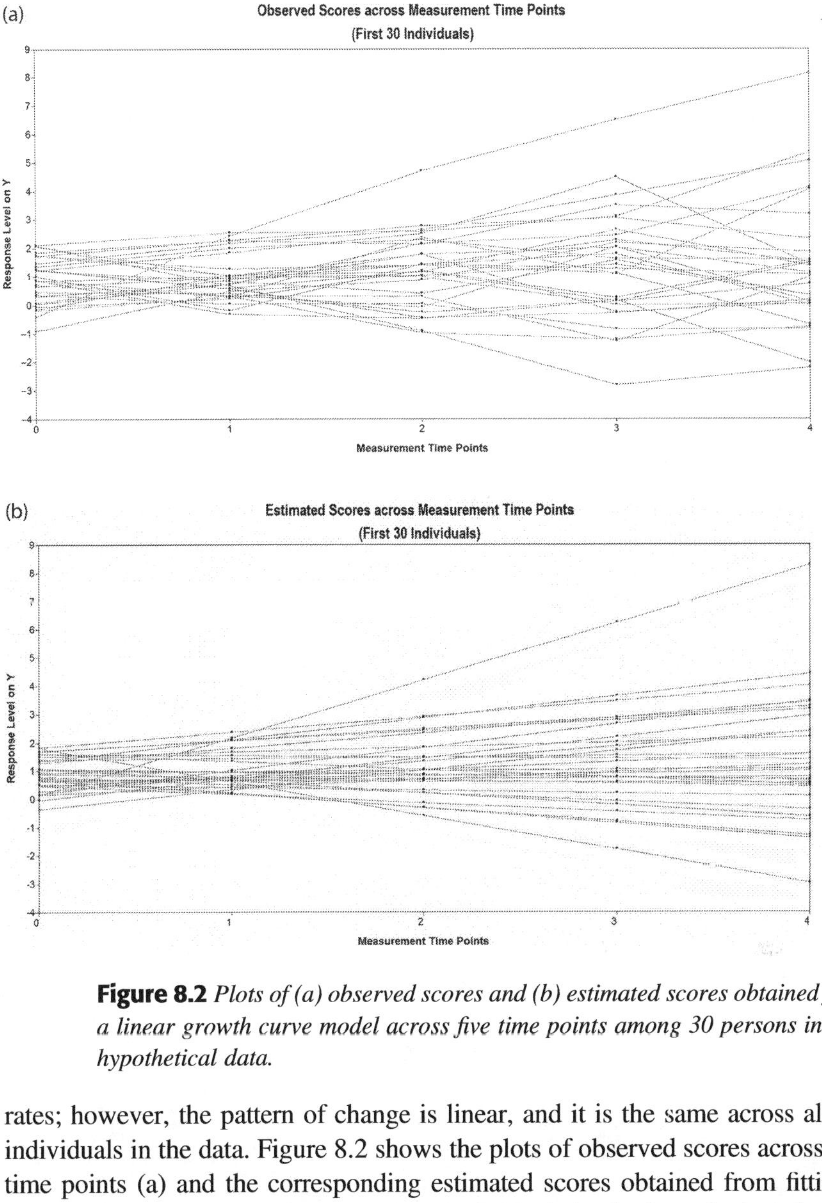

Figure 8.2 *Plots of (a) observed scores and (b) estimated scores obtained from a linear growth curve model across five time points among 30 persons in the hypothetical data.*

rates; however, the pattern of change is linear, and it is the same across all the individuals in the data. Figure 8.2 shows the plots of observed scores across five time points (a) and the corresponding estimated scores obtained from fitting a linear growth curve for a sample of 30 individuals in the hypothetical data. In panel (b), each straight line shows an individual person's trajectory estimated by the model. Different individuals have different magnitudes of the slope, but the functional form is all linear.

Growth Mixture Modeling

GMM (Muthén, 2001; Muthén & Muthén, 2000) combines the features of LGM and latent class growth analysis (LCGA). In LCGA, latent class membership is defined based on the trajectory shapes, using a single observed variable measured at multiple time points. For example, in a two-class model, one class may show linear growth, and the other may show quadratic growth. Posterior probabilities to be in each of the latent classes are computed for all individuals, and their most likely class membership is determined by each individual's highest posterior probability. In LCGA, means of the growth factors are estimated. However, within-class individual differences in the growth factors are not allowed, and the variances of the growth factors within each class are set to be 0 (Nagin, 2005). By comparison, GMM estimates both means and variances of the growth factors. Individuals in the same class are expected to show the same functional form of growth trajectory, but they are allowed to differ in their levels defined by the intercept factor and their change rates. Individuals in different classes are assumed to have different functional trajectory forms (e.g., linear vs. quadratic), and the variances and covariances of growth factors are also allowed to be different between the two latent classes.

When mixture modeling is conducted with longitudinal data, researchers should determine the functional form of change patterns. Deciding the functional form is important because it serves as the base for LGCA or GMM. Theory and prior studies can inform the functional forms. Inspecting the plots of individuals' observed scores can also provide insights about functional form. According to the plots in panel (a) in Figure 8.2, a linear trajectory may fit well for some individuals, but a quadratic trajectory may fit well for others. Thus, one may start with a linear trajectory and add a quadratic factor to the model. Once the trajectory shape is decided, the number of latent classes should be determined either based on theory and prior studies or taking an exploratory approach or both. Inspection of model fit statistics and classification diagnostics discussed for LCA and LPA models apply to GMM and LCGA as well.

Estimation of class membership can be quite complicated in GMM, with the increased number of parameters and the uncertainty of classification into group membership. Consequently, it is common to place additional parameter constraints to aid model estimation (Bauer & Curran, 2003; Muthén, 2001). The same functional form of change can be imposed across latent classes. Additionally, the variances and covariances of the growth factors and/or the residuals of the observed repeated measures can be equated across classes when the latent classes are expected to be different only in their trajectories (Muthén, 2001). Further, the variances of the growth factors can be constrained to be 0 across all classes, resulting in a LCGA model (Nagin, 2005). Imposing parameter constraints in the variances and covariances may help model identification; however, such constraints should be placed based on theory and prior studies.

Person-Centered Mediation Analysis

Mediation analysis is a family of methods suitable for assessing the underlying mechanisms of the relation between the predictor and the outcome

(MacKinnon, 2002; Sobel, 1982). The independent variable X is modeled to predict the mediator M ("a-path"), and the mediator is modeled to predict the outcome Y ("b-path") (see MacKinnon et al., 2002, for various approaches for testing mediation). In conventional mediation analysis, the population is assumed to be homogeneous for all variables in the mediation model, and the relations among X, M, and Y are assumed to hold for all individuals. When mediation analysis is conducted in a mixture modeling framework, it is assumed that distinctive subgroups of individuals exist that show different response patterns on the mediator and/or the outcome variables as a function of the independent variable. Latent class membership can be estimated using the models described in previous sections.

Studies applying LCA to mediation analysis (e.g., Hsiao et al., 2020; Witkiewitz et al., 2018) identified latent classes of the mediator and the outcome separately based on their response patterns on the relevant indicators. For example, to examine the latent classes of coping as a mediator in the relation between a combined behavioral intervention and AUD treatment outcomes, Witkiewitz et al. (2018) identified the latent classes of coping skills and the latent classes of drinking outcomes, using the data from the COMBINE (Combined Pharmacotherapies and Behavioral Interventions for Alcohol Dependence) study (Anton et al., 2006). Based on the endorsement patterns to 40 coping skills items, they identified three latent classes distinguished by the ranges and frequencies of coping skills used by individuals: narrow, moderate, and broad repertoire coping classes. Three drinking outcome classes were also identified: low heavy drinking/low consequence, occasional heavy drinking/moderate consequence, and frequent heavy drinking/high consequence. A series of multinomial regression analyses found that receiving the combined behavioral intervention (versus medication management) was associated with a higher likelihood of being in the broad coping repertoire class, as compared to the low repertoire class. Being in the broad repertoire class, in turn, predicted greater probability of being in the low heavy drinking/low consequences class or the occasional heavy drinking/moderate consequences class, rather than frequent heavy drinking/high consequences class.

Expanding the parallel process LGM approach to mediation (Cheong, 2011; Cheong et al., 2003), Cheong et al. (2009) applied GMM to mediation analysis using the data from a prevention study for adolescent drug use (Midwestern Prevention Project; Pentz et al., 1990). The mediator variable was peer norms of accepting alcohol use measured across three time points, and the outcome was monthly alcohol use measured across seven time points. Figure 8.3 presents the path diagram for GMM mediation model. The mediator latent classes and the outcome latent classes (denoted by C_M and C_Y) were identified based on the trajectory models as linear. For the mediator, two trajectory classes were identified: a risk trajectory class showing high peer alcohol norms at baseline with rapid increase and a low-risk trajectory class showing low peer norms at baseline with slow increase. Similar trajectory classes were identified for the outcome.

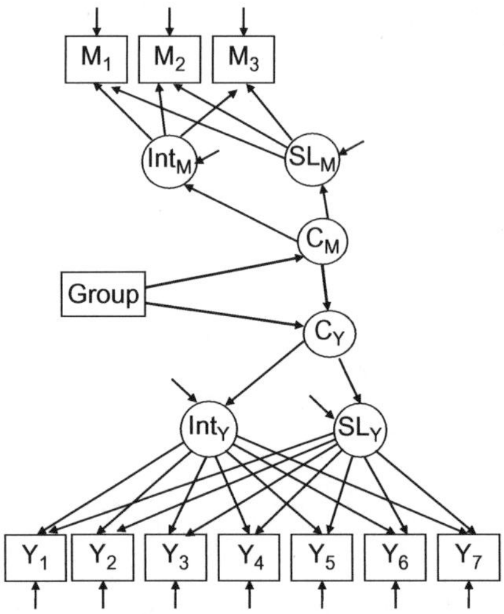

Figure 8.3 *Path diagram for growth mixture mediation model. Group: Treatment group (intervention vs. control); Int_M: Intercept factor of the mediator trajectory; SL_M: Slope factor of the mediator trajectory; Int_Y: Intercept factor of the outcome trajectory; SL_M: Slope factor of the outcome trajectory; C_M: Latent trajectory class of mediator; and C_Y: Latent trajectory class of outcome.*

The results showed that the adolescents in the treatment group, compared to those in the control group, were more likely to be in the low-risk mediator trajectory class than the risk trajectory class. In turn, adolescents in the low-risk mediator trajectory class were more likely to be in the low-risk outcome trajectory class than the risk trajectory class.

When mixture modeling is applied to mediation analysis, the mediational pathways are examined in the relations between the independent variable and the mediator class membership and the relation between the mediator class membership and the outcome class membership. In the two studies described above, the independent variable X was an observed variable, i.e., treatment group membership. One can hypothesize that receiving the treatment is expected to shift or change the class membership of the mediator, which, in turn, is expected to shift or change the class membership of the outcome. The key component here is to identify a "good" reference class representing the absence or lack of the influence of X. For example, with the data from intervention/prevention studies, it is desirable to identify a latent class representing the typical response patterns of the control group, so that the probability of being in the other class can be compared to the probability of being in the normative, control class. Obviously, as the number of latent classes increases, estimation of the mediated effect becomes quite intensive because many comparisons need to be made for testing both the a-paths and the b-paths. As with other mixture modeling applications, identifying the optimal number of latent classes that are meaningful is a critical part of mediation analysis as well, and the role of theory and prior studies becomes crucial. Finally, when estimating the a-paths and b-paths, the three-step methods (Bolck et al., 2004; Vermunt, 2010) can be used, as a series of simulation studies showed that they yield unbiased estimates of the mediated effects (Hsiao et al., 2020).

Conclusions and Recommendations

This chapter provided an overview of the finite mixture modeling approach and its application to both cross-sectional and longitudinal data analysis, as well as the application of mixture modeling to mediation analysis. The goal was to provide a basic foundational knowledge of finite mixture modeling and aid alcohol researchers in generating research questions and hypotheses that are suitable for person-centered analyses. For that reason, detailed technical aspects of mixture modeling were omitted. While finite mixture modeling has become quite popular as an analytic tool in addressing sophisticated research questions, methodologists have cautioned against the careless use of these methods, mainly because it is not possible to directly test whether there are distinctive subgroups in the population or to prove that the latent classes obtained in the analyses are true population classes (Bauer & Curran, 2003; Masyn, 2013). The role of theory and prior studies is therefore critically important in applying these methods.

Although the true classes cannot be tested directly, it is possible to identify the optimal number of meaningful and interpretable classes that could be replicated. One way to achieve this is to avoid insufficient sample sizes. Small samples can cause convergence problems, yield improper solutions, and/or fail to identify small but meaningful classes (Berlin, Parra et al., 2014). Determining sample size and achieving reasonable statistical power to identify true classes is complicated, as this is affected by a variety of factors, such as the degree of class separation (i.e., distinctiveness of latent classes), the number of classes in the population, the number of class indicators, and the reliability of the indicators (Berlin, Parra et al., 2014; Tein et al., 2013). Although methodological research is sparse to guide determining optimal sample sizes, a Monte Carlo simulation function has been implemented in some software programs (e.g., Mplus; Muthén & Muthén, 1998–2017). Thus, statistical power of a study at hand can be checked using the parameter estimates obtained from the data (Berlin, Williams et al., 2014).

Another practical consideration to improve class enumeration is the choice of latent class indicators. It is important to choose validated measures, i.e., established scales shown to have good psychometric properties, to reduce the measurement errors, as they tend to underestimate within-class parameters (Kim et al., 2020) and reduce the precision of estimates of growth parameters (Singer & Willet, 2003). In addition, the number of latent class indicators or the number of measurement occasions can be increased to more accurately estimate the latent classes based on the response patterns on the multiple indicators or repeated measures.

Interested readers are encouraged to review the literature cited in this overview chapter of finite mixture modeling. Mixture modeling may be a particularly useful tool for future research on recovery pathways, given the underlying concept that different subgroups of people may follow diverse and dynamic pathways to recovery. Recent research by Witkiewitz and colleagues has used latent profile analysis to study recovery profiles in the COMBINE Study and Project MATCH data (Witkiewitz et al., 2019, 2020), as summarized in Chapter 1 (Tucker & Witkiewitz, this volume). Expanding latent profiles of recovery to longitudinal data could provide more nuanced information on individual trajectories of recovery over time.

References

Akaike, H. (1987). Factor analysis and AIC. *Psychometrika, 52*(3), 317–332. https://doi.org/10.1007/BF02294359

Anton, R. F., O'Malley, S. S., Ciraulo, D. A., Cisler, R. A., Couper, D., Donovan, D. M., Gastfriend, D. R., Hosking, J., Johnson, B., LoCastro, J., Longabaugh, R., Mason, B., Mattson, M., Miller, W. R., Pettinati, H; Randall, C., Swift, R., Weiss, R., Williams, L., & Zweben, A. (2006). Combined pharmacotherapies and behavioral interventions for alcohol dependence the COMBINE study: A randomized controlled trial. *JAMA, 295*(17), 2003–2017. https://doi.org/10.1001/jama.295.17.2003

Asparouhov, T., & Muthén, B. (2014). Auxiliary variables in mixture modeling: Three-step approaches using Mplus. *Structural Equation Modeling, 21*(3), 329–341. https://doi.org/10.1080/10705511.2014.915181

Bakk, Z., Oberski, D. L., & Vermunt, J. K. (2016). Relating latent class membership to continuous distal outcomes: Improving the LTB approach and a modified three-step implementation. *Structural Equation Modeling, 23*(2), 278–289. https://doi.org/10.1080/10705511.2015.1049698

Bakk, Z., Tekle, F. B., & Vermunt, J. K. (2013). Estimating the association between latent class membership and external variables using bias adjusted three-step approaches. *Sociological Methodology, 43*(1), 272–311. https://doi.org/10.1177/0081175012470644

Bandeen-roche, K., Miglioretti, D. L., Zeger, S. L., & Rathouz, P. J. (1997). Latent variable regression for multiple discrete outcomes. *Journal of the American Statistical Association, 92*(440), 1375–1386. https://doi.org/10.1080/01621459.1997.10473658

Bauer, D. J., & Curran, P. J. (2003). Distributional assumptions of growth mixture models: Implications for over extraction of latent trajectory classes. *Psychological Methods, 8*(3), 338–363. https://doi.org/10.1037/1082-989X.8.3.338

Berlin, K. S., Parra, G. R., & Williams, N. A. (2014). An introduction to latent variable mixture modeling (part 2): Longitudinal latent class growth analysis and growth mixture models. *Journal of Pediatric Psychology, 39*(2), 188–203. https://doi.org/10.1093/jpepsy/jst085

Berlin, K. S., Williams, N. A., & Parra, G. R. (2014). An introduction to latent variable mixture modeling (part 1): Overview of cross-sectional latent class and latent profile analyses. *Journal of Pediatric Psychology, 39*(2), 174–187. https://doi.org/10.1093/jpepsy/jst084

Beseler, C. L., Taylor, L. A., Kraemer, D. T., & Leeman, R. F. (2012). A latent class analysis of DSM-IV alcohol use disorder criteria and binge drinking in undergraduates. *AlcoholismClinical & Experimental Research, 36*(1), 153–161. https://doi.org/10.1111/j.1530-0277.2011.01595.x

Bolck, A., Croon, M. A., & Hagenaars, J. A. (2004). Estimating latent structure models with categorical variables: One-step versus three-step estimators. *Political Analysis, 12*(1), 3–27. https://doi.org/10.1093/pan/mph001

Bollen, K. A., & Curran, P. J. (2005). *Latent curve models: A structural equation perspective*. John Wiley & Sons.

Cahalan, D. (1970). *Problem drinkers: A national survey*. Jossey-Bass.

Cheong, J. (2011). Accuracy of estimates and statistical power for testing mediation in latent growth modeling. *Structural Equation Modeling, 18*(2), 195–211. https://doi.org/10.1080/10705511.2011.557334

Cheong, J., Khoo, S. T., & MacKinnon, D. P. (2009). *Growth mixture modeling in mediation: An application of mixture modeling to evaluation of mediating mechanisms in a randomized prevention trial*. Paper presented at the Annual Convention of the Society for Prevention Research, Washington, DC.

Cheong, J., Mackinnon, D. P., & Khoo, S. T. (2003). Investigation of mediational processes using parallel process latent growth curve modeling. *Structural Equation Modeling, 10*(2), 238–262. https://doi.org/10.1207/S15328007SEM1002_5

Clogg, C. C. (1995). Latent class models. In G. Arminger, C. C. Clogg, & M. E. Sobel (Eds.), *Handbook of statistical modeling for the social and behavioral sciences* (pp. 311–359). Springer.

Collins, L. M. (2006). Analysis of longitudinal data: The integration of theoretical model, temporal design, and statistical model. *Annual Review of Psychology, 57*, 505–528. https://doi.org/10.1146/annurev.psych.57.102904.190146

Collins, L. M., & Lanza, S. T. (2009). *Latent class and latent transition analysis: With applications in the social, behavioral, and health sciences*. Wiley.

Grimm, K. J., Ram, N., & Hamagami, F. (2011). Nonlinear growth curves in developmental research. *Child Development, 82*(5), 1357–1371. https://doi.org/10.1111/j.1467-8624.2011.01630.x

Hsiao, Y. Y., Kruger, E. S., Van Horn, M. L., Tofighi, D., MacKinnon, D. P., & Witkiewitz, K. (2020). *Latent class mediation: A comparison of six approaches. Multivariate Behavioral Research.* Advance online publication. https://doi.org/10.1080/00273171.2020.1771674

Kim, M., Van Horn, M. L., Jaki, T., Vermunt, J., Feaster, D., Lichstein, K. L., Taylor, D., Riedel, B., & Bush, A. (2020). Repeated measures regression mixture models. *Behavior Research Methods, 52*(2), 591–606. https://doi.org/10.3758/s13428–019-01257-7

Lanza, S. T., & Cooper, B. R. (2016). Latent class analysis for developmental research. *Child Development Perspective, 10*(1), 59–64. https://doi.org/10.1111/cdep.12163

Lanza, S. T., Tan, X., & Bray, B. C. (2013). Latent class analysis with distal outcomes: A flexible model-based approach. *Structural Equation Modeling, 20*(1), 1–26. https://doi.org/10.1080/10705511.2013.742377

Lau-Barraco, C., Braitman, A. L., Stamates, A. L., & Linden-Carmichael, A. N. (2017). A latent profile analysis of drinking patterns among nonstudent emerging adults. *Addictive Behaviors, 62*(10), 14–19. https://doi.org/10.1016/j.addbeh.2016.06.001

Laursen, B., & Hoff, E. (2006). Person-centered and variable-centered approaches to longitudinal data. *Merrill-Palmer Quarterly, 52*(3), 377–389. https://doi.org/10.1353/mpq.2006.0029

Lo, Y., Mendell, N., & Rubin, D. B. (2001). Testing the number of components in a normal mixture. *Biometrika, 88*(3), 767–778. https://doi.org/10.1093/biomet/88.3.767

Lubke, G., & Neale, M. (2006). Distinguishing between latent classes and continuous factors: Resolution by maximum likelihood. *Multivariate Behavioral Research, 41*(4), 499–532. https://doi.org/10.1207/s15327906mbr4104_4

MacKinnon, D. P., Lockwood, C. M., Hoffman, J. M., West, S. G., & Sheets, V. (2002). A comparison of methods to test mediation and other intervening variable effects. *Psychological Methods, 7*(1), 83–104. https://doi.org/10.1037/1082-989x.7.1.83

Magnusson, D. (2003). The person approach: Concepts, measurement models, and research strategy. In S. C. Peck & R. W. Roeser (Eds.), *New directions for child and adolescent development: Person-centered approaches to studying development in context* (pp. 3–23). Jossey-Bass.

Masyn, K. E. (2013). Latent class analysis and finite mixture modeling. In T. Little (Ed.), *Oxford handbook of quantitative methods* (pp. 551–611). Oxford University Press.

McArdle, J. J., & Epstein, D. (1987). Latent growth curves within developmental structural equation models. *Child Development, 58*(1), 110–133. https://doi.org/10.2307/1130295

McLachlan, G., & Peel, D. (2000). *Finite mixture models*. Wiley.

Meredith, W., & Tisak, J. (1990). Latent curve analysis. *Psychometrika, 55*(1), 107–122. https://doi.org/10.1007/BF02294746

Muthén, B. (2001). Second-generation structural equation modeling with a combination of categorical and continuous latent variables: New opportunities for latent class-latent growth modeling. In L. M. Collins & A. G. Sayer (Eds.), *New methods for the analysis of change* (pp. 289–322). American Psychological Association.

Muthén, B., & Muthén, L. (1998–2017). Mplus user's guide: Statistical analysis with latent variables. 8th ed. Muthén & Muthén.

(2000). Integrating person-centered and variable-centered analyses: Growth mixture modeling with latent trajectory classes. *Alcoholism: Clinical & Experimental Research, 24*(6), 882–891. https://doi.org/10.1111/j.1530-0277.2000.tb02070.x

Nagin, D. S. (2005). *Group-based modeling of development*. Harvard University Press.

No, U., & Hong, S. (2018). A comparison of mixture modeling approaches in latent class models with external variables under small samples. *Educational and Psychological Measurement, 78*(6), 925–951. https://doi.org/10.1177/0013164417726828

Nylund, K., Asparouhov, T., & Muthén, B. (2007). Deciding on the number of classes in latent class analysis and growth mixture modeling: A Monte Carlo simulation study. *Structural Equation Modeling, 14*(4), 535–569. https://doi.org/10.1080/10705510701575396

Pentz, M. A., Trebow, E. A., Hansen, W. B., MacKinnon, D. P., Dwyer, J. H., Johnson, C. A., Flay, B. R., Daniels, S., & Cormack, C. (1990). Effects of program implementation on adolescent drug use behavior: The Midwestern Prevention Project (MPP). *Evaluation Review, 14*(3), 264–289. https://doi.org/10.1177/0193841X9001400303

Reboussin, B. A., Ip, E. H., & Wolfson, M. (2008). Locally dependent latent class models with covariates: An application to under-age drinking in the USA. *Journal of Royal Statistical Society: Series A, 171*(4), 877–897. https://doi.org/10.1111/j.1467-985X.2008.00544.x

Rinker, D. V., & Neighbors, C. (2015). Latent class analysis of DSM-5 alcohol use disorder criteria among heavy-drinking college students. *Journal of Substance Abuse Treatment, 57*, 81–88. https://doi.org/10.1016/j.jsat.2015.05.006

Rogosa, D. (1988). Myths about longitudinal research. In K. W. Schaie, R. T. Campbell, W. Meredith, & S. C. Rawlings (Eds.), *Methodological issues in aging research* (pp. 171–209). Springer.

Schwartz, G. (1978). Estimating the dimension of a model. *The Annals of Statistics, 6*(2), 461–464. https://doi.org/10.1214/aos/1176344136

Sclove, L. (1987). Application of model-selection criteria to some problems in multivariate analysis. *Psychometrika, 52*(3), 333–343. https://doi.org/10.1007/BF02294360

Singer, J. D., & Willet, J. B. (2003). *Applied longitudinal data analysis: Modeling change and event occurrence*. Oxford University Press.

Skinner, H. A., & Horn, J. L. (1984). *Alcohol Dependence Scale (ADS) user's guide*. Addiction Research Foundation.

Sobel, M. E. (1982). Asymptotic confidence intervals for indirect effects in structural equation models. In S. Leinhardt (Ed.), *Sociological methodology* (pp. 290–312). American Sociological Association.

Tein, J., Coxe, S., & Cham, H. (2013). Statistical power to detect the correct number of classes in latent profile analysis. *Structural Equation Modeling, 20*(4), 640–657. https://doi.org/10.1080/10705511.2013.824781

Titterington, D. M., Smith, A. F. M., & Makov, U. E. (1985). *Statistical analysis of finite mixture distributions*. Wiley.

Torrance-Rynard, V. L., & Walter, S. D. (1997). Effects of dependent errors in the assessment of diagnostic test performance. *Statistics in Medicine, 16*(19), 2157–2175. https://doi.org/10.1002/(sici)1097-0258(19971015)16:19<2157::aid-sim653>3.0.co;2-x

Tucker, J. A., Cheong, J., James, T. G., Jung, S., & Chandler, S. D. (2020). Preresolution drinking problem severity profiles associated with stable moderation outcomes of natural recovery attempts. *Alcoholism: Clinical & Experimental Research, 44*(3), 738–745. https://doi.org/10.1111/acer.14287

Tucker, J. A., Vuchinich, R. E., Black, B. C., & Rippens, P. D. (2006). Significance of a behavioral economic index of reward value in predicting drinking problem resolutions. *Journal of Consulting and Clinical Psychology, 74*(2), 317–326. https://doi.org/10.1037/0022-006X.74.2.317

Vacek, P. M. (1985). The effect of conditional dependence on the evaluation of diagnostic tests. *Biometrics, 41*(4), 959–968. https://doi.org/10.2307/2530967

Vermunt, J. K. (2010). Latent class modeling with covariates: Two improved three-step approaches. *Political Analysis, 18*(4), 450–469. https://doi.org/10.1093/pan/mpq025

Willet, J. B. (1989). Some results on reliability for the longitudinal measurement of change: Implications for the design of studies of individual growth. *Educational and Psychological Measurement, 49*(3), 587–602. https://doi.org/10.1177/001316448904900309

Witkiewitz, K., Roos, C. R., Tofighi, D., & Van Horn, M. L. (2018). Broad coping repertoire mediates the effect of the Combined Behavioral Intervention on alcohol outcomes in the COMBINE Study: An application of latent class mediation. *Journal of Studies on Alcohol and Drugs, 79*(2), 199–207. https://doi.org/10.15288/jsad.2018.79.199

Witkiewitz, K., Wilson, A. D., Pearson, M. R., Montes, K. S., Kirouac, M., Roos, C., Hallgren, K. A., & Maisto, S. A. (2019). Profiles of recovery from alcohol use disorder at three years following treatment: Can the definition of recovery be extended to include high functioning heavy drinkers? *Addiction, 114*(1), 69–80. https://doi.org/10.1111/add.14403

Witkiewitz, K., Wilson, A. D., Roos, C. R., Swan, J. E., Votaw, V. R., Stein, E. R., Pearson, M., Edwards, K., Tonigan, J. S., Hallgren, K., Montes, K., Maisto, S., & Tucker, J. A. (2020). Can individuals with alcohol use disorder sustain non-abstinent recovery? Non-abstinent outcomes 10 years after alcohol use disorder treatment. *Journal of Addiction Medicine. Advance online publication.* https://doi.org/10.1097/adm.0000000000000760

Yeater, E. A., Witkiewitz, K., López, G., Ross, R. S., Vitek, K., & Bryan, A. (2018). Latent profile analysis of alcohol consumption and sexual attitudes among college women: Associations with sexual victimization risk. *Violence against Women, 24*(11), 1279–1298. https://doi.org/10.1177/1077801218787926

PART II

Meso Level: Understanding and Promoting Individual Behavior Change within Natural Environments

9 Natural Recovery from Alcohol Use Disorder

Patterns, Contexts, and the Behavioral Economics of Change

Jalie A. Tucker

Natural Recovery from Alcohol Use Disorder: Patterns, Contexts, and the Behavioral Economics of Change

Over four decades ago, Room (1977) described the "two worlds of alcohol problems" represented in the then segregated empirical literatures derived from clinical studies examining individuals with alcohol use disorder (AUD) and population-level surveys of drinkers. Whereas individuals recruited in clinical samples tended to have more serious alcohol-related problems, surveys revealed the heterogeneous nature of harmful alcohol use in the population, ranging from mild to severe. Surveys also showed that seeking help for alcohol-related problems was uncommon and that many persons resolved their problems without treatment. These population level relationships have been replicated numerous times over the ensuing decades (e.g., Armor & Meshkoff, 1983; Dawson et al., 2005; Fan et al., 2019; Kelly et al., 2017; Sobell et al., 1996). Fewer than 25 percent of persons with problems utilize alcohol-focused services, and more than 70 percent of problem resolutions occur outside the context of treatment (e.g., Fan et al., 2019; Sobell et al., 1996). Moreover, stable low-risk drinking (i.e., moderation) is a relatively more common outcome in untreated samples, in part because treatment-seeking is associated with higher problem severity (Fan et al., 2019; Tucker, 2002), and most treatments emphasize abstinence.

"Natural recovery" is thus the dominant pathway to the resolution of AUD in the population of persons with alcohol-related problems. This chapter summarizes what is known about natural recovery based on (1) older descriptive studies that typically were cross-sectional or retrospective designs focused on persons who had achieved stable natural recovery and (2) more recent longitudinal studies of the natural recovery process as persons with AUD sought to change on their own, with emphasis on a research program guided by behavioral economics. Collectively, this body of work revealed the heterogeneity of pathways to stable positive change that can involve abstinence or low-risk drinking, a perspective often not obvious in clinical research focused on evaluating outcomes of a single treatment episode. Treatment-assisted change is an important component of understanding recovery but in isolation provides an incomplete picture of the diversity of change processes and outcomes and the different trajectories and temporal course involved in overcoming AUD. The chapter concludes with a discussion of the implications of natural recovery research for promoting positive change and future research directions.

Descriptive Research on Natural Recovery

Descriptive studies documenting the natural recovery phenomenon, the characteristics of persons who achieved it, and the surrounding life contexts have been accruing since the 1970s (reviewed by Fillmore, 1988; Klingemann & Sobell, 2007; Klingemann et al., 2001; Mariezcurrena, 1994; Roizen et al., 1977; Sobell et al., 2000; Smart, 1976; Stall & Biernacki, 1986; Tucker, 2002; Tucker & King, 1999; Watson & Sher, 1998). Studies typically were either large cross-sectional surveys that included a subset of persons with AUD who evidenced positive change without treatment (e.g., Sobell et al., 1996) or smaller retrospective studies of persons who achieved natural recovery, often compared to those who recovered with assistance from formal AUD treatment or Alcoholics Anonymous (AA) (e.g., King & Tucker, 2000; Sobell et al., 1993; Tucker & Gladsjo, 1993; Tucker et al., 2002a).

Taken together, research over the past four decades has found that the following features are associated with successful natural recovery:

- Persons who achieve natural recovery tend to be middle aged, middle income or higher, with relatively less serious problems compared to treatment-seekers. But the great majority fulfill clinical diagnostic criteria for AUD, and natural recovery occurs even among persons with serious alcohol-related problems (e.g., Sobell et al., 1996).
- Drinking pathways to natural resolution are variable (e.g., King & Tucker, 2000). Change can be abrupt or gradual and, in either case, can entail initial abstinence or low-risk drinking without problems that is maintained over time. In some cases, a period of initial abstinence is followed by resumption of stable low-risk drinking or, conversely, a period of initial low-risk drinking is followed by stable long-term abstinence. The number of quit attempts before stable recovery is achieved is quite variable (e.g., Kelly et al., 2017). Some individuals succeed on their first quit attempt, whereas others make many failed attempts before they succeed.
- Stable natural recovery is often associated with surrounding environmental contexts characterized by increased negative events before a recovery attempt followed by increased positive events during the first year or so of maintenance (e.g., Tucker, et al., 2002a). The negative events often occur in areas impaired by drinking (e.g., interpersonal relationships; work, legal, or health problems), whereas the positive events often reflect improved interpersonal relations and positive health habit changes (e.g., better nutrition, increased physical activity, smoking cessation). Moreover, changes in the macro environment (e.g., geographic re-location) that reduce access to alcohol or other drug-use opportunities can result in sustained cessation of harmful use (e.g., Robins, 1993).

- Many persons who recover on their own view their problem as a bad habit rather than a disease and as not serious enough to warrant treatment, even though they fulfill AUD diagnostic criteria and recognize that drinking is causing life-health problems (e.g., King & Tucker, 2000; Simpson & Tucker, 2002; Tucker et al., 2004). Treatment is often perceived as stigmatizing, and there are multiple barriers to treatment utilization, such as time, cost, and inconvenience. Many who recover and participate in research have not previously told anyone about their recovery experience.

Longitudinal Studies of Natural Recovery

Despite abundant evidence that natural recovery is common, prospective studies of the contexts and processes involved are a relatively recent development and are important for several reasons. First, they can advance understanding about successful change in the absence of the confounding effects of interventions. Whether acknowledged or not, all intervention approaches have a "program theory" about the change process and seek to guide and influence participants as they attempt to change. In the United States treatment system, the historically dominant change theory promotes abrupt abstinence typically by removing persons with AUD from the environments in which their problems occur (e.g., via hospital-based or residential treatment). Even if not acknowledged, this arrangement makes achieving and maintaining abstinence the focal goal of treatment, typically to the detriment of addressing non-drinking behavior patterns and life contexts that are intertwined with AUD. This contrasts with the program theory and treatment goals guiding behavioral treatments that explicitly aim to reduce substance use by increasing engagement in rewarding alcohol-free alternatives (e.g., Murphy et al., 2019; Murphy et al., Chapter 10 this volume; Petry et al., 2017), which are in line with findings from natural recovery research.

Second, natural recovery studies offer an opportunity to study low-risk drinking, which is a more common outcome of natural than treatment-assisted recovery attempts and a preferred goal of many persons with AUD. Facilitating stable moderation requires evidence concerning suitable candidates, supportive contexts, and the behavioral processes involved, about which there have been few advances since the 1980s. Early research conducted largely with clinical samples identified pre-treatment predictors of moderation drinking outcomes, including lower alcohol dependence levels, fewer psychosocial problems related to drinking, and younger age or shorter problem duration, which tend to be confounded (Rosenberg, 1993). While useful as prognostic indicators of suitable candidates for a moderation drinking goal, this work added little to understanding the contexts and behavior change processes involved in achieving stable moderation. This is important for informing intervention development to facilitate moderation drinking and thereby expand services beyond abstinence-oriented treatments suitable for those with more severe problems to reach the majority of the AUD population with mild to moderate problems (Tucker & Simpson, 2011). Such advances should help close the gap between population need and service utilization and improve overall recovery rates in the population with AUD.

Third, studying successful change departs from the longstanding focus on AUD relapse determinants using clinical samples and directs much needed attention toward investigating individual, social, and other contextual factors that support beneficial change. This shift aligns with a strength-based approach to AUD recovery that emphasizes the role of "recovery capital" in understanding and promoting lasting change (Best et al., Chapter 16 this volume; Klingemann et al., 2001). The forces promoting positive change versus relapse are not parallel, and recovery is not merely the absence of heavy drinking or remission of AUD symptoms. As discussed in Chapter 1 of this volume (Tucker & Witkiewitz), recovery is a dynamic change process in which improved biopsychosocial functioning and life satisfaction are fundamental (Tucker & Witkiewitz, 2020; Witkiewitz et al., 2020).

The remainder of this chapter summarizes a program of process-oriented research on natural recovery guided by behavioral economics, with emphasis on understanding moderation apart from abstinence and relapse. This work addresses the research issues outlined above and is consistent with a revised model of recovery that focuses not only on changing drinking practices, but encompasses concern with personal resources and natural environmental contexts that motivate and stabilize recovery over time. Behavioral economics and its utility for understanding harmful alcohol use and AUD recovery are described, followed by discussion of findings from five prospective studies of natural recovery that revealed the multi-dimensional contexts favorable and unfavorable to achieving stable positive change.

Behavioral Economics and Applications to Harmful Substance Use and Recovery

Behavioral economic theory combines principles of operant psychology with those from economics to explain choice behavior, defined in terms of how available resources such as time, money, and effort are allocated to available activities and commodities in the context of choice. A large body of research spanning the basic to applied continuum shows that choices and resource allocation are generally made in ways that maximize benefits and minimize costs (Rachlin et al., 1981). For humans, the benefits of certain choices and resource allocation may occur in family, social, emotional, health, financial, educational, and occupational domains, among others. Costs include the time, effort, and monetary expenditures necessary to obtain access to valuable alcohol and alcohol-free reinforcers, the opportunity costs that result from foregoing one reinforcer when another is chosen, and any associated physical or emotional discomfort.

A fundamental finding is that preference for a given activity or commodity depends on other available activities and commodities in the choice context and on the relative constraints on access to each of them. For example, alcoholic beverages are readily available with minimal constraints in most natural environments, whereas access to alcohol-free activities and commodities tend to be more variable at different costs and delays. Delay to reward availability is a critical determinant of choice. Referred to as delay discounting, this is a trans-species tendency to devalue delayed rewards according to a hyperbolic discount function (Ainslie & Herrnstein, 1981). This means that in choices between sooner smaller rewards (e.g., alcohol or drug use) and later larger rewards (e.g., valuable alcohol-free activities and commodities), the later larger reward will be preferred when both rewards are temporally distant. But when access to the sooner smaller reward becomes imminent, an abrupt preference shift typically occurs in favor of it. Moreover, some individuals, including those with AUD, tend to devalue delayed rewards to a greater extent than others, and their choice behavior is more sensitive to the effects of delay (Bickel et al., 2014).

This temporal dynamic and the choice context defined by reward availability and cost are central to the behavioral economic model of harmful substance use, which is characterized by preference shifts over time between substance use, harmful use, and abstinence (Vuchinich, 1995; Vuchinich & Heather, 2003). The perspective is well suited to studying harmful substance use because the primary problem is excessive demand for the substance over time. Harmful use is viewed as a reinforcer pathology (Bickel et al., 2014) that involves persistent preference for drug rewards that provide immediate reinforcement (euphoric, stimulant, anxiolytic, or analgesic effects) but longer-term costs in important life-health domains (e.g., good health, educational and vocational success). This can be contrasted with drug-free alternatives that typically have lower short-term but higher long-term value.

Conversely, behavioral economics conceptualizes recovery as foregoing the immediate rewarding *act* of drinking – and its attendant longer term negative consequences – in favor of *behavior patterns* that offer delayed alcohol-free rewards of higher value that in turn reinforce sobriety behaviors (Rachlin, 1995; Vuchinich, 1995; Vuchinich & Tucker, 1996). Research has shown that substance use is most likely when (1) the immediate costs of use are low with few constraints on access, (2) the choice environment offers limited rewarding substance-free alternatives, and (3) individuals have a relatively greater tendency to prefer immediate rather than delayed rewards (Bickel et al., 2014; Vuchinich, 1995; cf. Murphy et al., Chapter 10 and Yurasek et al., Chapter 15 this volume). In contrast, limiting access to substances and enriching the environment with rewarding substance-free alternatives reduces use (Carroll et al., 2001; Murphy et al., 2019). Furthermore, individuals who organize their choices over longer future intervals and engage in behavior patterns that increase the probability of receiving valuable delayed substance-free rewards should have a relatively higher probability of initiating and maintaining recovery (Tucker et al., 2012). This analysis leads to the overarching BE recovery hypothesis: *Recovery from alcohol problems requires a temporal shift from a shorter to a longer view of the future and entails shifts in resource allocation away from drinking and toward valuable delayed non-drinking rewards, which reinforce and stabilize the shifted recovery behavior patterns.*

Measurement Issues in a Behavioral Economic Analysis of Recovery

Another generalization from behavioral economic research is that preference for a given activity or commodity is inferred from the relative resources allocated to obtain it over time (Herrnstein, 1970; Vuchinich et al., 1988). This "molar" level of analysis focuses on identifying regularities between environmental conditions and behavior patterns over extended intervals and is well suited for conceptualizing and investigating addictive behaviors, which unfold over time and typically involve variable behavioral patterning spread over months to years as individuals transition through problem development, maintenance, remission, and, for some, relapse. Adopting a molar level of analysis with humans requires two measurement features: (1) Environment-behavior relationships should be assessed over sufficiently long intervals that encompass many relevant choices so that behavioral patterning can be discerned and (2) because different activities and commodities in people's lives vary considerably in their topographical characteristics, a common metric is needed that reflects relative resource allocation to and thus the relative reinforcement value of drinking compared to other substance-free choice alternatives.

Pursuing a behavioral economic analysis of recovery involved considerable methodological development to translate basic science findings into meaningful research questions in the natural environments in which human drinking problems occur. We developed a comprehensive measure of preference based on proportional resource allocation to alcohol versus other activities and commodities assessed over months to years. In early work, we focused on time allocation to different activities using daily prospective self-monitoring (Tucker et al., 1991). Because of the data collection burden this placed on participants, we also developed an interview-based retrospective data collection approach using an expanded Timeline Followback (TLFB) interview (Sobell & Sobell, 1992; Vuchinich & Tucker, 1996; Vuchinich et al., 1988). As used in our prospective natural recovery studies, the expanded TLFB comprehensively assessed participants' monetary allocation patterns during the year before and the year after a recent drinking quit attempt using commodity classes derived from US federal Consumer Expenditure Surveys (www.bls.gov/cex/). The assessment was based on financial records provided by participants, and additional interview reports were collected using TLFB interviewing techniques.

Income in dollars was reported by source (e.g., paid work, unemployment benefits, pensions, loans). Expenditures were reported in three general categories, each with subcategories. These included housing (e.g., mortgage, rent, utilities), consumable goods (e.g., food, tobacco, alcohol), and other expenditures (e.g., entertainment, transportation, loan payments, money saved). Reports in each commodity class typically involved many transactions throughout the assessment interval, which were summed to obtain category totals for analysis. In addition to direct verification using financial records (e.g., Vuchinich & Tucker, 1996), internal consistency and reliability checks on participants' reports of monetary allocation patterns supported their accuracy (e.g., Tucker et al., 2006, 2007).

This comprehensive measurement scheme added new information about problem severity and had incremental utility in predicting outcomes of resolution attempts (Tucker et al., 2009). The approach differs from the longstanding convention in the field to assess and represent drinking problem severity using topographical features of drinking practices (quantity/frequency indices) and associated symptoms that reflect direct negative consequences of heavy drinking (e.g., tolerance, dependence, psychosocial problems), per clinical diagnostic systems such as the *Diagnostic and Statistical Manual of Mental Disorders* (DSM-5, American Psychiatric Association, 2013).

Project ARC: Alcohol Recovery in Community

We used this measurement approach in five separate prospective studies of natural recovery attempts conducted over a 23-year data collection interval (Tucker et al., 2002b, 2006, 2008, 2012, 2016). Shared research features included the behavioral economic framework and methods, enrollment of community-dwelling problem drinkers attempting to recover on their own, and prospective designs that involved at least a 1-year follow-up after the initial onset of abstinence or low-risk drinking (NIAAA, 2005). The expanded TLFB interview conducted at enrollment and the 1-year follow-up assessed drinking practices, income, and expenditures covering the preceding year and produced detailed behavioral records covering the two years surrounding sobriety onset.

In addition to publications of individual study findings (e.g., Tucker et al., 2002b, 2006, 2007, 2008, 2012, 2016), we integrated the five studies to obtain sufficiently large groups of drinkers with different outcomes to address research questions aimed at understanding the contexts, processes, and patterns of behavior change associated with stable moderation outcomes compared to stable abstinence or unstable resolution involving relapse. We were guided by Marlatt's (1985; pp. 329–344) early theorizing that moderation involved a different behavioral regulation process compared to abstinence and relapse. Marlatt viewed abstinence and relapse as opposite ends of the same dynamic behavioral regulation process, reflecting over- and under-control of the daily act of drinking, respectively. In contrast, moderation depended on lifestyle balance and repetitive choices to drink well within the boundaries of extreme restraint or loss-of-control drinking. Translating this "differential regulation" hypothesis into behavioral economic terms, two primary hypotheses were evaluated using the integrated Project ARC data set:

- *Pre-resolution hypothesis:* Even when drinking heavily, the subset of persons with AUD who achieve stable moderation will exercise relatively more self-regulation of drinking and spending compared to other outcome groups.

- *Post-resolution hypothesis:* Recovery entails a shift in resource allocation away from drinking toward valuable delayed non-drinking rewards, which reinforce and stabilize the shifted recovery behavior patterns. Shifts will be distinctive for moderation drinkers compared to those who abstain or relapse, who will show similarities.

In all studies, community-dwelling problem drinkers in the Southeastern US were recruited using media advertisements and enrolled soon after stopping heavy drinking without treatment, either resolved abstinent (RA) or resolved non-abstinent (RNA) (Sobell et al., 1996). Eligibility screening included assessment of pre-resolution drinking practices, alcohol dependence levels, and alcohol-related life-health problems. More than 600 eligible participants were enrolled (N = 616, 67 percent male, 65 percent white, mean age = 46.5 years), and 73 percent had a 1-year follow-up assessment (n = 448). Almost all participants (99 percent) met then-current DSM criteria for alcohol dependence and had a mean problem duration of 16.6 years. Reports of drinking and help-seeking status were verified by collateral informants or internal reliability checks of participant reports. Expenditure reports were partially verified with financial records and were inflation-adjusted. Evidence of unreliable reporting was grounds for exclusion from the data analyses (< 1 percent).

Two sets of data analyses addressed the two main hypotheses. In both instances, drinking status codes were assigned based on the entire post-resolution year (i.e., terminal 1-year drinking status) as well as based on shorter intervals (e.g., 4-month quadrimesters) for select analyses. Terminal status codes at 1-year were: (1) unstable resolution (UR – 1 or more relapses defined as daily drinking in excess of NIAAA [2020] heavy drinking thresholds [4+/5+ drinks for women/men]; n = 140); (2) resolved non-abstinent (RNA – lower risk drinking only, no relapses to heavy drinking or alcohol-related problems; n = 80), and (3) resolved abstinent (RA – continuous abstinence, n = 273). The same criteria were used for drinking status codes for shorter post-resolution intervals. The UR and RNA 1-year outcome groups had good separation above or within low-risk drinking guidelines (NIAAA, 2005), respectively.

Pre-Resolution Predictors of 1-Year Drinking Outcomes

We hypothesized that even when drinking heavily, problem drinkers with more balanced monetary allocation patterns, indicative of greater sensitivity to longer-term contingencies, would be more successful in maintaining moderation than those with less-balanced patterns. To evaluate this hypothesis, participant reports of pre-resolution year expenditures were separated into obligatory and discretionary categories. Obligatory expenditures were for essential, ongoing, and largely fixed costs of living (e.g., for housing, transportation, health care, taxes and loans, automatic payroll deductions). Discretionary expenditures were for less essential commodities that could be purchased intermittently (i.e., entertainment, recreation, alcohol, tobacco, other consumable goods, gifts, and money saved

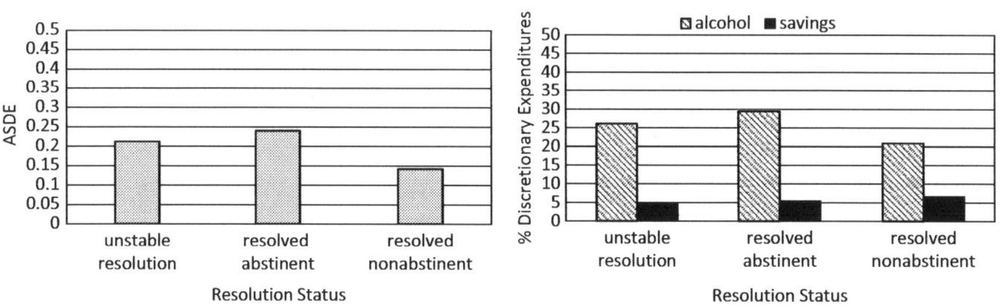

Figure 9.1 *Pre-resolution monetary expenditures as a function of drinking status at 1-year. The left panel shows the Alcohol-Savings Discretionary Expenditure (ASDE) index as a function of resolution status computed as the proportion of discretionary expenditures spent on drinking minus the proportion put into savings. Smaller ASDE values reflect longer time horizons as indexed by relatively greater proportional allocation to savings than to alcohol. The right panel shows the interaction among ASDE components (mean proportion allocated to alcohol vs. mean proportion allocated to savings).*

voluntarily) and were the focus of study because preferences for drinking should be readily expressed in this economic arena. Of primary interest were the proportions of pre-resolution discretionary spending on alcoholic beverages versus voluntary savings for future use, which were conceptualized as representing the value of rewards available over shorter and longer time horizons, respectively. The "Alcohol-Savings Discretionary Expenditure" (ASDE) index was computed for analysis as the proportion of discretionary expenditures spent on drinking minus the proportion of discretionary expenditures put into savings. Relatively greater allocation to savings than to drinking, reflected in lower ASDE values, was indicative of greater relative preferences for delayed rewards made possible by savings compared with more immediate drinking rewards.

As reported in Tucker et al. (2020) and shown in Figure 9.1, the pre-resolution ASDE hypothesis was supported ($p < 0.05$). Persons who maintained moderation drinking for one year (RNA group) had more balanced discretionary expenditure allocations to alcohol vs. savings and significantly lower ASDE values compared with those who abstained or relapsed (RA and UR groups, respectively), who did not differ significantly. This indicates greater sensitivity to future consequences among the RNA outcome group even when drinking heavily.

Additional Project ARC analyses evaluated whether multiple pre-resolution problem severity indicators formed distinctive latent profiles (Tucker et al., 2020) based on four problem severity indicators (drinking practices, alcohol dependence levels, alcohol-related life-health problems, and the ASDE index). Latent profile membership was then used to predict 1-year drinking outcomes. A 4-profile solution was obtained: (1) global low-risk on all indicators, (2) global high-risk on all indicators, (3) high-risk limited to drinking practices only, and

(4) high-risk limited to alcohol dependence and alcohol-related problems only. Outcomes differed by profile membership ($p < 0.01$). Multinomial logistic regression analyses showed that both the global low-risk profile and the heavy drinking risk only profile were associated with stable moderation during the post-resolution year. The high dependence and alcohol problems risk profile was associated with both abstinence and relapse during the 1-year follow-up ($ps < 0.05$).

Thus, consistent with prior clinical research (Rosenberg, 1993), moderation was associated with fewer alcohol-related problems and lower dependence levels, as well as with lower alcohol reinforcement value. Participants who simply drank heavily and did not have elevated risk on other indicators also had a higher probability of stable moderation. These findings suggest that greater alcohol consumption in isolation should not be used to predict failure to drink moderately, nor should lower consumption in isolation be used to predict successful moderation. Moderation was better predicted based on lower alcohol dependence, fewer functional problems related to drinking, and favorable financial allocation patterns per the ASDE index.

Contrary to clinical research, the composite quantity-frequency measure of drinking practices used in these analyses did not predict outcomes (i.e., "days well-functioning" defined as abstinent and gender-adjusted low-risk drinking days combined). Therefore, additional analyses examined different dimensions of drinking practices as predictors of 1-year outcomes (Cheong et al., 2020) that reflected either mean levels or variability in pre-resolution drinking practices (frequency of heavy drinking days, quantities consumed per drinking day, variability in days between heavy drinking days, and variability in quantities consumed per drinking day). Based on Marlatt's (1985) differential regulation hypothesis, relatively less variability in pre-resolution drinking patterns should predict low-risk drinking outcomes, even though mean consumption levels were high. This contrasts with conventional views that lower consumption levels prior to a quit attempt should predict low-risk drinking compared to abstinent or relapse outcomes.

Consistent with Marlatt's hypothesis, multinomial logistic regression models showed that variability in alcohol consumed per drinking day was the only significant predictor of 1-year outcomes when all dimensions were evaluated together. The RNA group showed less fluctuation in quantities consumed on pre-resolution drinking days compared to the groups that abstained or relapsed ($ps < 0.05$). Thus, problem drinkers who achieved stable moderation limited their quantities consumed prior to resolution within a relatively narrow range, a pattern they maintained post-recovery at much lower mean consumption levels. This suggests that assessing variability in quantities consumed may aid drinking goal selection.

Overall, the pre-resolution findings showed that the spending and drinking patterns of participants who maintained moderation differed from those of participants who maintained abstinence or relapsed and who exhibited similar behavior patterns. Even when drinking heavily, the RNA group showed relatively greater sensitivity to future outcomes with respect to proportional spending on alcohol vs. savings and kept their consumption quantities both pre- and post-resolution within a relatively tighter band of variability. By comparison, less balanced discretionary spending patterns and episodic heavy drinking (binging) were associated with both RA and UR outcomes.

Post-Resolution Shifts in Monetary Allocation and Associations with Drinking

Although all outcome groups were predicted to show some shifts in favor of spending on non-drinking rewards after stopping heavy drinking, the shifts in the moderation group were predicted to involve greater variability in spending and result in higher value "consumption bundles" that reinforced sobriety behaviors and included some limited drinking without problems. A consumption bundle refers to the collection of all goods and services consumed by an individual and generates a total utility function that measures the satisfaction a consumer receives from consumption of goods and services (Krugman & Well, 2012).

Although useful as a pre-resolution outcome predictor, the ASDE index is not as useful as a post resolution metric because most participants attempting recov ery greatly reduce their spending on alcohol, even those who relapse intermittently. Therefore, we used the pre-resolution year ASDE index as a covariate in longitudinal analyses that examined post-resolution monetary expenditures in all major commodity classes in relation to drinking. We identified the subset of classes that showed significant spending-drinking outcome associations with respect to 1-year outcomes and over shorter intervals during the post-resolution year (Tucker et al., 2021). Graphs showed the clearest associations between post-resolution drinking and spending using 4-month data aggregation intervals (quadrimesters). Longitudinal models evaluated whether changes in quadrimester spending predicted drinking status at 1-year using the RNA outcome group as the referent. Commodity classes with significant spending-outcome associations were further examined using cross-lagged models that identified when differences occurred during the post-resolution year.

Significant spending-outcome associations were found for alcoholic beverages, consumable goods, gifts, entertainment, financial/legal affairs, and housing/durable goods/insurance. Spending on alcoholic beverages decreased pre/post-resolution from 6 percent to $<$ 1 percent of all expenditures, as expected given that participants had initiated a serious quit attempt. Among the other commodity categories associated with drinking, the largest categories that together accounted for $>$ 80 percent of post-resolution expenditures were housing, durable goods, and associated insurance (45.7 percent of expenditures); financial/legal affairs (28.8 percent); and consumable goods other than alcohol (13.0 percent). Gifts given to others and entertainment each accounted for $<$ 5 percent of spending.

As hypothesized, the longitudinal analyses indicated that the spending patterns of RNA participants differed both interval-to-interval and over the entire post-resolution year from those of RA and UR participants, who were more similar.

The RNA group showed greater variability in spending patterns compared to other outcome groups. As noted earlier, their pre-resolution discretionary spending favored proportionately higher savings for the future than spending on alcohol compared to the RA and UR groups. But by mid-year after initial resolution, their overall spending was higher than the other outcome groups and had shifted in ways that entailed receipt of heretofore delayed large rewards (e.g., housing) that yield continued lifestyle benefits and involved some longer term financial commitments.

Compared to the RNA group, the RA and UR outcome groups had similar and less valuable post-resolution consumption bundles. Post-resolution, they spent relatively less overall and had less variability in their spending patterns. Furthermore, they tended to spend on smaller rewards (e.g., consumable goods, entertainment, gifts) throughout the post-resolution year, appearing to substitute alcohol with small, frequent substance-free rewards. But contrary to behavioral self-control programming, spending on small frequent rewards was not uniquely associated with stable resolution. Moreover, higher spending on consumable goods early in the post-resolution year was a negative prognostic indicator associated with UR status at one year.

Conclusions and Recommendations

The Project ARC findings are consistent with Marlatt's (1985) differential regulation hypothesis, framed here in behavioral economic terms, that the behavioral pathway to stable moderation is qualitatively different from the pathway to stable abstinence or relapse. In addition to the defining differences in drinking practices among outcome groups, moderation drinkers showed relatively more regulation of pre-resolution discretionary spending on alcohol and savings, but this pattern changed post-resolution after some initial success with moderation in ways that provided receipt of large, delayed rewards. Compared to the other outcome groups, the RNA group experienced higher value post-resolution consumption bundles that presumably served to reinforce and stabilize the shifted recovery behavior patterns while they engaged in some limited drinking without problems. This suggests that greater behavioral variability (flexibility) and its effective management distinguishes persons with AUD who can achieve stable moderation during a natural recovery attempt. Future research should investigate whether these relationships generalize to quit attempts made in the context of interventions, including interventions that seek to lengthen the time horizons for behavioral allocation. Some preliminary evidence suggests that such interventions promote drinking reductions generally (e.g., Murphy et al., 2019) and moderation drinking specifically (e.g., Tucker et al., 2012).

More generally, the Project ARC findings revealed multi-dimensional contexts defined in terms of economic behavior that were favorable and unfavorable to achieving stable recovery. Recovery coincided with and appears to be promoted by increased access to rewarding nondrug activities and commodities in both untreated and treated samples (e.g., Murphy et al., 2019; Moos & Moos, 2007; Tucker et al., 2020), and such enriched life contexts likely motivate and reinforce recovery processes and outcomes (Carroll et al., 2001). The research program highlighted the usefulness of the behavioral economic focus on molar behavioral patterns in illuminating recovery processes and showed the embeddedness of heavy drinking and its cessation in multiple areas of functioning using a common metric (money). The findings add to evidence that spending on substances predicts recovery outcomes in both treated and untreated samples (Belus et al., 2021; Murphy et al., 2015; Worley et al., 2015).

In Project ARC, different drinking outcomes were differentially associated with non-drinking behavior patterns and contexts before and after a quit attempt, indicating the importance of expanding the scope of outcome assessment in recovery research beyond drinking practices or problem severity indicators. As Project ARC demonstrated, behavioral economics offers measures and methods to expand research and practice in line with a broadened definition of recovery and the life contexts that support it (cf. Yurasek et al., Chapter 15 this volume). Further conceptual and empirical work to develop useful schemes and measures of functioning, well-being, and associated life contexts important in AUD recovery deserves priority in future research.

Project ARC added to evidence that there is no single pathway to recovery and highlighted the importance of investigating multiple pathways to positive change and how to promote them. Over the past four decades, moderation drinking has gained some qualified acceptance among treatment programs and providers for clients with less severe impairment who are typically treated in outpatient settings or as an intermediate step in the pursuit of abstinence (Rosenberg et al., 2020). This is a positive development that is responsive to the documented hetereogeneity in pathways to problem reduction or resolution and expands services to segments of the AUD population with mild to moderate problems.

Despite these salutary developments, efforts remain incomplete to improve service delivery systems in ways that are responsive to the hetereogeneity of AUD and support different pathways to problem reduction or resolution (Tucker & Simpson, 2011). Behavioral economics offers a framework for improving systems of care, including choice architecture interventions that seek to modify the environment to encourage beneficial choices and "nudge" people to make health-promoting decisions without mandating or forbidding any options (Lowenstein et al., 2007; Thaler & Sunstein, 2008). Such strategies can be applied across levels ranging from micro to macro to create contexts that promote beneficial choices and outcomes and can be used to promote help-seeking and reduce harmful substance use (Acuff et al., 2020; Tucker et al., 2017).

For example, some applications involve straightforward (micro-) environmental engineering (e.g., minimizing alcohol cues in local natural environments), whereas others explicitly arrange options so that people with greater choice biases make beneficial choices without constraining freedom of choice for less biased decision-makers (Loewenstein et al., 2007). Offering "treatment on demand" for harmful substance use or HIV/AIDS with minimal delays exemplifies the latter approach, which exploits delay discounting and capitalizes on the often-transitory motivational shifts in favor of pro-health behaviors over risky behaviors. Another example that has improved HIV testing rates is the change in default options for testing from an opt-in approach requiring consent to an opt-out approach requiring a request not to be tested (Chandisarewa et al., 2007). Choice architecture approaches are scalable and have potential for greater impact on overall population health than individual treatment interventions.

In conclusion, progress has been made in broadening definitions and investigations of recovery beyond the longstanding focus on drinking practices and symptom reduction, typically using clinical samples. Recent consideration of functioning and contextual factors surrounding recovery in both untreated and treated samples has advanced understanding of the recovery process and how such factors are intertwined with change. Project ARC demonstrated the utility of behavioral economic concepts and methods in understanding contextual factors in the natural recovery process, and related treatment research demonstrated that substance use can be reduced by increasing engagement in rewarding substance-free alternatives (e.g., Murphy et al., 2019; Petry et al., 2017). These lines of research have produced reliable and valid measures of alcohol and drug reward value as well as measures of rewarding alternatives to substance use that have utility to predict outcomes (Yurasek et al., Chapter 15). At the heart of this shift in focus is a now established fact: Drinking resolutions occur through several pathways, treatment is but one influence on successful change, and change attempts with or without the assistance of treatment occur in an ongoing, multivariate life context that warrant greater research and clinical attention.

Acknowledgments

The author thanks Rudy E. Vuchinich and Linda C. Sobell for their seminal generative research on the behavioral economics of harmful substance use and natural resolution of alcohol problems, respectively, and JeeWon Cheong for her data analytic work on Project ARC. The author's research was supported in part by NIH/NIAAA grants R01 AA08972, R01 AA017880, and R01 AA023657.

References

Acuff, S. F., Tucker, J. A., & Murphy, J. G. (2020). Behavioral economics of substance misuse: Understanding and reducing misuse during the COVID-19 pandemic. *Experimental and Clinical Psychopharmacology*. Advance online publication. https://doi.org/10.1037/pha0000431

Ainslie, G., & Herrnstein, R. J. (1981). Preference reversal and delayed reinforcement. *Animal Learning & Behavior*, *9*(4), 476–482. https://doi.org/10.3758/BF03209777

American Psychiatric Association (2013). *Diagnostic and statistical manual of mental disorders* (5th ed.). https://doi.org/10.1176/appi.books.9780890425596

Armor, D. J., & Meshkoff, J. E. (1983). Remission among treated and untreated alcoholics. *Advances in Substance Abuse*, *3*, 239–269.

Belus, J. M., Rose, A. L., Anderson, L. S. Joska, J. A. & Myers, B. (2021). The role of reward and reinforcement in understanding alcohol use among adults living with HIV in South Africa. *Psychology of Addictive Behaviors*, *35*(4), 424–431. https://doi.org/10.1037/adb0000728

Bickel, W. K., Johnson, M. W., Koffarnus, M. N., MacKillop, J., & Murphy, J. G. (2014). The behavioral economics of substance use disorders: Reinforcement pathologies and their repair. *Annual Review of Clinical Psychology, 10*, 641–677. https://doi.org/10.1146/annurev-clinpsy-032813-153724

Carroll, M. E., Bickel, W. K., & Higgins, S. T. (2001). Nondrug incentives to treat drug abuse: Laboratory and clinical developments. In M. E. Carroll & J. B. Overmier (Eds.), *Animal research and human psychological health: Advancing human welfare through behavioral science* (pp. 139–154). American Psychological Association.

Chandisarewa, W., Stranix-Chibanda, L., Chirapa, E., Miller, A., Simoyi, M., Mahomva, A., Maldonado, Y., & Shetty, A. K. (2007). Routine offer of antenatal HIV testing ("opt-out" approach) to prevent mother-to-child transmission of HIV in urban Zimbabwe. *Bulletin of the World Health Organization, 85*(11), 843–850. https://doi.org/10.2471/blt.06.035188

Cheong, J., Lindstrom, K., Chandler, S. D., & Tucker, J. A. (2020). Utility of different dimensional properties of drinking practices to predict stable low-risk drinking outcomes of natural recovery attempts. *Addictive Behaviors, 106*, 106387. https://doi.org/10.1016/j.addbeh.2020.106387

Dawson, B. F., Stinson, F. S., Chou, S. P., Huang, B., & Ruan, W. J. (2005). Alcohol dependence: United States, 2001–2002. *Addiction, 100*(3), 281–92. https://doi.org/10.1016/j.addbeh.2020.106387

Fan, A. Z., Chou, S. P., Zhang, H., Jung, J., & Grant, B. F. (2019). Prevalence and correlates of past-year recovery from DSM-5 alcohol use disorder: Results from National Epidemiologic Survey on Alcohol and Related Conditions – III. *Alcoholism: Clinical and Experimental Research, 43*(11), 2406–2420. https://doi.org10.1111/acer.14192

Fillmore, K. M. (1988). *Alcohol use across the life course: A critical review of 70 years of international longitudinal research.* Addiction Research Foundation.

Herrnstein, R. J. (1970). On the law of effect. *Journal of the Experimental Analysis of Behavior, 13*(2), 243–266. https://doi.org/10.1901/jeab.1970.13-243

Kelly, J. F., Bergman, B., Hoeppner, B. B., Bilsaint, C., & White, W. L. (2017). Prevalence and pathways of recovery from drug and alcohol problems in the United States population: Implications for practice, research, and policy. *Drug and Alcohol Dependence, 181*, 162–169. https://doi.org/10.1016/j.drugalcdep.2017.09.028

King, M. P., & Tucker, J. A. (2000). Behavior change patterns and strategies distinguishing moderation drinking and abstinence during the natural resolution of alcohol problems without treatment. *Psychology of Addictive Behaviors, 14*(1), 48–55. https://doi.org/10.1037//0893-164x.14.1.48

Klingemann, H., & Sobell, L. (Eds.) (2007). *Promoting self-change from addictive behaviors: Practical implications for policy, prevention, and treatment.* Springer Science+Business Media. https://doi.org/10.1007/978-0-387-71287-1

Klingemann, H., Sobell, L., Barker, J., Blomqviist, J., Cloud, W., Ellingstad, T., Fingfeld, D., Granfield, R., Hodgins, D., Hunt, G., Junker, C., Moggi, F., Peele, S., Smart, R., Sobell, M., & Tucker, J. (2001). *Promoting self-change from problem substance use: Practical implications, prevention, policy, and treatment* .Kluwer Academic.

Krugman, P., & Wells, R. (2012). *Economics and microeconomics* (3rd ed.). Worth Publishing.

Loewenstein, G., Brennan, T., & Volpp, K. G. (2007). Asymmetric paternalism to improve health behaviors. *Journal of the American Medical Association, 298* (20), 2415–2417. https://doi.org/10.1001/jama.298.20.2415

Mariezcurrena, R. (1994). Recovery from addictions without treatment: Literature review. *Scandinavian Journal of Behaviour Therapy, 23*(13), 1–154. https://doi.org/10.1080/16506079409455971

Marlatt, G. A. (1985). Lifestyle modification. In G. A. Marlatt & J. R. Gordon (Eds.), *Relapse prevention: Maintenance strategies in the treatment of addictive behaviors* (pp. 280–318). Guilford.

Moos, R. H., & Moos, B. S. (2007). Protective resources and long-term recovery from alcohol use disorders. *Drug and Alcohol Dependence, 86*(1), 46–54. https://doi.org/10.1016/j.drugalcdep.2006.04.015

Murphy, J. G., Dennhardt, A. A., Martens, M. P., Borsari, B. E., Witkiewitz, K., & Meshesha, L. Z. (2019). Randomized clinical trial evaluating the efficacy of a brief alcohol intervention supplemented with a substance-free activity session or relaxation training. *Journal of Consulting and Clinical Psychology, 87*(7), 657–669. https://doi.org/10.1037/ccp0000412

Murphy, J. G., Dennhardt, A. A., Martens, M. P., Yurasek, A. M., Skidmore, J. R., MacKillop, J., & McDevitt-Murphy, M. E. (2015). Behavioral economic predictors of brief alcohol intervention outcomes. *Journal of Consulting and Clinical Psychology, 83*, 1033–1043. https://doi.org/10.1037/ccp0000032

National Institute on Alcohol Abuse and Alcoholism (2005). *Helping patients who drink too much: A clinician's guide.* https://pubs.niaaa.nih.gov/publications/practitioner/cliniciansguide2005/guide.pdf

(2020). *Alcohol facts and statistics.* www.niaaa.nih.gov/alcohol-facts-and-statistics

Petry, N. M., Alessi, S. M., Olmstead, T. A., Rash, C. J., & Zajac, K. (2017). Contingency management treatment for substance use disorders: How far has it come, and where does it need to go? *Psychology of Addictive Behaviors, 31* (8), 897–906. https://doi.org/10.1037/adb0000287

Rachlin, H. (1995). Self-control: Beyond commitment. *Behavioral and Brain Sciences, 18*(1), 109–159. https://doi.org/10.1017/S0140525X00037602

Rachlin, H., Battalio, R., Kagel, J., & Green, L. (1981). Maximization theory in behavioral psychology. *Behavioral and Brain Sciences, 4*(3), 371–388. https://doi.org/10.1017/S0140525X00009407

Robins, L. N. (1993). The sixth Thomas James Okey memorial lecture. Vietnam veterans' rapid recovery from heroin addition: Fluke or normal expectation? *Addiction, 88* (8), 1041–1054. https://doi.org/10.1111/j.1360-0443.1993.tb02123.x

Rosenberg. H. (1993). Prediction of controlled drinking by alcoholics and problem drinkers. *Psychological Bulletin, 113*(1), 129–139. https://doi.org/10.1037/0033-2909.113.1.129

Rosenberg, H., Grant, J., & Davis, A. K. (2020). Acceptance of non-abstinence as an outcome goal for individuals diagnosed with substance use disorders: A narrative review of published research. *Journal of Studies on Alcohol and Drugs, 81* (4), 405–415. https://doi.org/10.15288/jsad.2020.81.405

Room, R. (1977). Measurement and distribution of drinking patterns and problems in general populations. In G. Edwards, M. S. Gross, M. Keller, J. Moser, & R. Room (Eds.), *Alcohol-related disabilities* (pp. 61–87). World Health Organization.

Simpson, C. A., Huang, J., Roth, D. L., Chandler, S. D., & Tucker, J. A. (2012). Predictors of utilization of an IVR self-monitoring program by problem drinkers with recent natural resolutions. *Drug and Alcohol Dependence, 126*(1–2), 111–117. https://doi.org/10.1016/j.drugalcdep.2012.04.022

Simpson, C. A., & Tucker, J. A. (2002). Temporal sequencing of alcohol-related problems, problem recognition, and help-seeking episodes. *Addictive Behaviors, 27* (5), 659–674. https://doi.org/10.1016/s0306–4603(01)00200-3

Smart, R. G. (1976). Spontaneous recovery in alcoholics: A review and analysis of the available research. *Drug and Alcohol Dependence, 1*(4), 277–285. https://doi.org/10.1016/0376-8716(76)90023-5

Sobell, L. C., Cunningham, J. A., & Sobell, M. B. (1996). Recovery from alcohol problems with and without treatment: Prevalence in two population studies. *American Journal of Public Health, 86*(7), 966–972. https://doi.org/10.2105/ajph.86.7.966

Sobell, L. C., Ellingstad, T. P., & Sobell, M. B. (2000). Natural recovery from alcohol and drug problems: Methodological review of the research with suggestions for future research. *Addiction, 95*(5), 749–764. https://doi.org/10.1046/j.1360-0443.2000.95574911.x

Sobell, L. C., & Sobell, M. B. (1992). Timeline Followback: A technique for assessing self reported alcohol consumption. In R. Litten & J. Allen (Eds.), *Measuring alcohol consumption* (pp. 41–72). Humana Press.

Sobell, L. C., Sobell, M. B., & Toneatto, T. (1992). Recovery from alcohol problems without treatment. In N. Heather, W. R. Miller, & J. Greeley (Eds.), *Self-control and addictive behaviors* (pp. 198–242). Macmillan.

Sobell, L. C., Sobell, M. B., Toneatto, T., & Leo, G. I. (1993). What triggers the resolution of alcohol problems without treatment? *Alcoholism: Clinical and Experimental Research, 17*(2), 217–224. https://doi.org/10.1111/j.1530-0277.1993.tb00752.x

Stall, R., & Biernacki, P. (1986). Spontaneous remission from the problematic use of substances: An inductive model derived from a comparative analysis of the alcohol, opiate, tobacco, and food/obesity literatures. *International Journal of the Addictions, 21*(1), 1–23. https://doi.org/10.3109/10826088609063434

Tucker, J. A. (2002). Natural resolution of alcohol-related problems. In J. P. Allen, M. Galanter, Deitrich, R., Gallant, D., Gottheil, E., Paredes, A., Rothschild,

M., Van Theil, D., Lagressa, D., Allen, J. P., Fuller, R., Litten, R., Eckardt, M., McCaul, M., & Monti, P. (Eds.), *Recent developments in alcoholism: Vol. 16. Research on alcoholism treatment* (pp. 77–90). Springer. https://doi.org/10.1007/0-306-47939-7_7

Tucker, J. A., Chandler, S. D., & Cheong, J. (2017). Role of choice biases and choice architecture in behavioral economic strategies to reduce addictive behaviors. In N. Heather & G. Segal (Eds.), *Addiction and choice: Rethinking the relationship* (pp. 346–364). Oxford University Press.

Tucker, J. A., Cheong, J., & Chandler, S. D. (2021). Shifts in behavioral allocation patterns as a natural recovery mechanism: Post-resolution expenditure patterns. *Alcoholism: Clinical and Experimental Research.* https://doi.org/10.1111/acer.14620

Tucker, J. A., Cheong, J., Chandler, S. D. Lambert, B. H., Pietrzak, B., & Kwok, H. (2016). Prospective analysis of behavioral economic predictors of stable moderation drinking among problem drinkers attempting natural recovery. *Alcoholism: Clinical and Experimental Research, 40*(12), 2676–2084. https://doi.org/10.1111/acer.13245

Tucker, J. A., Cheong, J., James, T. G., Jung, S., & Chandler, S. D. (2020). Pre-resolution drinking problem severity profiles associated with stable moderation outcomes of natural recovery attempts. *Alcoholism: Clinical and Experimental Research, 44*(3), 738–745. https://doi.org/10.1111/acer.14287

Tucker, J. A., Foushee, H. R., & Black, B. (2008). Behavioral economic analysis of natural resolution of drinking problems using IVR self-monitoring. *Experimental and Clinical Psychopharmacology, 16*(4), 332–340. https://doi.org/10.1037.a0012834

Tucker, J. A., Foushee, H. R., Black, B. C., & Roth, D. L. (2007). Agreement between prospective IVR self-monitoring and structured retrospective reports of drinking and contextual variables during natural resolution attempts. *Journal of Studies on Alcohol and Drugs, 68*(4), 538–542. https://doi.org/10.15288/jsad.2007.68.538

Tucker, J. A., & Gladsjo, J. A. (1993). Help-seeking and recovery by problems drinkers: Characteristics of drinkers who attended Alcoholics Anonymous, formal treatment, or recovered without assistance. *Addictive Behaviors, 18*(5), 529–542. https://doi.org/10.1016/0306-4603(93)90069-1

Tucker, J. A., & King, M. P. (1999). Resolving alcohol and drug problems: Influences on behavior change and help-seeking processes. In J. A. Tucker, D. M. Donovan, & G. A. Marlatt (Eds.), *Changing addictive behavior: Bridging clinical and public health strategies* (pp. 97–126). Guilford.

Tucker, J. A., Roth, D. L., Huang, J., Crawford, M. S., & Simpson, C. A. (2012). Effects of interactive voice response self-monitoring on natural resolution of drinking problems: Utilization and behavioral economic factors. *Journal of Studies on Alcohol and Drugs, 73*(4), 686–698. https://doi.org/10.15288/jsad.2012.73.686

Tucker, J. A., Roth, D. L., Vignolo, M., & Westfall, A. O. (2009). A behavioral economic reward index predicts drinking resolutions: Moderation re-visited and compared with other outcomes. *Journal of Consulting and Clinical Psychology,* 77(2), 219–228. https://doi.org/10.1037/a0014968

Tucker, J. A., & Simpson, C. A. (2011). The recovery spectrum: From self-change to seeking treatment. *Alcohol Research & Health, 33*(4), 371–379.

Tucker, J. A., Vuchinich, R. E., Black, B. C., & Rippens, P. D. (2006). Significance of a behavioral economic index of reward value in predicting problem drinking resolutions. *Journal of Consulting and Clinical Psychology, 74*(2), 317–326. https://doi.org/10.1037/0022-006X.74.2.317

Tucker, J. A., Vuchinich, R. E., Harris, C. V., Gavornik, M. G., & Rudd, E. J. (1991). Agreement between subject and collateral reports of alcohol consumption in older adults. *Journal of Studies on Alcohol, 52*(2), 148–155. https://doi.org/10.15288.jsa.1991.52.148

Tucker, J. A., Vuchinich, R. E., & Pukish, M. A. (1995). Molar environmental contexts surrounding recovery from alcohol problems by treated and untreated problem drinkers. *Experimental and Clinical Psychopharmacology, 3*, 195–204. https://doi.org/10.1037/1064-1297.3.2.195

Tucker, J. A., Vuchinich, R. E., & Rippens, P. D. (2002a). Predicting natural resolution of alcohol-related problems: A prospective behavioral economic analysis. *Experimental and Clinical Psychopharmacology*, 10(3), 248–257. https://doi.org/10.1037//1064-1297.10.3.248

(2002b). Environmental contexts surrounding resolution of drinking problems among problem drinkers with different help-seeking experiences. *Journal of Studies on Alcohol, 63*(3), 334–341. https://doi.org/10.15288/jsa.2002.63.334

(2004). A factor analytic study of influences on patterns of help-seeking among treated and untreated alcohol dependent persons. *Journal of Substance Abuse Treatment, 26*(3), 237–242. https://doi.org/10.1016/S0740–5472(03)00209-5

Vuchinich, R. E. (1995). Alcohol abuse as molar choice: An update of a 1982 proposal. *Psychology of Addictive Behaviors, 9*(4), 223–235. https://doi.org/10.1037/0893-164X.9.4.223

Vuchinich, R. E., & Heather, N. (Eds.). (2003). *Choice, behavioural economics, and addiction*. Pergamon/Elsevier Science Inc.

Vuchinich, R. E., & Tucker, J. A. (1996). Life events, alcoholic relapse, and behavioral theories of choice: A prospective analysis. *Experimental and Clinical Psychopharmacology, 4*(1), 19–28. https://doi.org/10.1016/B978–0-08-044056-9.X5040–4

Vuchinich, R. E., Tucker, J. A., & Harlee, L. (1988). Behavioral assessment. In D. M. Donovan & G. A. Marlatt (Eds.), *Assessment of addictive behaviours* (pp. 51–93). Guilford.

Watson, A. L., &, Sher, K. J. (1998). Resolution of alcohol problems without treatment: Methodological issues and future directions of natural recovery research. *Clinical Psychology: Science and Practice*, 5(1), 1–18. https://doi.org/10.1111/j.1468-2850.1998.tb00131.x

Witkiewitz, K., Montes, K. S., Schwebel, F. J., & Tucker, J. A. (2020). What is recovery? A narrative review of definitions of recovery from alcohol use disorder. *Alcohol Research: Current Reviews,* 40. https://doi.org/10.35946/arcr.v40.3.01

Witkiewitz, K., & Tucker, J. A. (2020). Abstinence not required: Expanding the definition of recovery from alcohol use disorder. *Alcoholism: Clinical and Experimental Research, 44*, 36–40. https://doi.org/10.1111/acer.14235

Worley, M. J., Shoptaw, S. J., Bickel, W. K., & Ling, W. (2015). Using behavioral economics to predict opioid use during prescription opioid dependence treatment. *Drug and Alcohol Dependence, 148*, 62–68. https://doi.org/10.1016/j.drugalcdep.2014.12.018

10 Individual Behavioral Interventions to Incentivize Sobriety and Enrich the Natural Environment with Appealing Alternatives to Drinking

James G. Murphy, Ashley A. Dennhardt, and Kathryn S. Gex

Individual Behavioral Interventions to Incentivize Sobriety and Enrich the Natural Environment with Appealing Alternatives to Drinking

Consistent with the guiding assumption of this book, we view recovery as the process of building a "life worth living." This process can be operationalized in a variety of ways, including engaging in meaningful and enjoyable work, family, social and leisure activities, experiencing a sense of autonomy (including control over drinking and drug use), positive affect, good health, and high life satisfaction (McKay, 2017). Although frequent and/or high quantity alcohol use can interfere with many aspects of health and life satisfaction (Levola et al., 2018), this is not always the case, particularly for young adults and individuals with mild to moderate levels of alcohol-related problems (Murphy, Correia et al., 2005; Witkiewitz et al., 2020). For example, moderate alcohol use can facilitate social bonding and positive experiences (Fairbairn et al., 2015), and many people maintain relatively high functioning across life-health domains despite meeting criteria for an alcohol use disorder (AUD) (Witkiewitz et al., 2018).

A corollary of this is that alcohol interventions can focus on building a life worth living even among individuals who are not interested in changing their drinking. This is an important development within the alcohol treatment paradigm given that an individual's desire to reduce drinking is often a prerequisite for participating in alcohol treatment, even though reducing or eliminating drinking may result in a sudden loss of reward (both from alcohol ingestion and from alcohol-related social activity) without any immediately available substitute rewards (Murphy, Correia et al., 2005). If, instead, treatment was viewed more holistically, individuals with an AUD could participate in treatments even without an initial desire to change their drinking, and they could instead use treatment to enhance other life-health domains and pursue more general wellness or life goals (McKay, 2017). Similarly, people who achieve initial drinking reductions, which often occur prior to treatment entry, could use treatment to focus on these same life enhancement goals rather than primarily focusing on avoiding relapse. Thus, alcohol treatment can facilitate recovery processes even without directly targeting alcohol use. It is also noteworthy that many people can experience recovery while still engaging in moderate levels of drinking that do not reduce their capacity for meaningful social relationships, autonomy/independence, health, and personally fulfilling work and leisure activities (Tucker et al., 2016).

Thus, the goal of this chapter is to describe alcohol intervention approaches that include elements that can help individuals build a life worth living. Although this would seem like an obvious goal for any effective alcohol treatment, historically alcohol treatment goals have been more narrowly focused on strategies to reduce or eliminate alcohol use and related problems (McKay, 2017; Witkiewitz et al., 2020). This is consistent with the prevailing theoretical models that have guided most forms of alcohol and other addiction treatment over the past 50 years, namely the disease or 12 Step model, and more recently, cognitive-behavioral and social-learning models. Although these theories are quite heterogeneous in some respects, and cognitive-behavioral and social-learning models explicitly incorporate environmental and affective risk factors, they all assume that the problem of excessive drug use lies primarily in the interaction between the chemical properties of the drug, situational triggers, and unique internal vulnerabilities of the individual (e.g., personality features, negative affect/stress, cognitive biases about the effects of the drug, elevated craving) that result in excessive motivation to use the drug (Vuchinich & Heather, 2003). From this perspective, a primary emphasis on reducing or eliminating alcohol use is logical and parsimonious and has led to a variety of relatively efficacious psychosocial and pharmacological intervention approaches (Ray et al., 2019; Witkiewitz et al., 2020). These approaches generally assume that effective treatment must begin with abstinence or drinking reduction that may then be followed by secondary treatment elements that seek to enhance positive affect and more general social and health functioning. For example, cognitive behavioral therapy (CBT) includes some specific modules on reducing negative affect and increasing pleasant alcohol-free activities, but these elements reflect a relatively small proportion of the overall treatment approach as it is typically administered (Hendershot et al., 2011). Additionally, involvement with Alcoholics Anonymous (AA) often provides individuals with alcohol-free social support and activities, which are established mechanisms of change and likely to enhance quality of life. However, enhancing social support is viewed as secondary to the primary goal of AA, which is to support abstinence and complete the 12 recovery steps, and the amount of social support an individual experiences is predicated on their compatibility with other group members and their commitment to the AA recovery model (Kelly et al., 2012).

In contrast, two highly effective behavioral therapies – community reinforcement and contingency management – attempt to reduce alcohol use by systematically increasing both (a) the response cost of alcohol use (social and tangible rewards are administered contingent upon verified abstinence) and (b) the availability of rewarding alternatives that are incompatible with use (Higgins et al., 2004). These treatments have a robust evidence base but until recently have not been widely disseminated in treatment settings (Crescenzo et al., 2018). Additionally, they are intensive treatments that often require an upfront commitment to abstinence, and this may reduce treatment initiation for some.

Over the past two decades, the ascendance of the harm reduction movement, along with theoretical accounts of addiction emphasizing that alcohol and other drug use is more likely when few drug-free alternative rewards are available in the environment, has contributed to more flexible and holistic alcohol treatment models (Tucker & Simpson, 2011). There are now many harm reduction treatments that are opportunistic and brief and thus well suited for the vast majority of individuals who do not present for formal treatment, many of whom have mild to moderate AUD symptoms (Hennessy et al., 2019). Nevertheless, a significant barrier to widespread dissemination is that many individuals who report heavy drinking express very little interest in intervention approaches that directly target alcohol use reductions (including even those with harm reduction goals; Fucito et al., 2017). Consequently, outside of mandated situations such as arrests or alcohol policy violation sanctions, individuals with mild to moderate alcohol problems may be unlikely to voluntarily complete alcohol-focused brief interventions (Buscemi et al., 2010). Thus, prevention and intervention programs that address alcohol use indirectly in the context of an overall focus on wellness, mood enhancement, and goal setting may have greater appeal and potential for dissemination than traditional alcohol brief interventions. As described next, behavioral economic theory is a more recent extension of behavioral theories of addiction that has led to a range of brief intervention approaches that are well-suited to the goal of encouraging patterns of meaningful and enjoyable alternatives to alcohol and drug use even among those who may not be motivated to make immediate reductions in their alcohol consumption (Fazzino et al., 2019; Murphy et al., 2019).

Behavioral Economic Theory as a Framework for Guiding Alcohol Interventions that Enrich the Environment with Alternative Reinforcers

Behavioral economic theory suggests that low levels of substance-free reward will increase the relative reinforcing value of alcohol, leading to increases in drinking, particularly among persons with elevated impulsivity or comorbid conditions such as depression and anxiety (Bickel et al., 2014; Vuchinich & Heather, 2003). These risk factors often interact to contribute to the persistently high valuation of brief, high-intensity reinforcers such as alcohol relative to reinforcers derived from patterns of activities that serve to advance future goals (e.g., work, educational attainment, hobbies, relationships). This *reinforcer pathology* process is recursive because frequent alcohol and drug use can result in diminished sensitivity to the reinforcing effects of non-drug stimuli such as sex, food, or exercise, thereby reducing the reinforcing efficacy of salient alternatives and further increasing the relative preference for alcohol and drugs (Field et al., 2020).

Experimental laboratory studies have shown that: (a) high rates of substance use are most likely in contexts devoid of substance-free sources of reinforcement, (b) extensive and persistent substance use is associated with diminished dopamine response to naturally occurring substance-free reinforcers, and (c) substance use will generally decrease if access to alternative reinforcers is increased (Bickel et al., 2014; Higgins et al., 2004; Vuchinich & Heather, 2003). For example, we found that a measure of environmental reward deprivation predicted AUD symptoms among young adults, independent of mood and drinking level (Joyner et al., 2016). In contrast, having next-day responsibilities (e.g., employment, classes, volunteer work) was linked to lower alcohol demand (motivation to drink), as measured by a behavioral economic task that quantifies hypothetical alcohol consumption and alcohol-related expenditures as a function of drink price (Joyner et al., 2019). Another study found that emerging adults who were instructed to increase either exercise or creative activities reported doing so, and they also reduced their drinking compared to control participants (Correia et al., 2005). Other research suggests that emerging adults who reduced their drinking showed increased reinforcement from substance-free activities at follow up, and changes in proportionate reinforcement related to substance-free activities mediated the relation between a brief alcohol intervention and reductions in alcohol use (Murphy et al., 2019).

Individuals who drink heavily may under-engage in constructive alternatives to drinking because the benefits of these activities are generally delayed, relative to the immediately reinforcing effects of alcohol (Bickel et al., 2014). Although the perceived value of all reinforcers decreases with delay, substantial individual differences exist in the degree to which delayed reinforcers lose value. Individuals who sharply discount the value of delayed health and career outcomes may be less likely to engage in the behaviors consistent with success in these areas (e.g., seeking and maintaining employment, exercising, investing in long-term relationships and health), and instead may allocate their behavior toward immediately reinforcing activities such as drinking. Indeed, numerous studies have demonstrated that individuals who misuse substances discount the value of delayed reinforcers more steeply than control participants (Kluwe-Schiavon et al., 2020). This “delay discounting” phenomenon appears to be a core yet potentially malleable process associated with harmful substance use (Amlung & McKillop, 2011).

Behavioral economic or reinforcer pathology models have three clear implications for the assessment and treatment of AUD. First, the assessment of alcohol problem severity and response to treatment should include measurement of the relative availability and valuation of alcohol-related and alcohol-free rewards (Acuff et al., 2019; Tucker et al., 2016; see Yurasek et al., Chapter 15 this volume for relevant behavioral economic assessment approaches). Second, treatment should attempt to reduce the availability or increase the response cost of alcohol and other drug use. Third, treatment should attempt to increase the salience of personally meaningful goals and facilitate patterns of substance-free activities that are organized around pursuing those goals (Fazzino et al., 2019; McKay, 2017).

A central assumption of behavioral economic theory is that alcohol intervention approaches should attempt to reduce the relative reinforcing value of alcohol by increasing engagement in future-oriented positive alternatives to drinking. Behavioral economic laboratory research suggests that increasing the salience of the delayed outcomes of behavior can reduce impulsive response patterns and increase future orientation (Ashe & Wilson, 2020). For example, laboratory studies have demonstrated that focused thinking/writing about potential positive future events (episodic future thinking) can reduce delay discounting and alcohol demand and may promote positive health behavior change (Patel & Amlung, 2020; Snider et al., 2016). Additional evidence suggests that if future events were framed as part of a temporally extended behavior pattern leading to delayed rewards ("reward bundling"), then their value was discounted less steeply than if they were presented as independent events or discrete choices (Rung & Madden, 2018). This suggests that interventions should encourage those who use substances to think about desired future outcomes and to view their daily behaviors as part of a larger pattern of behavior necessary to achieve those outcomes (Ashe & Wilson, 2020). This shift in perspective may be promoted by the personalized substance use feedback included in most brief alcohol intervention approaches (e.g., quantitative information reflecting meaningful tallies of alcohol/drug use decisions, like instances of drug use per week and money spent on drug use during a month/year). A unique implication of behavioral economic theory is that interventions should encourage individuals to view their day-to-day decisions and activities (both substance-related and substance-free) as patterns that have implications for and connections with desired future outcomes and goals (Murphy et al., 2019). Alcohol intervention approaches that do not attempt to increase substance-free activities and future orientation may be missing a key opportunity to support the initiation and/or maintenance of reductions in drinking (McKay, 2017; Meshesha et al., 2020), particularly for individuals whose drinking may be related to a lack of behavioral alternatives to alcohol or steep discounting of the future, as well as for individuals who are not initially receptive to reducing their drinking.

As described next and as presented in Table 10.1, there are now multiple intervention approaches that address behavioral economic mechanisms (Daughters et al., 2018; Fazzino et al., 2019). Some of these interventions focus directly on these mechanisms, while others include elements that clinicians can

Table 10.1. *Behavioral economic intervention elements that enrich the environment with alternative reinforcers*

Behavioral Economic Target	Example	Lower Threshold Interventions	Comprehensive AUD/SUD Treatments
Reduce the reward value of alcohol or other drugs by increasing the associated response costs	• Increase the salience of potential substance use costs or actual response costs by discussing, thinking about, or receiving feedback on the financial, social, and health costs of patterns of substance use over time	• Substance-free Activity Session • Episodic Future Thinking • Motivational Interviewing & Motivational Enhancement Therapy	• Contingency Management • Community Reinforcement Approach • Behavioral Couples Therapy • Cognitive Behavioral Therapy • Mindfulness-Oriented Recovery Enhancement • Mindfulness-Based Relapse Prevention
Enhance alternative reinforcement/ emphasize general wellness	• Increase awareness of or participation in rewarding substance-free activities by generating ideas for enjoyable and goal-consistent activities and committing to a specific plan to engage in those activities	• Substance-free Activity Session	• Contingency Management • Community Reinforcement Approach • Behavioral Activation • 12-Step Facilitation • Behavioral Couples Therapy

			• Cognitive Behavioral Therapy • Mindfulness-Oriented Recovery Enhancement • Mindfulness-Based Relapse Prevention • Network Support Treatment • Exercise-based interventions • Acceptance & Commitment Therapy
Increase future orientation	• Make future goals and benefits of change more salient by vividly describing positive future outcomes associated with reductions in substance use and increases in substance-free activities	• Substance-free Activity Session • Episodic Future Thinking • Implementation Intentions • Motivational Interviewing & Motivational Enhancement Therapy	• Acceptance & Commitment Therapy • Behavioral Activation

Note. Low threshold interventions can be offered to individuals who are not seeking clinical care or added as an adjunct to a comprehensive treatment. Comprehensive alcohol or drug use treatments are intended for individuals who present for clinical care. AUD = Alcohol Use Disorder. SUD = Substance Use Disorder.

prioritize in order to more explicitly enhance alternatives to drinking, future orientation, and general wellness. These approaches may enhance overall well-being and quality of life even among individuals who are not initially interested in changing their alcohol use. They are organized around whether they are (a) low threshold interventions that can be offered to individuals who are not seeking clinical care or can added as an adjunct to a comprehensive treatment, or (b) more comprehensive alcohol or drug use treatments intended for individuals who present for clinical care.

Low Threshold Interventions that Enrich the Environment with Alternative Reinforcers

Substance-Free Activity Session (SFAS)

The SFAS is a single session intervention that has been used as a supplement to standard alcohol or drug focused interventions with both college students (Murphy et al., 2012, 2019) and adults in alcohol treatment (Meshesha et al., 2020).

The SFAS combines motivational interviewing elements with a personalized feedback approach to target the behavioral economic mechanisms of substance-free reinforcement and delay discounting (Murphy et al., 2013). Specific session elements include a discussion of future goals, the benefits of achieving those goals, and the congruence between substance use and achieving those goals. The SFAS includes personalized feedback on recent time allocation across a variety of activities (e.g., drinking, exercising, time with family, volunteering) to highlight potential discrepancies in how the individual spends their time and personal goals or values. Additionally, individuals receive personalized feedback on specific locally available substance-free activities that are consistent with their interests. The SFAS also targets depression and anxiety via an overall focus on increasing enjoyable and goal-directed activities (consistent with behavioral activation) and by providing feedback on coping skills (Murphy et al., 2013). The primary focus is on identifying general life goals and accompanying patterns of activities, and the SFAS thus does not require interest in changing alcohol use. When combined with a brief alcohol intervention, the SFAS has been associated with significant reductions in alcohol use and problems out to 16-month post-intervention in college students (Murphy et al., 2012, 2019). The SFAS has also showed promising results in a small pilot trial when used as a booster session for adults participating in outpatient alcohol treatment (Meshesha et al., 2020).

Episodic Future Thinking (EFT)

EFT is the act of vividly imagining one's future, which involves imagining a future alcohol and drug-free event in great detail including associated feelings, sensations, and emotions (Patel & Amlung, 2020; Snider et al., 2016). As noted earlier, individuals with AUD often have shortened time horizons for behavioral choice and are more likely to discount the value of delayed rewards, and this approach is intended to make those future rewards more salient (Bickel et al., 2014). Several studies support the efficacy of EFT for reducing hypothetical alcohol demand and delay discounting in college students and individuals with AUD (Mellis et al., 2019; Patel & Amlung, 2020). Patel and Amlung (2020) found that continued practice of EFT produced greater magnitude reductions in various demand indices at the one-week follow-up compared to a control task, among individuals enrolled in inpatient AUD treatment. Meshesha et al. (2020) integrated EFT into the SFAS session, although the design did not allow determination of the unique efficacy of EFT. This incipient body of research provides initial support for the utility of EFT as an element of a more comprehensive approach to enhance positive goal-pursuit and future orientation but to date there is no evidence that EFT can reduce drinking as a stand-alone intervention (Voss et al., 2021).

Implementation Intentions (II)

II is a self-regulatory, behavioral intervention that attempts to reduce "habitual" drinking behaviors by linking high-risk drinking situations with alternative, healthier responses (Moody et al., 2018). Thus, the approach could be useful to facilitate follow-through with plans to increase engagement in rewarding alternatives to drinking, although this has not yet been well studied. Several studies have demonstrated reductions in alcohol use related to II, including in a general community sample of adult drinkers (Armitage, 2009). In a study of college students, those who were asked to form an II to drink within safe limits reported consuming fewer drinks at the 1-month follow-up than control participants (Hagger et al., 2012). Although there is less evidence of their use with adults with AUD, one study found that while individuals with AUD did not reduce their number of drinking days, they reported greater reductions in drinks per drinking day than those in the control condition (Moody et al., 2018).

Comprehensive Alcohol or Drug Use Treatments Delivered in Clinical Care Settings that Enrich the Environment with Alternative Reinforcers

Behavioral Activation (BA)

BA is an evidence-based treatment for depression that focuses on increasing access to environmental rewards and engagement in enjoyable and goal-directed activities (Lejuez et al., 2001). Given that behavioral economic and other models of addiction highlight the role of reward deprivation in addiction as well as depression (Joyner et al., 2016), BA has been adapted as a treatment for alcohol and drug use disorders. BA treatments for substance use have primarily taken two forms: Brief Behavioral Activation for Depression (BATD; Lejuez et al., 2001) and Life Enhancement Treatment for Substance Use (Let's Act; Daughters et al., 2018). These two BA-based treatments have shown promise in increasing environmental reward and reducing depression and substance use in treatment-seeking populations (Daughters et al., 2018; Martinez-Vispo et al., 2018). These treatments have also been effective among non-treatment-seeking populations that reported risky alcohol and/or drug use, including urban homeless individuals in the United States (Satnisky et al., 2020), individuals living with HIV in South Africa (Magidson et al., 2020), and US college students with comorbid ADHD and heavy drinking (Meinzer et al., 2021). These promising outcomes, in addition to the already robust empirical support for BA for depression, suggest that BA may offer a sound approach to enhance substance-free rewards and quality of life even for individuals who have no interest in changing their substance use.

Cognitive Behavioral Treatments (CBT)

Several CBT approaches are efficacious in reducing harmful substance use and promoting abstinence (Ray et al., 2019). Although not their primary focus or goal, some CBT protocols include components or goals that are relevant to enhancing engagement in alternative reinforcing activities and reducing the reward value of the target substance. One example is Cognitive Behavioral Coping Skills Therapy, which focuses on teaching coping skills of distress tolerance, interpersonal effectiveness, and emotion regulation. The treatment also includes modules that emphasize increasing engagement in substance-free pleasant activities, social support, and building job-seeking skills. Although meta-analyses suggest the treatment overall is associated with reliable, albeit small, magnitude effects that exceed supportive counseling (Magill et al, 2020), no research to date has teased apart the effects of these additional components on harm reduction or abstinence outcomes, or sought to evaluate changes in these domains following treatment.

Mindfulness- and Acceptance-Based Treatments

Mindfulness-Oriented Recovery Enhancement (MORE) was adapted from Mindfulness-Based Cognitive Therapy as an integrative treatment for addiction, stress, physical and emotional pain, and diminished ability to experience natural (substance-free) reward (Garland et al., 2016). The three primary components of MORE are: (a) mindfulness exercises that help individuals shift focus from addictive cues and stressors to mindful breathing; (b) reappraisal of maladaptive thoughts contributing to negative emotions and addictive behaviors; and (c) savoring to focus attention on naturally rewarding experiences and the enjoyment of these experiences (Garland et al., 2019). MORE has been shown to reduce total substance craving compared to a CBT intervention (Garland et al., 2016), and is efficacious in reducing opiate use (Garland et al., 2019), but more research is needed to assess its efficacy in increasing positive reward and reducing alcohol use and problems in individuals with AUD. MORE is a very promising addiction treatment and stands out for its unique focus on reducing stress and pain and enhancing one's capacity to experience substance-free reward. Similarly,

Mindfulness-Based Relapse Prevention (MBRP) has a focus on increasing engagement in nourishing activities and bringing greater present moment awareness to substance-free rewards, and has been shown to be more effective than CBT and treatment as usual in preventing substance use and decreasing craving (Bowen et al., 2014).

Acceptance and Commitment Therapy (ACT) is well known for its emphasis on mindfulness, acceptance, and values-based committed action to manage psychological distress adaptively. ACT focuses on identifying core values and establishing goals and behavior patterns that are consistent with those values (Levin & Hayes, 2009), which is highly consistent with the behavioral economic concepts of reward bundling and increased engagement in substance-free rewarding alternatives. A review of 12 studies of ACT for substance use found that ACT had significant but small effects on abstinence and reductions in substance use compared to control/comparison conditions (Lee et al., 2015). ACT also has been found to improve depression and anxiety outcomes among individuals with comorbid substance use disorder (SUD) and affective disorder (Thekiso et al., 2015).

Network Support Treatment (NST) and Twelve Step Facilitation (TSF)

Several naturalistic studies of AA revealed that reductions in drinking were found to be partially mediated by changes in social networks, particularly reductions in network support for drinking (Bond, 2003). NST utilizes the 12 Step treatment model as basic infrastructure and focuses on surrounding oneself with the right people, places, and things, and increasing pleasant substance-free activities (Litt et al., 2009). Each session includes homework that aims to expand the patient's social network to be supportive of recovery and includes engagement in rewarding substance-free activities related to family, recreation, and employment. Studies of NST have shown favorable reductions in drinking days and consequences compared to case management (Litt et al., 2009) and a packaged CBT (Litt et al., 2016) at 2-years post-treatment. The effects were mediated by changes in abstinence self-efficacy, the proportion of non-drinkers in the social network, and AA attendance. Given the centrality of substance-free activities and social support to building a life worth living, this seems to be an ideal treatment approach for individuals who are motivated to engage in a relatively intensive intervention. Moreover, elements of NST can easily be applied as part of briefer treatments that might support a variety of treatment goals, including moderate drinking and examining one's social network and systematically attempting to increase the number of individuals who are supportive of drinking changes.

Also focused on building on AA attendance, TSF therapy provides resources to begin and maintain involvement in AA or other 12 Step and self-help organizations and, as a result, functionally provides a peer-support network for recovery. A 2020 Cochrane review indicated that AA/TSF interventions are comparable to other AUD interventions (e.g., CBT) in their efficacy to reduce harmful alcohol use and actually out-perform these treatments in terms of continuous abstinence and healthcare cost savings (Kelly et al., 2020). For individuals who are motivated to pursue abstinence and appreciate the AA model, this approach may be optimal for enhancing social support and providing meaningful substance-free activities (e.g., AA meetings, social activities with one's sponsor or other members).

Exercise-Based Interventions

Exercise-based interventions for addiction emerged in part due to the realization that individuals who recover from a SUD, with or without participating in treatment, often make other health behavior changes, including increasing exercise (King & Tucker, 2000). Much like social activity, exercise is a highly potent natural reward that reliably enhances mood (Penedo & Dahn, 2005) and may serve as a viable substitute for alcohol and drug-related reward (Correia et al., 2005). Several recent meta-analyses suggest that physical exercise is beneficial in improving quality of life in individuals with a history of SUD (Giménez-Meseguer et al., 2020). Exercised-based interventions may be used as a stand-alone wellness-based approach in non-treatment-seeking populations or as an adjunct to SUD treatment. One study found an exercise intervention significantly reduced alcohol use in a dose dependent manner (Brown et al., 2014), and a second study found large effect size increases in exercise for the intervention condition relative to control and equal reductions in drinking and consequences over time (Weinstock et al., 2020). These studies suggest that targeting exercise may enhance wellness, though this may not have specific effects on alcohol use without additional treatment elements.

Contingency Management (CM)

Meta-analyses and systematic reviews spanning several decades suggest that CM is consistently effective in reducing substance use and increasing abstinence by providing abstinence-contingent reinforcement in the form of money, prizes, vouchers, or other tangible incentives (Crescenzo et al., 2018). Further, consistent with this book's holistic perspective on recovery, one study of CM evaluated the treatment's effects on engagement in non-drug reinforcing activities (Rogers et al., 2008). In a small sample of cocaine and heroin users, take-home methadone plus money vouchers (THM+V) for negative drug screens resulted in more reported engagement in non-drug reinforcing activities, as measured by the Pleasant Events Schedule, compared to THM only. This suggests that there is an important and unique opportunity within CM interventions to not only incentivize abstinence but also to facilitate increased access to non-drug sources of reinforcement (e.g., employment; Subramaniam et al., 2018). For example, CM interventions should also attempt to increase reinforcement derived from alternative, non-substance sources, by including therapeutic components focused on increasing rewarding alternatives to substance use (e.g., vocational counseling, social/leisure activity planning) and by helping individuals select voucher rewards that provide viable alternatives to substance use (e.g., movie tickets, sporting equipment, family activities, tuition for classes).

More specific to CM treatment approaches for AUD, advancements in technology and remote biometric assessment of alcohol use provide the opportunity to extend CM beyond the traditionally time- and labor-intensive in-person approach. For example, transdermal alcohol monitoring devices (e.g., SCRAM; Barnett et al., 2017) and remote objective breath tests (Koffarnus et al., 2018) may make it possible to continue to provide immediately available extrinsic rewards in a more naturalistic setting and may also encourage increased engagement in substance-free activities through voucher-based (vs. monetary) rewards.

Community Reinforcement Approach (CRA)

The CRA focuses on enhancing life areas that are pleasurable, health-promoting, and incongruent with substance use (Hunt & Azrin, 1973). Comprehensive reviews and meta-analyses over the past three decades have consistently supported the effectiveness of CRA for AUD and other SUDs including for individuals with psychiatric comorbidity, across a variety of rural and urban populations, and for individuals with differing goals related to substance use (e.g., abstinence, harm reduction; Meyers et al., 2011). Of note, for those attempting recovery from cocaine and/or opioid use, inclusion of CM vouchers early on in the treatment process has been shown to provide initial and immediate reinforcement while the individual works to build up and re-engage in reinforcement from community sources (Garcia-Rodriquez et al. 2009; Higgins et al., 2004). Despite these findings, however, it remains unclear in the CRA and CM literature the degree to which these treatment approaches increase engagement in substance-free rewarding activities above and beyond standard treatments or how this increased engagement may provide incremental effects on substance use outcomes.

Importance of Dissemination to High-Risk and Underserved Populations

A review of social and cultural contexts of alcohol use (Sudhinaraset et al., 2016) highlighted that neighborhoods characterized by poverty, inferior building conditions, and low-quality water and sanitation have higher levels of heavy drinking than more affluent and resourced neighborhoods. AUD does not impact all individuals equally, and several factors influence rates of treatment seeking, engagement, and ultimately successful change for individuals in the general population with AUD and those from underserved populations (Vaeth et al., 2017; see Chapter 1 this volume). AUD and other SUDs continue to be highly stigmatized conditions for all demographic groups but in particular for Black, indigenous, and people of color, who have been and continue to be oppressed by a criminal justice system that historically takes a punitive approach to alcohol and other drug problems (James & Jordan, 2018). These population subgroups have lower odds of receiving and completing treatment (Vaeth et al., 2017), and many minority individuals in need of mental health services report that stigma plays a significant role in preventing them from seeking voluntary treatment services when a problem is identified (James & Jordan, 2018). Given the substantial literature showing the role of environmental factors in AUD development and response to treatment (Higgins et al., 2004), the more limited access that ethnic minority and low SES populations have to quality professional treatments like those described in this chapter is especially concerning.

Appropriately addressing AUD treatment disparities from a wellness and environmental enrichment perspective requires understanding of the social, cultural, and other contextual influences on alcohol use, the perception of alcohol problems and perceived need for treatment, and perceptions of access to and the experience of alcohol treatment. In the larger population, fewer than 25 percent of individuals with a SUD receive treatment, and self-reported reasons for *not* receiving treatment, even when there was a perceived need for it, include "not being ready to stop using," "not knowing where to go for treatment," and "having no health care coverage and not being able to afford the cost of treatment" (Substance Abuse and Mental Health Services Administration, 2020). This situation is exacerbated by the likelihood that people of color and other marginalized populations are not only more likely to experience discrimination and stigma but also to live in an under-resourced community (James & Jordan, 2018). Given the differing social and environmental experiences directly related to skin color, psychosocial and behavioral interventions targeting the enrichment of these life areas to incentivize sobriety or harm reduction should be sensitive and responsive to cultural differences. This might include providing a variety of culturally tailored treatment options, using less stigmatizing person-first/person-centered language, and increasing the diversity of treatment providers (Alvanzo et al., 2014). Individuals from marginalized groups who are struggling with AUD/SUD may be more likely to benefit from larger community-based efforts to implement and disseminate culturally tailored evidence-based treatments that promote a more holistic approach to recovery (Kristjansson et al., 2020; Subramaniam et al., 2018).

Conclusions and Recommendations

In this chapter, we presented the conceptual and empirical bases that indicate alcohol treatments should include a significant focus on helping individuals increase access to and the ability to experience personally meaningful and/or enjoyable substance-free activities. These activity patterns have the potential to: (a) provide viable sources of alternative reinforcement to replace the rewards previously experienced from alcohol and other drug use; (b) increase positive affective states; (c) facilitate progress toward valued life goals; and (d) enhance overall health, wellness, and quality of life. We reviewed specific treatment approaches that include components to enhance substance-free activities and reward experience, many of which are appropriate for individuals even if they are not ready to make a change in their drinking practices. The evidence suggests that these approaches have the potential to increase treatment engagement and efficacy and broaden the scope of interventions beyond a limited focus on changing drinking practices and avoiding relapse to include life enhancement goals that can reinforce and maintain recovery. Life enhancing alcohol treatment approaches may be especially helpful for individuals who are members of marginalized communities (see also Collins et al.; Best et al.; Snell-Rood et al., Chapters 12, 16, and 17 this volume).

Acknowledgments

The author's research on behavioral economic approaches to understanding risk for alcohol problems was supported in part by NIH/NIAAA grant R01AA024930.

References

Acuff, S. F., Dennhardt, A. A., Correia, C. J., & Murphy, J. G. (2019). Measurement of substance-free reinforcement in addiction: A systematic review. *Clinical Psychology Review, 70*, 79–90. https://doi- org.ezproxy.memphis.edu/10.1016/j.cpr.2019.04.003

Alvanzo, A. A., Storr, C. L., Mojtabai, R., Green, K. M., Pacek, L. R., La Flair, L. N., Cullen, B. A., & Crum, R. M. (2014). Gender and race/ethnicity differences for initiation of alcohol-related service use among persons with alcohol dependence. *Drug and Alcohol Dependence, 140*, 48–55. https://doi.org/10.1016/j.drugalcdep.2014.03.010

Amlung, M., & MacKillop, J. (2011). Delayed reward discounting and alcohol misuse: The roles of response consistency and reward magnitude. *Journal of Experimental Psychopathology*, *2*(3), 418–431. http://doi.org/10.5127/jep.017311

Armitage, C. J. (2009). Effectiveness of experimenter-provided and self-generated implementation intentions to reduce alcohol consumption in a sample of the general population: A randomized exploratory trial. *Health Psychology, 28*(5), 545–553. https://doi.org/10.1037/a0015984

Ashe, M. L., & Wilson, S. J. (2020). A brief review of choice bundling: A strategy to reduce delay discounting and bolster self-control. *Addictive Behaviors Reports, 11*, 100262. https://doi.org 10.1016/j.abrep.2020.100262

Barnett, N. P., Celio, M. A., Tidey, J. W., Murphy, J. G., Colby, S. M., & Swift, R. M. (2017). A preliminary randomized controlled trial of contingency management for alcohol use reduction using a transdermal alcohol sensor. *Addiction, 112*(6), 1025–1035. https://doi.org/10.1111/add.13767

Bickel, W. K., Johnson, M. W., Koffarnus, M. N., MacKillop, J., & Murphy, J. G. (2014). The behavioral economics of substance use disorders: Reinforcement pathologies and their repair. *Annual Review of Clinical Psychology, 10*(1), 641–677. https://doi.org/10.1146/annurev-clinpsy-032813-153724

Bond, J., Kaskutas, L. A., & Weisner, C. (2003). The persistent influence of social networks and Alcoholics Anonymous on abstinence. *Journal of Studies on Alcohol, 64*(4), 579–588. https://doi.org/10.15288/jsa.2003.64.579

Bowen, S., Witkiewitz, K., Clifasefi, S. L., Grow, J., Chawla, N., Hsu, S. H., Carroll, H. A., Harrop, E., Collins, S. E., Lustyk, M. K., & Larimer, M. E. (2014). Relative efficacy of mindfulness-based relapse prevention, standard relapse prevention, and treatment as usual for substance use disorders: A randomized clinical trial. *JAMA Psychiatry, 71*(5), 547–556. https://doi.org/10.1001/jamapsychiatry.2013.4546

Brown, R. A., Abrantes, A. M., Minami, H., Read, J. P., Marcus, B. H., Jakicic, J. M., & Stuart, G. L. (2014). A preliminary, randomized trial of aerobic exercise for alcohol dependence. *Journal of Substance Abuse Treatment, 47,*1–9. http://doi .org/10.1016/j.jsat.2014.02.004

Buscemi, J., Murphy, J. G., Martens, M. P., McDevitt-Murphy, M. E., Dennhardt, A. A., & Skidmore, J. R. (2010). Help-seeking for alcohol-related problems in college students: Correlates and preferred resources. *Psychology of Addictive Behaviors, 24*(4), 571–580. https://doi.org/10.1037/a0021122

Correia, C. J., Benson, T. A., & Carey, K. B. (2005). Decreased substance use following increases in alternative behaviors: A preliminary investigation. *Addictive Behaviors, 30*(1), 19–27. https://doi.org/10.1016/j.addbeh.2004.04.006

Crescenzo, F. D., Ciabattini, M., D'Alò, G. L., Giorgi, R. D., Giovane, C. D., Cassar, C., Janiri, L., Clark, N., Ostacher, M. J., & Cipriani, A. (2018). Comparative efficacy and acceptability of psychosocial interventions for individuals with cocaine and amphetamine addiction: A systematic review and network meta-analysis. *PLOS Medicine, 15*(12), e1002715. https://doi.org/10.1371/journal .pmed.1002715

Daughters, S. B., Magidson, J. F., Anand, D., Seitz-Brown, C. J., Chen, Y., & Baker, S. (2018). The effect of a behavioral activation treatment for substance use on post-treatment abstinence: A randomized controlled trial. *Addiction, 113*(3), 535–544. https://doi.org/10.1111/add.14049

Fairbairn, C. E., Sayette, M. A., Aalen, O. O., & Frigessi, A. (2015). Alcohol and emotional contagion: An examination of the spreading of smiles in male and female drinking groups. *Clinical Psychological Science, 3*(5), 686–701. https:// doi.org/10.1177/2167702614548892

Fazzino, T. L., Bjorlie, K., & Lejuez, C. W. (2019). A systematic review of reinforcement-based interventions for substance use: Efficacy, mechanisms of action, and moderators of treatment effects. *Journal of Substance Abuse Treatment, 104*, 83–96. https://doi.org/10.1016/j.jsat.2019.06.016

Field, M., Heather, N., Murphy, J. G., Stafford, T., Tucker, J. A., & Witkiewitz, K. (2020). Recovery from addiction: Behavioral economics and value-based decision making. *Psychology of Addictive Behaviors, 34*(1), 182–193. https://doi .org/10.1037/adb0000518

Fucito, L. M., Demartini, K. S., Hanrahan, T. H., Yaggi, H. K., Heffern, C., & Redeker, N. S.. (2017). Using sleep interventions to engage and treat heavy-drinking college students: A randomized pilot study. *Alcoholism: Clinical and Experimental Research, 41*(4), 798–809. http://doi.org/10.1111/acer.13342

García-Rodríguez, O., Secades-Villa, R., Higgins, S., Fernández Hermida, J., Carballo, J., Errasti Perez, J. M., & Al-Halabí, S. (2009). Effects of voucher-based intervention on abstinence and retention in an outpatient treatment for cocaine addiction: A randomized controlled trial. *Experimental and Clinical Psychopharmacology, 17*(3), 131–138. https://doi.org/10.1037/a0015963

Garland, E. L. (2016). Mindfulness-Oriented Recovery Enhancement versus CBT for co-occurring substance dependence, traumatic stress, and psychiatric disorders: Proximal outcomes from a pragmatic randomized trial. *Behaviour Research and Therapy, 77*, 7–16. https://doi.org/10.1016/j.brat.2015.11.01210

Garland, E. L., Hanley, A. W., Riquino, M. R., Reese, S. E., Baker, A. K., Salas, K., Yack, B. P., Bedford, C. E., Bryan, M. A., Atchley, R., Nakamura, Y., Froeliger, B., & Howard, M. O. (2019). Mindfulness-oriented recovery enhancement reduces opioid misuse risk via analgesic and positive psychological mechanisms: A randomized controlled trial. *Journal of Consulting and Clinical Psychology, 87*(10), 927–940. https://psycnet.apa.org/doi/10.1037/ccp0000390

Giménez-Meseguer, J., Tortosa-Martínez, J., & Cortell-Tormo, J. M. (2020). The benefits of physical exercise on mental disorders and quality of life in substance use disorders patients: Systematic review and meta-analysis. *International Journal of Environmental Research and Public Health, 17*(10), 3680. https://doi.org/10.3390/ijerph17103680

Hagger, M. S., Lonsdale, A., Koka, A., Hein, V., Pasi, H., Lintunen, T., & Chatzisarantis, N. L. (2012). An intervention to reduce alcohol consumption in undergraduate students using implementation intentions and mental simulations: A cross-national study. *International Journal of Behavioral Medicine, 19*(1), 82–96. http://doi.org/10.1007/s12529–011-9163-8

Hennessy, E. A., Tanner-Smith, E. E., Mavridis, D., & Grant, S. P. (2019). Comparative effectiveness of brief alcohol interventions for college students: Results from a network meta-analysis. *Prevention Science, 20*(5), 715–740. https://doi.org/10.1007/s11121–018-0960-z

Higgins, S. T., Heil, S. H., & Lussier, J. P. (2004). Clinical implications of reinforcement as a determinant of substance use disorders. *Annual Review of Psychology, 55*(1), 431–461. https://doi.org/10.1146/annurev.psych.55.090902.142033

Hunt, G. M., & Azrin, N. H. (1973). A community-reinforcement approach to alcoholism. *Behavior Research and Therapy, 11*(1), 91–104. https://doi.org/10.1016/0005-7967(73)90072-7

James, K., & Jordan, A. (2018). The opioid crisis in black communities. *Journal of Law, Medicine & Ethics, 46*, 404–421. https://doi.org/10.1177/1073110518782949

Joyner, K. J., Meshesha, L. Z., Dennhardt, A. A., Borsari, B., Martens, M. P., & Murphy, J. G. (2019). High opportunity cost demand as an indicator of weekday drinking and distinctly severe alcohol problems: A behavioral economic analysis. *Alcoholism: Clinical and Experimental Research, 43*(12), 2607–2619. https://doi.org/10.1111/acer.14206

Joyner, K. J., Pickover, A. M., Soltis, K. E., Dennhardt, A. A., Martens, M. P., & Murphy, J. G. (2016). Deficits in access to reward are associated with college student alcohol use disorder. *Alcoholism: Clinical and Experimental Research, 40*(12), 2685–2691. https://doi.org/10.1111/acer.13255

Kelly, J. F., Abry, A., Ferri, M., & Humphreys, K. (2020). Alcoholics Anonymous and 12 Step facilitation treatments for alcohol use disorder: A distillation of a 2020 Cochrane review for clinicians and policy makers. *Alcohol and Alcoholism*, 1–12. https://doi.org/10.1093/alcalc/agaa050

Kelly, J. F., Hoeppner, B., Stout, R. L., & Pagano, M. (2012). Determining the relative importance of the mechanisms of behavior change within Alcoholics Anonymous: A multiple mediator analysis. *Addiction, 107*(2), 289–299. http://doi.org/10.1111/j.1360-0443.2011.03593.x

King, M. P., & Tucker, J. A. (2000). Behavior change patterns and strategies distinguishing moderation drinking and abstinence during the natural resolution of alcohol problems without treatment. *Psychology of Addictive Behaviors, 14,* 48–55. https://doi.org/10.1037/0893-164X.14.1.48

Kluwe-Schiavon, B., Viola, T. W., Sanvicente-Vieira, B., Lumertz, F. S., Salum, G. A., Grassi-Oliveira, R., & Quednow, B. B. (2020). Substance related disorders are associated with impaired valuation of delayed gratification and feedback processing: A multilevel meta-analysis and meta-regression. *Neuroscience and Biobehavioral Reviews, 108*, 295–307. https://doi-org.ezproxy.memphis.edu/10.1016/j.neubiorev.2019.11.016

Koffarnus, M. N., Bickel, W. K., & Kablinger, A. S. (2018). Remote alcohol monitoring to facilitate incentive-based treatment for alcohol use disorder: A randomized trial. *Alcoholism: Clinical and Experimental Research, 42*(12), 2423–2431. https://doi.org/10.1111/acer.13891

Kristjansson, A.L., Mann, M.J., Sigfusson, J., Thorisdottir, I.E., Allegrante, & J.P., Sigfusdottir, I.D. (2020) Development and guiding principles of the Icelandic model for preventing adolescent substance use. *Health Promotion Practice, 21* (1), 62–69. https://doi.org/10.1177/1524839919849032

Lejuez, C. W., Hopko, D. R. & Hopko, S. D. (2001). A brief behavioral activation treatment for depression: Treatment manual. *Behavior Modification, 25,* 255–286. https://doi.org/10.1177/0145445501252005

Levin, M., & Hayes, S. C. (2009). ACT, RFT, and contextual behavioral science. In J. T. Blackledge, J. Ciarrochi, & F. P. Deane (Eds.), *Acceptance and commitment therapy: Contemporary theory, research and practice* (pp. 1–40). Australian Academic Press.

Levola, J., Pitkänen, T., Kampman, O., & Aalto, M. (2018). The association of alcohol use and quality of life in depressed and non-depressed individuals: A cross-sectional general population study. *Quality of Life Research, 27*(5), 1217–1226. https://doi.org/10.1007/s11136–017-1741-z

Litt, M. D., Kadden, R. M., Kabela-Cormier, E., & Petry, N. M. (2009). Changing network support for drinking: Network support project 2-year follow-up. *Journal of Consulting and Clinical Psychology, 77*(2), 229–242. https://doi.org/10.1037/a0015252

Litt, M. D., Kadden, R. M., Tennen, H., & Kabela-Cormier, E. (2016). Network support II: Randomized controlled trial of network support treatment and cognitive behavioral therapy for alcohol use disorder. *Drug and Alcohol Dependence, 165*, 203–212. https://doi.org/10.1016/j.drugalcdep.2016.06.010

Magidson, J. F., Andersen, L. S., Satinsky, E. N., Myers, B., Kagee, A., Anvari, M., & Joska, J. A. (2020). "Too much boredom isn't a good thing": Adapting behavioral activation for substance use in a resource-limited South African HIV care setting. *Psychotherapy, 57*(1), 107–118. https://doi.org/10.1037/pst0000257

Magill, M., Ray, L., Kiluk, B., Hoadley, A., Bernstein, M., Tonigan, J.S., & Carroll, K. (2020). A meta-analysis of cognitive-behavioral therapy for alcohol or other drug use disorders: Treatment efficacy by contrast condition. *Journal of Consulting and Clinical Psychology, 87*(12), 1093–1105. https://doi.org/10.1037/ccp0000447

Martínez-Vispo, C., Martínez, Ú., López-Durán, A., del Río, E. F., & Becoña, E. (2018). Effects of behavioural activation on substance use and depression: A systematic review. *Substance Abuse Treatment, Prevention, and Policy 13*, 36 (2018). https://doi.org/10.1186/s13011–018-0173-2

Meinzer, M. C., Oddo, L. E., Vasko, J. M., Murphy, J. G., Iwamoto, D., Lejuez, C. W., & Chronis-Tuscano, A. (2021). A novel intervention to reduce alcohol-related negative consequences in college students with ADHD. *Psychology of Addictive Behaviors.* https://doi.org/10.1037/adb0000663

Mellis, A. M., Snider, S. E., Deshpande, H. U., LaConte, S. M., & Bickel, W. K. (2019). Practicing prospection promotes patience: Repeated episodic future thinking cumulatively reduces delay discounting. *Drug and Alcohol Dependence, 204*, 107507. https://doi.org/10.1016/j.drugalcdep.2019.06.010

Meshesha, L. Z., Soltis, K. E., Wise, E. A., Rohsenow, D. J., Witkiewitz, K., & Murphy, J. G.. (2020). Pilot trial investigating a brief behavioral economic intervention as an adjunctive treatment for alcohol use disorder. *Journal of Substance Abuse Treatment, 113,* 108002. http://doi.org/10.1016/j.jsat.2020.108002

Meyers, R. J., Roozen, H. G., & Smith, J. E. (2011). The community reinforcement approach: An update of the evidence. *Alcohol Research & Health, 33*(4), 380–388.

McKay, J. R. (2017). Making the hard work of recovery more attractive for those with substance use disorders. *Addiction, 112*(5), 751–757. https://doi.org/10.1111/add.13502

Moody, L. N., Tegge, A. N., Poe, L. M., Koffarnus, M. N., & Bickel, W. K. (2018). To drink or to drink less? Distinguishing between effects of implementation intentions on decisions to drink and how much to drink in treatment-seeking individuals with alcohol use disorder. *Addictive Behaviors, 83*, 64–71. https://doi.org/10.1016/j.addbeh.2017.11.010

Murphy, J. G., Correia, C. J., Colby, S. M., & Vuchinich, R. E. (2005). Using behavioral theories of choice to predict drinking outcomes following a brief intervention. *Experimental and Clinical Psychopharmacology, 13,* 93–101. https://doi.org/10.1037/1064-1297.13.2.93

Murphy, J. G., Dennhardt, A. A., Martens, M. P., Borsari, B., Witkiewitz, K., & Meshesha, L. Z. (2019). A randomized clinical trial evaluating the efficacy of a brief alcohol intervention supplemented with a substance-free activity session or relaxation training. *Journal of Consulting and Clinical Psychology, 87*(7), 657–669. https://doi.org/10.1037/ccp0000412

Murphy, J. G., Dennhardt, A. A., Skidmore, J. R., Borsari, B., Barnett, N. P., Colby, S. M., & Martens, M. P. (2012). A randomized controlled trial of a behavioral economic supplement to brief motivational interventions for college drinking. *Journal of Consulting and Clinical Psychology, 80*(5), 876–886. http://doi.org/10.1037/a0028763

Murphy, J. G., McDevitt-Murphy, M. E., & Barnett, N. P. (2005). Drink and be merry? Gender, life satisfaction, and alcohol consumption among college students. *Psychology of Addictive Behaviors, 19*(2), 184. https://doi.org/10.1037/0893-164X.19.2.184

Murphy, J. G., Yurasek, A. M., Dennhardt, A. A., Skidmore, J. R., McDevitt-Murphy, M. E., MacKillop, J., & Martens, M. P. (2013). Symptoms of depression and PTSD are associated with elevated alcohol demand. *Drug and Alcohol Dependence, 127*(1–3), 129–136. https://doi.org/10.1016/j.drugalcdep.2012.06.022

Patel, H., & Amlung, M. (2020). Acute and extended exposure to episodic future thinking in a treatment seeking addiction sample: A pilot study. *Journal of Substance Abuse Treatment*, 108046. http://doi.org/10.1016/j.jsat.2020.108046

Penedo, F. J., & Dahn, J. R. (2005). Exercise and well-being: A review of mental and physical health benefits associated with physical activity. *Current Opinion in Psychiatry, 18*(2), 189–193. https://doi.org/10.1097/00001504-200503000-00013

Powers, M. B., Vedel, E., & Emmelkamp, P. M. G. (2008). Behavioral couples therapy (BCT) for alcohol and drug use disorders: A meta-analysis. *Clinical Psychology Review, 28*(6), 952–962. https://doi.org/10.1016/j.cpr.2008.02.002

Ray, L. A., Bujarski, S., Grodin, E., Hartwell, E., Green, R., Venegas, A., & Miotto, K. (2019). State-of-the-art behavioral and pharmacological treatments for alcohol use disorder. *American Journal of Drug and Alcohol Abuse*, *45*(2), 124–140. https://doi.org/10.1080/00952990.2018.152826

Rung, J. M., & Madden, G. J. (2018). Experimental reductions of delay discounting and impulsive choice: A systematic review and meta-analysis. *Journal of Experimental Psychology: General*, *147*(9), 1349–1381. https://doi.org/10.1037/xge0000462

Sancho, M., De Gracia, M., Rodríguez, R. C., Mallorquí-Bagué, N., Sánchez-González, J., Trujols, J., Sánchez, I., Jiménez-Murcia, S., & Menchón, J. M. (2018). Mindfulness-based interventions for the treatment of substance and behavioral addictions: A systematic review. *Frontiers in Psychiatry, 9*. https://doi.org/10.3389/fpsyt.2018.00095

Spillane, N. S., Smith, G. T., & Kahler, C. W. (2013). Perceived access to reinforcers as a function of alcohol consumption among one First Nation group. *Alcoholism: Clinical and Experimental Research*, *37*, E314–E321. https://doi.org/10.1111/j.1530-0277.2012.01864.x

Subramaniam, S., Holtyn, A. F., Jarvis, B. P., Koffarnus, M. N., Leoutsakos, J. S., & Silverman, K. (2018). Illicit drug use and work in a model therapeutic workplace. *Drug and Alcohol Dependence, 191*, 110–116. https://doi.org/10.1016/j.drugalcdep.2018.06.019

Substance Abuse and Mental Health Services Administration (2020). *Key substance use and mental health indicators in the United States: Results from the*

2019 National Survey on Drug Use and Health (HHS Publication No. PEP20–07-01-001, NSDUH Series H-55). Center for Behavioral Health Statistics and Quality, Substance Abuse and Mental Health Services Administration. www.samhsa.gov/data/

Sudhinaraset, M., Wigglesworth, C., & Takeuchi, D. T. (2016). Social and cultural contexts of alcohol use. *Alcohol Research: Current Reviews, 38*(1), 35–45.

Thekiso, T. B., Murphy, P., Milnes, J., Lambe, K., Curtin, A., & Farren, C. K. (2015). Acceptance and commitment therapy in the treatment of alcohol use disorder and comorbid affective disorder: A pilot matched control trial. *Behavior Therapy, 46*(6), 717–728. https://doi.org/10.1016/j.beth.2015.05.005

Tucker, J. A., Cheong, J., Chandler, S. D., Lambert, B. H., Pietrzak, B., Kwok, H., & Davies, S. L. (2016). Prospective analysis of behavioral economic predictors of stable moderation drinking among problem drinkers attempting natural recovery. *Alcoholism: Clinical and Experimental Research, 40*(12), 2676–2684. https://doi.org/10.1111/acer.13245

Tucker, J. A., Cheong, J., James, T. G., Jung, S., & Chandler, S. D. (2020). Preresolution drinking problem severity profiles associated with stable moderation outcomes of natural recovery attempts. *Alcoholism: Clinical and Experimental Research, 44*(3), 738–745. https://dx.doi.org/10.1111/acer.14287

Tucker, J. A., & Simpson, C. A. (2011). The recovery spectrum: From self-change to seeking treatment. *Alcohol Research & Health, 33*(4), 371–379.

Vaeth, P. A. C., Wang-Schweig, M., & Caetano, R. (2017). Drinking, alcohol use disorder, and treatment access and utilization among US racial/ethnic groups. *Alcoholism: Clinical and Experimental Research, 41*(1), 6–19. https://doi.org/10.1111/acer.13285

Voss, A., Jorgensen, R., & Murphy J. G. (2021). Episodic future thinking as a brief alcohol intervention for heavy drinking college students: A pilot feasibility study. *Experimental and Clinical Psychopharmacology*. https://doi.org/10.1037/pha0000451

Weinstock, J., Petry, N. M., Pescatello, L. S., Henderson, C. E., & Nelson, C. R. (2020). Randomized clinical trial of exercise for nontreatment seeking adults with alcohol use disorder. *Psychology of Addictive Behaviors, 34*(1), 65–75. https://doi.org/10.1037/adb0000506

Witkiewitz, K., Kranzler, H. R., Hallgren, K. A., O'Malley, S. S., Falk, D. E., Litten, R. Z., Hasin, D. S., Mann, K. F., & Anton, R. F. (2018). Drinking risk level reductions associated with improvements in physical health and quality of life among individuals with alcohol use disorder. *Alcoholism: Clinical and Experimental Research, 42*(12), 2453–2465. https://doi.org/10.1111/acer.13897

Witkiewitz, K., Pearson, M. R., Wilson, A. D., Stein, E. R., Votaw, V. R., Hallgren, K. A., Maisto, S. A., Swan, J. E., Schwebel, F. J., Aldridge, A., Zarkin, G. A., & Tucker, J. A. (2020). Can alcohol use disorder recovery include some heavy drinking? A replication and extension up to 9 years following treatment. *Alcoholism: Clinical and Experimental Research, 44*(9), 1862–1874. https://doi.org/10.1111/acer.14413

11 Family and Social Processes in Recovery from Alcohol Use Disorder

Amber M. Jarnecke, Delisa G. Brown, and
Alexander J. Melkonian

Family and Social Processes in Recovery from Alcohol Use Disorder

Social relationships and processes are integral to the development and maintenance of, as well as recovery from, alcohol use disorder (AUD). Individuals with AUD tend to have relatively few social support resources and poor social functioning (Groh et al., 2007; Le Berre, 2019). Positive social support, however, can have a powerful impact on recovery from AUD (Brooks et al., 2017; Buckman et al., 2008; Groh et al., 2007). As this chapter reviews, social support and social networks have considerable influence on AUD and AUD recovery, and both general social support and specific support for recovery are beneficial for positive behavior change. The chapter first considers family and social processes that may be particularly relevant to AUD. Next, background on how these processes can contribute to the development and maintenance of AUD is discussed, which is crucial for understanding the trajectory of AUD and identifying potential targets for interventions. The chapter then reviews research on how family and other sources of social support can contribute to recovery and concludes by identifying directions for future clinical practice and research.

Family and Social Processes Relevant to AUD

The literature examining the role of family and social processes on AUD and AUD recovery is vast and has been studied through the lens of multiple disciplines, such as psychology, sociology, human development, family studies, and genetics, among others. This chapter focuses on several familial and social mechanisms that impact AUD development, maintenance, and recovery. Given the heterogeneity in the development and trajectories of AUD, we briefly review the intergenerational transmission of AUD, along with how early childhood and family factors and relationships can be associated with AUD; discuss the influence of peers in the development and maintenance of AUD; and evaluate how life transitions such as marriage, parenting, and the transition into retirement and older adulthood contribute to AUD. This chapter crucially highlights how social factors influence AUD recovery and how social networks and relationships can be modified and enhanced through mutual help groups, psychotherapies, and other resources to aid recovery.

For the family and social processes considered in this chapter, it is necessary to examine how the nature and quality of social relationships influence AUD and AUD recovery. Historically, researchers have defined social support in various ways. Relevant to the literature on AUD and AUD recovery, two dimensions are general and individual specific social support and social support sources that can include people (e.g., family, friends, pastors, clinicians) or places (e.g., sober living houses, AA, church groups) often encountered in life and throughout the recovery process. General social support measures assess structural (i.e., number of people in social networks) and functional (i.e., quality of social support) dimensions of support; specific social support refers to the actual type of support received by an individual in AUD recovery (i.e., support for drinking vs. support for abstinence) (Groh et al., 2007). The four most commonly studied forms of specific social support include: (1) emotional support – expressions of empathy, love, trust, and caring, often measured as "moral" support; (2) instrumental support – tangible aid and service (e.g., housing, assistance finding a job); (3) informational support – advice, suggestions, and information one may receive related to AUD recovery; and (4) appraisal support – information that is useful for self-evaluation that informs decisions on recovery (Brooks et al., 2017). Regardless of the type of social support, research indicates that social support is important throughout the AUD recovery process and can have desirable effects on drinking outcomes including drinking rates, entry into treatment, and maintenance of treatment gains following treatment (Brooks et al., 2017; Groh et al., 2007).

Family and Social Processes in the Development and Maintenance of AUD

Family Factors Predicting or Protecting against the Development of AUD

It has long been established that there is intergenerational transmission of AUD. Considerable evidence from twin and family data shows that AUD is transmitted among close family lines and that both genetic and environmental factors are at play in the development of AUD (Verhulst et al., 2015). Rearing environments often set the stage for future behavioral and psychosocial outcomes. Drinking norms and attitudes, interpersonal relationship dynamics, and coping skills are all factors that are first established in early childhood rearing environments and may become so entrenched that they affect later alcohol use and AUD recovery. Studies have found that childhood stressors (e.g., disrupted family environment, neglect), insecure parent-child attachment, and witnessing parental intoxication mediate the link between parental AUD and offspring AUD (Kerr et al., 2012; Lee et al., 2016; Sher et al., 1997). Other social factors are associated with the development of AUD in offspring as well. Children who are abused or neglected are at increased risk for later harmful alcohol use, and poor parental monitoring has frequently been linked to greater alcohol use and AUD in later life (Meque et al., 2019; Sher et al., 1997).

Conversely, strong, positive family and community relationships have a substantial role in preventing AUD, particularly among youths and emerging adults. Research has found that more harmonious family relationships, clearly defined family rules, and parental reinforcement for positive behaviors all lower the risk for AUD (Guo et al., 2001). Among Yup'ik Alaska Native adolescents, connections to adults and elders protect against AUD, and community-level factors have a greater impact on AUD outcomes than individual-level factors (Philip et al., 2016). Greater familism (i.e., placing family values ahead of individual values) is associated with reduced alcohol and drug use among adolescents, even after controlling for race and ethnicity (Ewing et al., 2015). This suggests that family values may be particularly relevant for AUD outcomes among multiple ethno-racial groups. In Black youths and emerging adults, parental support buffers against the effect that racial discrimination has on harmful alcohol use (Zapolski et al., 2016). Parents may also have the potential to mitigate the influence of peers, even into early adulthood. Both parental and peer influence is often exerted through perceived norms and attitudes regarding drinking. Among emerging adults who perceive low permissiveness for drinking from their parents, the association between peer influence and harmful alcohol use is weakened (Wood et al., 2004). Thus, enhancing engagement with norm-based education may represent one malleable treatment target through which emerging adult harmful alcohol use can be decreased or prevented.

Siblings can significantly influence alcohol use as well, with some studies showing that sibling alcohol use may have as much of or an even greater impact on adolescent alcohol use than parental alcohol use (Scholte et al., 2008). Older siblings, in particular, may model substance use behaviors for their younger siblings, perhaps normalizing use. Further, siblings may increase access to use for their siblings. Same gender siblings with shared friend groups tend to show more similarity in their alcohol use attitudes and behaviors relative to different gender siblings, siblings with fewer friends in common, or siblings who report trying to be different from one another (Whiteman et al., 2014).

Peer Factors Predicting or Protecting Against the Development of AUD

Peer factors in the development of AUD have been studied extensively, particularly among adolescents and emerging adults. Alcohol-using peers are consistently found to predict alcohol use, and the more peers in a social network that use alcohol further increases risk (Leung et al., 2014). In a sample of Latino adolescents, alcohol use expectancies were found to mediate the association between peer and adolescent alcohol use, such that adolescents who believed alcohol would enhance their social behavior around peers drank more (Segura et al., 2004). There is also evidence from a longitudinal sample of adolescents that suggests deviant peer affiliation is associated with adolescent alcohol use, which further predicts lower levels of positive parenting at a later time point, rather than the other way around (Trucco et al., 2014). It may be that parent-child communication can erode when adolescents use alcohol or engage with delinquent peers rather than this association necessarily being a result of poor parenting.

Emerging adults' drinking has also been strongly correlated with peer substance use, perceived norms, and attitudes about drinking (Reid & Carey, 2018; Tucker et al., 2015). There may be a bidirectional influence between perceived drinking norms and alcohol consumption in certain subpopulations. Among emerging adult lesbian and bisexual women, one study found that women perceived that lesbian and bisexual women drank more than straight women, and perceived drinking norms and alcohol consumption influenced one another in a reciprocal pattern (Talley et al., 2016). Importantly, patterns of peer influence are often studied among college samples; however, similar effects of peer relationships on alcohol use are also observed for non-college emerging adults (Lau-Barraco & Collins, 2011).

Because interpersonal relationships are dynamic, the extant literature has also looked at peer selection effects and alcohol use. There is increasing evidence to support that adolescents who use alcohol or are at high-risk for using alcohol tend to select friends with similar levels of alcohol use or risk (Osgood et al., 2013). Research shows that this may point to a shared genetic liability, wherein the genetic factors associated with one's alcohol use are also associated with affiliation with peers who use alcohol (Hill et al., 2008). Further, familial and genetic risk for AUD has been found to interact with peer influences to drink and increase the likelihood of harmful alcohol use and AUD in some samples (Guo et al., 2009). However, in one sample of African American college students, peer deviance did not interact with an AUD polygenic risk score nor family history of harmful alcohol use to predict AUD symptoms (Su et al., 2018).

Positive social support and peer networks consisting of members who do not drink or engage in harmful alcohol use may decrease risk for AUD, even among individuals with a familial history of AUD. The link between paternal substance use and childhood use has shown to be mitigated when children are not exposed to friends who use substances (Henry et al., 2018). Likewise, among Black college students, global social support and support from friends weaken the association between parental AUD and offspring AUD (Pittman et al., 2019). For lesbian, gay, bisexual, transgender, queer, intersex, and asexual (LGBTQIA+) youth, Gay-Straight Alliances and explicit anti-homophobic policies have been associated with lower odds of drinking and heavy drinking episodes, particularly among girls (Talley et al., 2016).

Social Processes Maintaining AUD among Adults

Social factors remain one of the most consistent predictors of an individual's alcohol use into adulthood and maintenance of AUD. As in adolescence and emerging adulthood, social networks play a key role in alcohol use among adults.

Longitudinal research has shown that having expectations that alcohol will enhance social facilitation accounts for the association between drinking peers and alcohol use (including harmful use) among adults, although this effect appears to be stronger for men than women (Lau-Barraco et al., 2012). Further, peers who drink alcohol shape an individual's expectations for the effects that alcohol will have on social facilitation (Lau-Barraco et al., 2012). Having individuals in one's social network that use alcohol increases one's likelihood of alcohol use and relapse after treatment for AUD. Some research has found that following treatment for AUD, the composition of social networks may not change substantially (Min et al., 2013). This may be because some members of the social network include family members with whom an individual is not willing to break ties. Thus, the influence of social network members who drink may hold even after AUD treatment and contribute to the maintenance of AUD.

The role of adult intimate relationships and marriage are social factors that have long been identified as associated with alcohol use and extensively studied with respect to AUD (Leonard & Eiden, 2007). As individuals transition throughout life stages into adulthood, the marital relationship may become a more important influence on alcohol use than peer relationships. For many, the transition to marriage is associated with decreases in hazardous drinking, even among those with prior AUD, and marriage represents a strong protective factor against alcohol use (Leonard & Eiden, 2007; Rodriguez et al., 2014). Controlling for genetic variation, twin studies also indicate a decrease in drinking for married individuals compared to their single twins (Dinescu et al., 2016). Furthermore, this decrease is consistent across a wide range of racially diverse individuals and appears similar regardless of age of marriage, suggesting that marriage may provide a unique benefit on drinking beyond age-related maturity changes alone. Although further research is needed to explain these patterns, some theories suggest that individuals may be more likely to pair with individuals who are similar to them in drinking patterns ("assortative mating") and also that marriage may result in a change in behavior patterns and attitudes about drinking (Bachman et al., 2014).

Marriage, however, is not universally associated with decreases in alcohol use. Social learning theory provides a framework for understanding how some partners' drinking behaviors may maintain drinking or result in increases in drinking in the other partner. Partner influence models suggest that within a couple, partners' substance use behaviors influence one another's over time. For some, one partner's pre-marriage drinking can predict future drinking for the other, and development of AUD is more likely when one partner has been diagnosed with or has risk factors for AUD (Leonard & Mudar, 2003; Salvatore et al., 2020). Many researchers have highlighted the importance of assessing patterns of drinking concordance between partners. Beyond individual levels of drinking, agreement between partners' drinking patterns and harmful alcohol use has implications for relationship health. Even when alcohol use is elevated, drinking levels that are more consistent with a partner are associated with fewer relationship problems. Greater discrepancies in alcohol use have been associated with poorer relationship health, greater dissatisfaction, and greater risk for divorce in both cross-sectional and longitudinal studies (Holden & Rollins, 2019; Leonard & Eiden, 2007).

The association between intimate partners' drinking and relationship distress is more complex than simply considering drinking concordance. In general, intimate relationship distress increases alcohol use and risk for AUD, even among married individuals who did not have AUD at the start of marriage (Whisman et al., 2006). Greater relationship distress and maladaptive conflict resolution can contribute to increased cravings for alcohol, and ultimately divorce is associated with greater alcohol use (Flanagan et al., 2020; Kretsch & Harden, 2014). Harmful alcohol use may also have negative consequences for the relationship, including decreased relationship satisfaction, intimate partner violence, and divorce (Leonard & Eiden, 2007; Rodriguez et al., 2014). Overall, there is significant interplay between intimate partners' drinking, stress, and conflict.

Other family factors have been examined for their role in AUD in adulthood. The transition to parenthood marks another social process that influences alcohol use and AUD for some individuals. In general, studies have found that heavy drinking in both men and women decreases from pre-pregnancy to pregnancy. For men, this decrease in drinking is primarily explained by marital status, employment, and living arrangements, whereas for women, the reduction appears to be more directly linked to the pregnancy (Bachman et al., 2013). For women, drinking tends to return to near pre-pregnancy levels approximately one year after giving birth (Bachman et al., 2013). Likewise, parenthood itself tends to decrease frequency of drinking and heavy drinking, particularly for women and custodial parents (Fergusson et al., 2012). Family cohesion may play a key process in maintaining or protecting against AUD in adulthood as well. For instance, among Hispanic adults, family cohesion increases perceptions of social support and decreases risk of AUD (Caetano et al., 2017; Cano et al., 2018).

Historically, data have suggested that as individuals age, alcohol use and harmful alcohol use declines; however, this may not be true for all older adults (Barrick & Connors, 2002). As adults transition into older age, another host of social factors play a role in AUD. For some, the transition from work to retirement may cause a change in routine, responsibilities, and social interactions and can contribute to harmful alcohol use (Barrick & Connors, 2002). Social networks for older adults may also shrink over time as children leave the home and close friends and family members pass away. Research has shown that both social connectedness and social isolation are positively associated with alcohol use in older adults. For example, one study found that older women who drank heavily reported more social support than older women who did not drink heavily; however, older men who drank heavily reported lower social support than older men who did not drink heavily (Choi & DiNitto, 2011). Older women tend to have a larger social network than older men, and thus older women may be more likely to drink in the presence of others compared to older men who may be more likely to drink in social isolation. Other research has found that LGBTQIA+ populations may also be at unique risk for AUD in older adulthood. In a large United States sample of lesbian, gay, and bisexual (LGB) adults, approximately one-fifth of older LGB adults reported high-risk drinking (Bryan et al., 2017). Greater social support and perceived drinking norms were associated with greater drinking for LGB women, but not for men. Discrimination-related stress was a strong predictor of drinking for men.

Family and Social Processes in AUD Recovery

Social Connectedness as a Key Factor in AUD Recovery

In addition to the previously discussed impact that social support and social network members can have on AUD development and maintenance, social connectedness can be a critical factor in the AUD recovery process. Isolation has an overwhelming effect on AUD, with many studies demonstrating that individuals who feel more socially isolated tend to report more mental health disorders and substance use disorders, including AUD (Chou et al., 2011). Further, social isolation may have a greater negative effect on AUD recovery for some ethno-racial groups compared to others; for example, individuals who identify as Black, Indigenous, or people of color (BIPOC) tend to value social connectedness to a greater extent than white individuals (Constantine et al., 2003). Regardless of ethno-racial group, however, the process by which social isolation can influence alcohol use can be understood through research on belonging and loneliness. A lack of sense of belonging can lead to loneliness, which in turn is associated with negative self-perception, and research has shown that both negative perception and a sense of loneliness are associated with increased alcohol use (Chou et al., 2011). Hence, social connectedness with family, friends, neighbors, and/or religious leaders, or connections with individuals via organizations (e.g., treatment centers, self-help groups) are a critical part of the recovery process and can amplify specific forms of social support for recovery.

Family and Social Processes in AUD Recovery

Social support is important during all phases of AUD recovery, and having support early in recovery may be most critical. Qualitative research has shown that individuals in recovery identify service providers, siblings, and/or caring peers as among the most helpful social network members for initiating the recovery process (Pettersen et al., 2019). For individuals who pursue inpatient treatment or intensive outpatient treatment as a step in the recovery process, the transition from treatment back into their community may be particularly challenging. While in the "safe zone" of a treatment facility, individuals are surrounded by helpful staff, clinicians, and like-minded others who are working toward recovery. Individuals in inpatient and intensive outpatient treatment settings may be exposed to fewer triggering situations and may be held more accountable for decisions related to drinking. However, when individuals leave these treatment settings, aspects of the structure and routine they had in treatment dissipate or change. Brooks and colleagues (2017) analyzed the social networks of individuals with severe AUD throughout their recovery process from early recovery (i.e., inpatient treatment) through their transition back into the community. Results pointed to the importance of helping individuals in AUD recovery choose social networks that are most conducive to recovery so that gains made in treatment could be adequately reinforced. Thus, bolstering support for recovery in a structured environment and gradually allowing individuals to transition back into their communities may lead to more sustained recovery. Brooks et al. (2017) also demonstrated the role of sober living houses for individuals early in recovery to avoid an abrupt transition from the inpatient setting back into the community. These structured living environments not only provide quasi-safe zones, but they allow individuals early in recovery to develop social networks conducive to the recovery process and ease the transition back into the community.

Participation in AUD mutual help groups like Alcoholics Anonymous (AA) and Self-Management and Recovery Training (SMART) can also increase social support for individuals in AUD recovery and may be particularly helpful when individuals are early in the process. These groups have been shown to decrease drinking, increase constructive pro-abstinent social interactions, and decrease social ties with drinking peers (Brooks et al., 2017; Humphreys et al., 2014; Stevens et al., 2015). Research indicates that AA affiliation is associated with greater abstinence among men residing in sober living homes, and increased AA meeting attendance is associated with abstinence in both early and longer-term recovery (Humphreys et al., 2014; Stevens et al., 2015). Research on the efficacy of SMART in AUD recovery is limited. Nevertheless, over 3,000 meetings are held weekly worldwide (Tucker et al., 2020), which suggests that SMART is a commonly sought-after resource for alcohol-related problems. As with group therapy, the social and peer support aspects of mutual help group participation seem important in AUD recovery (Barrick & Connors, 2002).

Evidence also suggests that online support forums may be beneficial in reducing alcohol use (Liu et al., 2020). More recently, novel digital tools such as smartphone applications have been developed and tested. Some include digital sensors such as breathalyzers, text messaging services, and recovery-focused social networking sites. One study found that making more connections with other users on an AUD recovery-focused social networking application was positively associated with length of sobriety, though more "check-ins" on the application was associated with shorter length of sobriety and a greater number of relapses (Ashford et al., 2020). This may suggest that individuals struggling more with the recovery process are seeking out online support more frequently. Further, this study found generational differences in the use of the application such that Baby Boomers and Generation X users had more connections and activity on the application than Millennials. Additionally, Baby Boomers were more likely than Millennials to report longer periods of sobriety and fewer relapses.

AUD Treatments that Incorporate Close Others

As discussed earlier, not all social relationships have positive associations with AUD recovery. Certain family members or close friends can serve as triggers for craving and use, or individuals may not know how to provide proper support to their loved one in recovery. Group psychotherapies for AUD have long been used, and groups may uniquely stimulate therapeutic mechanisms of change while promoting feelings of support (Yalom, 1995). Beyond this, professionals working with individuals in AUD recovery may want to consider including family members, friends, or additional close others in the recovery process. For instance, clinicians may want to occasionally have individuals in AUD recovery invite close others to individual psychotherapy sessions to learn about AUD recovery and discover techniques for bolstering their support.

Evidence of the importance of involving social network members in AUD treatment has led to the development of novel evidence-based couple and family psychotherapies for AUD and other substance use disorders. These psychotherapies seek to bolster AUD recovery by integrating the support of family members or friends while addressing relationship dynamics that may affect the recovery process. These psychotherapies not only focus on addressing alcohol use and how close others can help the individual with AUD recover, but also aim to help repair damage in relationship related to harmful alcohol use. Over the past 40 years, research has found that family and partner involvement in treatment leads to reduced alcohol use and improved marital and family functioning compared to individual therapy alone (Klostermann & O'Farrell, 2021). This research encouraged the Joint Commission on Accreditation of Health Care Organizations to modify standards for substance use treatment in the United States requiring "... an adult family member to be included, at minimum in the initial assessment phase of the treatment process" (Klostermann & O'Farrell, 2021).

It is important to note that the definition of family varies across cultures and belief systems, which also vary by race. Thus, the definition of family continues to evolve and, as defined by Klostermann and O'Farrell (2021), may include any of the following configurations:

> (a) [A] traditional nuclear family in which members are cohabiting in the household; (b) a single-parent household; (c) a "blended" family resulting from divorce, separation, or remarriage; (d) lesbian or gay couples with or without custodial children; (e) a multigenerational household including grandparents, parents, and children; or (e) long-term cohabiting partners who are not romantically linked, but define themselves as a family. (p. 448)

Some ethno-racial groups (e.g., African Americans) often have expanded definitions of family, and special consideration for social support systems should include, in addition to those listed above, friends, coworkers, counselors, religious leaders, and church and other community members (Hall, 2007; Pittman et al., 2019). Depending on the individual's conceptualization of family and treatment needs, any of these configurations can and should be involved in treatment.

A number of psychotherapies that integrate different family configurations into AUD treatment have been found to be efficacious. Alcohol-focused Behavioral Couple Therapy (ABCT) is a cognitive-behavioral therapy (CBT) that assumes multiple factors maintain the drinking, including individual, dyadic, familial, and other social/environmental variables (McCrady et al., 2016). The intervention combines three major components to affect change in drinking behavior and negative interactions developed among couples, including (1) targeting drinking in the individual with AUD, (2) enhancing the significant other's role in supporting change in their partner's drinking behavior, and (3) enhancing relationship functioning (McCrady et al., 2016). ABCT is an effective family-integrated intervention for couples, and outcome data show substantial decreases in drinking and significant improvements in relationship outcomes across follow-up periods from immediate to 30 months post-treatment (McCrady et al., 2016). Behavioral Couples Therapy (BCT) for substance use disorders is another evidence-based manualized therapy, developed on the foundation of social learning theory, which assumes that couples who engage in harmful substance use also engage in reciprocal patterns of interactions of punishment as opposed to beneficial reinforcing behaviors (Klostermann & Mignone, 2019). BCT has two objectives, including reducing alcohol use and altering the dyadic or family dynamics in the promotion of healthier couples relationships, which should then serve as healthy support for AUD recovery (Klostermann & Mignone, 2019). In a meta-analysis of BCT compared to individual therapy alone, results revealed a clear overall advantage for BCT for reducing frequency of alcohol use and consequences of use and improving relationship satisfaction (Powers et al., 2008).

Community Reinforcement and Family Training (CRAFT) and A Relational Intervention Sequence for Engagement (ARISE) are pre-treatment techniques designed to help family members encourage individuals to seek AUD treatment in a non-confrontational way. CRAFT practitioners use manualized procedures focused on improvement of an individual's awareness of negative consequences, reinforcement of sober behavior, and improvement of familial communication skills (Roozen et al., 2010). ARISE practitioners utilize multiple meetings to engage the individual with AUD as well as family members who are acting as motivational enhancers to encourage treatment; however, nothing is done among family members without the individual's awareness so as not to create mistrust (Landau & Garrett, 2008). Both CRAFT and ARISE have yielded favorable outcomes with over 70 percent of individuals with AUD attending treatment (Landau & Garrett, 2008; Roozen et al., 2010).

Finally, other treatments have focused on increasing social network support for individuals in recovery. For instance, Network Support treatment (Litt et al.,

2015) is an individual-focused treatment that seeks to help individuals with AUD alter their social network in ways that support recovery instead of continued drinking. This is accomplished by encouraging AA or other mutual help group attendance, exploring ways to change one's social network, and teaching social skills. Some evidence suggests that individuals who receive this treatment demonstrate increases in support for abstinence, self-efficacy, and AA involvement, which in turn is associated with more days abstinent (Litt et al., 2009).

Conclusions and Recommendations

As reviewed in this chapter, considerable research has been conducted on how social factors can contribute to or protect against AUD and how specific and general social support from multiple sources can be harnessed to aid AUD recovery. The literature highlights how family history and environment as well as other childhood factors contribute to the development of AUD. As individuals transition into adolescence and then adulthood, peer influences, intimate relationships, and parenthood become more salient influences on the AUD trajectory. During older adulthood, other social factors relevant to AUD include retirement, widowhood, and network changes that increase social isolation. Depending on an individual's stage of development, some or all of these social factors may be relevant to consider, and they may represent individual vulnerabilities that need to be addressed during the recovery process. Fortunately, numerous resources, programs, and treatment options have been developed to enhance social support and bolster relationships, therefore addressing some of these individual vulnerabilities. Many of these options have a solid evidence base indicating they can aid tremendously in one's recovery process.

Although extensive work has been done to understand family and social processes in AUD and to develop options to address deficits in support for recovery, there is much work left to do. More longitudinal studies are needed to understand the dynamic interplay of various relationships and alcohol use, particularly in adult and older adult populations. Many studies that explore AUD recovery tend to focus on early recovery and neglect longer term recovery. This makes it difficult to ascertain how social relationships and social support affect recovery at different stages in the process. The lack of studies focused on long-term recovery limits inferences about which subpopulations and at which time points in the dynamic recovery process social relationships or general versus specific types of social support may be particularly relevant. Likewise, more longitudinal studies that examine the long-term effects of programs and treatments that aim to enhance social support for AUD recovery are necessary. Some studies have follow-up assessments that examined intervention outcomes a few months to a couple of years post-treatment, but longer-term follow-up assessments are rare. This is critical to informing whether social support "booster" sessions would be useful to individuals as they traverse the recovery process. Relatedly, development of a guideline for a stepped-care approach for integrating social supports into the AUD recovery process at various stages is needed.

More work is also needed to examine how family and social processes influence AUD and AUD recovery as a function of personal identity and cultural context. Much of the research examining social factors in AUD has had a lens on the dominant culture, and the resulting findings from the dominant culture have been the basis for developing interventions that incorporate close others and bolster social support. There is a need to increase relevant research with individuals of various identities and cultural backgrounds and develop culturally-sensitive interventions that incorporate close others for various populations. For instance, many existing couples and family focused treatments for AUD have not explicitly addressed expanded definitions of family or focused on integrating other community members (e.g., religious leaders, friends) into treatment. Additionally, although some efforts and interventions specifically focus on building communities of support for individuals in recovery, future work should aim to create novel and inclusive programs, treatments, and resources that bolster communities of support for individuals in recovery throughout different stages of the process. Much of the research literature and many existing resources and programs emphasize recovery through an abstinence-based approach, and more research and interventions are needed that are focused on or adapted for individuals pursuing recovery using a harm reduction approach.

Finally, more efforts are needed to disseminate and utilize evidence-based social support-focused recovery resources. Not all individuals in a community can be expected to ascribe to one pathway to AUD recovery; thus, communities may need multiple resources to provide support for individuals in recovery. For instance, in some communities only AA groups may be available, and other mutual help groups for recovery (e.g., SMART) are lacking. Likewise, few professionals provide couples- and family-focused treatments in real-world clinical settings. Despite enthusiasm for these treatments on the part of individuals, families, and clinicians, major barriers exist for their implementation (McCrady et al., 2019), including a lack of training for or time to train clinicians; clinician concerns about confidentiality, billing, and documentation of the family members; and difficulty with transportation and scheduling of more than one person in a family or couple for appointments. Additional dissemination and training efforts, including web-based and virtual trainings for professionals, may help providers become more comfortable integrating social network members into treatment. Further, advocacy, policy, and funding decisions can ameliorate barriers to treatment. For example, with increased support and funding, childcare services can be integrated into treatment centers to make it easier for couples and families to engage in AUD treatment. Fostering a corporate culture that encourages self-care and mental health treatment-seeking could motivate companies and businesses to offer time off for such services.

In summary, a solid empirical foundation exists for understanding how family and social processes contribute to AUD development, maintenance, and recovery processes. It is evident that even though AUD and AUD recovery are very heterogeneous, the role of close others is crucial regardless of AUD trajectory. Research to date on social and family processes in AUD has been used to develop programs, interventions, and resources that integrate social support for individuals recovering from AUD. Additional work from multiple disciplines is needed to advance understanding of the dynamic social factors involved in AUD and AUD recovery and to integrate social supports into the recovery process for individuals with AUD across subpopulations with various cultural backgrounds, identities, and goals for recovery.

Acknowledgments

This chapter is the result of work supported, in part, by the National Institute on Alcohol Abuse and Alcoholism (K23AA027307), the Office of Research on Women's Health (U54DA016511), and the Department of Veterans Affairs Office of Academic Affiliations Advanced Fellowship Program in Mental Illness Research and Treatment (MIRECC).

References

Ashford, R. D., Giorgi, S., Mann, B., Pesce, C., Sherritt, L., Ungar, L., & Curtis, B. (2020). Digital recovery networks: Characterizing user participation, engagement, and outcomes of a novel recovery social network smartphone application. *Journal of Substance Abuse Treatment*, *109*, 50–55. https://doi.org/https://doi.org/10.1016/j.jsat.2019.11.005

Bachman, J. G., O'Malley, P. M., Schulenberg, J. E., Johnston, L. D., Bryant, A. L., & Merline, A. C. (2014). *The decline of substance use in young adulthood: Changes in social activities, roles, and beliefs*. Psychology Press.

Bachman, J. G., Wadsworth, K. N., O'Malley, P. M., Johnston, L. D., & Schulenberg, J. E. (2013). *Smoking, drinking, and drug use in young adulthood: The impacts of new freedoms and new responsibilities*. Psychology Press.

Barrick, C., & Connors, G. J. (2002). Relapse prevention and maintaining abstinence in older adults with alcohol use disorders. *Drugs & Aging*, *19*(8), 583–594. https://doi.org/10.2165/00002512-200219080-00004

Brooks, A. T., Magaña Lòpez, M., Ranucci, A., Krumlauf, M., & Wallen, G. R. (2017). A qualitative exploration of social support during treatment for severe alcohol use disorder and recovery. *Addictive Behaviors Reports*, *6*, 76–82. https://doi.org/https://doi.org/10.1016/j.abrep.2017.08.002

Bryan, A. E. B., Kim, H.-J., & Fredriksen-Goldsen, K. I. (2017). Factors associated with high-risk alcohol consumption among LGB older adults: The roles of gender, social support, perceived stress, discrimination, and stigma. *The Gerontologist, 57*(suppl_1), S95–S104. https://doi.org/10.1093/geront/gnw100

Buckman, J. F., Bates, M. E., & Morgenstern, J. (2008). Social support and cognitive impairment in clients receiving treatment for alcohol and drug use disorders: A replication study. *Journal of Studies on Alcohol and Drugs, 69*(5), 738–746. https://doi.org/10.15288/jsad.2008.69.738

Caetano, R., Vaeth, P. A., & Canino, G. (2017). Family cohesion and pride, drinking and alcohol use disorder in Puerto Rico. *American Journal of Drug and Alcohol Abuse, 43*(1), 87–94. https://doi.org/10.1080/00952990.2016.1225073

Cano, M. Á., Sánchez, M., Rojas, P., Ramírez-Ortiz, D., Polo, K. L., Romano, E., & De La Rosa, M. (2018). Alcohol use severity among adult Hispanic immigrants: Examining the roles of family cohesion, social support, and gender. *Substance Use & Misuse, 53*(4), 668–676. https://doi.org/10.1080/10826084.2017.1356333

Choi, N. G., & DiNitto, D. M. (2011). Heavy/binge drinking and depressive symptoms in older adults: Gender differences. *International Journal of Geriatric Psychiatry, 26*(8), 860–868. https://doi.org/https://doi.org/10.1002/gps.2616

Chou, K. L., Liang, K., & Sareen, J. (2011). The association between social isolation and DSM-IV mood, anxiety, and substance use disorders: Wave 2 of the National Epidemiologic Survey on Alcohol and Related Conditions. *Journal of Clinical Psychiatry, 72*(11), 1468–1476. https://doi.org/10.4088/JCP.10m06019gry

Constantine, M. G., Gainor, K. A., Ahluwalia, M. K., & Berkel, L. A. (2003). Independent and interdependent self-construals, individualism, collectivism, and harmony control in African Americans. *Journal of Black Psychology, 29*(1), 87–101. https://doi.org/10.1177/0095798402239230

Dinescu, D., Turkheimer, E., Beam, C. R., Horn, E. E., Duncan, G., & Emery, R. E. (2016). Is marriage a buzzkill? A twin study of marital status and alcohol consumption. *Journal of Family Psychology, 30*(6), 698. https://doi.org/10.1037/fam0000221

Ewing, B. A., Osilla, K. C., Pedersen, E. R., Hunter, S. B., Miles, J. N. V., & D'Amico, E. J. (2015). Longitudinal family effects on substance use among an at-risk adolescent sample. *Addictive Behaviors, 41*, 185–191. https://doi.org/https://doi.org/10.1016/j.addbeh.2014.10.017

Fergusson, D. M., Boden, J. M., & John Horwood, L. (2012). Transition to parenthood and substance use disorders: Findings from a 30-year longitudinal study. *Drug and Alcohol Dependence, 125*(3), 295–300. https://doi.org/https://doi.org/10.1016/j.drugalcdep.2012.03.003

Flanagan, J. C., Jarnecke, A. M., Leone, R. M., & Oesterle, D. W. (2020). Effects of couple conflict on alcohol craving: Does intimate partner violence play a role? *Addictive Behaviors, 109*, 106474. https://doi.org/https://doi.org/10.1016/j.addbeh.2020.106474

Groh, D. R., Jason, L. A., Davis, M. I., Olson, B. D., & Ferrari, J. R. (2007). Friends, family, and alcohol abuse: An examination of general and alcohol-specific social support. *American Journal on Addictions, 16*(1), 49–55. https://doi.org/10.1080/10550490601080084

Guo, G., Elder, G. H., Cai, T., & Hamilton, N. (2009). Gene–environment interactions: Peers' alcohol use moderates genetic contribution to adolescent drinking behavior. *Social Science Research*, *38*(1), 213–224. https://doi.org/10.1016/j.ssresearch.2008.04.002

Guo, J., Hawkins, J. D., Hill, K. G., & Abbott, R. D. (2001). Childhood and adolescent predictors of alcohol abuse and dependence in young adulthood. *Journal of Studies on Alcohol*, *62*(6), 754–762. https://doi.org/10.15288/jsa.2001.62.754

Hall, J. (2007). Kinship ties: Attachment relationships that promote resilience in African American adult children of alcoholics. *Advances in Social Work*, *8*, 130–140. https://doi.org/10.18060/136

Henry, K. L., Fulco, C. J., Agbeke, D. V., & Ratcliff, A. M. (2018). Intergenerational continuity in substance abuse: Does offspring's friendship network make a difference? *Journal of Adolescent Health*, *63*(2), 205–212. https://doi.org/https://doi.org/10.1016/j.jadohealth.2018.02.014

Hill, J., Emery, R. E., Harden, K. P., Mendle, J., & Turkheimer, E. (2008). Alcohol use in adolescent twins and affiliation with substance using peers. *Journal of Abnormal Child Psychology*, *36*(1), 81–94. https://doi.org/10.1007/s10802–007-9161-0

Holden, C. L., & Rollins, P. (2019). Discrepant alcohol use, conflict, and couples satisfaction in a community sample. *The American Journal of Family Therapy*, *47*(5), 311–327. https://doi.org/10.1080/01926187.2019.1658554

Humphreys, K., Blodgett, J. C., & Wagner, T. H. (2014). Estimating the efficacy of Alcoholics Anonymous without self-selection bias: An instrumental variables re-analysis of randomized clinical trials. *Alcoholism: Clinical and Experimental Research*, *38*(11), 2688–2694. https://doi.org/10.1111/acer.12557

Kerr, D. C., Capaldi, D. M., Pears, K. C., & Owen, L. D. (2012). Intergenerational influences on early alcohol use: Independence from the problem behavior pathway. *Developmental Psychopathology*, *24*(3), 889–906. https://doi.org/10.1017/s0954579412000430

Klostermann, K., & Mignone, T. (2019). Behavioral couples therapy for substance use disorders. *Social Behavior Research and Practice*, *3*(1), 25–27. https://doi.org/10.17140/SBRPOJ-3-113

Klostermann, K., & O'Farrell, T. J. (2021). Couple and family therapy in treatment of alcoholism and drug abuse. In N. el-Guebaly, G. Carrà, M. Galanter, & A. M. Baldacchino (Eds.), *Textbook of Addiction Treatment: International Perspectives* (pp. 447–458). Springer International Publishing. https://doi.org/10.1007/978-3-030-36391-8_31

Kretsch, N., & Harden, K. P. (2014). Marriage, divorce, and alcohol use in young adulthood: A longitudinal sibling-comparison study. *Emerging Adulthood*, *2*(2), 138–149. https://doi.org/10.1177/2167696813513260

Landau, J., & Garrett, J. (2008). Invitational intervention: The ARISE model for engaging reluctant alcohol and other drug abusers in treatment. *Alcoholism Treatment Quarterly*, *26*(1-2), 147–168. https://doi.org/10.1300/J020v26n01_08

Lau-Barraco, C., Braitman, A. L., Leonard, K. E., & Padilla, M. (2012). Drinking buddies and their prospective influence on alcohol outcomes: Alcohol expectancies as a mediator. *Psychology of Addictive Behaviors*, *26*(4), 747–758. https://doi.org/10.1037/a0028909

Lau-Barraco, C., & Collins, R. L. (2011). Social networks and alcohol use among nonstudent emerging adults: A preliminary study. *Addictive Behaviors*, *36*(1-2), 47–54. https://doi.org/10.1016/j.addbeh.2010.08.017

Le Berre, A.-P. (2019). Emotional processing and social cognition in alcohol use disorder. *Neuropsychology, 33*(6), 808–821. https://doi.org/10.1037/neu0000572

Lee, J. Y., Brook, J. S., Nezia, N., & Brook, D. W. (2016). Adolescent predictors of alcohol use in adulthood: A 22-year longitudinal study. *American Journal on Addictions, 25*(7), 549–556. https://doi.org/10.1111/ajad.12438

Leonard, K. E., & Eiden, R. D. (2007). Marital and family processes in the context of alcohol use and alcohol disorders. *Annual Review of Clinical Psychology, 3*(1), 285–310. https://doi.org/10.1146/annurev.clinpsy.3.022806.091424

Leonard, K. E., & Mudar, P. (2003). Peer and partner drinking and the transition to marriage: A longitudinal examination of selection and influence processes. *Psychology of Addictive Behaviors, 17*(2), 115–125. https://doi.org/10.1037/0893-164X.17.2.115

Leung, R. K., Toumbourou, J. W., & Hemphill, S. A. (2014). The effect of peer influence and selection processes on adolescent alcohol use: A systematic review of longitudinal studies. *Health Psychology Review, 8*(4), 426–457. https://doi.org/10.1080/17437199.2011.587961

Litt, D. M., Lewis, M. A., Rhew, I. C., Hodge, K. A., & Kaysen, D. L. (2015). Reciprocal relationships over time between descriptive norms and alcohol use in young adult sexual minority women. *Psychology of Addictive Behaviors, 29*(4), 885–893. https://doi.org/10.1037/adb0000122

Litt, M. D., Kadden, R. M., Kabela-Cormier, E., & Petry, N. M. (2009). Changing network support for drinking: Network support project 2-year follow-up. *Journal of Consulting and Clinical Psychology, 77*(2), 229–242. https://doi.org/10.1037/a0015252

Liu, Y., Kornfield, R., Shaw, B. R., Shah, D. V., McTavish, F., & Gustafson, D. H. (2020). Giving and receiving social support in online substance use disorder forums: How self-efficacy moderates effects on relapse. *Patient Education and Counseling, 103*(6), 1125–1133. https://doi.org/https://doi.org/10.1016/j.pec.2019.12.015

McCrady, B., Wilson, A., Muñoz, R., Fink, B., Fokas, K., & Borders, A. (2016). Alcohol-focused behavioral couple therapy. *Family Process, 55*(3), 443–459. https://doi.org/10.1111/famp.12231

McCrady, B. S., Wilson, A., Fink, B., Borders, A., Muñoz, R., & Fokas, K. (2019). A consumer's eye view of family-involved alcohol treatment. *Alcoholism Treatment Quarterly, 37*(1), 43–59. https://doi.org/10.1080/07347324.2018.1482245

Meque, I., Salom, C., Betts, K. S., & Alati, R. (2019). Predictors of alcohol use disorders among young adults: A systematic review of longitudinal studies. *Alcohol and Alcoholism, 54*(3), 310–324. https://doi.org/10.1093/alcalc/agz020

Min, M. O., Tracy, E. M., Kim, H., Park, H., Jun, M., Brown, S., McCarty, C., & Laudet, A. (2013). Changes in personal networks of women in residential and outpatient substance abuse treatment. *Journal of Substance Abuse Treatment, 45*(4), 325–334. https://doi.org/10.1016/j.jsat.2013.04.006

Osgood, D. W., Ragan, D. T., Wallace, L., Gest, S. D., Feinberg, M. E., & Moody, J. (2013). Peers and the emergence of alcohol use: Influence and selection processes in adolescent friendship networks. *Journal of Research on Adolescence*, *23*(3), 500–512. https://doi.org/https://doi.org/10.1111/jora.12059

Pettersen, H., Landheim, A., Skeie, I., Biong, S., Brodahl, M., Oute, J., & Davidson, L. (2019). How social relationships influence substance use disorder recovery: A collaborative narrative study. *Substance Abuse: Research and Treatment*, *13*, 1178221819833379. https://doi.org/10.1177/1178221819833379

Philip, J., Ford, T., Henry, D., Rasmus, S., & Allen, J. (2016). Relationship of social network to protective factors in suicide and alcohol use disorder intervention for rural Yup'ik Alaska native youth. *Psychosocial Intervention*, *25*(1), 45–54. https://doi.org/10.1016/j.psi.2015.08.002

Pittman, D. M., Quayson, A. A., Rush, C. R., & Minges, M. L. (2019). Revisiting resilience: Examining the relationships between stress, social support, and drinking behavior among black college students with parental substance use disorder histories. *Journal of Ethnicity in Substance Abuse*, 1–22. https://doi .org/10.1080/15332640.2019.1707142

Powers, M. B., Vedel, E., & Emmelkamp, P. M. (2008). Behavioral couples therapy (BCT) for alcohol and drug use disorders: A meta-analysis. *Clinical Psychology Review*, *28*(6), 952–962. https://doi.org/10.1016/j.cpr.2008.02.002

Reid, A. E., & Carey, K. B. (2018). Why is social network drinking associated with college students' alcohol use? Focus on psychological mediators. *Psychology of Addictive Behaviors*, *32*(4), 456. https://doi.org/10.1037/adb0000374

Rodriguez, L. M., Neighbors, C., & Knee, C. R. (2014). Problematic alcohol use and marital distress: An interdependence theory perspective. *Addiction Research & Theory*, *22*(4), 294–312. https://doi.org/10.3109/16066359.2013.841890

Roozen, H. G., de Waart, R., & van der Kroft, P. (2010). Community reinforcement and family training: An effective option to engage treatment-resistant substance-abusing individuals in treatment. *Addiction*, *105*(10), 1729–1738. https://doi .org/10.1111/j.1360-0443.2010.03016.x

Salvatore, J. E., Larsson Lönn, S., Sundquist, J., Sundquist, K., & Kendler, K. S. (2020). Disentangling social-genetic from rearing-environment effects for alcohol use disorder using Swedish national data. *Psychological Science*, *31*(9), 1140–1149. https://doi.org/10.1177/0956797620931542

Scholte, R. H. J., Poelen, E. A. P., Willemsen, G., Boomsma, D. I., & Engels, R. C. M. E. (2008). Relative risks of adolescent and young adult alcohol use: The role of drinking fathers, mothers, siblings, and friends. *Addictive Behaviors*, *33*(1), 1–14. https://doi.org/10.1016/j.addbeh.2007.04.015

Segura, Y. L., Page, M. C., Neighbors, B. D., Nichols-Anderson, C., & Gillaspy, S. (2004). The importance of peers in alcohol use among Latino adolescents: The role of alcohol expectancies and acculturation. *Journal of Ethnicity in Substance Abuse*, *2*(3), 31–49. https://doi.org/10.1300/J233v02n03_02

Sher, K. J., Gershuny, B. S., Peterson, L., & Raskin, G. (1997). The role of childhood stressors in the intergenerational transmission of alcohol use disorders. *Journal of Studies on Alcohol*, *58*(4), 414–427. https://doi.org/10.15288/jsa.1997.58.414

Stevens, E., Jason, L. A., Ram, D., & Light, J. (2015). Investigating social support and network relationships in substance use disorder recovery. *Substance Abuse*, *36* (4), 396–399. https://doi.org/10.1080/08897077.2014.965870

Su, J., Kuo, S. I. C., Meyers, J. L., Guy, M. C., & Dick, D. M. (2018). Examining interactions between genetic risk for alcohol problems, peer deviance, and interpersonal traumatic events on trajectories of alcohol use disorder symptoms among African American college students. *Developmental Psychopathology*, *30*(5), 1749–1761. https://doi.org/10.1017/S0954579418000962

Talley, A. E., Gilbert, P. A., Mitchell, J., Goldbach, J., Marshall, B. D. L., & Kaysen, D. (2016). Addressing gaps on risk and resilience factors for alcohol use outcomes in sexual and gender minority populations. *Drug and Alcohol Review*, *35*(4), 484–493. https://doi.org/10.1111/dar.12387

Trucco, E. M., Colder, C. R., Wieczorek, W. F., Lengua, L. J., & Hawk Jr., L. W., (2014). Early adolescent alcohol use in context: How neighborhoods, parents, and peers impact youth. *Developmental Psychopathology*, *26*(2), 425–436. https://doi.org/10.1017/s0954579414000042

Tucker, J. A., Chandler, S. D., & Witkiewitz, K. (2020). Epidemiology of recovery from alcohol use disorder. *Alcohol Research : Current Reviews*, *40*(3), 02. https://doi.org/10.35946/arcr.v40.3.02

Tucker, J. A., Cheong, J., Chandler, S. D., Crawford, S. M., & Simpson, C. A. (2015). Social networks and substance use among at-risk emerging adults living in disadvantaged urban areas in the southern United States: A cross-sectional naturalistic study. *Addiction*, *110*(9), 1524–1532. https://doi.org/10.1111/add.13010

Verhulst, B., Neale, M. C., & Kendler, K. S. (2015). The heritability of alcohol use disorders: A meta-analysis of twin and adoption studies. *Psychological Medicine*, *45*(5), 1061–1072. https://doi.org/10.1017/s0033291714002165

Whisman, M. A., Uebelacker, L. A., & Bruce, M. L. (2006). Longitudinal association between marital dissatisfaction and alcohol use disorders in a community sample. *Journal of Family Psychology*, *20*(1), 164–167. https://doi.org/10.1037/0893-3200.20.1.164

Whiteman, S. D., Jensen, A. C., & Maggs, J. L. (2014). Similarities and differences in adolescent siblings' alcohol-related attitudes, use, and delinquency: Evidence for convergent and divergent influence processes. *Journal of Youth and Adolescence*, *43*(5), 687–697. https://doi.org/10.1007/s10964–013-9971-z

Wood, M. D., Read, J. P., Mitchell, R. E., & Brand, N. H. (2004). Do parents still matter? Parent and peer influences on alcohol involvement among recent high school graduates. *Psychology of Addictive Behaviors*, *18*(1), 19. https://doi.org/10.1037/0893-164X.18.1.19

Yalom, I. D. (1995). *The theory and practice of group psychotherapy* (4th ed). Basic Books.

Zapolski, T. C., Fisher, S., Hsu, W. W., & Barnes, J. (2016). What can parents do? Examining the role of parental support on the negative relationship between racial discrimination, depression, and drug use among African American youth. *Clinical Psychological Science*, *4*(4), 718–731. https://doi.org/10.1177/2167702616646371

12 Community-Based Harm Reduction Approaches for Alcohol Use Disorder

Susan E. Collins, Seema L. Clifasefi, Grover "Will" Williams, Lovella Black Bear, and The LEAP Community Advisory Board

Community-Based Harm Reduction Approaches for Alcohol Use Disorder

At the beginning of every harm reduction training we conduct, we ask the audience, "What comes to mind when you hear the term 'harm reduction'?" Over the past decade of our trainings, the first response shouted out is typically "Needle exchange!" In the past couple of years, however, we have heard a much more differentiated set of responses from our audience, which now includes case managers, nurses, housing providers, physicians, social workers, licensed mental health professionals, and psychologists. At our most recent training, participants called out, "Working with your client where they are at," "Providing a menu of options ranging from abstinence-based treatment to low-barrier Housing First programs," and simply, "Being compassionate."

In this chapter, we speak to this ever-evolving operationalization of harm reduction in the specific context of alcohol use disorder (AUD) and how it is applied in community-based settings with marginalized populations (i.e., specific groups of people who are affected by structural inequities that result in disproportionate harm and exclusion from the dominant culture's social, economic, or political privileges). We also discuss its current evidence base, provide community perspectives, and point out future directions within this defined scope. The emphasis on *community* in the chapter title acknowledges that the approaches we are emphasizing are deeply embedded in the communities they serve, have often been developed within the community, are delivered in community settings, and are implemented at the community level. Although this chapter has a very specific focus on AUD, harm reduction approaches can and have been applied in various settings and levels of intervention and can benefit people across the lifespan and in different communities, socioeconomic strata, and health-related behaviors.

The What's and Why's of Community-Based Harm Reduction Approaches for AUD

As applied to alcohol use, the umbrella term "harm reduction" refers to a compassionate stance and a set of pragmatic strategies that minimize alcohol-related harm and enhance quality of life for people who use alcohol and their communities. As its name suggests, harm reduction breaks with traditional abstinence-based approaches in that it does not require or even particularly elevate abstinence or use reduction as the ultimate goals (Collins et al., 2011). As harm reductionists, we neither preclude nor deny the healing power of abstinence-based approaches, but instead view harm reduction approaches as necessary additions to the spectrum of service options to ensure greater reach and effectiveness of our existing treatment and public health systems.

Drawing on ecological systems theory (Bronfenbrenner, 1979), harm reduction approaches for AUD may be applied at various levels, ranging from the microsystem level (i.e., individual-level treatment) to the mesosystem level (i.e., community-level interventions) to the exosystem level (i.e., population-based approaches) to the macrosystem level (i.e., law and public policy; Collins et al., 2011). Taking the widest lens, exo- and macrosystem levels comprise population-based approaches (e.g., public service announcements discouraging drinking and driving) and policy change (e.g., decriminalizing public intoxication, government regulations requiring warning labels on alcoholic beverages; Marlatt & Witkiewitz, 2010). In this chapter, we focus on approaches to harm reduction for AUD that are delivered in community-based settings on either the individual (e.g., community-codesigned harm-reduction treatment delivered in community-based settings) or community (e.g., low-barrier housing programs that do not require abstinence) levels. In this section, we operationalize community-based harm reduction in practice and provide its rationale.

Community-Based Harm Reduction Fills a Treatment Service Gap

When abstinence-based approaches are not optimally reaching and treating marginalized community members, community-based harm reduction approaches can fill the gap. Abstinence-based approaches are simply not relevant to the vast majority of Americans with AUD. In the National Survey on Drug Use and Health, the Substance Abuse and Mental Health Services Administration (SAMHSA, 2019) showed that 15.5 million Americans needed treatment for AUD (i.e., either meet criteria for AUD or had attended treatment in the past year), but only about 9 percent received it. Among those who met criteria for AUD but did not receive treatment, 96 percent reported they did not need treatment (SAMHSA, 2019). Abstinence-based treatments are thus not engaging the vast majority of the general United States (US) population affected by AUD, and the same treatment gap exists in nearly all countries around the globe.

Within the general population, marginalized communities often have access to treatment through systemic facilitators (e.g., state-provided case management and treatment options) and systemic pressures (e.g., court-mandated treatment). However, abstinence-based treatment attendance and completion is likewise poor, and among those who do complete treatment, subsequent outcomes are modest at best (Orwin et al., 1999). In other words, our current treatment systems are failing many. Qualitative research has indicated that abstinence-based treatment is often not considered desirable, relevant, or effective by groups that have been marginalized in the existing treatment system, including communities of color, people who are socioeconomically marginalized, and people who are experiencing homelessness (Collins, Clifasefi, Andrasik et al., 2012; Collins, Clifasefi, Dana et al., 2012; Collins et al., 2016; Crabtree et al., 2018; Lee & Petersen, 2009; Vaeth et al., 2017).

In contrast, harm reduction approaches are often viewed as the "only thing that works" by both staff and marginalized community members who have been afforded the opportunity to practice harm reduction in community-based settings (Collins, Clifasefi, Andrasik et al., 2012; Collins, Clifasefi, Dana et al., 2012; Collins et al., 2016; Crabtree et al., 2018; Lee & Petersen, 2009). In this case, context matters. Those who are working in community-based settings versus typical AUD treatment settings are not waiting for abstinence-ready clients to present to their clinic; they must serve all clients, even those not ready, willing, or able to stop using substances. In this case, harm reduction approaches are preferred even among staff who, as chemical dependency counselors, were steeped in the abstinence-based treatment traditions. As a chemical dependency counselor in one of our qualitative studies put it: "I would like to see abstinence. But that's an unrealistic hope for our population ... That's an option that will only do more harm than good. So, you want them to have the liberty to drink, but not hurt themselves or anyone else" (Collins, Clifasefi, Dana et al., 2012).

Focusing on Harm Reduction Instead of Use Reduction Is Theoretically Parsimonious

Community-based harm reduction recognizes that a focus on harm reduction rather than use reduction is more parsimonious. Abstinence-based approaches are predicated on the belief that the more one uses alcohol, the more alcohol-related harm one experiences. The corollary is that the more one reduces use, with the perceived ultimate success culminating in abstinence, the more one's alcohol-related harm will decrease. While this assumption is rarely explicitly acknowledged, it forms the foundation of treatment systems in the United States. Alcohol treatment is typically reserved for people who are experiencing enough alcohol-related harm to disrupt the systems they live in. Thus, the common belief is that, if a person simply goes to treatment and stops drinking, they will stop experiencing alcohol-related harm, and they will stop disrupting the systems they live in.

Unfortunately, this assumed one-to-one correlation between use reduction and harm reduction does not consistently hold. Research conducted around the world has consistently shown that larger familial, community-wide, and even geopolitical forces create disparities that precipitate and maintain a disproportionate level of alcohol-related harm in more marginalized and vulnerable populations (Collins, 2016). Conversely, people from dominant classes (e.g., in the United States, white, male, heterosexual, cisgender, higher socioeconomic status) can consume larger quantities of alcohol with far fewer consequences (Collins, 2016). These findings underscore the greater importance of systems inequities over individuals' alcohol use in shaping their experience of and others' perceptions of the extent of their alcohol-related harm.

There are also individual-level, biological factors that contradict an assumption that use reduction is synonymous with harm reduction. For people who are physiologically dependent, use reduction can even fuel alcohol-related harm. The kindling effect provides a clear example of this phenomenon, i.e., repeated cycles through the revolving door of self-induced or treatment-required abstinence alternating with heavy drinking can precipitate increasingly severe and deadly withdrawal symptoms (Becker, 1998). Thus, for those who are physiologically dependent, drinking some alcohol every day and thereby avoiding withdrawal and its kindling effect is less harmful than circling the revolving door. Despite this known medical phenomenon and grassroots efforts to educate community members on harm reduction to address it, our existing treatment systems do not allow for patients to use alcohol to "get well" or avoid withdrawal, and self-led alcohol tapers are not considered viable options.

Because the assumed one-to-one relationship between use reduction and harm reduction does not hold, particularly in marginalized communities, harm reductionists apply the Occam's razor or law of parsimony. We set aside the middle men – the proxy of abstinence and the insistence on abstinence-based and clinic-based treatment as the pathway to it. We focus instead on the most relevant and parsimonious solution for the individual, their families, their communities, and public health – reduction in alcohol-related harm and improvement in quality of life and more local community-based means of achieving it.

Community-Based Harm Reduction Respects Individual and Community-Level Autonomy

Given its grassroots affiliation and person-driven stance, harm reduction centers show respect for the autonomy of people who use substances (Harm Reduction Coalition, 2020). This stance is, however, also pragmatic. Providers cannot realistically force behavior change outside of highly structured inpatient treatment settings (Denning & Little, 2012). Indeed, it stands to reason that only the affected individual fully understands the personal context in which they would enact change and, given that, what means of alcohol-related harm reduction and quality-of-life improvement will be feasible and effective for them (Denning & Little, 2012). In support of this autonomous approach, research with people experiencing homelessness has shown that people's intrinsic motivation for change is a stronger predictor than the external pressures of abstinence-based treatment attendance in the amelioration of alcohol-related harm (Collins et al., 2012).

Community-Based Harm Reduction Works Best When It Is Community-Driven

When asked how they would redesign AUD approaches in their own vision, people in marginalized communities have indicated they want AUD programs in which (a) more providers share their racial, ethnic, and cultural affiliation; (b) their values, goals, and cultural traditions are centered; (c) abstinence is not the sole or primary emphasis because meeting basic needs must be prioritized (e.g., housing, food, managing withdrawal); and (d) providers honor their own pathways to healing (Clifasefi et al., 2016; Collins, Clifasefi, Andrasik et al. 2012; Collins, Clifasefi, Dana et al., 2012; Collins et al., 2016; Crabtree et al., 2018; Lee & Petersen, 2009). Such community-driven approaches have been shown to better engage marginalized community members, reduce their alcohol-related harm, and improve their quality of life (Clifasefi, Collins, & The LEAP Advisory Board, 2020; Collins et al., 2019; Collins, Duncan et al., 2021). In a recent study, we found that the more community members are leading and shaping community-based harm-reduction approaches, the more their alcohol outcomes improve (Collins, Goldstein et al., 2020).

The Evidence Base for Community-Based Harm Reduction Approaches

Harm reduction approaches are often embedded into communities that include networks of people more severely affected by AUD. Community-level applications that have received the greatest research attention include low-barrier supportive housing often referred to as the "Housing First" approach, managed alcohol programs, and harm reduction programming for community-based service sites.

Housing First

Housing First entails the provision of immediate, permanent, low-barrier, non-abstinence-based supportive housing to chronically homeless individuals (Malone et al., 2015; Tsemberis, 2010). Supportive service provision (including outreach; intensive case management; psychiatric, medical and/or nursing care; substance-use counseling; connections to external service providers; and assistance with basic needs) is predicated on assertive engagement, not coercion, and uses a harm reduction approach in addressing substance use. Specifically, residents are housed as quickly as possible and are not required to achieve abstinence, attend treatment, engage with services, or achieve psychiatric stability before receiving housing. This low-barrier approach contrasts with the housing approach widely used in the decades leading up to the 2000s, known variously as the linear, "continuum-of-care," or "treatment-first" approach, in which increasingly permanent housing (i.e., moving from a shelter to transitional housing to permanent housing) is contingent on fulfilling various criteria, including psychiatric stability, treatment adherence, and abstinence from alcohol and other drug use (Kertesz, 2009).

Two primary types of Housing First, differentiated principally by the separation (scattered-site) or clustering (single-site or project-based) of housing units, have been evaluated. The scattered-site approach has been in use since the early 1990s (Tsemberis & Eisenberg, 2000). In this approach, residents are offered a choice of housing units scattered throughout a larger community and can access supportive services via an assertive community treatment model.

Research on the scattered site approach has accumulated for two decades. In the early 2000s, randomized controlled trials conducted in the United States showed that, compared to the linear model of housing, scattered-site Housing First was associated with less time to housing, improved housing retention and stability, higher perceived choice, and no differences in substance use outcomes (Tsemberis & Eisenberg, 2000; Tsemberis, Gulcur, & Nakae, 2004; Tsemberis, Kent, & Respress, 2012). Larger multisite randomized controlled trials were subsequently conducted in Canada and have largely supported and extended the US research findings. Compared to participants who received the linear housing approach, scattered-site Housing First participants overall have shown strong, positive, long-term effects, including greater housing stability, improved community functioning, and reduced alcohol-related harm and money spent on alcohol (Kirst et al., 2015; Stergiopoulos et al., 2015).

In the single-site Housing First approach, residents are provided with individual units within a single building and can elect to receive on-site supportive services (Malone et al., 2015). A nonrandomized controlled evaluation, which used propensity score weighting to accommodate potential group imbalance, showed that single-site Housing First was associated with reduced utilization of publicly funded services (i.e., shelter, jail, ER, emergency medical services, sleep-off facilities, safety-net hospital) and associated costs (i.e., $4 million in cost offsets during the first year; Larimer et al., 2009). Subsequent studies have shown significant longer-term reductions in county jail bookings and time incarcerated (Clifasefi, Malone, & Collins, 2013), decreased alcohol use and alcohol-related harm (Collins, Malone, Clifasefi, et al., 2012), and strong housing retention in a population traditionally characterized as unmotivated for and unsuccessful in housing (Collins, Malone, & Clifasefi, 2013; Malone, 2009). Additional qualitative studies have indicated that moving into single-site

Housing First improves residents' connection to service providers, increases their sense of stability, and strengthens community-building (Collins, Clifasefi, Andrasik et al., 2012; Collins, Clifasefi, Dana et al., 2012). Other single-site Housing First programs have been evaluated alone or alongside scattered-site Housing First programs and have shown similarly positive effects on psychiatric and housing stability (Brown et al., 2016; Somers et al., 2017). Considering its effectiveness in addressing homelessness and other issues affecting this population, Housing First has become an important component in national and international policy efforts to end homelessness (National Alliance to End Homelessness, 2012)

Managed Alcohol Programs

Housing First programs, as well as certain shelters, drop-in programs, and case management programs, have embraced a harm reduction approach that often includes a tolerance of onsite drinking (Grazioli et al., 2017; Thornquist et al., 2002; Tsemberis et al., 2004), and in some cases, providers plan together with program participants a scheduled distribution of program participants' pre-purchased alcohol (Collins, Clifasefi, Dana et al., 2012). These types of harm-reduction programs have been shown to be successful in encouraging program participation, reducing alcohol-related harm, increasing housing retention, and reducing publicly funded service utilization (Clifasefi et al., 2013; Collins et al., 2013; Collins, Malone, Clifasefi et al., 2012; Grazioli et al., 2017; Larimer et al., 2009; Mackelprang et al., 2014; Tsemberis et al., 2004).

Embedded in Housing First programs, shelters and other community-based settings, managed alcohol programs (MAPs) go further than tolerance of or planning with participants regarding distributing pre-purchased alcohol to them. Instead, MAPs involve medically supervised and often prescribed provision of beverage alcohol at regular intervals to program participants who are physiologically dependent on alcohol. The goal of MAPs is to avoid extreme and medically dangerous intoxication/withdrawal cycles, stabilize participants' day-to-day functioning, and reduce use of high cost publicly funded services. They are often administered in the context of other supportive services as well (i.e., clinical management, access to food, money management, meaningful activities, and social connection; Pauly et al., 2018).

Such services do not currently exist in the United States but are relatively prevalent in Canada. For over a decade, a handful of smaller pilot studies have established the promise of this approach, notably showing MAP participants' decreased contact with law enforcement and use of high cost publicly funded services (e.g., emergency departments, emergency medical services, shelters, detox; Pauly et al., 2013; Podymow et al., 2006; Vallance et al., 2016). None of these studies were randomized controlled trials, and thus the findings are more suggestive than conclusive (Muckle et al., 2012). More recently, however, a larger nonrandomized controlled study indicated that longer term (> 2 months in program) MAP participants drank more frequently but substantially less alcohol per day (−7.1 standard drinks) and were significantly less likely to report alcohol-related harm (i.e., medical, interpersonal, housing, legal problems) compared to matched controls (Stockwell et al., 2018). Newer arrivals to the MAP programs (< 2 months in program) evinced better alcohol outcomes than control participants but had less positive outcomes than longer term participants (Stockwell et al., 2018). Taken together, findings to date indicate that MAPs are well-positioned to achieve program goals of greater stability and harm reduction for participants. Randomized controlled trials are needed to ascribe causality to MAPs for the observed improvements. Nevertheless, the accumulating pilot work on MAPs is promising for community-based harm reduction.

Meaningful Activities Programming

Nestled within community-based settings, client-driven meaningful activities programming can serve as an important adjunct to more traditional treatment and service provision. Its perceived importance in community-based harm reduction is underscored by its inclusion as a key component of Housing First interventions (Gilmer et al., 2013; Malone et al., 2015; Tsemberis, 2010; Watson et al., 2013). Specifically, it is recommended that programming be meaningful to residents and resident-driven, and can include individual/group outings, creative activities, and regular tenant-input meetings (Gaetz et al., 2013).

This recommendation has been echoed in a qualitative study documenting Housing First residents' expressed interest in programming that incorporates their input, improves their health and well-being, helps them reconnect to their own values and goals, and contributes to the community (Clifasefi et al., 2016). Studies conducted in other social services and clinical settings have shown an association between participation in meaningful activities (e.g., art therapy, gardening-based interventions, music therapy) and improved housing, psychiatric, and substance use outcomes (Clatworthy et al., 2013; Dingle et al., 2008; Slayton et al., 2010). However, only one controlled trial to date has tested the implementation of community-based harm reduction programming (Clifasefi et al., 2020).

The Life Enhancing Alcohol-management Program (LEAP) was developed and evaluated together with residents, staff, and management in a Housing First setting in the context of a multiphase community-based participatory research project. In the first phase, interviews and focus groups were conducted to determine what programming was considered desirable by residents and feasible by staff. Residents expressed an interest in collaboratively developed harm reduction programming that comprised meaningful activities and support for community-defined pathways to recovery (Clifasefi et al., 2016). Using the qualitative data, a community advisory board comprised of academic researchers as well as Housing First residents, staff, and management developed the LEAP using a community-based participatory research process (Collins et al., 2018).

A subsequent nonrandomized controlled trial (using propensity score weighting to balance groups) compared alcohol and quality of life outcomes for the Housing First program that received the LEAP versus two Housing First programs that received services as usual (Clifasefi et al., 2020). Findings indicated that LEAP participants engaged in significantly more meaningful activities than participants who received services as usual in their Housing First settings during a 6-month timeframe. Additional within-subjects analyses of LEAP participants showed significant decreases in alcohol-related harm and typical alcohol quantity (Clifasefi et al., 2020). This within-subjects finding was dose-dependent. During the 6-month follow-up, participants who regularly attended LEAP activities ($\geq$ 2 activities per month) reported drinking 16 percent less in typical alcohol quantity and experiencing 10 percent less alcohol-related harm for each month that passed compared to people who did not regularly attend activities (i.e., $<$ 3 activities during the entire 6-month period). An ongoing cluster randomized trial will provide a stronger test of the effectiveness of such a community-level, harm reduction-based meaningful activities program.

Community-Based Harm Reduction Approaches Applied at the Individual Level

Individual level, community-based harm reduction approaches for AUD have primarily entailed treatment that meets people "where they're at" in both their motivation for change and in their community settings. It assumes the same ecological systems framework discussed in prior sections, which holds that substance use is not only influenced by individual-level factors, but also broader familial, community, and even geopolitical factors (Bronfenbrenner, 1979). Because AUD is not viewed as residing solely within the individual, harm reduction counselors and clinicians avoid pathologizing or placing moral value on substance use (Denning & Little, 2012). Instead, they provide community members with the information they need to make scientifically but also personally informed decisions to reduce their alcohol-related harm and improve their quality of life – for themselves, their families, and their communities.

There has been some disagreement about what differentiates harm reduction treatment from other treatment approaches (Heather, 2006). It is, however, the primary therapeutic intention – harm reduction versus use reduction or abstinence – that provides the clearest point of differentiation (Collins et al., 2011; Heather, 2006). Even in its name, the therapeutic intention of harm reduction is transparent and explicit, whereas abstinence or use-reduction treatment goals are often assumed or implied in most other approaches in practice. Finally, harm reduction treatment is less directive in its style than other AUD treatments, which typically utilize different strategies to engage people with provider-guided goals, most often abstinence or moderate drinking. While the name does convey its agenda, harm reduction treatment is flexible and thus can easily and must necessarily accommodate any patient-driven goals that can reduce substance-related harm (e.g., reduced blackouts, avoiding withdrawal, abstinence) and/or improve quality of life within a person's own context and community (Collins et al., 2015).

Harm reduction approaches applied on the individual level have garnered an evidence base in the context of other substance use disorders (e.g., opioids; Des Jarlais et al., 2013; Nielsen et al., 2016) and for risky drinking in nonclinical populations (e.g., college drinkers; Marlatt et al., 1998; Pearson, 2013). Additionally, work has been done in alcohol research and treatment to begin to broaden the definition of recovery (e.g., Witkiewitz et al., 2020). Best treatment practices, however, still indicate abstinence as the recommended goal and desired treatment outcome for people with AUD (NIAAA, 2005; Willenbring, 2014), and abstinence is the required focus of most publicly funded AUD treatment in the United States.

Despite these traditions in AUD treatment, some states and localities have begun to institute mandates that harm reduction be included in the spectrum of treatment service provision. Alcohol researchers have also long noted the need for harm-reduction treatment approaches to AUD (Marlatt & Witkiewitz, 2002), and the importance of honoring client-directed change (Sobell et al., 2000). Respected colleagues in the harm reduction field have developed explicit harm reduction psychotherapeutic practices, clinician manuals, and self-help guides (Anderson, 2010; Denning & Little, 2012, 2017; Tartarsky, 2002). Thus, the tradition of individual-level harm reduction approaches and the acknowledgment of the need for individual-level harm reduction approaches for AUD is not new.

These efforts, however, have resulted in few empirical trials of harm-reduction treatment. This dearth of research has resulted, in part, from the long-standing controversy around the appropriateness of harm reduction for clinically affected populations (people with AUD versus "risky drinkers") and barriers to accessing research funding explicitly for harm reduction treatment. Further, there are few AUD treatments that have been co-created with marginalized communities and are implemented in community-based versus clinic-based settings. In the next section, we describe the only two known empirical studies of community-based harm reduction treatment for AUD. These studies were conceptualized and co-designed with community members who would be the treatment recipients, and services were delivered in community-based versus traditional substance use treatment clinic settings to non-treatment-seeking community members.

Community-Based Behavioral Harm Reduction Treatment for AUD

Recently, our team developed a community-based behavioral harm reduction treatment for individuals with AUD using a multiphase community-based participatory research approach similar to that discussed in the earlier section on meaningful activities LEAP programming (Collins et al., 2018). Initially, interviews were conducted with 50 people with lived experience of homelessness and AUD to understand community perspectives on existing abstinence-based treatment and the community's vision for redesigning AUD treatment to be more relevant, acceptable, desirable, and effective (Collins et al., 2016). The findings indicated a lack of interest in existing abstinence-based approaches, which were considered to be institutionally oppressive, overly focused on abstinence, physically removed from their community, and mismatched to their own experience of AUD and larger life context (Collins et al., 2016). Instead, participants preferred client-driven, community-based, nonjudgmental, nonabstinence-based approaches that emphasize engagement in meaningful activities, personal goal-setting, and discussions of safer-drinking strategies. These findings echoed those of prior qualitative studies with people with lived experience of homelessness and AUD regarding their preferences on programming content and treatment goals (Clifasefi et al., 2016; Collins, Clifasefi, Dana, et al., 2012; Collins et al., 2015; Crabtree et al., 2018; Lee & Petersen, 2009).

Based on these stated preferences, researchers worked together with staff, management, and clients at community-based non-profits to co-develop a community-based, behavioral Harm Reduction Treatment for AUD (HaRT-A). The resulting treatment entailed a community-driven and pragmatic mindset that prioritized client-driven harm reduction and quality of life improvement over abstinence achievement or use reduction goal-setting. HaRT-A also entailed a compassionate approach, founded in the spirit, processes, and communication skills of motivational interviewing (Miller & Rollnick, 2012), with the difference being that it is explicitly directed toward a harm reduction end. HaRT-A interventionists used only strengths-based reflections and affirmations and did not engage in advice-giving or judgment about alcohol use (Miller & Rollnick, 2012). HaRT-A-specific components included (1) collaborative assessment and tracking of client-preferred alcohol metrics, (2) elicitation of client-driven harm reduction and quality of life goals, and (3) discussion of community-crowdsourced safer-drinking strategies. The latter included ways to buffer alcohol's effects on the body (e.g., taking B-complex vitamins, eating before/during drinking), make changes in the manner of drinking (e.g., drinking in a safer place, moving from nonbeverage alcohol [e.g., hand sanitizer] to beverage alcohol [beer, wine, or liquor]), and/or safely change the amount consumed (e.g., engaging in some nondrinking activities, tapering toward abstinence while preventing withdrawal, replacing alcohol with cannabis to avoid further liver damage).

Findings showed strong participant engagement. Among the 184 non-treatment-seekers who were screened for participation, 99 percent consented, and 98 percent attended the baseline assessment. In keeping with the low-barrier, harm reduction approach, inclusion and exclusion criteria were minimal; thus, 92 percent of people who completed the baseline assessment were included in the trial. At the final, 3-month follow-up, 74 percent of participants completed data collection. The vast majority (92 percent) of HaRT-A participants reported a positive treatment experience, whereas 8 percent had mixed or neutral perceptions of HaRT-A. No participants reported a negative perception of HaRT-A.

HaRT-A participants showed clinically meaningful reductions in peak alcohol quantity (−66 percent), alcohol-related harm (−71 percent), and number of AUD symptoms (−63 percent) across the 3-month study period, which translated into statistically significant differences between the HaRT-A and services-as-usual control conditions. Despite the fact that abstinence is not a priority or stated goal in harm reduction, HaRT-A participants evinced significantly fewer positive alcohol biomarker tests (−20 percent) over the course of the study compared to control participants (+19 percent) (Collins et al., 2019)

Combined Pharmacotherapy and Behavioral Treatment for Harm Reduction in AUD

Extending the HaRT-A approach, we also conducted an additional randomized controlled trial to test the efficacy of combining pharmacotherapy (i.e., extended-release naltrexone) and community-based behavioral harm reduction treatment for people experiencing homelessness and AUD (Collins, Duncan, et al., 2021). Participants were 308 adults experiencing homelessness and AUD who were receiving shelter and drop-in services at one of three community-based, non-profit agencies in downtown Seattle, WA. Participants were randomized to one of four treatment arms: (1) behavioral harm reduction treatment for AUD framed for medical providers working in community-based service provision (HaRT-A) plus extended-release naltrexone (XR-NTX), (2) HaRT-A plus placebo injections, (3) HaRT-A only, and (4) supportive services treatment as usual (TAU) at their community-based setting.

Of those approached, nearly all (97 percent) were interested in participation, and over three-fourths of participants in the HaRT-A+XR-NTX arm attended the final Week 12 treatment session. Participants' stated goals focused on increasing meeting basic needs (27 percent), changing alcohol use (26 percent), enhancing quality of life (21 percent), and improving health (16 percent), among others (10 percent); only 4 percent of participants' stated goals were to attain or maintain abstinence from alcohol.

Compared to services as usual, the HaRT-A+XR-NTX arm evinced significant, baseline-to-posttreatment improvements across five of six outcomes: peak alcohol quantity, alcohol frequency, alcohol-related harm, alcohol biomarker tests, and physical health-related quality of life (HR-QoL). After treatment discontinuation at 12 weeks, improvements were maintained through the 36-week follow-up. Participants receiving HaRT-A+Placebo and HaRT-A alone showed improvements across three of six outcomes compared to TAU. Overall, findings indicated that combining behavioral harm reduction treatment and XR-NTX resulted in decreased alcohol use and alcohol-related harm and improved physical HR-QoL for people experiencing homelessness and severe AUD compared to existing community-based services as usual. Future studies are needed to see if a maintenance treatment approach can extend these positive outcomes.

Community Perspectives on Harm Reduction Approaches

There is an ever-increasing evidence base for community-based harm reduction interventions, suggesting that they are effective in reducing alcohol-related harm, improving quality of life, and decreasing use of high cost publicly funded services. However, a deeper understanding of the impact of community-based approaches is imparted by community members involved in the work. To place community-based harm reduction approaches in context, the co-authors of this chapter had a series of conversations about the importance and meaning of this work given their own intergenerational and personal lived experience of AUD and alcohol-related harm. The resulting conversations provided key themes for researchers and clinicians to consider in community-based harm reduction efforts. Table 12.1 presents quotes to illustrate these themes.

First, we all reflected on the experience and pain of intergenerational alcohol-related harm and its deep, long-lasting impact on families and communities. Making space to acknowledge and share about this intergenerational pain without shame is key to personal recovery and to productive engagement in

Table 12.1. *Perceptions of key elements to success in community-based harm reduction*

Theme	Illustrative quotes from co-authors
Acknowledging intergenerational alcohol-related harm	My mother started drinking when I was 13. It came to a point that I was drinking with her, and these things I carry within me. These things I would like to share, because a lot of people withhold their inner feelings and what they have lived through. Not sharing or talking about these hurts or whatever it is we go through in life and using alcohol and drugs—that hurt my children deeply. It hurt my family. It hurt my community. And these things I need to talk about.
	My father recently shared a picture of three men, smiling, holding up whiskey in a toast. It was my great grandfather—tavern owner and prohibition bootlegger—behind his bar serving my grandfather and my great uncle. The latter two men would go on to commit years of domestic violence. In their wake, too many of the next generation's lives were lost violently and prematurely. I finally decided that harm reduction meant I needed to stop drinking. But I think I did it mostly because I needed to know my daughter would be able to see a different pathway forward for herself, four generations later.
Collaborating and co-learning with community	Working on the community advisory board keeps you grounded, and then you get to meet grounded people. It is a meeting of the minds coming together at the round table. My favorite part was meeting all of the different people and knowing that people were interested in what was going on in the community. They were interested in what we were talking about and what we were trying to do.

Table 12.1. (*cont.*)

Theme	Illustrative quotes from co-authors
	It allows for connections. I may not always agree with everyone, but people can learn from me, and I can learn from them. This is about being heard. Sitting around a table with other people, people can hear me.
Meeting community members where they are at	I think of the Come As You Are [harm reduction treatment] Group. I think about [one of the founding members] all the time. Whenever she said, "Hey, just come as you are!" People did come! It's about being educational without being preachy. We wanted our population to have options, not just one thing to try. We wanted them to have multiple options, in case one didn't work for them. We wanted to see if there would be progress—change in their health and habits. For those who stuck with the program, the results were satisfying.
	If one is motivated—self-motivated, perhaps by having "hit bottom"—abstinence is possible under the ideal circumstances. However, many in the homeless community are not living under ideal circumstances. It's not the option of abstinence that does more harm than good, it's the *requirement* that makes it more difficult and unrealistic... Community-based harm reduction, with its less rigid structure, allows for some flexibility. This seems appropriate in cases where, due to chaotic circumstances such as homelessness, people have less ability to keep to a strictly defined routine. It can help fill the gap.
Not leaving anyone behind	I have been there. Once you have been there, you can't leave them behind. Just because I don't have a drink this hour, I can help my fellow man. I have had experiences in my past that can benefit others. When I see a person who is suffering and needing help, I know that I can open my door and offer help when they are in a time of need. Working on our community-based harm reduction programs has helped me to understand that when other people are in need, I can open my door to help someone else. By allowing me to be on the board and share my ideas and build on others' ideas, I've learned that I can bring that home to my community to help others.

harm-reduction efforts. Another key theme is the importance of working together with communities – community members and other stakeholders – to co-design and co-lead community-based harm-reduction programming. Community collaboration ensures the effort is desirable to those it means to serve, builds community investment and sustainability, supports co-learning, and builds community capacity for future efforts. Next, community-based harm-reduction efforts need to focus on nonjudgmentally accepting people "wherever they're at." This openness and flexibility of harm-reduction programming is what makes an initial connection possible and then helps forge a trusting connection over time. Finally, community members said that the effort toward harm reduction must continue, even in the face of obstacles, because we "can't leave people behind." Embracing a harm-reduction perspective through this work has given us the mindset, "heartset," tools, and networks to share recovery more broadly as we move forward together.

Conclusions and Recommendations

Community-based harm reduction for AUD is nothing new to communities, but it is a newer area of focus in AUD research and intervention. In this chapter, we defined community-based harm reduction for AUD, reviewed the existing evidence base, and shared community members' thoughts on the process and findings.

Community-based harm reduction services delivered on both the community and individual levels are well-positioned to fill the gap where abstinence-based approaches are not optimally reaching and treating marginalized community members. In practice, harm reductionists recognize the importance, desirability, and parsimony of moving our intervention focus from abstinence to harm reduction and quality of life enhancement. Community-based harm reduction respects individual and community-level autonomy, and it works best when it is community-driven.

The existing literature indicates strong support for immediate, permanent, low-barrier, non-abstinence-based Housing First for people experiencing homelessness. Other community-level harm-reduction approaches, including managed alcohol programs and meaningful activities programming, show promise in nonrandomized controlled trials and will benefit from future, larger, and more rigorous studies of their effectiveness. There is a small but growing literature showing the efficacy of community-based, individual-level harm reduction behavioral and combined pharmacotherapy and behavioral treatment when offered to non-treatment-seekers in community settings. Overall, community-based harm reduction is a needed addition to our existing menu of options for AUD, so that "no one is left behind."

Acknowledgments

We acknowledge the many years of contributions of the LEAP community advisory board members, both past and present. Current members include Lovella BlackBear*, Shawn Buffalomeat, Todd Cole*, Diane Davis, Roger Field*, Shannon "Star" Jones, John Knudson*, Michael Landman, Jeffrey Lumsden*, John Sutherland*, Doug Wicklander, and Mike Zachary. The asterisk denotes members who actively contributed perspectives for this chapter. We dedicate this chapter to our late employee and long-time community consultant, Joey Stanton, who showed us how to advocate for communities and live in a harm-reduction way.

References

Anderson, K. (2010). *How to change your drinking: A harm reduction guide to alcohol.* HAMS Harm Reduction Network.

Becker, H. C. (1998). Kindling in alcohol withdrawal. *Alcohol Health & Research World, 22*, 25–33.

Bronfenbrenner, U. (1979). *The ecology of human development.* Harvard University Press.

Brown, M. M., Jason, L. A., Malone, D. K., Srebnik, D., & Sylla, L. (2016). Housing first as an effective model for community stabilization among vulnerable individuals with chronic and nonchronic homelessness histories. *Journal of Community Psychology, 44*, 384–390. https://doi.org/10.1002/jcop.21763

Clatworthy, J., Hinds, J., & Camic, P. M. (2013). Gardening as a mental health intervention: A review. *Mental Health Review Journal, 18*, 214–225. https://doi.org/10.1108/MHRJ-02-2013-0007

Clifasefi, S. L., Collins, S. E., & The LEAP Advisory Board. (2020). The life enhancing alcohol-management program (LEAP): Results from a 6-month nonrandomized controlled pilot study assessing a community-based participatory research program in Housing First. *Journal of Community Psychology, 48*, 763–776. https://doi.org/10.1002/jcop.22291

Clifasefi, S. L., Collins, S. E., Torres, N. I., Grazioli, V. S., & Mackelprang, J. L. (2016). Housing First, but what comes second? A qualitative study of resident, staff, and management perspectives on single-site Housing First program enhancement. *Journal of Community Psychology, 44*, 845–855. https://doi.org/10.1002/jcop.21812

Clifasefi, S. L., Malone, D., & Collins, S. E. (2013). Associations between criminal history, Housing First exposure, and jail outcomes among chronically homeless individuals with alcohol problems. *International Journal of Drug Policy, 24*, 291–296. https://doi.org/10.1016/j.drugpo.2012.10.002

Collins, S. E. (2016). Associations between socioeconomic factors and alcohol outcomes. *Alcohol Research: Current Reviews, 38*, 83–94.

Collins, S. E., Clifasefi, S. L., Andrasik, M. P., Dana, E. A., Stahl, N. E., Kirouac, M., Welbaum, C., King, M., & Malone, D. K. (2012). Exploring transitions within a project-based Housing First setting: Qualitative evaluation and practice implications. *Journal of Health Care for the Poor and Underserved, 23*, 1678–1697. https://doi.org/10.1353/hpu.2012.0187

Collins, S. E., Clifasefi, S. L., Dana, E. A., Andrasik, M. P., Stahl, N. E., Kirouac, M., Welbaum, C., King, M., & Malone, D. K. (2012). Where harm reduction meets Housing First: Exploring alcohol's role in a project-based Housing First setting. *International Journal of Drug Policy, 23*, 111–119. https://doi.org/10.1016/j.drugpo.2011.07.010

Collins, S. E., Clifasefi, S. L., Logan, D. E., Samples, L., Somers, J., & Marlatt, G. A. (2011). Chapter 1–Harm reduction: Current status, historical highlights, and basic principles. In G. A. Marlatt, K. Witkiewitz, & M. E. Larimer (Eds.), *Harm reduction: Pragmatic strategies for managing high-risk behaviors.* (2nd ed.) (pp. 3-35). Guilford.

Collins, S. E., Clifasefi, S. L., Nelson, L. A., Stanton, J., Goldstein, S. C., Taylor, E. M., Hoffmann, G., King, V. L., Hatsukami, A. S., Cunningham, Z. L., Taylor, E., Mayberry, N., Malone, D. K., & Jackson, T. R. (2019). Randomized controlled trial of harm reduction treatment for alcohol (HaRT-A) for people experiencing homelessness and alcohol use disorder. *International Journal of Drug Policy, 67*, 24–33. https://doi.org/10.1016/j.drugpo.2019.01.002

Collins, S. E., Clifasefi, S. L., Stanton, J., The LEAP Advisory Board, Straits, K. J. E., Gil-Kashiwabara, E., Nicasio, A. V., Hawes, S. M., Nelson, L. A., Duran, B. M., & Wallerstein, N. (2018). Community-based participatory research (CBPR): Towards equitable involvement of community in psychology research. *American Psychologist, 73*, 884–898. https://doi.org/10.1037/amp0000167

Collins, S. E., Duncan, M. H., Saxon, A. J., Taylor, E. M., Mayberry, N., Merrill, J. O., Hoffmann, G. E., Clifasefi, S. L., & Ries, R. K. (2021). Combining extended-release naltrexone and behavioral harm-reduction treatment for people experiencing homelessness and alcohol use disorder in the USA: A randomized clinical trial. *The Lancet Psychiatry*. https://doi.org/10.1016/S2215-0366(20)30489-2

Collins, S. E., Goldstein, S. C., King, V. L., Orfaly, V. E., Gu, J., Clark, A., Vess, A., Lee, G., Taylor, E. M., Fentress, T., Braid, A. K., & Clifasefi, S. L. (2020). Characterizing components of and attendance at resident-driven Housing First programming in the context of community-based participatory research. *Journal of Community Psychology,* 1–17. https://doi.org/10.1002/jcop.22491

Collins, S. E., Grazioli, V., Torres, N., Taylor, E., Jones, C., Hoffman, G., Haelsig, L., Zhu, A., Hatsukami, A. S., Koker, M. J., Herndon, P., Greenleaf, S. M., & Dean, P. (2015). Qualitatively and quantitatively evaluating harm-reduction goals among chronically homeless individuals with alcohol dependence. *Addictive Behaviors, 45*, 184–190. https://doi.org/10.1016/j.addbeh.2015.02.001

Collins, S. E., Jones, C. B., Hoffmann, G., Nelson, L. A., Hawes, S. M., Grazioli, V. S., Mackelprang, J. L., Holttum, J., Kaese, G., Lenert, J., Herndon, P., & Clifasefi, S. L. (2016). In their own words: Content analysis of pathways to recovery among individuals with the lived experience of homelessness and alcohol use disorders. *International Journal of Drug Policy, 27*, 89–96. https://doi.org/10.1016/j.drugpo.2015.08.003

Collins, S. E., Malone, D. K., & Clifasefi, S. L. (2013). Housing retention in single-site Housing First for chronically homeless individuals with severe alcohol problems. *American Journal of Public Health, 103*, S269–S274. https://doi.org/10.2105/AJPH.2013.301312

Collins, S. E., Malone, D. K., Clifasefi, S. L., Ginzler, J. A., Garner, M. D., Burlingham, B., Lonczak, H. S., Dana, E. A., Kirouac, M., Tanzer, K., Hobson, W., Marlatt, A., & Larimer, M. E. (2012). Project-based Housing First for chronically homeless individuals with alcohol problems: Within-subjects analyses of two-year alcohol-use trajectories. *American Journal of Public Health, 102*, 511–519. https://doi.org/10.2105/AJPH.2011.300403

Collins, S. E., Malone, D. K., & Larimer, M. E. (2012). Motivation to change and treatment attendance as predictors of alcohol-use outcomes among project-based housing first residents. *Addictive Behaviors, 37*, 931–939. https://doi.org/10.1016/j.addbeh.2012.03.029

Crabtree, A., Latham, N., Morgan, R., Pauly, B., Bungay, V., & Buxton, J. A. (2018). Perceived harms and harm reduction strategies among people who drink non-beverage alcohol: Community-based qualitative research in Vancouver, Canada. *International Journal of Drug Policy, 59*, 85–93. https://doi.org/10.1016/j.drugpo.2018.06.020

Denning, P., & Little, J. (2012). *Practicing harm reduction psychotherapy: An alternative approach to addictions* (2nd ed.). Guilford.

Denning, P., & Little, J. (eds.). (2017). *Over the influence: The harm reduction guide for managing drugs and alcohol.* Guilford.

Des Jarlais, D. C., Feelemyer, J. P., Modi, S. N., Abdul-Quader, A., & Hagan, H. (2013). High coverage needle/syringe programs for people who inject drugs in low and middle income countries: A systematic review. *BMC Public Health, 13*, 53. https://doi.org/10.1186/1471-2458-13-53

Dingle, G. A., Gleadhill, L., & Baker, F. A. (2008). Can music therapy engage patients in group cognitive behavior therapy for substance abuse treatment? *Drug and Alcohol Review, 27*, 190–196. https://doi.org/10.1080/09595230701829371

Gaetz, S., Scott, F., & Gulliver, T. (2013). *Housing First in Canada: Supporting communities to end homelessness.* Canadian Homelessness Research Network Press.

Gilmer, T. P., Stefancic, A., Sklar, M., & Tsemberis, S. (2013). Development and validation of a Housing First fidelity survey. *Psychiatric Services, 64*, 911–914. https://doi.org/10.1176/appi.ps.201200500

Grazioli, V. S., Collins, S. E., Paroz, S., Graap, C., & Daeppen, J. B. (2017). Six-month outcomes among socially marginalized alcohol and drug users attending a drop-in center allowing alcohol consumption. *International Journal of Drug Policy, 41*, 65–73. https://doi.org/10.1016/j.drugpo.2016.12.015

Harm Reduction Coalition (2020). *Principles of Harm Reduction.* Retrieved from https://harmreduction.org/about-us/principles-of-harm-reduction/

Heather, N. (2006). Controlled drinking, harm reduction and their roles in the response to alcohol-related problems. *Addiction Research and Theory, 14*, 7–18. https://doi.org/10.1080/16066350500489170

Kertesz, S. G., Crouch, K., Milby, J. B., Cusimano, R. E., & Schumacher, J. E. (2009). Housing First for homeless persons with active addiction: Are we overreaching? *Milbank Quarterly, 87*, 495–534. https://doi.org/10.1111/j.1468-0009.2009.00565.x

Kirst, M., Zerger, S., Misir, V., Hwang, S., & Stergiopoulos, V. (2015). The impact of a Housing First randomized controlled trial on substance use problems among homeless individuals with mental illness. *Drug and Alcohol Dependence, 146*, 24–29. https://doi.org/10.1016/j.drugalcdep.2014.10.019

Larimer, M., Malone, D., Garner, M., Atkins, D., Burlingham, B., Lonczak, H., Tanzer, K., Ginzler, J., Clifasefi, S. L., Hobson, W. G., & Marlatt, G. A. (2009). Health care and public service use and costs before and after provision of housing for chronically homeless persons with severe alcohol problems. *JAMA, 301*, 1349–1357. https://doi.org/10.1001/jama.2009.414

Lee, H. S., & Petersen, S. R. (2009). Demarginalizing the marginalized in substance abuse treatment: Stories of homeless, active substance users in an urban harm reduction based drop-in center. *Addiction Research & Theory, 17*, 622–636. https://doi.org/10.3109/16066350802168613

Mackelprang, J. L., Collins, S. E., & Clifasefi, S. L. (2014). Housing First is associated with reduced use of emergency medical services. *Prehospital Emergency Care, 18*, 478–482. https://doi.org/10.3109/10903127.2014.916020

Malone, D. K. (2009). Assessing criminal history as a predictor of future housing success for homeless adults with behavioral health disorders. *Psychiatric Services, 60*, 224–230. https://doi.org/10.1176/appi.ps.60.2.224

Malone, D. K., Collins, S. E., & Clifasefi, S. L. (2015). Single-site Housing First for chronically homeless people. *Housing, Care and Support, 18*, 62–66. https://doi.org/10.1108/HCS-05-2015-0007

Marlatt, A., & Witkiewitz, K. (2002). Harm reduction approaches to alcohol use: Health promotion, prevention, and treatment. *Addictive Behaviors, 27*, 867–886. https://doi.org/10.1016/S0306-4603(02)00294-0

Marlatt, G. A., Baer, J. S., Kivlahan, D. R., Dimeff, L. A., Larimer, M., Quigley, L., Somers, J. M., & Williams, E. (1998). Screening and brief intervention for high-risk college student drinkers: Results from a 2-year follow-up assessment. *Journal of Consulting and Clinical Psychology, 66*, 604–615. https://doi.org/10.1037//0022-006X.66.4.604

Marlatt, G. A., & Witkiewitz, K. (2010). Update on harm-reduction policy and intervention research. *Annual Review of Clinical Psychology, 6*, 591–606. https://doi.org/10.1146/annurev.clinpsy.121208.131438

Miller, W. R., & Rollnick, S. (2012). *Motivational interviewing: Helping people change* (3rd ed.). Guilford.

Muckle, W., Muckle, J., Welch, V., & Tugwell, P. (2012). Managed alcohol as a harm reduction intervention for alcohol addiction in populations at high risk for substance abuse. *Cochrane Database of Systematic Reviews, 12*, CD006747. https://doi.org/10.1002/14651858.CD006747.pub2

National Alliance to End Homelessness. (2012). *Solutions: Housing First*. www.endhomelessness.org/pages/solutions

NIAAA. (2005). *Helping patients who drink too much: A clinician's guide*. https://pubs.niaaa.nih.gov/publications/practitioner/cliniciansguide2005/guide.pdf

Nielsen, S., Larance, B., Degenhardt, L., Gowing, L., Kehler, C., & Lintzeris, N. (2016). Opioid agonist treatment for pharmaceutical opioid dependent people. *Cochrane Database of Systematic Reviews,* 5. https://doi.org/10.1002/14651858.CD011117.pub2

Orwin, R. G., Garrison-Mogren, R., Jacobs, M. L., & Sonnefeld, L. J. (1999). Retention of homeless clients in substance abuse treatment: Findings from the National Institute on Alcohol Abuse and Alcoholism Cooperative Agreement Program. *Journal of Substance Abuse Treatment, 17,* 45–66. https://doi.org/10.1016/s0740-5472(98)00046-4

Pauly, B., Vallance, K., Wettlaufer, A., Chow, C., Brown, R., Evans, J., Gray, E., Krysowaty, B., Ivsins, A., Schiff, R., & Stockwell, T. (2018). Community managed alcohol programs in Canada: Overview of key dimensions and implementation. *Drug and Alcohol Review, 37,* S132–S139. https://doi.org/10.1111/dar.12681

Pauly, B. M., Stockwell, T., Chow, C., Gray, E., Krysowaty, B., & Vallance, K. (2013). *Towards alcohol harm reduction: Preliminary results from an evaluation of a Canadian managed alcohol program.* Centre for Additions Research of British Columbia.

Pearson, M. R. (2013). Use of alcohol protective behavioral strategies among college students: A critical review. *Clinical Psychology Review, 33.* https://doi.org/10.1016/j.cpr.2013.08.006

Podymow, T., Turnbull, J., Coyle, D., Yetisir, E., & Wells, G. (2006). Shelter-based managed alcohol administration to chronically homeless people addicted to alcohol. *Canadian Medical Association Journal, 174,* 45–49. https://doi.org/10.1503/cmaj.1041350

Substance Abuse and Mental Health Services Administration (2019). *Key substance use and mental health indicators in the United States: Results from the 2018 National Survey on Drug Use and Health (NSDUH).* www.samhsa.gov/data/sites/default/files/cbhsq-reports/NSDUHNationalFindingsReport2018/NSDUHNationalFindingsReport2018.pdf

Slayton, S. C., D'Archer, J., & Kaplan, F. (2010). Outcome studies on the efficacy of art therapy: A review of findings. *Art Therapy, 27,* 108–118. https://doi.org/10.1080/07421656.2010.10129660

Sobell, L. C., Ellingstad, T. P., & Sobell, M. B. (2000). Natural recovery from alcohol and drug problems: Methodological review of the research with suggestions for future directions. *Addiction, 95,* 749–764. https://doi.org/10.1046/j.1360-0443.2000.95574911.x

Somers, J. M., Moniruzzaman, A., Patterson, M., Currie, L., Rezansoff, S. N., Palepu, A., & Fryer, K. (2017). A randomized trial examining Housing First in congregate and scattered site formats. *PLoS ONE, 12,* e0168745. https://doi.org/10.1371/journal.pone.0168745

Stergiopoulos, V., Gozdzik, A., Misir, V., Skosireva, A., Connelly, J., Sarang, A., Whisler, A., Hwang, S. W., O'Campo, P., & McKenzie, K. (2015). Effectiveness of Housing First with intensive case management in an ethnically diverse sample of homeless adults with mental illness: A randomized controlled trial. *PLoS ONE, 10,* e0130281. https://doi.org/10.1371/journal.pone.0130281

Stockwell, T., Pauly, B., Chow, C., Erickson, R. A., Krysowaty, B., Roemer, A., Vallance, K., Wettlaufer, A., & Zhao, J. (2018). Does managing the consumption of people with severe alcohol dependence reduce harm? A comparison of participants in six Canadian managed alcohol programs with locally recruited controls. *Drug and Alcohol Review, 37*, S159-S166. https://doi.org/10.1111/dar.12618

Tartarsky, A. (2002). *Harm reduction psychotherapy: A new treatment for drug and alcohol problems*. Rowman &Littlefield.

Thornquist, L., Biros, M., Olander, R., & Sterner, S. (2002). Health care utilization of chronic inebriates. *Academic Emergency Medicine, 9*, 300–308. https://doi.org/10.1111/j.1553-2712.2002.tb01323.x

Tsemberis, S. (2010). *Housing First: The pathways model to end homelessness for people with mental illness and addiction*. Hazelden Publishing.

Tsemberis, S., & Eisenberg, R. F. (2000). Pathways to Housing: Supported housing for street-dwelling homeless individuals with psychiatric disabilities. *Psychiatric Services, 51*, 487–493. https://doi.org/10.1176/appi.ps.51.4.487

Tsemberis, S., Gulcur, L., & Nakae, M. (2004). Housing First, consumer choice, and harm reduction for homeless individuals with a dual diagnosis. *American Journal of Public Health, 94*, 651–656. https://doi.org/10.2105/AJPH.94.4.651

Tsemberis, S., Kent, D., & Respress, C. (2012). Housing stability and recovery among chronically homeless people with co-occurring disorders in Washington DC. *American Journal of Public Health, 102*, 13–16. https://doi.org/10.2105/AJPH.2011.300320

Vaeth, P. A., Wang-Schweig, M., & Caetano, R. (2017). Drinking, alcohol use disorder, and treatment access and utilization among US racial/ethnic groups. *Alcoholism: Clinical and Experimental Research, 41*, 6–19. https://doi.org/10.1111/acer.13285

Vallance, K., Stockwell, T., Pauly, B., Chow, C., Gray, E., Krysowaty, B., Perkin, K., & Zhao, J. (2016). Do managed alcohol programs change patterns of alcohol consumption and reduce related harm? A pilot study. *Harm Reduction Journal,* 13, *13. https://doi.org/10.1186/s12954-016-0103-4*

Watson, D. P., Orwat, J., Wagner, D. E., Shuman, V., & Tolliver, R. (2013). The Housing First model (HFM) fidelity index: Designing and testing a tool for measuring integrity of housing programs that serve active substance users. *Substance Abuse Treatment, Prevention and Policy, 8*, 1–16. https://doi.org/10.1186/1747-597X-8-16

Willenbring, M. L. (2014). Treatment of heavy drinking and alcohol use disorder. In R. K. Ries, D. A. Fiellin, S. C. Miller, & R. Saitz (Eds.), *The ASAM principles of addiction medicine* (5th ed.) (pp. 375–388). Wolters Kluwer.

Witkiewitz, K., Montes, K. S., Schwebel, F. J., & Tucker, J. A. (2020). What is recovery? *Alcohol Research: Current Reviews, 40*, 01–01. https://doi.org/10.35946/arcr.v40.3.01

13 Use of Mobile Technology to Understand and Improve Recovery from Alcohol Use Disorder

Matthew R. Pearson, Noah N. Emery, and
Frank J. Schwebel

Use of Mobile Technology to Understand and Improve Recovery from Alcohol Use Disorder

For the past two decades, an increasingly relevant question is how can mobile technology be used to understand and improve recovery from alcohol use disorder (AUD). Presently, we would argue the question has become how can one understand and improve AUD recovery *without* the use of mobile technology? In this chapter, the ways in which mobile technology can be leveraged to study change in alcohol use and related mechanisms of behavior change (MOBC) are described, with reference to several related chapters in this book. In the book's introduction, Tucker and Witkiewitz highlighted the importance of offering interventions outside of the traditional healthcare system as a means to reduce the gap between treatment need and treatment seeking, and to improve rates of recovery. This chapter discusses how mobile technology offers an imminently feasible solution to reach greater numbers of individuals with AUD who are on a variety of recovery pathways that may or may not involve treatment or mutual help groups.

In 2002, 62 percent of US adults owned a cell phone and, by 2019, 96 percent owned a cell phone, and 81 percent owned a smartphone (Pew Research Center, 2019). In the past decade, there has been exponential growth in computational power, leading to the proliferation of near continuous and ecologically valid data streams collected via mobile technology. Despite this rapid technological progress, researchers' ability to conduct well-designed studies that capitalize on these technologies has lagged behind, and only a small fraction of the potential benefits of using mobile technology to probe alcohol-related recovery processes has been realized. Although most of the mobile technologies covered in this chapter can be applied to a wide range of addictive behaviors and other areas of mental health, we focus on alcohol and AUD recovery outcomes given the purpose of this volume. We discuss distinct applications of both active and passive technology-assisted data collection to assess alcohol use as well as the antecedents, mechanisms of behavior change, and broader AUD recovery outcomes. Further, we discuss both assessment and intervention approaches that take advantage of ubiquitous mobile technology.

Ecological Momentary Assessment

Ecological momentary assessment (EMA) involves the use of intensive repeated assessments to capture moment-to-moment fluctuations in emotional, cognitive, and behavioral experiences using mobile technology (Shiffman, 2009; Shiffman et al., 2008). The simplest form of EMA is the daily diary design in which a single assessment is captured each day. Just as one recruits a sample of participants to generalize to the population of interest, the next stage of design complexity is the experience sampling design, which involves use of random or quasi-random prompts to obtain a sample of assessments throughout the day. As technology has advanced, more complicated EMA protocols have become common, which integrate use of event-contingent and time-based assessments that can either be prompted or self-initiated several times a day.

These intensive longitudinal methods offer numerous advantages relative to more commonly used cross-sectional retrospective surveys or more traditional longitudinal (i.e., panel) designs. Since these assessments occur in real time (i.e., event-level) while participants are in their natural environment (i.e., *in vivo*) via smartphones or wearable devices, experiences can be modeled as they unfold with temporal ordering. EMA also maximizes generalizability given the nature of collecting data on dynamic processes in the "real world" that more accurately reflect the lived experience of individuals with AUD in ways that directly inform AUD research and practice.

EMA also enhances the generalizability of findings by reducing recall bias that can affect more conventional global or single occasion measures that rely exclusively on retrospective reporting. For example, affective states are a central context in which alcohol use occurs and a focal variable of interest to both etiological and treatment researchers. However, recall of affective experiences for periods longer than a week shows considerable bias because individuals tend to draw upon their stable beliefs about the types of affect they generally tend to experience (Tugade et al., 2007).

EMA also has the advantage that multiple in-the-moment assessments (e.g., affect experienced in specific moments and context) can be captured and aggregated across time points to make reliable measures of emotional functioning or other dynamic processes (Emery & Simons, 2020; Simons et al., 2014). Thus, EMA allows for the disentanglement of within- and between-person processes. Given that theoretical accounts of substance use are largely based on within-person processes (e.g., learning), this feature of intensive longitudinal methods is critical. However, the majority of research has focused on between-person designs (Colder et al., 2010; Curran & Bauer, 2011). Another important quality of EMA methods is they can be used to measure a broad array of processes and contextual factors, many of which cannot be simulated in the laboratory, such as the subjective intoxicating effects of alcohol in underage drinkers or the impact of alcohol use on self-injurious behaviors.

Ecological Momentary Assessment of Alcohol Use

Perhaps the most basic reason for using EMA in alcohol research is that it allows the collection of alcohol use data in an ecologically valid manner that is less subject to retrospective memory biases. While individuals can often recall their average levels of drinking with reasonable accuracy, they tend to find it difficult to retrospectively describe the contingencies of drinking behavior that are crucial to effectively understand the stimulus-response chain (e.g., Carney et al., 1998). Research has shown that retrospective memory biases for self-reported alcohol consumption are significant with an assessment window as short as seven days (Ekholm, 2004; Gmel & Daeppen, 2007). Improving the accuracy of alcohol use data provides more precise outcomes in the context of studying drinking behavior change over time, including evaluating treatment efficacy or capturing "natural recovery" in the absence of treatment (Tucker et al., 2007). Further, in the face of continuously falling costs of mobile technology, EMA designs offer an efficient solution that can enhance statistical power and reduce research expenses (Carpenter et al., 2020).

We consider three non-mutually exclusive EMA methods for assessing alcohol use, each with their own strengths and limitations. First, a daily "end of day" report and/or a morning "past 24 hours" report (e.g., Beckjord & Shiffman, 2014; Emery & Simons, 2020; Simons et al., 2015) of alcohol consumption is a simple method that reduces the length of the retrospective recall period while minimizing participant burden. Second, "random" prompts throughout the day can be used to assess alcohol use "since the previous report" and provides data with higher temporal resolution, which can be helpful to distinguish antecedents and consequences of alcohol consumption (Stevenson et al., 2019). Third, self-initiated, event-contingent reporting can be used to obtain a high level of temporal resolution as participants can record each drink that they consume in real time (Miranda et al., 2014a). With this approach, researchers can calculate more precise alcohol variables, including duration of the drinking episode, pacing of consumption of drinks, and an estimation of the blood alcohol concentration (BAC) curve. This type of information supports quantification of how an individual or group of individuals consume alcohol in the moment, and which use patterns confer greater risk. For example, research shows youths in the company of peers or who have more AUD symptoms had significantly steeper increases in estimated BAC during drinking episodes (i.e., they drank faster; Carpenter et al., 2019). While individual acts of consumption may seem small in and of themselves, this work suggests that they hold important information about the development of harmful patterns of use.

The drawback of event-contingent reporting is the prospective memory burden placed on participants to complete these reports (i.e., they forget), and the potential challenges involved in promoting reporting compliance, especially given that increased alcohol consumption may be systematically related to missingness. The cognitive-behavioral impairments caused by alcohol intoxication can contribute to the timeliness and accuracy of drinking reports diminishing throughout a drinking episode. To address this concern, some researchers have begun to limit assessments to just before participants begin drinking and after the first four standard drinks on any given day. The rationale for four drinks comes from evidence that subjective effects of alcohol require a minimum BAC of 0.04. By capturing four drinks, which occurs regularly, youths can cross this BAC threshold, but are not too intoxicated to complete assessments (Miranda et al., 2014a, 2014b).

Ambulatory Assessment of Alcohol Use

Although self-reported EMA measures of alcohol use tend to be more precise than retrospective self-reports, they are still self-reports and are influenced by a range of factors that can make them less reliable and accurate. Beyond EMA, the rapid proliferation of sensor technology available in the modal smartphone as well as the increasing number of wearable technologies to collect physiological data provide opportunities for passive data collection in the alcohol field. When EMA is used in combination with such technologies, the broader term "ambulatory assessment" is often used (Trull & Ebner-Priemer, 2013, 2014). In the alcohol field, transdermal alcohol sensors and mobile breathalyzers are worth considering.

Transdermal alcohol sensors provide a means of objective, unobtrusive, and continuous assessment of alcohol consumption in the natural environment. A small amount of alcohol is secreted continuously through the skin, which can be measured via an electrochemical sensor. These devices are commonly used in the criminal justice system to monitor enforced abstinence (Marques & McKnight, 2009; McKnight et al., 2012). The Wrist Transdermal Alcohol Sensor (WrisTAS) is a device about the size of a watch that provides continuous readings of alcohol secreted through the skin. In addition, it contains temperature and skin conductance sensors that are used to determine that the device is being worn to prevent tampering given its applications in criminal justice settings. Using the WrisTAS, researchers have demonstrated young adults with relatively more AUD symptoms tend to have drinking episodes characterized by higher peak BAC and faster time to reach peak BAC (Simons et al., 2015). This study also provided validation of self-reported alcohol consumption through biochemical verification and showed that random EMA assessments (i.e., time-based assessment) of alcohol consumption were more likely to miss low level drinking events compared to daily next morning reports.

A current limitation of these sensors is that they cannot determine exact quantities consumed by an individual without personalized calibrations that are both cost and time prohibitive. Another barrier is that transdermal alcohol concentration data are systematically different from more traditional measures such as BAC or breath alcohol concentrations (BrAC). First, there is a time delay between onset of consumption and when alcohol is secreted through the skin making exact timing difficult to ascertain. Factors such as individual differences in skin thickness and variation in device characteristics introduce even more complexity and can moderate the device output (Luczak & Rosen, 2014; Swift, 2000). Also, transdermal alcohol curves tend to be skewed and have lower peaks relative to BAC and BrAC (Sakai et al., 2006). Thus, there are practical and financial reasons that qualify and limit the use of transdermal alcohol sensors. However, continued technological development might help increase the utility of these sensors, and further research is merited.

Mobile breathalyzers leverage Bluetooth-enabled smartphones as a data collection hub, with recordings from other devices/wearables sent to the smartphone. To do this, a personal smart breathalyzer device and smartphone application are paired together to collect BrAC. One version of this pairing is the BACtrack Mobile Pro personal mobile breathalyzer and its associated BACtrack mobile application (www.bactrack.com). BACtrack is the first, and currently the only, company to have obtained FDA approval to manufacture and market breathalyzers for personal consumer use. Through an attached mouthpiece of the device, a user can blow and record their BrAC on the BACtrack app. The app can also record GPS-based location with an additional comment area that allows the user to take notes. The user can retrieve and compare the information over time. Depending on the BrAC level, the app also displays appropriate suggestions along with the BAC reading. In addition, the app provides the user an estimated time when their BrAC level is expected to drop to zero. The app also contains convenience features, such as calling for a ride from a rideshare app.

Most of these features are designed to be consumer-facing (i.e., for the individual consumer). However, researchers have begun to capitalize on the rich data stream these features provide. For example, Lauckner et al. (2019) found that it was feasible to use this technology with high compliance and that participants reported favorable attitudes about using it. They also demonstrated associations between binge drinking frequency at baseline and measures of alcohol consumption derived from the mobile breathalyzer (e.g., average BrAC, percent drinking days). Although not passive, given that the relationship between BrAC and BAC is well-characterized, mobile breathalyzers offer an opportunity to obtain objective measures of alcohol consumption.

Selecting an Intensive Longitudinal Assessment Method

When deciding to use any of these intensive longitudinal methods to obtain alcohol data, researchers should consider the quality of the collected data, relative burden on participants, and cost of the methodology, among other concerns. For instance, daily self-report assessments minimize participant burden and can be accomplished without sophisticated technology; e.g., simple text messaging (short message service, aka SMS) can be used to collect such data. In contrast, transdermal alcohol sensors can be used to obtain objective data with high temporal resolution, but data loss and data inconsistency from technical difficulties can arise, and the technology is presently expensive. The strengths and limitations of each of these methods should be carefully weighed given the primary purpose of their use when embarking on an intensive longitudinal study of drinking practices and related variables (for a review, see Wray et al., 2014).

Technology-Assisted Measurement of AUD Recovery Outcomes and Mechanisms of Behavior Change

In addition to assessing drinking practices, EMA can provide highly accurate assessment of broader AUD recovery outcomes. As summarized in this volume (see Chapter 1) and elsewhere (Witkiewitz et al., 2020), AUD recovery entails more than abstinence from alcohol; thus, even the most precise assessment of alcohol use will fail to capture essential features of AUD recovery. An increasing number of definitions of recovery emphasize "improvements in physical and mental health, quality of life, and other dimensions of well-being" (National Institute on Alcohol Abuse and Alcoholism, 2020). EMA data have advantages in the assessment and monitoring of many of these domains. For example, Ebner-Priemer and Trull (2009) highlighted major benefits of using EMA to study mood (dys)regulation, which include reducing retrospective biases, identifying setting- or context-specific relationships, and enhancing generalizability. De Vries et al. (2020) reviewed EMA studies of subjective well-being, quality of life, happiness, and satisfaction with life, and illustrated how EMA data provide insights into fluctuations and patterns of well-being that cannot be captured with retrospective self-report measures. The potential for EMA to enhance the study of these domains in the context of AUD recovery has not yet been realized, but represents an important area for continued development.

EMA can also be used to probe many recovery-relevant processes and contexts described in other chapters in this book. For example, Witkiewitz and Maisto (Chapter 2) highlighted the role of negative affect and craving in drinking behavior change processes and outcomes, two constructs known to fluctuate over time. Assessing these processes is one of the most common uses of EMA in the alcohol field (Serre et al., 2015). Roos, Bowen, and Kober (Chapter 3) described self-regulation strategies that are executed to pursue drinking behavior change goals, including cognitive reappraisal, problem solving, mindful awareness, and seeking social support. Elsewhere, Roos et al. (2020) discussed the unique contribution of EMA "to enhance our understanding of the dynamic, intra-individual process in which self-regulation strategies facilitate substance use behavior change over time" (p. 313). Bates, Price, and Buckman (Chapter 4) reviewed psychophysiological risk and protective factors for harmful alcohol use, including the baroreflex. They documented how the baroreflex can be manipulated "in the moment" using resonance breathing, and they are currently conducting trials using an iPhone app to both encourage resonance breathing and assess heart rate variability via photo plethysmography.

These chapters and others provide examples of diverse variable domains and processes of change that could benefit from technology-assisted data collection such as EMA and advance understanding of alcohol use and AUD dynamics. Not only do EMA methods support precise assessment of alcohol-related outcomes, but this can be extended to a wide range of cognitive, emotional, physiological, and contextual antecedents to alcohol and AUD recovery outcomes – as well as consequences of alcohol use/AUD – considered important in different conceptual models of etiology and behavior change. These methods support examination of the within-subject processes that are theorized to lead to the development and escalation of AUD, as well as those theorized to lead to behavior change on a timescale closer to which these processes operate.

For example, ambulatory assessment using passive technology-assisted data collection can be used to probe physiological mechanisms of behavior change or to identify physiological correlates of promising psychological mechanisms of behavior change. Ambulatory assessment can be used to obtain more objective assessments of putative mechanisms of behavior change often with much greater temporal resolution. These continuous objective assessments can be used to gain a clear assessment of the temporal sequencing among the variables of interest. In the case of the baroreflex, for instance, Buckman et al. (2018) described dynamic physiological processes that support behavior change and involve a well-characterized neuro-cardiac feedback loop. They further discussed how heart rate variability serves as a non-invasive probe of baroreflex functioning, which is strongly implicated in the stress response. Periodic (with smartphone only) or continuous (with wearable technology) measures can be obtained to evaluate this hypothesized mechanism of behavior change.

Other research has taken advantage of unobtrusive sensors to collect proxy variables for more complicated behavior patterns. For example, Bae and colleagues (2018) collected data from 56 sensor features related to time (e.g., day of week), movement (e.g., accelerometry, rotation), communication (e.g., phone calls, texting), and psychomotor impairment (e.g., typing speed – Android only). Using a Random Forest model (a machine learning algorithm), they were able to detect high-risk drinking periods within 30 minutes after drinking onset with 90 percent accuracy after only 10 days of data collection. More recently, Suffoletto et al. (2020) used accelerometer data from smartphones to detect alcohol intoxication-related gait impairments. Although this study was conducted under controlled laboratory conditions, the findings offer a glimpse of the potential for ways that sensor data can be utilized.

Treatment of Time in EMA Data Analyses

Previous reviews have summarized the many uses of EMA to study drinking-related variables and AUD recovery (e.g., Morgenstern et al., 2014; Wray et al., 2014). Building on a review of EMA studies in the smoking literature (Shiffman, 2014), below we describe how distinct research questions can be examined using EMA data based on how time is conceptualized in the analyses. To simplify, the illustrative example uses EMA data in which only three variables were assessed: (1) a binary variable of context (alone vs. with others), (2) a continuous variable of craving, and (3) a count variable of number of standard alcohol drinks consumed.

A simple multilevel model can be used to calculate an intraclass correlation coefficient (ICC), which could express the overall degree of variability in craving that is between-persons (ICC) vs. within-persons (1-ICC). This simple model shows the degree to which craving is trait-like (i.e., high level of variability between persons) as well as state-like (i.e., high level of variability within-persons). By considering how to center time (i.e., before and after a drinking episode), how craving changes before and/or after a drinking episode can be examined. The pattern of alcohol use across time of day and days of the week can be investigated, and timing between drinking episodes can be modeled using survival analysis.

Given that intensive longitudinal data provide a relatively new way in which data are structured, methods to advance analyses in this area are developing rapidly. Based on models like dynamical systems theory, models like the Bayesian Hierarchical Ornstein-Uhlenbeck Model (BHOUM, Oravesz et al., 2016) and recurrence quantification analysis (Danvers et al., 2020) can be used to study how the temporal dynamics of a particular variable relate to outcomes. For example, the BHOUM can identify three variables that summarize the temporal dynamics of craving and examine how they relate to outcomes: (1) the attractor state (i.e., typical/baseline levels of craving), (2) within-person variability in craving, and (3) attractor strength (i.e., auto-regressive component reflective of self-regulatory processes). Models like Time-Varying Effect Models (TVEMs; Li et al., 2017; Linden-Carmichael et al., Chapter 7 this volume) and dynamic structural equation models (DSEM; Hamaker et al., 2018) allow more flexibility to determine if the associations between variables change over time. Although these novel sophisticated quantitative methods have seldom been applied in the alcohol field, they hold great promise to better understand the heterogeneous processes of recovery from AUD.

Improving AUD Treatment Outcomes and Promoting Recovery

The use of mobile and wireless technology to improve health falls within the rapidly advancing field of mHealth (Nahum-Shani et al., 2018), which includes classic telehealth approaches as well as advanced ecological momentary interventions. We next consider the primary motivations for using mHealth interventions, review some key dimensions on which mHealth interventions differ, discuss a few intervention examples, and offer suggestions concerning the future of mHealth interventions.

Despite the widespread prevalence of AUD, there are several individual-level and system-level barriers to receiving treatment. Interrelated barriers include stigma, cost of services, and limited availability of services, among many others (Browne et al., 2016). If someone cannot make it to the clinic, perhaps the clinic can be brought to them. Mobile-delivered interventions offer a means of providing care that can be more cost-effective and easier to disseminate compared to face-to-face interventions. Further, at least a subset of individuals with AUD experience it as a chronic, relapsing condition (Cunningham & McCambridge, 2012; O'Brien, 1994), yet the dominant AUD treatment model in the United States is an acute care model that offers time-limited services only. Mobile interventions provide the opportunity to deliver long-term continuity-of-care and can be used in a stepped care fashion; e.g., ongoing monitoring through mobile technology can be used to initiate a higher level of care if risk factors increase or the problem behavior re-emerges. For example, quarterly post-treatment Recovery Management Check-ups have been shown to improve treatment outcomes among individuals with substance use disorders (Dennis et al., 2003; Scott & Dennis, 2009). More frequent and automated check-ins can be facilitated using mobile technology. Another comparative strength of technology-delivered interventions is that they can be provided with high fidelity, unlike many face-to-face therapies in which so-called therapist effects abound (Miller, 2016).

Classic Telehealth

Classic telehealth approaches deliver traditional face-to-face treatments virtually using technology, which may involve mobile or other computer/communication technology (e.g., interactions via a desktop computer). Overall, telehealth approaches have been demonstrated to be efficacious in treating individuals with AUD (Kruse et al., 2020). At the time of writing this chapter, the world is in the midst of the COVID-19 pandemic, and many health care providers have migrated to telehealth approaches out of necessity as providers and clients alike are sheltering in place, quarantining, and/or practicing physical distancing. Typical telehealth approaches can help address barriers to treatment access by removing physical and geographical barriers (i.e., for rural populations), while retaining the classic one-to-one or small group format of treatment. As such, telehealth is a useful but incomplete method to broaden the base of AUD services to reach a larger segment of the affected population with problems.

Ecological Momentary Interventions

Fortunately, rapid advances in mobile computing makes ecological momentary interventions (EMIs) increasingly feasible (Heron & Smyth, 2010). EMIs refer to interventions that can be delivered in one's natural environment (i.e., ecological) in real time (i.e., momentary) through the use of mobile technology. Not only can EMIs be delivered in real time and in natural settings, but they can also deliver intervention content repeatedly over time and in times of greatest need. Thus, EMIs can be used to optimize the timing and context of the intervention, as well as increase the dose of the intervention at little or no additional cost. EMIs can vary from offering simple, non-tailored text message reminders to a complicated mobile application that monitors a wide range of self-reported and sensor-based inputs that can be used to tailor the timing and content of interventions, often referred to as Just-In-Time Adaptive Interventions (JITAIs) (Nahum-Shani et al., 2018).

A modified version of a framework offered by Litvin et al. (2013) can be used to describe and organize technology-based interventions and highlight ways in which mobile interventions differ from one another. Litvin et al. (2013) identified four primary design considerations: accessibility, usage, amount of human contact, and intervention content. Within the context of mobile interventions, accessibility describes the potential reach based on the technological elements employed for the EMI. Usage includes the frequency and intensity of the intervention, whether and how app usage data are collected, whether individuals are reminded to complete the intervention, and the pattern of attrition. EMIs can be delivered as a standalone treatment, as an adjunct to face-to-face treatments, or any blend between these two extremes. Intervention content can be divided into at least three categories that are important for designing EMIs: (1) the degree to which intervention content is tailored, (2) the type of intervention content that is delivered, and (3) the theoretical model guiding intervention development.

These elements are interrelated, and the development of an efficacious EMI will likely depend on carefully selecting optimal features for the target recipients. Accessibility is highest when using SMS given that 96 percent of individuals in the United States have cellular phones. Given that 81 percent of individuals in the United States have smartphones (Pew Research Center, 2019), accessibility remains high but it is appreciably lower for mobile applications. To use a smartphone app, it must be downloaded onto a smartphone. App downloading for research purposes occurs at relatively low rates, possibly because of lack of participant motivation, knowledge (e.g., not knowing how to download the application), or capacity/ability (e.g., not having a smartphone) to interact with the technology (Berry et al., 2017; Bucci et al., 2019; Lord et al., 2016; Ramsey et al., 2016). As wearable technology has been introduced (e.g., Fitbit, transdermal alcohol sensors), the opportunity to tailor intervention content based on continuous data streams has increased, but accessibility has decreased because of concomitant financial and technical constraints. As Litvin et al. (2013) noted, it is important to consider the trade-off between using the latest technology and ensuring the broadest level of compatibility across devices and service providers.

Although a fully automated standalone treatment likely provides the greatest opportunity to broaden intervention reach, EMIs delivered in conjunction with conventional treatment are likely to have the highest level of efficacy, and such EMIs can offer continuity of care among those who have sought face-to-face treatment. Although the application of EMIs targeting alcohol problems is in its infancy, a brief summary of available applications is shown in Table 13.1 and illustrates the diversity of approaches evaluated to date. EMIs have targeted college students who co-use alcohol and tobacco (Witkiewitz et al., 2014), hazardous drinking among young adults recruited from emergency departments (Suffoletto et al., 2012, 2014), military personnel with subclinical psychological problems (Kizakevich et al., 2018), and individuals with AUD (Gustafson et al., 2014; Moody et al., 2017). Intervention content has ranged widely from mindfulness techniques (Kizakevich et al., 2018; Witkiewitz et al., 2014), normative feedback (Witkiewitz et al., 2014), educational messages (Suffoletto et al., 2014), goal setting (Moody et al., 2018; Suffoletto et al., 2014), and care management (Gustafson et al., 2014).

Capitalizing on the modality with the largest potential reach, Suffoletto and colleagues pilot-tested (2012) and then fully evaluated (2014) the efficacy of a text message intervention targeting hazardous-drinking in young adults recruited from a hospital emergency department. Across both trials, they delivered 1–2 text messages per week for 12 weeks, which involved responses to a small number of questions via text with a small degree of tailoring based on participant goals and whether they endorsed low-risk vs. high-risk drinking. Gustafson et al. (2014) demonstrated the efficacy of the Addiction-Comprehensive Health Enhancement Support System (A-CHESS) as a long-term, mobile application-delivered treatment, providing this intervention for eight months following residential treatment. This comprehensive mobile application uses GPS technology to send an alert if someone approaches a high-risk area (e.g., a drinking establishment), has a "panic" button that connects them with social support if one is about to relapse, and provides graphs based on weekly functioning data that can be sent to one's counselor.

Although efficacy testing is incomplete, one of the most comprehensive mobile applications was built upon the Personal Health Intervention Toolkit (PHIT) framework (Eckhoff et al., 2015) to target stress reduction, sleep improvement, and alcohol moderation. The PHIT for Duty JITAI tailors content ranging from recommending one consult with their primary care provider to recommending mindfulness, sleep, and/or alcohol-related interventions (Kizakevich et al., 2018). Tailoring variables included heart rate variability determined with a pulse sensor on the earlobe, wrist, or chest; sleep monitoring determined with actigraphy data; and anxiety and depression determined via a self-report, among other data sources.

Table 13.1. *Ecological momentary interventions targeting alcohol use and alcohol use disorder*

Examples: SMS-Delivered Ecological Momentary Interventions (estimated potential reach in the USA = 96 percent)					
	Duration	Adjunct vs. Stand-alone	Intervention Content	Theoretical Background	Population
Moody et al. (2018)	Daily for 2 weeks	Stand-alone	Implementation intentions	Mindset Theory of Action Phases	Adults with AUD
Suffoletto et al. (2012)	12–24 messages for 12 weeks	Stand-alone	Safe-drinking guidelines, goal setting, strategies for cutting down, decisional balance	Unspecified	Young adult hazardous drinkers from emergency department
Suffoletto et al. (2014)	12–24 messages for 12 weeks	Stand-alone	Intentions to binge drink, knowledge of risks, norms, skills, and goal commitment	Health Belief Model, Information Motivation Behavior model, Theory of Reasoned Action, Motivational Interviewing	Young adult hazardous drinkers from emergency department
Examples: Mobile Application-Delivered Ecological Momentary Interventions (estimated potential reach in the USA = 81 percent)					
	Duration	Adjunct vs. Stand-alone	Intervention Content	Theoretical Background	Population
Gonzalez & Dulin (2015)	7 modules in 6 weeks	Stand-alone	Assessment/feedback, high-risk locations, selecting/using supportive people for change, cravings, problem-solving skills, communication/drink refusal skills, pleasurable/non-drinking activities	Cognitive Behavioral	Individuals with AUD

Gustafson et al. (2014)	8 months	Adjunct	Relaxation exercises, GPS for "rescue" reminders, healthy event newsletter, care management	Self-Determination Theory	Individuals with AUD
Kizakevich et al. (2018)	Various	Stand-alone	Mindfulness-based stress reduction, sleep intervention, relaxing music and sounds to enhance sleep, alcohol education, heart-rate variability biofeedback	Unspecified	Military personnel with subclinical psychological problems
Witkiewitz et al. (2014)	Up to 31 modules in 14 days (median = 24)	Stand-alone	Norms, health information, protective behavioral strategies, alternative activities, urge-surfing, decisional balance	Cognitive Behavioral, Mindfulness	College student drinkers/ smokers

Note. SMS = short message service (i.e., text messages), US = United States, AUD = alcohol use disorder, GPS = global positioning system.

Importantly, with the exception of one intervention currently undergoing evaluation (Kizakevich et al., 2018), both individually and in a broader meta-analysis (Wang & Miller, 2020) these interventions have demonstrated efficacy in terms of pre-post improvements in alcohol outcomes as well as between-group improvements relative to control groups.

Next Generation mHealth Interventions

Smartphones represent a powerful tool for delivering technology-based interventions for substance use and other behavioral health disorders. Smartphones contain a range of sensors that can be leveraged by apps to facilitate active or passive data collection and interventions and to track the daily lives of people. These sensors include but are not limited to: accelerometers, gyroscope, GPS, barometer, pedometer, battery, screen, Bluetooth, and Wi-Fi. Although utilized more frequently in other areas of study (e.g., computer science), using sensor-based data to predict behavior is beginning to be applied in substance-related research and practice (Bae et al., 2017, 2018; Suffoletto et al., 2017, 2020).

The AWARE framework is an open-source tool that can be downloaded as an Android or iOS app to collect data actively and passively using sensors and EMA methods. Although functionality varies slightly between the Android and iOS versions due to operating system restrictions and limitations, the app uses sensors and EMA data to collect large amounts of information with relative ease. As mentioned earlier, sensor data gleaned from the AWARE app detected high-risk drinking periods within 30 minutes after drinking onset with 90 percent accuracy after only 10 days of data collection (Bae et al., 2018). Although further research is needed to understand and replicate these findings, the preliminary results are encouraging for use of sensor data for advanced adaptive interventions (e.g., JITAIs).

Although JITAIs represent an important advancement of technology-delivered interventions, we foresee that the second or third generation of interventions will incorporate machine learning methods that will greatly individualize intervention content. We assume that there is great inter-individual and intra-individual heterogeneity in the relative strengths of specific antecedents to harmful alcohol use and, further, that the most effective interventions will acknowledge and incorporate these sources of heterogeneity to individualize the intervention. As the computational power and diversity of unobtrusive data streams continue to increase exponentially, we envision EMIs will be able to tailor and adjust intervention content in a fully personalized manner to achieve individualized intervention optimization (i.e., precision medicine).

Conclusions and Recommendations

By no means do we view mobile technology as a panacea that will uncover all that is unknown about AUD recovery, nor will it address all the unmet needs of individuals suffering directly or indirectly from this debilitating disorder. Nevertheless, researchers and treatment providers are far from realizing the full potential benefits of mobile technology to understand and facilitate AUD recovery. Despite many advances in mobile technology-assisted assessment (EMA and ambulatory assessment), determining how to maximize the utility of information gathered using both active and passive data streams is an active research area. This chapter demonstrates how intensive longitudinal data can be used to investigate the dynamic processes, contexts, and outcomes of AUD described in other chapters in this book.

Although there are numerous technological (Burke et al., 2017) and implementation (Kim et al., 2019) challenges involved in incorporating EMA and EMIs into complicated health care systems, mobile technology offers opportunities to broaden the reach of services and support for individuals during their AUD recovery journey. To date, several EMIs have shown promise in assisting individuals during recovery. For example, the evidence-based A-CHESS application has been integrated with the evidence-based Computer Based Training for Cognitive Behavioral Therapy (Carroll et al., 2008), and rebranded as the Connections app (www.chess.health). In the United Kingdom, the SURE Recovery app (www.kcl.ac.uk/research/sure-recovery-app) includes a recovery tracker based on the validated patient-reported outcome measure, the Substance Use Recovery Tracker (Neale et al., 2016), among other recovery support options (see Chapter 21). These mobile-based recovery support services represent a small portion of the apps on the market, and we expect their capabilities will be greatly enhanced with the continuing advancements in machine learning and artificial intelligence. We anticipate the next generation of EMIs will more closely approximate personalized treatment, or precision medicine.

Acknowledgments

This research was supported in part by a grant (R01-AA022328, PI, Witkiewitz) from the National Institute on Alcohol Abuse and Alcoholism (NIAAA). MRP is supported by a career development grant (K01-AA023233) from the NIAAA. FJS is supported by a training grant (T32-AA018108) from the NIAAA. These agencies had no role in study design, data collection and analysis, decision to publish, or preparation of the manuscript.

References

Bae, S., Chung, T., Ferreira, D., Dey, A. K., & Suffoletto, B. (2018). Mobile phone sensors and supervised machine learning to identify alcohol use events in young adults: Implications for just-in-time adaptive interventions. *Addictive Behaviors*, *83*, 42–47. https://doi.org/10.1016/j.addbeh.2017.11.039

Bae, S., Ferreira, D., Suffoletto, B., Puyana, J. C., Kurtz, R., Chung, T., & Dey, A. K. (2017). Detecting drinking episodes in young adults using smartphone-based sensors. *Proceedings of the ACM on interactive, mobile, wearable and ubiquitous technologies*, *1*(2), 1–36. https://doi.org/10.1145/3090051

Beckjord, E., & Shiffman, S. (2014). Background for real-time monitoring and intervention related to alcohol use. *Alcohol Research: Current Reviews*, *36*(1), 9–18. https://pubmed.ncbi.nlm.nih.gov/26258996

Berry, N., Bucci, S., & Lobban, F. (2017). Use of the internet and mobile phones for self-management of severe mental health problems: Qualitative study of staff views. *JMIR Mental Health*, *4*(4), e52. https://doi.org/10.2196/mental.8311

Browne, T., Priester, M. A., Clone, S., Iachini, A., Dehart, D., & Hock, R. (2016). Barriers and facilitators to substance use treatment in the rural south: A qualitative study. *Journal of Rural Health*, *32*(1), 92–101. https://doi.org/10.1111/jrh.12129

Bucci, S., Schwannauer, M., & Berry, N. (2019). The digital revolution and its impact on mental health care. *Psychology and Psychotherapy: Theory, Research and Practice*, *92*(2), 277–297. https://doi.org/10.1111/papt.12222

Buckman, J. F., Vaschillo, E. G., Fonoberova, M., Mezic, I., & Bates, M. E. (2018). The translational value of psychophysiology methods and mechanisms: Multilevel, dynamic, personalized. *Journal of Studies on Alcohol and Drugs*, *79*, 229–238. https://doi.org/10.15288/jsad.2018.79.229

Burke, L. E., Shiffman, S., Music, E., Styn, M. A., Kriska, A., Smailagic, A., Siewiorek, D., Ewing, L. J., Chasens, E., French, B., Mancino, J., Mendez, D., Strollo, P., & Rathbun, S. L. (2017). Ecological momentary assessment in behavioral research: Addressing technological and human participant challenges. *Journal of Medical Internet Research*, *19*(3), e77. https://doi.org/10.2196/jmir.7138

Carney, M. A., Tennen, H., Affleck, G., del Boca, F. K., & Kranzler, H. R. (1998). Levels and patterns of alcohol consumption using timeline follow-back, daily diaries, and real time "electronic interviews." *Journal of Studies on Alcohol*, *59*(4), 447-454. https://doi.org/10.15288/jsa.1998.59.447

Carpenter, R. W., Squeglia, L. M., Emery, N. N., & McClure, E. A. (2020). Making pharmacotherapy trials for substance use disorder more efficient: Leveraging real-world data capture to maximize power and expedite the medication development pipeline. *Drug and Alcohol Dependence*, *209*, 107897. https://doi.org/10.1016/j.drugalcdep.2020.107897

Carpenter, R. W., Treloar Padovano, H., Emery, N. N., & Miranda, R. (2019). Rate of alcohol consumption in the daily life of adolescents and emerging adults. *Psychopharmacology*, *236*(11), 3111–3124. https://doi.org/10.1007/s00213-019-05262-8

Carroll, K. M., Ball, S. A., Martino, S., Nich, C., Babuscio, T. A., Nuro, K. F., Gordon, M. A., Portnoy, G. A., & Rounsaville, B. J. (2008). Computer-assisted delivery of cognitive-behavioral therapy for addiction: A randomized trial of CBT4CBT. *American Journal of Psychiatry*, *165*(7), 881–888. https://doi.org/10.1176/appi.ajp.2008.07111835

Colder, C. R., Chassin, L., Lee, M. R., & Villalta, I. K. (2010). Developmental perspectives: Affect and adolescent substance use. In J. D. Kassel (Ed.), *Substance abuse and emotion* (pp. 109–135). American Psychological Association. https://doi.org/10.1037/12067-005

Cunningham, J. A., & McCambridge, J. (2012). Is alcohol dependence best viewed as a chronic relapsing disorder? *Addiction*, *107*(1), 6–12. https://doi.org/10.1111/j.1360-0443.2011.03583.x

Curran, P. J., & Bauer, D. J. (2011). The disaggregation of within-person and between-person effects in longitudinal models of change. *Annual Review Of Psychology*, *62*, 583–619. https://doi.org/10.1146/annurev.psych.093008.100356

Danvers, A. F., Sbarra, D. A., & Mehl, M. R. (2020). Understanding personality through patterns of daily socializing: Applying recurrence quantification analysis to naturalistically observed intensive longitudinal social interaction data. *European Journal of Personality*, *34*, 777–793. https://doi.org/10.1002/per.2282

De Vries, L. P., Baselmans, B. M. L., & Bartels, M. (2020). Smartphone-based ecological momentary assessment of well-being: A systematic review and recommendations for future studies. *Journal of Happiness Studies*, *22*, 2361–2408. https://doi.org/10.1007/s10902–020-00324-7

Dennis, M., Scott, C. K., & Funk, R. (2003). An experimental evaluation of recovery management check-ups (RMC) for people with chronic substance use disorders. *Evaluation and Program Planning*, *26*(3), 339–352. https://doi.org/10.1016/S0149–7189(03)00037-5

Ebner-Priemer, U. W., & Trull, T. J. (2009). Ecological momentary assessment of mood disorders and mood dysregulation. *Psychological Assessment*, *21*(4), 463–475. https://doi.org/10.1037/a0017075.

Eckhoff, R. P., Kizakevich, P. N., Bakalov, V., Zhang, Y., Bryant, S. P., & Hobbs, M. A. (2015). A platform to build mobile health apps: The personal health intervention toolkit (PHIT). *JMIR MHealth and UHealth*, *3*(2), e4202. https://doi.org/10.2196/mhealth.4202

Ekholm, O. (2004). Influence of the recall period on self-reported alcohol intake. *European Journal of Clinical Nutrition*, *58*, 60–63. https://doi.org/10.1038/sj.ejcn.1601746

Emery, N. N., & Simons, J. S. (2020). The role of affect, emotion management, and attentional bias in young adult drinking: An experience sampling study. *Psychopharmacology*, *237*(5), 1557–1575. https://doi.org/10.1007/s00213–020-05480-5

Gmel, G., & Daeppen, J.-B. (2007). Recall bias for seven-day recall measurement of alcohol consumption among emergency department patients: Implications for case-crossover designs. *Journal of Studies on Alcohol and Drugs*, *68*(2), 303–310. https://doi.org/10.15288/jsad.2007.68.303

Gustafson, D. H., McTavish, F. M., Chih, M. Y., Atwood, A. K., Johnson, R. A., Boyle, M. G., Levy, M. S., Driscoll, H., Chisholm, S. M., Dillenburg, L., Isham, A., & Shah, D. (2014). A smartphone application to support recovery from alcoholism: A randomized clinical trial. *JAMA Psychiatry*, *71*(5), 566–572. https://doi.org/10.1001/jamapsychiatry.2013.4642

Hamaker, E. L., Asparouhov, T., Brose, A., Schmiedek, F., & Muthén, B. (2018). At the frontiers of modeling intensive longitudinal data: Dynamic structural equation models for the affective measurements from the COGITO study. *Multivariate Behavioral Research*, *53*(6), 820–841. https://doi.org/10.1080/00273171.2018.1446819

Heron, K. E., & Smyth, J. M. (2010). Ecological momentary interventions: Incorporating mobile technology into psychosocial and health behavior treatments. *British Journal of Health Psychology*, *15*(1), 1–39. https://doi.org/10.1348/135910709X466063

Kim, J., Marcusson-Clavertz, D., Yoshiuchi, K., & Smyth, J. M. (2019). Potential benefits of integrating ecological momentary assessment data into mHealth care systems. *BioPsychoSocial Medicine*, *13*(1), 19. https://doi.org/10.1186/s13030–019-0160-5

Kizakevich, P. N., Eckhoff, R., Brown, J., Tueller, S. J., Weimer, B., Bell, S., Weeks, A., Hourani, L. L., Spira, J. L., & King, L. A. (2018). PHIT for Duty, a mobile application for stress reduction, sleep improvement, and alcohol moderation. *Military Medicine*, *183*, 353–363. https://doi.org/10.1093/milmed/usx157

Kruse, C. S., Lee, K., Watson, J. B., Lobo, L. G., Stoppelmoor, A. G., & Oyibo, S. E. (2020). Measures of effectiveness, efficiency, and quality of telemedicine in the management of alcohol abuse, addiction, and rehabilitation: Systematic review. *Journal of Medical Internet Research*, *22*(1), 1–8. https://doi.org/10.2196/13252

Lauckner, C., Taylor, E., Patel, D., & Whitmire, A. (2019). The feasibility of using smartphones and mobile breathalyzers to monitor alcohol consumption among people living with HIV/AIDS. *Addiction Science & Clinical Practice*, *14*(1), 43. https://doi.org/10.1186/s13722–019-0174-0

Li, R., Dziak, J. J., Tan, X., Huang, L., Wagner, A. T., & Yang, J. (2017). *TVEM (time-varying effect model) SAS macro users' guide* (Version 3.1.1). The Methodology Center, Pennsylvania State University. Retrieved from http://methodology.psu.edu

Litvin, E. B., Abrantes, A. M., & Brown, R. A. (2013). Computer and mobile technology-based interventions for substance use disorders: An organizing framework. *Addictive Behaviors*, *38*(3), 1747–1756. https://doi.org/10.1016/j.addbeh.2012.09.003

Lord, S., Moore, S. K., Ramsey, A., Dinauer, S., & Johnson, K. (2016). Implementation of a substance use recovery support mobile phone app in community settings: Qualitative study of clinician and staff perspectives of facilitators and barriers. *JMIR Mental Health*, *3*(2), e24. https://doi.org/10.2196/mental.4927

Luczak, S. E., & Rosen, I. G. (2014). Estimating BrAC from transdermal alcohol concentration data using the BrAC estimator software program. *Alcoholism: Clinical and Experimental Research*, *38*(8), 2243–2252. http://dx.doi.org/10.1111/acer.12478

Marques, P. R., & McKnight, A. S. (2009). Field and laboratory alcohol detection with two types of transdermal devices. *Alcoholism: Clinical and Experimental Research*, *33*(4), 703–711. https://doi.org/10.1111/j.1530-0277.2008.00887.x

McKnight, A. S., Fell, J. C., & Auld-Owens, A. (2012). *Transdermal alcohol monitoring: Case studies* (Report No. DOT HS 811 603). US Department of Transportation, National Highway Traffic Safety Administration. www.adtsea.org/webfiles/fnitools/documents/nhtsa-transdermal-alcohol-monitoring.pdf

Miller, W. R. (2016). Sacred cows and greener pastures: Reflections from 40 years in addiction research. *Alcoholism Treatment Quarterly*, *34*(1), 92–115. https://doi.org/10.1080/07347324.2015.1077637

Miranda, R., Monti, P. M., Ray, L., Treloar, H. R., Reynolds, E. K., Ramirez, J., Chun, T., Gwaltney, C. J., Justus, A., Tidey, J., Blanchard, A., & Magill, M. (2014a). Characterizing subjective responses to alcohol among adolescent problem drinkers. *Journal of Abnormal Psychology*, *123*(1), 117–129. https://doi.org/10.1037/a0035328

Miranda, R., Ray, L., Blanchard, A., Reynolds, E. K., Monti, P. M., Chun, T., Justus, A., Swift, R. M., Tidey, J., Gwaltney, C. J., & Ramirez, J. (2014b). Effects of naltrexone on adolescent alcohol cue reactivity and sensitivity: An initial randomized trial. *Addiction Biology*, *19*(5), 941–954. https://doi.org/10.1111/adb.12050

Moody, L. N., Tegge, A. N., Poe, L. M., Koffarnus, M. N., & Bickel, W. K. (2018). To drink or to drink less? Distinguishing between effects of implementation intentions on decisions to drink and how much to drink in treatment-seeking individuals with alcohol use disorder. *Addictive Behaviors*, *83*, 64–71. https://doi.org/10.1016/j.addbeh.2017.11.010

Morgenstern, J., Kuerbis, A., & Muench, F. (2014). Ecological momentary assessment and alcohol use disorder treatment. *Alcohol Research: Current Reviews*, *36*(1), 101–110. https://arcr.niaaa.nih.gov/alcohol-research-and-ehealth-technology/ecological-momentary-assessment-and-alcohol-use-disorder

Nahum-Shani, I., Smith, S. N., Spring, B. J., Collins, L. M., Witkiewitz, K., Tewari, A., & Murphy, S. A. (2018). Just-in-time adaptive interventions (JITAIs) in mobile health: Key components and design principles for ongoing health behavior support. *Annals of Behavioral Medicine*, *52*(6), 446–462. https://doi.org/10.1007/s12160–016-9830-8

National Institute on Alcohol Abuse and Alcoholism (2020). *NIAAA recovery research definitions*. www.niaaa.nih.gov/research/niaaa-recovery-from-alcohol-use-disorder/definitions

Neale, J., Vitoratou, S., Finch, E., Lennon, P., Mitcheson, L., Panebianco, D., Rose, D., Strang, J., Wykes, T., & Marsden, J. (2016). Development and validation of "SURE": A patient reported outcome measure (PROM) for recovery from drug and alcohol dependence. *Drug and Alcohol Dependence*, *165*, 159–167. https://doi.org/10.1016/j.drugalcdep.2016.06.006

O'Brien, C. P. (1994). Treatment of alcoholism as a chronic disorder. *Alcohol*, *11*(6), 433–437. https://doi.org/10.1016/0741-8329(94)90063-9

Oravecz, Z., Tuerlinckx, F., & Vandekerckhove, J. (2016). Bayesian data analysis with the bivariate hierarchical Ornstein-Uhlenbeck process model. *Multivariate Behavioral Research*, *51*(1), 106–119. https://doi.org/10.1080/00273171.2015.1110512

Pew Research Center (2019). *Mobile fact sheet*. www.pewresearch.org/internet/fact-sheet/mobile/

Ramsey, A., Lord, S., Torrey, J., Marsch, L., & Lardiere, M. (2016). Paving the way to successful implementation: Identifying key barriers to use of technology-based therapeutic tools for behavioral health care. *Journal of Behavioral*

Health Services & Research, *43*(1), 54–70. https://doi.org/10.1007/s11414–014-9436-5

Roos, C. R., Kober, H., Trull, T. J., MacLean, R. R., & Mun, C. J. (2020). Intensive longitudinal methods for studying the role of self-regulation strategies in substance use behavior change. *Current Addiction Reports*, *7*(3), 301–316. https://doi.org/10.1007/s40429–020-00329-5

Sakai, J. T., Mikulich-Gilbertson, S. K., Long, R. J., & Crowley, T. J. (2006). Validity of transdermal alcohol monitoring: Fixed and self-regulated dosing. *Alcoholism: Clinical and Experimental Research*, *30*(1), 26–33. https://doi.org/10.1111/j.1530-0277.2006.00004.x

Scott, C. K., & Dennis, M. L. (2009). Results from two randomized clinical trials evaluating the impact of quarterly recovery management check-ups with adult chronic substance users. *Addiction*, *104*(6), 959–971. https://doi.org/10.1111/j.1360-0443.2009.02525.x

Serre, F., Fatseas, M., Swendsen, J., & Auriacombe, M. (2015). Ecological momentary assessment in the investigation of craving and substance use in daily life: A systematic review. *Drug and Alcohol Dependence*, *148*, 1–20. https://doi.org/10.1016/j.drugalcdep.2014.12.024

Shiffman, S. (2009). Ecological momentary assessment (EMA) in studies of substance use. *Psychological Assessment*, *21*(4), 486–497. https://doi.org/10.1037/a0017074

(2014). Conceptualizing analyses of ecological momentary assessment data. *Nicotine and Tobacco Research*, *16*(SUPPL2), 76–87. https://doi.org/10.1093/ntr/ntt195

Shiffman, S., Stone, A. A., & Hufford, M. R. (2008). Ecological momentary assessment. *Annual Review of Clinical Psychology*, 4, 1–32. https://doi.org/10.1146/annurev.clinpsy.3.022806.091415

Simons, J. S., Wills, T. A., Emery, N. N., & Marks, R. M. (2015). Quantifying alcohol consumption: Self-report, transdermal assessment, and prediction of dependence symptoms. *Addictive Behaviors*, *50*, 205–212. https://doi.org/10.1016/j.addbeh.2015.06.042

Simons, J. S., Wills, T. A., & Neal, D. J. (2014). The many faces of affect: A multilevel model of drinking frequency/quantity and alcohol dependence symptoms among young adults. *Journal of Abnormal Psychology*, *123*(3), 676–694. https://doi.org/10.1037/a0036926

Stevenson, B. L., Dvorak, R. D., Kramer, M. P., Peterson, R. S., Dunn, M. E., Leary, A. V., & Pinto, D. (2019). Within- and between-person associations from mood to alcohol consequences: The mediating role of enhancement and coping drinking motives. *Journal of Abnormal Psychology*, *128*(8), 813–822. https://doi.org/10.1037/abn0000472

Suffoletto, B., Callaway, C., Kristan, J., Kraemer, K., & Clark, D. B. (2012). Text-message-based drinking assessments and brief interventions for young adults discharged from the emergency department. *Alcoholism: Clinical and Experimental Research*, *36*(3), 552–560. https://doi.org/10.1111/j.1530-0277.2011.01646.x

Suffoletto, B., Dasgupta, P., Rayuymatiao, B. S., Huber, J., & Flickinger, K. (2020). A preliminary study using smartphone accelerometers to sense gait impairments due to alcohol intoxication. *Journal of Studies on Alcohol and Drugs, 81*, 505–510. https://doi.org/10.15288/jsad.2020.81.505

Suffoletto, B., Kristan, J., Callaway, C., Kim, K. H., Chung, T., Monti, P. M., & Clark, D. B. (2014). A text message alcohol intervention for young adult emergency department patients: A randomized clinical trial. *Annals of Emergency Medicine, 64*(6), 664–672. e4. https://doi.org/10.1016/j.annemergmed.2014.06.010

Swift, R. (2000). Transdermal alcohol measurement for estimation of blood alcohol concentration. *Alcoholism: Clinical and Experimental Research, 24*(4), 422–423. https://doi.org/10.1111/j.1530-0277.2000.tb02006.x

Trull, T. J., & Ebner-Priemer, U. (2013). Ambulatory assessment. *Annual Review of Clinical Psychology, 9*, 151–176. https://doi.org/10.1146/annurev-clinpsy-050212-185510

(2014). The role of ambulatory assessment in psychological science. *Current Directions in Psychological Science, 23*(6), 466–470. https://doi.org/10.1177/0963721414550706

Tucker, J. A., Foushee, H. R., Black, B. C., & Roth, D. L. (2007). Agreement between prospective interactive voice response self-monitoring and structured retrospective reports of drinking and contextual variables during natural resolution attempts. *Journal of Studies on Alcohol and Drugs, 68*(4), 538–542. https://doi.org/10.15288/jsad.2007.68.538

Tugade, M. M., Conner, T., & Barrett, L. F. (2007). Assessment of mood. In S. Ayers, A. Baum, C. McManus, S. Newman, K. Wallston, J. Weinman, & R. West (Eds.), *The Cambridge handbook of psychology, health, and medicine* (2nd ed.), pp. 278–286. Cambridge University Press.

Wang, L., & Miller, L. C. (2020). Just-in-the-moment adaptive interventions (JITAI): A meta-analytical review. *Health Communication, 35*(12), 1531–1544. https://doi.org/10.1080/10410236.2019.1652388

Witkiewitz, K., Desai, S. A., Bowen, S., Leigh, B. C., Kirouac, M., & Larimer, M. E. (2014). Development and evaluation of a mobile intervention for heavy drinking and smoking among college students. *Psychology of Addictive Behaviors, 28*(3), 639–650. https://doi.org/10.1037/a0034747

Witkiewitz, K., Montes, K. S., Schwebel, F. J., & Tucker, J. A. (2020). What is recovery? *Alcohol Research: Current Reviews, 40*(3), 1–12. https://doi.org/10.35946/arcr.v40.3.01

Wray, T. B., Merrill, J. E., & Monti, P. M. (2014). Using ecological momentary assessment (EMA) to assess situation-level predictors of alcohol use and alcohol-related consequences. *Alcohol Research: Current Reviews, 36*(1), 19–28. https://arcr.niaaa.nih.gov/alcohol-research-and-ehealth-technology/using-ecological-momentary-assessment-ema-assess-situation

14 Studying Recovery in the Social Context

A Primer on Methods for Measuring and Modeling Social Network Data in Applied Recovery Research

Kevin A. Hallgren

Studying Recovery in the Social Context: A Primer on Methods for Measuring and Modeling Social Network Data in Applied Recovery Research

Social environments play a crucial role in the processes of developing, sustaining, treating, and recovering from substance use disorders (SUDs; Groh et al., 2007; McCrady et al., 2004), and numerous prevention, treatment, and recovery models emphasize the importance of the social environment. Many individuals who successfully recover do so in part by reducing their contact with people who use substances in unhealthy ways, increasing their contact with people who do not use substances or use them in smaller quantities and frequencies, engaging with people in mutual help groups, building social networks that can offer general support and comfort, and/or changing their interactions with the people in their social environments. These social environmental changes may not only help individuals increase the likelihood of reducing their substance use, but may also be critical components of recovery itself. Healthy and supportive social relationships are fundamental components of health, wellness, and functioning that are cornerstones of contemporary definitions of recovery (White, 2007).

Measuring and analyzing social network data can allow researchers to understand more precisely the dynamic roles that social environments may serve in recovery and offer opportunities to understand recovery at multiple levels of analysis. Social environments can be modeled as both a characteristic of individuals (e.g., what is the social environment like for individuals who seek recovery?) and as characteristics of communities as a whole (e.g., what are the social environments like within various types of recovery-oriented communities?).

Approaches to measuring and analyzing social network data often differ from the methods used in most psychosocial research. This chapter therefore aims to provide a primer on methods that researchers may use to measure and analyze social network data in SUD recovery research. The chapter is divided into two major sections that describe *egocentric* and *sociocentric* approaches to studying social networks (terms that are described in the following section), with overviews of introductory issues related to measurement and data analysis for each type of approach, along with exemplar applications in SUD research that illustrate the types of insights that may be obtained using the methods described. The focus is primarily conceptual, and computational details are generally omitted except when they aid with conceptual understanding. References that provide more in-depth explanations of the methods and computational details are provided throughout the chapter.

Egocentric and Sociocentric Approaches

A social network typically refers to a set of individuals who are socially connected, either formally through designated relationships (e.g., people who are friends or family members) or informally through shared interactions (e.g., people within the same organizations or communities) or activities (e.g., people who co-use substances or who offer advice to one another). Approaches to measuring and analyzing social network data are often classified as either egocentric or sociocentric. The *egocentric* approach usually focuses on the people with direct social connections to participants within a study, where information about the people directly connected to a participant is aggregated into a set of variables meant to summarize one or more aspects of each participant's social environment (McCarty et al., 2019). For example, a study using the egocentric approach may ask each participant to identify individuals who are in their social network (e.g., close friends, family), collect information about each of those identified individuals (e.g., typical drinking frequency of each network member), and then aggregate that information into a summary variable meant to encapsulate a relevant aspect of each participant's social environment (e.g., the percentage of people with heavy drinking within each participant's social network). "Complete" network information is not required; for example, the researcher need not know whether participants identify other participants in the study as their close friends. Individual participants are retained as the unit of analysis, and statistical analyses typically model aggregate summary variables describing each person's social environment similarly to how they would model other personal characteristics (e.g., entered as independent, dependent, moderator, or mediator variables in statistical models).

The *sociocentric* approach focuses on the structures of entire social networks – that is, the network of relationships among all (or most) individuals within a defined community or population (Wasserman & Faust, 1994). Analyses may characterize the egocentric networks of individuals, but are uniquely able to also characterize full network-level characteristics, such as how the network is structured, how relationships form or dissolve over time, how information and behaviors spread across the network, and whether certain individuals occupy more influential roles. The sociocentric approach often focuses on a full network as the unit of analysis and often uses social network analytic approaches that may differ from statistical methods used in non-network related psychosocial research.

Methods for Studying Egocentric Social Networks

Measuring Egocentric Social Networks

As described above, studies using an *egocentric* approach typically identify sets of individuals with whom research participants have direct social ties, then collect relevant information about each identified network member, and then compute summary variables meant to characterize one or more aspects of each participant's social environment. The participants in the study are sometimes called *egos* and the individuals they identify as having a relationship with are often called *alters* (McCarty et al., 2019).

Key measurement considerations include (1) defining the type of alters to query participants about (e.g., friends vs. important people vs. people from whom they seek advice), (2) the preferred number of alters and closeness of the alters that participants should identify (e.g., small number of close alters vs. many alters with varying closeness), (3) the type of information to be queried for each alter (e.g., substance use vs. encouragement for substance use vs. co-use of substances by the participant and alter), and (4) clarifying how that information will be aggregated into summary measures (e.g., average frequency of drinking among alters vs. percentage of alters who drink daily). Numerous factors may guide these decisions, including psychometric and validation studies; theoretical, clinical, and practical considerations; and the extent to which summary measures will be meaningful to research stakeholders.

One of the most well described and commonly used tools for measuring egocentric networks in SUD treatment and recovery research is the Important People instrument (IP; Clifford & Longabaugh, 1991). In its usual format (e.g., Longabaugh et al., 2010), participants identify up to 10 alters who they consider important or with whom they have had recent contact. Then for each identified alter, participants answer 10 to 15 questions about their relationship to the alter (e.g., friend, sibling, etc.), the alter's general supportiveness to the participant, the alter's reactions to the participant's drinking or drug use, and the alter's typical drinking or drug use behavior. The IP has been validated in interview, paper-and-pencil, and computer-based questionnaire formats (Hallgren et al., 2013), and several revisions of the measure have been used to characterize egocentric social networks with respect to drinking (Clifford & Longabaugh, 1991), other drug use (Owens & McCrady, 2014; Zywiak et al., 2009), and tobacco use (Roberts et al., 2015). It has also been validated in populations of college students (e.g., DeMartini et al., 2013; Hallgren et al., 2013; Orford et al., 2004), adults in outpatient SUD treatment (e.g., Groh et al., 2007, 2011; Longabaugh et al., 2010; Zywiak et al., 2002), and in criminal justice populations (e.g., Nargiso et al., 2014; Owens & McCrady, 2014).

Psychometric studies have generally supported the reliability, concurrent validity, and predictive validity of numerous summary measures derived from the IP (Hallgren et al., 2013; Longabaugh et al., 1998). However, factor analytic studies that have tried to combine summary indices into more general higher-level constructs have yielded inconsistent findings (e.g., 2–6 latent factors; Groh et al., 2007; Hallgren et al., 2013; Longabaugh et al., 1998, 2010; Zywiak et al., 2009). Substance-related measures derived from the IP (DeMartini et al., 2013; Groh et al., 2007, 2011; Hallgren et al., 2013; Owens & McCrady, 2014; Zywiak et al., 2002) and similar social network scales (e.g., Tucker et al., 2015) that aggregate substance use *behaviors* and *encouragement* of substance use among network members have often found stronger concurrent and predictive associations with participants' substance use behaviors compared to summary indices of network characteristics unrelated to substance use (e.g., network size, general network supportiveness).

The full IP may require participants to answer up to 100-150 questions, depending on the version being used – for example, participants may nominate up to 10 alters, then answer 10-15 follow-up questions per alter. Fortunately, shorter versions have been validated that may significantly reduce assessment burden by asking participants to identify fewer alters and answer fewer follow-up questions per alter. The IP-5 (Hallgren & Barnett, 2016) asks participants to nominate up to five important people with three follow-up questions per alter and yielded only minor loss of reliability and validity for measuring egocentric network drinking behavior in college students relative to a full 10-person instrument (Hallgren & Barnett, 2016). Likewise, the Brief Alcohol Social Density Assessment (BASDA; Levitt et al. 2019) asks participants to identify four nonbiologically related alters with five follow-up questions per alter and yielded strong reliability and concurrent validity among a general population of adults with any past-year drinking. These briefer instruments may reduce assessment burden and free up time to administer other measures or allow network constructs to be measured more frequently (e.g., in longitudinal studies).

Analysis and Example Applications of Egocentric Networks in Recovery Research

Egocentric network summary indices aim to characterize the social environments for each participant in a study. Statistical analyses of these indices therefore frequently utilize approaches similar to those used for modeling other participant characteristics. For example, descriptive statistics of network indices should be evaluated and reported, and descriptive statistics of network characteristics may often be interesting in their own right – particularly if the indices are computed in a manner that is intuitively understandable to clinical and community stakeholders. For example, in a longitudinal study of individuals who had contact with alters who use drugs, Buchanan and Latkin (2008) reported a large reduction in the percentage of alters who used drugs (from 40 percent to 16 percent) over a nine-month period among participants who stopped using heroin, cocaine, or both compared to participants who continued using these drugs over the same time period (from 44 percent to 38 percent).

Egocentric network measures may be modeled as predictors, outcomes, mediators, and moderators of interventions using many of the existing statistical tools that would be used for modeling other personal characteristics. For example, Groh et al. (2008) provided an in-depth review of studies on social networks for people involved in 12 Step programs and reported that individuals who participate in 12 Step programs tend to maintain larger numbers of friends in their networks by replacing previous friends with other 12 Step group members. They also tend to report more general social support, more encouragement for abstinence, and less substance use among the friends in their egocentric networks, which in turn predict a higher likelihood of abstinence. Others have shown that the degree of heavy drinking within the pre-treatment networks of people entering alcohol use disorder treatment may moderate the effectiveness of pharmacological and behavioral interventions, suggesting the potential for matching patients to specific treatments based in part on their pre-treatment social environments (Longabaugh et al., 1998; Worley et al., 2015).

There are likely numerous additional creative and unexplored ways to measure and analyze egocentric networks in recovery research, including with ideographic approaches, data visualization methods, and by utilizing the assessment of networks as an intervention. For example, Beckwith et al. (2019) extended the IP to create a Social Identity Mapping in Addiction Recovery procedure (SIM-AR) in which participants identified alters who they considered important and then grouped the alters into distinct social subgroups using a visual map. Individual alters and alter subgroups were graphically annotated on the map using Post-it notes, stickers, and colored pens to characterize recovery-related features (e.g., importance, compatibility or conflict with the participant; risk for alcohol and drug use) to facilitate the measurement of specific sub-communities (rather than individual alters) and help patients better understand their social environments. Using this procedure in a sample of individuals entering therapeutic communities, Beckwith et al. (2019) found that reductions in the proportion of high-risk subgroups over a six-month period were associated with reductions in participants' substance use, reduced substance use identity, and increased recovery identity six months later.

Methods for Studying Sociocentric Social Networks

Measuring Sociocentric Social Networks

As described earlier, studies that use a *sociocentric* approach typically measure the complete (or mostly complete) set of social connections within a defined group of individuals (e.g., in specific classrooms, organizations, communities, etc.). The individuals being studied are often called *nodes* or *actors*; the relationships between them are often called *edges*, *arcs*, or *ties*.

Measurement considerations include (1) identifying groups, communities, or populations of actors that have clear enough boundaries to define whether individuals are considered to be a part of that group, community, or population (e.g., "classrooms" where students are considered in the network if enrolled in the class); (2) specifying the nature and strength of the relationship required to indicate whether a social tie between actors is present; (3) choosing a method for collecting data about the presence and absence of social ties (e.g., will participants identify alters from a list of names or a photo roster? Will ties be measured passively based on who interacts with whom online?); and (4) identifying which actor-level covariates should be measured and how they will be measured (e.g., will actors self-report their own drinking and drug use frequency?). Additional considerations are often necessary depending on the study design and the types of networks being studied (see the later discussion about various types of network data that may be collected); researchers should refer to additional sources to identify particular requirements that match the specific approaches they will use. For example, stochastic actor-oriented models (described at the end of this chapter) perform optimally when the number of ties between actors is relatively limited (e.g., less than ~20 ties per actor). Studies can be designed to conform to this requirement by allowing participants to identify only their "closest friends" as opposed to all friends and by using data collection instruments that clearly indicate the intended range of alters that should be identified (e.g., data collection forms could show a maximum of 20 fields for identifying alters).

Types of Social Ties

In addition to the considerations above, researchers may measure various types of social ties that in turn affect the analytic approaches used. Social ties may be *directed*, in which case a relationship can be extended by an actor without being reciprocated (i.e., actor *i* can identify actor *j* as their friend, regardless of whether *j* considers *i* their friend), or *undirected*, where relationships are always considered mutual (i.e., *i* and *j* are considered friends and any directionality in the relationship cannot be determined). Panels A and B in Figure 14.1 illustrate hypothetical directed and undirected networks, with arrows indicating the directionality of ties and the lack of arrows indicating undirected ties. Ties may also be *weighted*, where the strength of some social ties are stronger than others, or *unweighted*, where a tie is simply present or absent. Panels B and C in Figure 14.1 depict examples of networks with unweighted and weighted ties, respectively; in both cases, ties are also undirected.

Ties may also form between qualitatively different types of nodes, creating *two-mode* or *bipartite networks*. For example, rather than directly asking participants to identify their friends, a researcher could link participants to another type of entity – such as the clubs they participate in, police reports in which the actors are named, or recovery communities in which actors participate. Panel D in Figure 14.1 illustrates a bipartite network with actors presented as circles and the

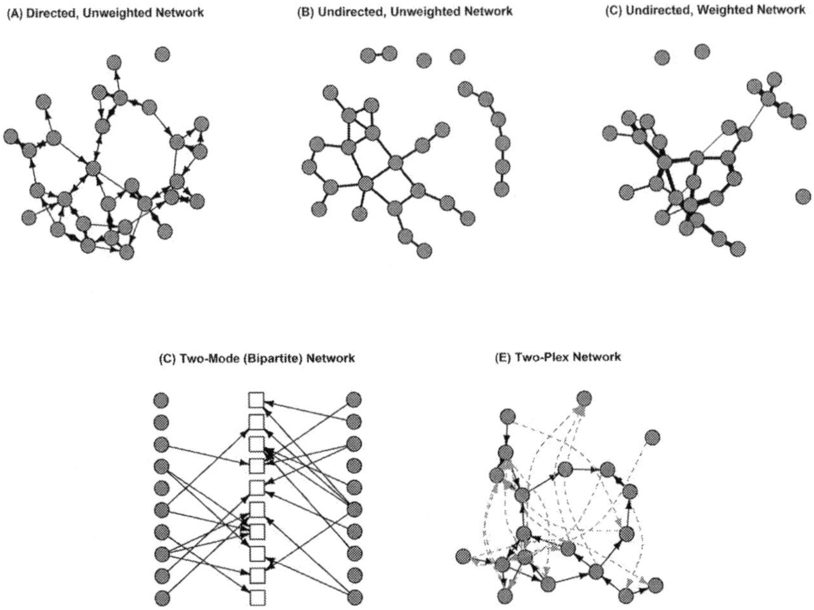

Figure 14.1 *Graphs illustrating varying types of social ties that may be measured in social networks.*

entities they connect to presented as squares. Notably, actors only extend ties to the entities they are associated with – actors do not extend ties to other actors. However, bipartite networks may be transformed to represent single-mode networks with direct ties between actors, for example, by assuming direct ties exist between actors tied to the same entity. This approach may provide a means of obtaining network information without requiring participants to self-report who they share social ties with. For example, Aaronson et al. (2020) utilized electronic health record data to create a bipartite network of connections between medical patients who use opioids and the healthcare providers who provided services to them, with patients and providers each reflected as different types of nodes. These bipartite network data could then be collapsed into a one-mode network; e.g., a one-mode network consisting of only healthcare providers could be created by modeling ties between healthcare providers who provided services to the same patients.

Researchers may also choose to measure two or more qualitatively different types of social ties within the same network (e.g., ties associated with friendships and ties associated with advice-seeking). These are known as *multiplex* networks, and they allow researchers to compare how different types of social structures may be present within the same group or community. A hypothetical example is illustrated in panel E of Figure 14.1.

For brevity, the following sections that focus on representing sociocentric data and modeling actor- and network-level attributes focus only on directed, unweighted, single-mode networks that measure only one type of tie (i.e., like those in panel A in Figure 14.1). However, readers are referred to other sources for discussion of

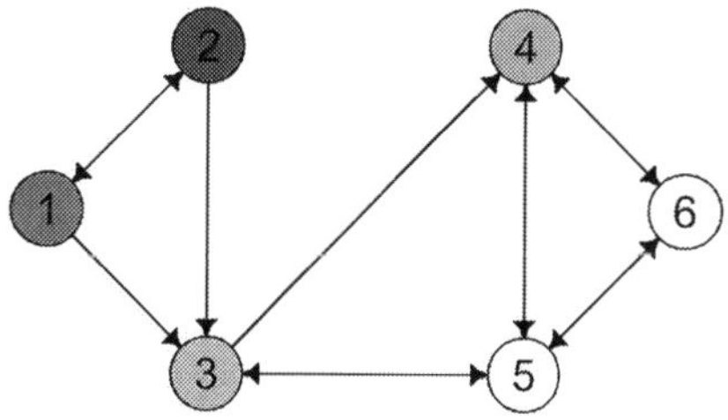

Figure 14.2 *Graph for a hypothetical directed network with six actors, corresponding to network **X*** described in text.

measurement and analytic issues of the other types of networks described above (McCulloh et al., 2013; Scott & Carrington, 2011; Wasserman & Faust, 1994).

Representing Sociocentric Networks

Social ties in sociocentric networks can be represented as network graphs, edge lists, and adjacency matrices. Network graphs are visual representations that display actors as nodes and social ties as lines or arrows between nodes. Examples of network graphs are shown in Figure 14.1; another example is shown in Figure 14.2 and will be used to illustrate the measurement and analytic topics discussed below. The shading, colors, shapes, and sizes of nodes and arrows in network graphs may be changed to help illustrate different attributes of actors and social ties (e.g., darker nodes in Figure 14.2 may indicate more past-month heavy drinking days).

Edge lists can be used to identify social ties in a way that is both easily readable and convenient for data entry. Usually, an edge list is a two-column data structure that indicates which egos (column 1) extend ties to which alters (column 2). A third column may be included for weighted networks to indicate the strength of ties. The network in Figure 14.2 can be represented by the following edge list:

$$\begin{bmatrix} 1 & 2 \\ 1 & 3 \\ 2 & 1 \\ 2 & 3 \\ 3 & 4 \\ 3 & 5 \\ 4 & 5 \\ 4 & 6 \\ 5 & 3 \\ 5 & 4 \\ 5 & 6 \\ 6 & 4 \\ 6 & 5 \end{bmatrix}$$

An adjacency matrix may also be used to represent social ties and is typically used for computational purposes. The adjacency matrix, which will be called $\boldsymbol{X}$ in this chapter, is an $n \times n$ matrix where n is the number of actors in the network. For an unweighted and directed network, the value in row i, column j (referred to as $X_{i,j}$) equals one if actor i extends a tie to actor j and equals zero if they do not extend such a tie. Notably, all values along the diagonal are usually zero because actors do not extend ties to themselves. The graph in Figure 14.2 and the edge list above can be represented by the following adjacency matrix:

$$X = \begin{bmatrix} 0 & 1 & 1 & 0 & 0 & 0 \\ 1 & 0 & 1 & 0 & 0 & 0 \\ 0 & 0 & 0 & 1 & 1 & 0 \\ 0 & 0 & 0 & 0 & 1 & 1 \\ 0 & 0 & 1 & 1 & 0 & 1 \\ 0 & 0 & 0 & 1 & 1 & 0 \end{bmatrix}$$

Characterizing Actor-Level Attributes with Sociocentric Data

Encoding social ties in an adjacency matrix enables the use of matrix algebra to compute several interesting network-related characteristics. For example, the number of outgoing ties extended by each actor can be computed by summing values in each row of X (e.g., rows 1 and 2 each sum to a value of two, indicating that actors 1 and 2 each nominate two other actors as friends). Similarly, the number of incoming ties received from other actors can be computed by summing the values in each column (e.g., actors 1 and 2 are each identified as friends by one actor).

Squaring the adjacency matrix via matrix multiplication produces a new $n \times n$ matrix, where each value indicates the number of paths between actor pairs that are exactly two degrees apart (see Weisstein, 2020 for brief review of matrix multiplication). For example, the matrix X^2 shown below has a value of 2 in the 3rd row, 6th column ($X^2{}_{3,6}$). This indicates that there are exactly 2 two-degree pathways from actor 3 to actor 6, which as shown in Figure 14.1, occur through actors 4 and 5.

$$X^2 = \begin{bmatrix} 0 & 1 & 1 & 0 & 0 & 0 \\ 1 & 0 & 1 & 0 & 0 & 0 \\ 0 & 0 & 0 & 1 & 1 & 0 \\ 0 & 0 & 0 & 0 & 1 & 1 \\ 0 & 0 & 1 & 1 & 0 & 1 \\ 0 & 0 & 0 & 1 & 1 & 0 \end{bmatrix} \begin{bmatrix} 0 & 1 & 1 & 0 & 0 & 0 \\ 1 & 0 & 1 & 0 & 0 & 0 \\ 0 & 0 & 0 & 1 & 1 & 0 \\ 0 & 0 & 0 & 0 & 1 & 1 \\ 0 & 0 & 1 & 1 & 0 & 1 \\ 0 & 0 & 0 & 1 & 1 & 0 \end{bmatrix} = \begin{bmatrix} 1 & 0 & 1 & 1 & 1 & 0 \\ 0 & 1 & 1 & 1 & 1 & 0 \\ 0 & 0 & 1 & 1 & 1 & 2 \\ 0 & 0 & 1 & 2 & 1 & 1 \\ 0 & 0 & 0 & 2 & 3 & 1 \\ 0 & 0 & 1 & 1 & 1 & 2 \end{bmatrix}$$

This use of matrix multiplication can be helpful for identifying pathways within a network – for example, which actors are friends-of-friends of each actor. Unlike with matrix X, the values along the diagonal of X^2 are not always zero, as it is possible to trace a path from an actor back to them themselves (e.g., through reciprocated ties). The values in X^3 would likewise indicate the number of unique paths that are exactly three degrees apart (e.g., friends-of-friends-of-friends), and so on.

Measures of *centrality* may also be computed for individual actors to understand their relative "importance" based on their position within the network. For example, *outdegree centrality* and *indegree centrality* can be measured by counting the number of ties extended from or received by a given actor, which as described above, can be computed by summing the values in $\boldsymbol{X}$ across rows or columns, respectively. Actors with higher centrality may have relatively higher importance, influence, or prestige within a network, particularly when the number of incoming ties is high (i.e., high indegree centrality), since it indicates that many other actors have nominated the individual as serving a particular social role for them (e.g., friend, someone they seek advice from, etc.). Another index of centrality, *betweenness centrality*, reflects how many times the shortest paths between all combinations of actor pairs in the network goes through an individual actor. For example, actor 3 has the largest betweenness centrality in network $\boldsymbol{X}$, which may be clarified by examining Figure 14.1. Actor 3 is the only actor who bridges two smaller subsets of actors (actors 1–2 and 4–6), so the shortest path between numerous combinations of actor pairs in network $\boldsymbol{X}$ necessarily goes through actor 3. Individuals with high betweenness centrality may hold key positions in networks; for example, they may serve as "brokers" between other actors in the network (Spiro et al., 2013) who can control the transmission of information or behaviors between subgroups. Their connectedness with members of different subgroups may place them in positions of power where they also can control the facilitation of connections or matchmaking between members of unconnected subgroups.

Actor-level covariates may also be used in combination with the adjacency matrix to describe the behaviors, beliefs, and other characteristics across all the alters connected to a specific actor (i.e., the egocentric networks of an actor). For example, suppose $\boldsymbol{v}$ is an $n \times 1$ matrix, where the value in position i reflects the number of past-month heavy drinking days for actor i (e.g., actor 1 has 21 past-month heavy drinking days, actor 2 has 30 past-month heavy drinking days, etc.):

$$\boldsymbol{v} = \begin{bmatrix} 21 \\ 30 \\ 10 \\ 12 \\ 0 \\ 0 \end{bmatrix}$$

Matrix multiplication of $\boldsymbol{X} \times \boldsymbol{v}$ will yield an $n \times 1$ matrix, the values of which contain the summed number of heavy drinking days amongst the alters who receive social ties from each actor – or in other words, the summed number of heavy drinking days for each actor's egocentric network. For example, actor 1 extends ties actors 2 and 3, who have a sum of 40 past-month heavy drinking days $(30 + 10)$ and actor 2 extends ties to actors 1 and 3, who have a sum of 31 past-month heavy drinking days $(21 + 10)$:

$$Xv = \begin{bmatrix} 0 & 1 & 1 & 0 & 0 & 0 \\ 1 & 0 & 1 & 0 & 0 & 0 \\ 0 & 0 & 0 & 1 & 1 & 0 \\ 0 & 0 & 0 & 0 & 1 & 1 \\ 0 & 0 & 1 & 1 & 0 & 1 \\ 0 & 0 & 0 & 1 & 1 & 0 \end{bmatrix} \begin{bmatrix} 21 \\ 30 \\ 10 \\ 12 \\ 0 \\ 0 \end{bmatrix} = \begin{bmatrix} 40 \\ 31 \\ 12 \\ 0 \\ 22 \\ 12 \end{bmatrix}$$

Transposing matrix X (i.e., flipping it with respect to its diagonal) and performing the same operation likewise provides an $n \times 1$ matrix reflecting the summed number of drinking days based on *incoming* ties to each actor. For example, actor 3 receives friendship ties from actors 1, 2, and 5, who have a sum of 51 heavy drinking days $(21 + 30 + 0)$:

$$X^T v = \begin{bmatrix} 0 & 1 & 0 & 0 & 0 & 0 \\ 1 & 0 & 0 & 0 & 0 & 0 \\ 1 & 1 & 0 & 0 & 1 & 0 \\ 0 & 0 & 1 & 0 & 1 & 1 \\ 0 & 0 & 1 & 1 & 0 & 1 \\ 0 & 0 & 0 & 1 & 1 & 0 \end{bmatrix} \begin{bmatrix} 21 \\ 30 \\ 10 \\ 12 \\ 0 \\ 0 \end{bmatrix} = \begin{bmatrix} 30 \\ 21 \\ 51 \\ 10 \\ 22 \\ 12 \end{bmatrix}$$

If vector v were a binary variable (e.g., *any* past-month heavy drinking), the operations above could be used to indicate the number of alters connected to each actor who have any past-month heavy drinking. The resulting values could be divided by the outdegree or indegree centrality of each actor (i.e., number of outgoing or incoming ties) to obtain indices reflecting the *average* number of past-month heavy drinking days for each actor's alters or the *proportion* of each actor's alters with any past-month heavy drinking.

Characterizing Network-Level Attributes with Sociocentric Data

In addition to characterizing attributes of individual actors, sociocentric data can be modeled to understand characteristics of entire networks, including various aspects of how networks are structured (e.g., How connected are actors? How hierarchical are relationships? Are actors organized into sub-communities?). This section describes some network-level structural characteristics that may be of interest in SUD treatment and recovery research; however, only a limited number of these characteristics are discussed for brevity (see Scott & Carrington, 2011; and Wasserman & Faust, 1994 for more in-depth discussion). Each of the network-level characteristics described in this section can be modeled using cross-sectional or longitudinal data.

The *density* of a network describes how connected individuals within a network are to each other. Formally, density is often computed as the proportion of ties present out of the number of possible ties. For networks that are directed and unweighted, this is equal to the summed number of ties indicated in X, divided by the potential number of ties, $n(n\text{-}1)$. For example, network X above has 13 out of 30 possible ties, or a density of 0.43, indicating an average tendency for actors to extend ties to 43 percent of the other actors in the network. In general, larger networks tend to have lower densities because as the number of potential ties increases, actors generally limit the number of ties they extend (i.e., maintaining relationships imposes costs, so people tend to limit the number of ties they have). However, when networks are similar in size to one another, the networks with greater density may have greater cohesiveness and, potentially, a higher propensity for information, behaviors, or other socially transmissible attributes to spread more easily throughout the network.

In a directed network, *reciprocity* describes the extent to which ties between actor pairs are reciprocated – that is, if actor i extends a tie to actor j, how often does j extend a tie back to i? One index of reciprocity is computed by dividing the number of reciprocated ties by the total number of ties present. For example, in network $\boldsymbol{X}$ above, there are 10 reciprocated ties (this is equal to the sum of values along the diagonal of $\boldsymbol{X}^2$; it can also be seen by the five double-headed arrows in Figure 14.2, each of which reflects two reciprocated ties) and three non-reciprocated ties (i.e., single-headed arrows in Figure 14.2). Reciprocity is therefore 0.77, meaning that outgoing ties are reciprocated 77 percent of the time by the actors who receive them. Reciprocity can offer insights into the direction ality of relationships in a network and the degree of agreement between actors about the presence of social relationships. Low reciprocity may indicate the presence of hierarchy within a social structure (e.g., low reciprocity among advice-seeking ties may indicate that advice is sought unidirectionally within a community) or a high proportion of potentially "weaker" ties that might be less stable than a reciprocated tie (e.g., a one-sided friendship may be "weaker" or less stable over time than a mutual friendship). Higher reciprocity may indicate more equal views of relationships and the presence of "stronger" relationships (e.g., mutuality within friendship ties, more equitable "giving and taking" within advice-seeking ties).

Transitivity describes the extent to which actors extend ties to individuals who are tied to their own alters – for example, if actor i is friends with actor $j(i \rightarrow j)$ and actor j is friends with actor $k(j \rightarrow k)$, then does actor i also tend to nominate actor k as their friend $(i \rightarrow k)$? An example transitive triplet is shown between actors 1, 2, and 3 in network $\boldsymbol{X}(1 \rightarrow 2, 2 \rightarrow 3, 1 \rightarrow 3)$; triplets are also present between actors 3–6. Several formulas are available to characterize the degree of transitivity within a network; one involves identifying the number of combinations of actor triads where a 2nd-degree connection is present (i.e., $i \rightarrow j$ and $j \rightarrow k$), and among them, determining the proportion of times transitive closure is obtained (i.e., $i \rightarrow k$). In network $\boldsymbol{X}$ above, there are 19 triads with a 2nd-degree connection (i.e., sum of values in $\boldsymbol{X}^2$ excluding values on the diagonal). Eleven of these obtain transitive closure, yielding a transitivity index of 0.58. The degree of transitivity can provide insights into the larger network structure. For example, high transitivity may indicate that connections among actors may tend to be consolidated into well-connected communities or subgroups, whereas low transitivity can indicate that networks may be structured more hierarchically (e.g., actor *i* advises actors *j, k,* and *l*, but the latter actors do not advise each other) or that network members form long paths (e.g., *i* advises *j*, who in turn advises *k*, who in turn advises *l*) as opposed to more completely-connected clusters (e.g., *i, j, k,* and *l* all advise each other). High transitivity may also indicate a tendency for actors to be in positions where they can act as brokers – that is, many actors may mediate the links between other actor pairs, and therefore help control the flow of information across the network.

Researchers may also be interested in identifying subgroups or sub-communities within social networks, for example, to understand if recovery-related beliefs or behaviors differ between members of different sub-communities. Members of sub-communities often exhibit more similarities with other members of their sub-community compared to individuals outside of their sub-community. For example, actors may self-organize into sub-communities based on similarity in pre-existing attributes (e.g., sex, race, age, substance use behaviors), and simultaneously, readily transmit the information, beliefs, and behaviors within a particular sub-community to other members of the sub-community since individuals within the sub-community are well connected.

A *clique* is a type of sub-community in which all possible social ties are present between all the actors within the clique. For example, all actors in a clique may identify all other actors in the clique as their friend. Actors 4–6 in Figure 14.2 meet this definition.

A *cluster* is a group of actors who share ties with most other actors in the cluster while having relatively few ties to actors outside the cluster. Actors 1–3 and 3–6 in Figure 14.2 represent two clusters. (Of note, there are many community detection algorithms that identify clusters differently; Bedi & Sharma, 2016.) The degree of clustering across an entire network may be measured to understand how subdivided a network is or to understand whether networks with more or less clustering may differ on outcomes of interest (e.g., does clustering into sub-communities help individuals obtain higher quality support and/or contribute to health inequities?). One measure of network-level clustering involves taking a single actor, identifying all the alters connected to that actor (i.e., that actor's "neighborhood"), and measuring the average density within that neighborhood. This process is repeated for each actor and the average density of each actor's neighborhood provides an index of clustering. For network ***X***, this clustering coefficient is 0.82, indicating on average, the alters in each actor's local neighborhood are connected to 82 percent of the other actors in that neighborhood. In contrast, actors are only connected to 43 percent of other actors across the full network (i.e., density = 0.43), and thus the 0.82 clustering coefficient may indicate much higher connectedness within neighborhoods than within the full network.

A *component* describes a group of actors who are directly or indirectly connected to all other actors within the same component but are completely disconnected from actors in other components. In other words, the number of components in a network indicates how many isolated subgroups there are with no ties between any members of the different components. Network ***X*** above only has one component because all actors are connected to each other directly or indirectly; however, if the ties that actors 1 and 2 extend to actor 3 were removed, actors 1 and 2 would form a single component (i.e., isolated from the other actors), and actors 3–6 would form a second component. Because different components are socially isolated from each other, information, behaviors, beliefs, and other socially transmitted characteristics may be unlikely to travel to other components until one or more actors serves as a bridge (i.e., connector) between the components.

Analysis and Example Applications of Cross-Sectional Sociocentric Networks

Individual- and network-level summary indices described above may provide valuable information about the roles of social environments in SUD and recovery. Network-level descriptive statistics are often of interest in their own right as they can provide insights about network structure. For example, Jason et al. (2020) characterized three types of social ties reflecting friendship, trust, and mentoring (i.e., a three-plex network) among 10 residents of an Oxford House located on Native American tribal territory and found different network structures for each type of tie. Density and reciprocity were highest within friendship networks (.52 and .55, respectively), somewhat lower within trust networks (.42 and .32), and lowest within mentoring networks (.18 and .25), indicating that residents tended to trust and obtain mentorship from relatively fewer individuals than they were friends with and that trusting and mentoring relationships were more likely to be unidirectional rather than mutual. Collectively, these findings suggest that friendships, trusted relationships, and mentoring comprised separate aspects of social connections and that networks reflecting each type of relationship were structured differently within the Oxford House community.

Individual-level attributes derived from sociocentric data may also be utilized to help understand how one's positioning within a social network relates to their recovery-related outcomes. For example, Patterson et al. (2020) studied 40 students in a collegiate recovery community and collected data on the social ties between actors based on who each student felt that they could turn to for personal matters. They found that a longer length of abstinence was associated with higher in-degree centrality, suggesting that students with longer periods of abstinence may be more often turned to for social support by individuals in the recovery community. As a result, this placed individuals with longer periods of sobriety in a more central location within the recovery community network structure.

Analysis and Example Applications of Longitudinal Sociocentric Networks

Often, researchers study networks longitudinally to characterize temporal and causal effects that occur within networks. For example, while cross-sectional analyses may demonstrate that heavier drinking individuals tend to have more heavy-drinking friends, longitudinal data may be used to indicate how that network structure came to exist. That is, it is possible that (1) actors could have transmitted their drinking behavior to their friends (i.e., actors *socially influenced* other actors); (2) actors tended to self-select into friendships with other actors who drank similarly to themselves (i.e., actors *socially selected* friendships based on similarity in drinking); (3) one or more third variables drove friendship formation and drinking behaviors simultaneously (e.g., the clubs and activities in which actors are involved facilitated friendship formation and changes in drinking); or (4) multiple versions of these causal effects occurred simultaneously.

Stochastic actor-oriented models (SAOMs, Snijders, 1996, Snijders et al., 2010) provide one framework for modeling longitudinal sociocentric networks and may help researchers identify and untangle these multiple underlying causal effects. In brief, SAOMs examine changes in social networks as stochastic processes (i.e., at any given time, the likelihood of an actor changing their social ties can be modeled as a probabilistic function) and as Markov processes (i.e., at any time, the probability of an actor changing any of their friendships can be modeled based on the state of the network at that time). Models may be fit using RSiena software (Ruth et al., 2020) with social ties represented by two or more adjacency matrices ($\boldsymbol{X}$) at two or more fixed longitudinal time points. Actor-level attributes at those time points may likewise be represented by two or more vectors ($\boldsymbol{v}$), or a single vector if the attribute is invariant over time. Researchers may specify models that include a number of effects that can simultaneously influence how actors change their friendships and/or behaviors over time. For example, friendship formation may be influenced by a tendency for networks to maintain particular levels of density, reciprocity, and transitivity, and by the tendencies for actors to self-select into friendships with people who drink or smoke similarly to themselves (e.g., Huang et al., 2014). Likewise, changes in actor behaviors (e.g., drinking, smoking) may be influenced by multiple factors simultaneously, including the extent to which the behavior is self-reinforcing (e.g., a mild amount of smoking at time t may predict a higher amount of smoking at time $t + 1$) and the tendency for actors to be influenced by the behavior of their friends. A simulation-based algorithm in the RSiena program can be used to estimate the magnitude, direction, and statistical significance of these multiple effects that may operate simultaneously and account for the differences in social ties observed across the observed time points. This may yield, for example, estimates of how strongly actors are influenced by the smoking of their friends, while controlling for other network effects, including the tendency for actors to self-select into friendships with others who smoke similarly to themselves. Computational details are not provided here; however, Snijders et al. (2010) provide a very approachable introduction to SAOM methodology.

Several studies have used SAOMs to better understand whether correlations between one's substance use and the substance use of their alters is attributable to social influence, social selection, third variables, or a combination of these factors. Many of these studies have utilized non-SUD populations of adolescent classroom or school networks (e.g., Huang et al., 2014; Mundt et al., 2012), and fewer studies have used these approaches in populations of people with SUDs or in recovery-focused networks. Kreager et al. (2019) used SAOMs to study longitudinal sociocentric networks in a prison-based therapeutic community, with social ties defined according to the residents with whom they "get along with the most" and engagement with the treatment program as the primary outcome of interest. They found that residents' engagement with the treatment program did not influence the degree of engagement among the prison community members with whom they were tied (i.e., no evidence of social influence). These findings were inconsistent with a hypothesized mechanism of change for that intervention, which posited that engaged members may facilitate greater engagement among other members of the community with whom they got along most. Instead, residents tended to form ties with others who had similar levels of engagement with the treatment program as themselves (i.e., evidence of social selection), resulting in sub-communities within the larger network that varied in their degree of engagement. Further, it was found that the tendency to self-select into these communities was driven by a tendency for residents to form ties to other residents of similar race, age, education, and time within the unit, suggesting that resident ties were more likely segregated based on these factors, rather than driven by engagement with the treatment program.

Conclusions and Recommendations

A large and growing range of methods for measuring and modeling social networks can help shed light on how network-based interventions and recovery communities help individuals with SUD seek, achieve, and maintain recovery. Many studies have utilized egocentric network approaches to understand the role of social networks in recovery, and recent developments of briefer, psychometrically validated egocentric network measurement instruments may facilitate more in-depth research in this area among people who use a range of different substances. Additionally, briefer psychometrically validated instruments may facilitate more frequent longitudinal measurement, which when paired with other methods for testing prediction, mediation, and moderation, may help articulate more precisely how one's immediate social environment affects (and is affected by) their recovery outcomes. Advances in sociocentric data analysis may further advance understanding of how larger network-level structures may promote or hinder recovery efforts, with cross-sectional and longitudinal sociocentric analyses providing valuable insights about the structure and formation of recovery-related communities, respectively. To date, SUD-related research using sociocentric approaches has lagged behind research using egocentric approaches. However, both approaches hold considerable promise for informing the development of community-based interventions, clarifying how and for whom those interventions work, and understanding them within the context of complex social structures and social processes. Opportunities to study these topics deeper will likely continue to grow as recovery-oriented communities are developed and supported and as opportunities to collect social network data passively through technology become increasingly available (e.g., via social media, online recovery community interactions, electronic health records, etc.).

Acknowledgments

This work was supported by National Institute on Alcoholism and Alcohol Abuse of the National Institutes of Health, award numbers F31AA021031 and K01AA024796. The content is solely the responsibility of the author and does not necessarily represent the official views of the National Institutes of Health.

References

Aronson, B., Yang, K. C., Odabas, M., Ahn, Y. Y., & Perry, B. L. (2020). Comparing measures of centrality in bipartite social networks: A study of drug seeking for opioid analgesics. https://osf.io/preprints/socarxiv/hazvs/

Beckwith, M., Best, D., Savic, M., Haslam, C., Bathish, R., Dingle, G., Mackenzie, J., Staiger, P. K., & Lubman, D. I. (2019). Social identity mapping in addiction recovery (SIM-AR): Extension and application of a visual method. *Addiction Research & Theory*, *27*(6), 462–471. https://doi.org/10.1080/16066359.2018.1544623

Bedi, P., & Sharma, C. (2016). Community detection in social networks. *Wiley interdisciplinary reviews: Data mining and knowledge discovery,* *6*(3), 115–135. https://doi.org/10.1002/widm.1178

Buchanan, A. S., & Latkin, C. A. (2008). Drug use in the social networks of heroin and cocaine users before and after drug cessation. *Drug and Alcohol Dependence*, *96*(3), 286–289. https://doi.org/10.1016/j.drugalcdep.2008.03.008

Clifford, P. R., & Longabaugh, R. (1991). *Manual for the administration of the Important People and Activities Instrument.* Adapted for Project MATCH for NIAAA R01AA06698–05, R. Longabaugh, Principal Investigator. https://pubs.niaaa.nih.gov/publications/AssessingAlcohol/InstrumentPDFs/39_IPA.pdf

DeMartini, K. S., Prince, M. A., & Carey, K. B. (2013). Identification of trajectories of social network composition change and the relationship to alcohol consumption and norms. *Drug and Alcohol Dependence*, *132*(1-2), 309–315. https://doi.org/10.1016/j.drugalcdep.2013.02.020

Groh, D. R., Jason, L. A., Davis, M. I., Olson, B. D., & Ferrari, J. R. (2007). Friends, family, and alcohol abuse: An examination of general and alcohol-specific social support. *American Journal on Addictions*, *16*(1), 49–55. https://doi.org/10.1080/10550490601080084

Groh, D., Jason, L. A., Ferrari, J., & Halpert, J. (2011). A longitudinal investigation of the predictability of the three-factor model of the Important People

Inventory. *American Journal of Drug and Alcohol Abuse*, *37*(4), 259–263. https://doi.org/10.3109.00952990.2011.591017

Groh, D. R., Jason, L. A., & Keys, C. B. (2008). Social network variables in alcoholics anonymous: A literature review. *Clinical Psychology Review*, *28*(3), 430–450. https://doi.org/10.1016/j.cpr.2007.07.014

Hallgren, K. A., & Barnett, N. P. (2016). Briefer assessment of social network drinking: A test of the Important People Instrument–5 (IP-5). *Psychology of Addictive Behaviors*, *30*(8), 955. https://doi.org/10.1037/adb0000218

Hallgren, K. A., Ladd, B. O., & Greenfield, B. L. (2013). Psychometric properties of the Important People Instrument with college student drinkers. *Psychology of Addictive Behaviors*, *27*(3), 819–825. https://doi.org/10.1037/a0032346

Hallgren, K. A., Greenfield, B. L., & Ladd, B. O. (2016). Psychometric properties of the adolescent reinforcement survey schedule-alcohol use version with college student drinkers. *Substance Use & Misuse*, *51*(7), 812–822. https://doi.org/10.3109/10826084.2016.1155609

Huang, G. C., Unger, J. B., Soto, D., Fujimoto, K., Pentz, M. A., Jordan-Marsh, M., & Valente, T. W. (2014). Peer influences: The impact of online and offline friendship networks on adolescent smoking and alcohol use. *Journal of Adolescent Health*, *54*(5), 508–514. https://doi.org/10.1016/j.jadohealth.2013.07.001

Jason, L. A., Stevens, E., Kassanits, J., Reilly, A., Bobak, T., Guerrero, M., & Doogan, N. J. (2020). Recovery homes: A social network analysis of Oxford Houses for Native Americans. *Journal of Ethnicity in Substance Abuse*, *19*(2), 174–189. https://doi.org/10.1080/15332640.2018.1489748

Kreager, D. A., Schaefer, D. R., Davidson, K. M., Zajac, G., Haynie, D. L., & De Leon, G. (2019). Evaluating peer-influence processes in a prison-based therapeutic community: A dynamic network approach. *Drug and Alcohol dependence*, *203*, 13–18. https://doi.org/10.1016/j.drugalcdep.2019.05.018

Levitt, E. E., Oshri, A., Clifton, A., Stout, R., Costello, M. J., VanDellen, M., Kelly, J. F., & MacKillop, J. (2019). Psychometric validation of the brief alcohol social density assessment in an adult community. *Alcoholism: Clinical and Experimental Research, 44*(1), 212–218. https://doi.org/10.1016/j.jsat.2019.12.009

Longabaugh, R., Wirtz, P. W., Zweben, A., & Stout, R. L. (1998). Network support for drinking, Alcoholics Anonymous, and long-term matching effects. *Addiction*, *93*(9), 1313–1333. https://doi.org/10.1046/j.1360-0443.1998.93913133.x

Longabaugh, R., Wirtz, P. W., Zywiak, W. H., & O'Malley, S. S. (2010). Network support as a prognostic indicator of drinking outcomes: The COMBINE study. *Journal of Studies on Alcohol and Drugs*, *71*(6), 837–846. https://doi.org/10.15288/jsad.2010.71.837

McCarty, C., Lubbers, M. J., Vacca, R., & Molina, J. L. (2019). *Conducting personal network research: A practical guide*. Guilford.

McCrady, B. S. (2004). To have but one true friend: Implications for practice of research on alcohol use disorders and social network. *Psychology of Addictive Behaviors*, *18*(2), 113. https://doi.org/10.1037/0893-164X.18.2.113

McCulloh, I., Armstrong, H., & Johnson, A. (2013). *Social network analysis with applications*. John Wiley & Sons.

Mundt, M. P., Mercken, L., & Zakletskaia, L. (2012). Peer selection and influence effects on adolescent alcohol use: A stochastic actor-based model. *BMC Pediatrics, 12* (1), 115. https://doi.org.10.1186/1471-2431-12-115

Nargiso, J. E., Kuo, C. C., Zlotnick, C., & Johnson, J. E. (2014). Social support network characteristics of incarcerated women with co-occurring major depressive and substance use disorders. *Journal of psychoactive drugs*, *46*(2), 93–105. https://doi.org/10.1080/02791072.2014.890766

Orford, J., Krishnan, M., Balaam, M., Everitt, M., & Van der Graaf, K. (2004). University student drinking: The role of motivational and social factors. *Drugs: Education, Prevention and Policy*, *11*(5), 407–421. https://doi.org/10.1080.09687630310001657944

Owens, M. D., & McCrady, B. S. (2014). The role of the social environment in alcohol or drug relapse of probationers recently released from jail. *Addictive Disorders & Their Treatment*, *13*(4), 179. https://doi.org/10.1097/ADT.0000000000000039

Patterson, M. S., Russell, A. M., Nelon, J. L., Barry, A. E., & Lanning, B. A. (2020). Using social network analysis to understand sobriety among a campus recovery community. *Journal of Student Affairs Research and Practice*, 1–16. https://doi.org/10.1080/19496591.2020.1713142

Ripley, R. M., Snijders, T. A. B., Boda, Z., Voros, A., & Preciado, P. (2020). *Manual for RSiena* (Version 4.0, R package Version 1.2-23). [Computer software] www.cran.r-project.org/web/packages/RSiena/

Roberts, M. E., Nargiso, J. E., Gaitonde, L. B., Stanton, C. A., & Colby, S. M. (2015). Adolescent social networks: General and smoking-specific characteristics associated with smoking. *Journal of Studies on Alcohol and Drugs*, *76*(2), 247–255. https://doi.org/10.15288/jsad.2015.76.247

Scott, J., & Carrington, P. J. (2011). *The SAGE handbook of social network analysis*. SAGE Publications.

Snijders, T.A.B. (1996). Stochastic actor-oriented models for network change. *Journal of Mathematical Sociology*, *21*(1-2), 149–172. https://doi.org/10.1080/0022250X.1996.9990178

Snijders, T. A. B., Van de Bunt, G. G., & Steglich, C. E. (2010). Introduction to stochastic actor-based models for network dynamics. *Social Networks*, *32*(1), 44–60. https://doi.org/10.1016/j.socnet.2009.02.004

Spiro, E. S., Acton, R. M., & Butts, C. T. (2013). Extended structures of mediation: Re-examining brokerage in dynamic networks. *Social Networks*, *35*(1), 130–143. https://doi.org/10.1016/j.socnet.2013.02.011

Tucker, J. A., Cheong, J., Chandler, S. D., Crawford, M. S., & Simpson, C. A. (2015). Social networks and substance use among at-risk emerging adults living in disadvantaged urban areas in the southern United States: A cross-sectional naturalistic study. *Addiction, 110*(9), 1524–1532. https://doi.org/10.1111/add.13010

Wasserman, S., & Faust, K. (1994). *Social network analysis: Methods and applications.* Cambridge University Press. https://doi.org/10.1017/CBO9780511815478

Weisstein, E. W. *Matrix multiplication*. Wolfram MathWorld – A Wolfram Web Resource. https://mathworld.wolfram.com/MatrixMultiplication.html

White, W. L. (2007). Addiction recovery: Its definition and conceptual boundaries. *Journal of Substance Abuse Treatment*, *33*(3), 229–241. https://doi.org/10.1016/j.jsat.2007.04/015

Worley, M. J., Witkiewitz, K., Brown, S. A., Kivlahan, D. R., & Longabaugh, R. (2015). Social network moderators of naltrexone and behavioral treatment effects on heavy drinking in the COMBINE study. *Alcoholism: Clinical and Experimental Research*, *39*(1), 93–100. https://doi.org/10.1111/acer.12605

Zywiak, W. H., Longabaugh, R., & Wirtz, P. W. (2002). Decomposing the relationships between pre-treatment social network characteristics and alcohol treatment outcome. *Journal of Studies on Alcohol*, *63*(1), 114–121.

Zywiak, W. H., Neighbors, C. J., Martin, R. A., Johnson, J. E., Eaton, C. A., & Rohsenow, D. J. (2009). The Important People Drug and Alcohol interview: Psychometric properties, predictive validity, and implications for treatment. *Journal of Substance Abuse Treatment*, *36*(3), 321–330. https://doi.org/10.1016/j.jsat.2008.08.001

15 Measuring Substance Use Contexts and Substance-Free Reinforcement

Ali M. Yurasek, Samuel F. Acuff, and Meredith S. Berry

Measuring Substance Use Contexts and Substance-Free Reinforcement

A major theme that has emerged in theory and research on addictive behavior change is the importance of assessing and monitoring contextual features of substance use throughout treatment and recovery (Donovan, 2013). To this end, this chapter summarizes contextual, substance-involved, and substance-free measurement procedures that are commonly used in human studies. This work is guided by behavioral economics, described below (cf. Chapters 9 and 10 this volume), which provides useful concepts and methods to characterize and measure the contexts surrounding substance use.

Overview of Behavioral Economic Theory and Relative Reinforcing Efficacy

Behavioral economics is a merger of approaches from consumer demand theory in micro-economics with methods of behavior analysis to understand and "nudge" choice behavior, operationally defined as how limited resources (e.g., time, money, effort) are allocated to obtain access to commodities and activities in the context of choice (Bickel et al., 2014; Johnson & Bickel, 2006; Vuchinich & Heather, 2003). The diversity of behavioral economic approaches allows for a flexible and multifaceted approach to understanding and targeting elements of unhealthy behaviors (e.g., cigarette smoking, harmful alcohol consumption, physical inactivity) that can be altered to promote health. Choice plays a central role in behavioral economic concepts and applications, such as "nudging" behavior by arranging the environment or choice presentation to influence and promote healthy decisions (Thaler & Sunstein, 2008; Tucker et al., 2017).

Relative value or reinforcing efficacy refers to the behavior-maintaining or behavior-strengthening property of a reinforcer (e.g., drug, food, socializing opportunity) when compared to the value of another reinforcer under a range of different conditions (Griffiths et al., 1979; Johnson & Bickel, 2006). Modern iterations of reinforcement surveys for measuring the relative reinforcing efficacy of substance use are grounded in the matching law, which indicates that the reinforcement an individual receives from a given activity is directly proportional to the resources allocated to this commodity or activity (Herrnstein, 1970). Given this established relationship, one can ascertain reinforcing efficacy of a given activity by examining allocation of behavior or resources to obtain it. Behavioral or resource allocation is considered zero sum because resources (e.g., money, time, effort) are finite and constrained, and allocation to a given activity is thus "subtracted" from the available resource pool. As a result, activity engagement depends on other available activities and commodities in the choice context and on the relative constraints on access to them. Importantly, preference is inferred from the level of resource allocated to obtain a given reinforcer relative to allocations to other reinforcers (Herrnstein, 1970).

One example of a behavioral economic approach used to study relative reinforcing efficacy is the demand function framework that uses hypothetical or real reinforcers (e.g., drugs or money). As discussed later, the demand framework describes how consumption of a reinforcer declines with increases in its "price" (e.g., the cost or effort required to obtain it; Hursh, 1984; Reed et al., 2013). Demand can also serve to evaluate how value for one commodity may increase or decrease based on the availability and price of another commodity. Thus, reinforcing efficacy of one commodity depends on numerous factors, including how expensive or difficult it is to obtain the other available options.

A related behavioral economic approach that has proven useful in the study of substance use is delay discounting, which refers to the loss of reinforcer value as a function of delay to its receipt (Bickel et al., 2014; Johnson et al., 2007). The delay discounting framework, with origins in the matching law, evaluates how reinforcer efficacy is diminished with delay to its receipt (e.g., Ainslie & Herrnstein, 1981; Mazur, 1987). Intervening to reduce delay discounting has been explored as a potential intervention to reduce preference for smaller, more immediate rewards (e.g., cigarette smoking) and increase preference for larger, more delayed outcomes (e.g., a long term healthy lifestyle; e.g., Berry et al., 2014, 2015; Koffarnus, et al., 2013; Stein et al., 2017).

These approaches highlight the influence of contextual factors in drug use, rather than focusing on a fixed property of the drug itself or a characteristic of the person who uses the drug. Through this contextual lens, a well-supported generalization is that preference for drug use increases as constraints on drug use decrease (e.g., lower price, ready availability; e.g., Tucker et al., 2006; Vuchinich & Tucker, 1988, 1996). Preference for drug use is also likely to increase as availability of alternative non-drug reinforcers (e.g., social interactions) declines. Conversely, preference for drug use is likely to decrease with increased constraints on drug use (e.g., price increases), as well as with increased availability of non-drug reinforcers (e.g., social reinforcement, enjoyable activities such as sports or hiking). Although behavioral economics focuses heavily on contextual factors of drug use, these approaches further interface with other variables relevant to drug use, including biobehavioral factors such as neurological or genetic contributions (Bickel et al., 2014), or state variables such as craving or stress levels.

These findings highlight the importance of assessing and monitoring contextual features surrounding substance use and targeting contextual features associated with substance use in interventions. We next summarize contextual, substance-related, and substance-free measurement procedures common in human studies and useful for this purpose. These include techniques to assess the interaction of the environment and the person, including aspects of enjoyment and contextual situations associated with drug-taking, rating scale measures of drug and drug-free rewards, and relative reinforcement value measures.

Assessment of Substance Use Context and Reinforcement

Reinforcement Surveys

Reinforcement surveys are based on the matching law concerning relative resource allocation patterns among multiple commodities in a context of choice. They are self-report behavioral inventories of two widely accepted parameters of reinforcement: the amount of time spent engaged in the activity and the subjective enjoyment of the activity. Research suggests that these two facets of reinforcement (frequency and enjoyment) may be divergent (Magidson et al., 2016; Murphy et al., 2007), although both are theoretically relevant to understanding choice behavior. Both approaches are variations of important factors of reinforcement commonly studied in basic research, namely reinforcement frequency (i.e., rate of reward receipt; Davison & Baum, 2000; Schneider, 1973) and magnitude (i.e., strength of the reinforcer; Davison & Baum, 2003; Young, 1981). Frequency and enjoyment ratings are multiplied together to create cross-products that quantify substance-free and substance-related reinforcement based on both facets of activity engagement.

Reinforcement surveys used in research on substance use are modifications of early reinforcement surveys that focused on general reinforcement in relation to psychological disorders (e.g., depression and anxiety) and did not account for the relative nature of behavioral allocation. More recent surveys assess the reinforcing efficacy of a substance relative to reinforcement from all other activities and are useful in research on substance use (Correia et al., 1998). Participants complete two sets of frequency and enjoyment ratings for each activity – one for instances when the activity occurred while drinking or using drugs (substance-related reinforcement), and one for instances that occurred when the participant was not drinking or using drugs (substance-free reinforcement). A reinforcement ratio is then calculated by dividing the substance-related cross-product by the total reinforcement received (substance-related + substance-free), which represents reinforcement received from substances *relative to* substance-free reinforcement.

The 320-item *Pleasant Events Schedule* (PES; MacPhillamy & Lewinsohn, 1982) is a reinforcement survey that covers a wide range of activities – including social and nonsocial, passive and active, and discretionary and required activities – and has demonstrated test-retest reliability and concurrent and predictive validity. The PES has proven useful as a means of monitoring the reinforcing activities of depressed patients participating in behavior therapy (Lewinsohn et al., 1980), and it also accurately predicts future behavior (MacPhillamy & Lewinsohn, 1982). *The Adolescent Reinforcement Survey Schedule* (ARSS; Holmes et al., 1987; Holmes et al., 1991) is another well-validated measure that has been widely used in research on substance use among teens and young adults. The ARSS includes 45 items that are primarily social in nature (e.g., dating, peer and family interactions). Psychometric evaluation has established the test-retest reliability and concurrent validity of the measure in a college sample (Hallgren et al., 2016).

Reinforcement surveys are the most widely used measures to assess the relative value of rewards available in different contexts and are well validated (Correia et al., 2002; Hallgren et al., 2016; Lewinsohn, 1974; Lewinsohn et al., 1980). Higher reinforcement ratios indicating higher relative substance-related reinforcement are associated with substance use outcomes among college students (Acuff et al., 2018a; Correia et al., 1998), teenagers (Andrabi et al., 2017), individuals in psychiatric outpatient treatment (Correia & Carey, 1999), and general adult samples (Meshesha et al., 2020; Morris et al., 2017). These surveys demonstrate strong psychometric properties, robust relations across various forms of drug use, and can be used to inform treatment planning (e.g., to provide feedback on the relative reinforcement ratio and to identify potential alternatives to drinking) and as a secondary treatment outcome variable.

Measures of Resource Allocation

Resource allocation measures are also derived directly using principles of the matching law by examining the ratio of a single class of resource (e.g., time, money) allocated to substance-related activities relative to resources allocated to other activities. Two such measures are the *Alcohol-Savings Discretionary Expenditure* index and the *Time Allocation* measure.

Alcohol-Savings Discretionary Expenditure (ASDE) Index

The ASDE index was developed by Tucker and colleagues (2002, 2009, Chapter 9 this volume) in prospective research on natural recovery from alcohol problems and is a measure of the relative reinforcement value of alcohol based on patterns of resource allocation in the natural environment over long time periods (up to a year or more). Tucker et al. reasoned that, for persons with fixed recurring expenditures and discretionary income, the spending pattern of discretionary funds on alcohol versus savings would reflect relative preference for alcohol compared to delayed rewards offered by savings (Tucker et al., 2009).

The ASDE index is the ratio of discretionary money spent on alcohol versus savings aggregated over many choices. The index thus compares actual resource allocation to a short-term reward (alcohol) to delayed, alternative rewards made possible by savings and involves intertemporal decision-making (delay discounting), a robust risk factor for harmful substance use (Bickel et al., 2014).

The original ASDE index was based on an expanded Timeline Followback (TLFB; Sobell & Sobell, 1992) interview that used data from a review of financial records provided by participants and additional interview reports collected using standard TLFB interviewing techniques. In addition to direct verification using financial records, internal consistency and reliability checks on participants' reports of monetary allocation patterns supported their accuracy (e.g., Tucker et al., 2006, 2007). Other simpler iterations asked participants to estimate alcohol versus saving expenditures, which reduces participant burden but increases error. These versions have been used primarily with college students, and the index was significantly associated with drinks per week, but not with alcohol-related problems (Murphy et al., 2009, 2015; Skidmore et al., 2014). Although studies suggest that the ASDE provides a valid index of the relative value of alcohol versus delayed alternative rewards in middle class community and college student samples, the measure may need to be modified for samples that do not regularly allocate money to savings, such as low SES samples.

Time Allocation

Given that time is a finite and "zero sum" resource for all, the amount of time allocated to one activity relative to others expressed as a proportion of total time in a week or day is an objective measure of reinforcing value (Baum & Rachlin, 1969; Herrnstein, 1970). Studies measuring time allocation using questionnaires typically ask participants to estimate the total number of hours spent in various activities during a typical week in the past month. For example, Meshesha and colleagues (2015) assessed time spent in the following activities using a sample of college students: (a) class, (b) doing homework, (c) participating in social fraternity or sorority activities, (d) participating in other university organizations, (e) internship or volunteer activity related to major or potential career, (f) paid employment, (g) exercise or sports, (h) time with family, (i) religious activity, (j) drinking, (k) using drugs, and (l) using the internet for non-academic purposes (e.g., social media). More detailed daily reports of time allocation to multiple activities (including alcohol consumption) over weeks to months have been collected via prospective self-monitoring with high reliability of participant reports when compared to recall reports of participants and collateral informants (Samo et al., 1989; Tucker et al., 1991).

Generally, substance use is associated with lower time spent engaged in alternative activities (Acuff et al., 2017; Meshesha et al., 2015, 2017, 2018). Comparing differences in time allocation in heavy drinkers who did and did not also use cannabis or other substances (Meshesha et al., 2015), those who used multiple substances reported significantly less time allocated to exercise, extracurricular activities, and academics compared to heavy drinkers who did not use other drugs. These results have been extended prospectively among college students who reported non-medical prescription opioid use (Meshesha et al., 2017). Compared to non-drug users, those reporting opioid use spent less time engaged in academic activities and extracurricular activities over a 12-month period. These findings suggest that time allocation is a useful method to measure reinforcement value in substance use research.

Purchase Tasks

Purchase tasks are another widely used measure of relative reinforcing efficacy. Purchase tasks emulate progressive ratio tasks that have been used in animal and laboratory human research on reinforcer strength (Bickel et al., 2014). Because actual laboratory purchase tasks can be costly and time consuming, researchers have developed hypothetical purchase tasks that are both cost- and time-effective to administer. In a typical alcohol purchase task, individuals report how many drinks they would purchase during a hypothetical drinking scenario at each price in a series of escalating prices. Responses across prices reflect the impact of a specific constraint (i.e., monetary cost) on choice behavior, thus capturing a contextualized index of alcohol value. Purchase task data can be plotted to create a demand curve, and various parts of the curve represent different aspects of motivation to consume alcohol. The most common indices of alcohol demand are: intensity (consumption when alcohol is free, or unconstrained consumption), breakpoint (the first price at which consumption is fully suppressed), O_{max} (maximum monetary expenditure across the full task), P_{max} (the price at which O_{max} occurs) and elasticity (the rate of change in consumption as a function of price). Research has shown that data from hypothetical alcohol purchase tasks correspond to real purchasing behavior (Amlung & MacKillop, 2015; Amlung et al., 2012; MacKillop et al., 2010a) and that demand indices demonstrate good one-month test-retest reliability, with the strongest reliability demonstrated among persons whose drinking does not change (Acuff & Murphy, 2017). These findings suggest that changes in alcohol demand correspond to real world changes in drinking.

Although hypothetical consumption generally decreases as monetary constraints increase, individuals differ in their rates of responding, which theoretically reflect person-level differences in the reinforcing efficacy of alcohol. Behavioral economics suggests that those with higher levels of alcohol demand will also evidence greater alcohol use and related problems. Indeed, alcohol demand indices have robust correlations with alcohol consumption (Lemley et al., 2016; Murphy & MacKillop, 2006), alcohol problems (Acuff et al., 2018a), and Alcohol Use Disorder (Bertholet et al., 2015). Demand indices are also robust prospective predictors of drinking behavior even after controlling for past alcohol consumption, suggesting that this contextual measure of drinking behavior, which aggregates a series of hypothetical drinking decisions across escalating constraints, has predictive utility over and above measures of drinking practices. These findings support the utility of purchase tasks and other contextual approaches to measuring alcohol-related decision making.

Despite their utility, standard alcohol purchase tasks only manipulate one form of cost constraint and thus miss other aspects of the context. Researchers have begun to address this critical gap by administering state-like hypothetical purchase tasks that ask about purchasing behavior based on how the participant feels right now following an experimental manipulation. For example, MacKillop and colleagues (2010b) compared responding on a purchase task following presentation of a neutral cue condition (looking at a cup of water and smelling it) and an alcohol cue exposure (looking at a cup of beer and smelling it). The alcohol cue condition increased demand intensity, breakpoint, and O_{max} to a significantly greater degree than the neutral condition.

Other studies manipulated the hypothetical scenario used in the purchase task. For example, Acuff et al. (2020a) administered two modified hypothetical alcohol purchase tasks, one in which the participant would be drinking with two friends and one in which the individual would be drinking alone. The results suggested a roughly 40 percent increase in alcohol demand in the social than the solitary condition, which speaks to the impact social context can have on motivation to drink. A meta-analysis aggregated the effects of other contextual factors that influenced demand (Acuff et al., 2020b) and found that manipulations increasing stress (Owens et al., 2015) and reinforcer magnitude (Benson et al., 2009) also increase demand and that introducing an opportunity cost (such as a next day responsibility) decreases demand (Gilbert et al., 2014; Joyner et al., 2019). The meta-analysis further revealed consistent reductions in alcohol demand resulting from some behavioral and pharmacotherapies, although considerable heterogeneity in effects were found (likely due to differences in therapies). Other factors, such as increased sexual arousal (Spelman & Simons, 2018) and pain (Moskal et al., 2018), have also been studied but lack enough studies to be meta-analyzed. In the studies that do exist, sexual arousal increases alcohol demand (Spelman & Simons, 2018), whereas pain had no effect on alcohol demand (Moskal et al., 2018).

Rating Scale Measures of Reward

General Contextual Substance Use Surveys

Measures that assess the discrete choice context associated with substance use, including negative and positive emotions and the immediate social environment, can help identify situations likely to increase the value of substances, overall substance use, and risk of relapse. One common tool used to assess specific contexts associated with heavy drinking is the *Inventory of Drinking Situations* (IDS; Annis et al., 1987). The IDS is a 100-item questionnaire that measures the frequency of heavy drinking in relation to eight high-risk situations (e.g., unpleasant emotions, physical discomfort). Research using the IDS suggests that individuals who experience more problems related to their drinking tend to consume alcohol following negative situations (Marlatt & Gordon, 1985; Turner et al., 1997), whereas those who experience fewer alcohol-related consequences tend to consume alcohol following positive and social situations (Lau-Barraco et al., 2016; Victorio-Estrada & Mucha, 1997).

Similarly, the *Inventory of Drug-Taking Situations* (IDTS; Annis et al., 1992) is a 50-item questionnaire used to identify contexts associated with use of various illicit drugs and tobacco. Comparable to drinking outcomes, the experience of unpleasant emotions was associated with higher levels of use of a variety of drugs, including methamphetamine, cocaine, and polysubstance use (Halkitis et al., 2003; Kelly & Parsons, 2008; Palamar et al., 2008; Waldrop et al., 2007). Pleasant and social situations were related to polysubstance and cocaine use (Kelly & Parsons, 2008; Palamar et al., 2008). Both the IDS and IDTS have been examined with adults and college student populations and their subscales demonstrate high internal consistency and good content, construct, and concurrent validity (Annis et al., 1987; Turner et al., 1997).

In addition to assessing the situations associated with substance use, questionnaires are available that assess individuals' confidence in their ability to *resist* using substances in those situations. The *Situational Confidence Questionnaire* (Annis & Graham, 1988), *Alcohol Abstinence Self-Efficacy Scale* (DiClemente et al., 1994), and *Drug-Taking Confidence Questionnaire* (Annis et al., 1992) are examples of common questionnaires used to assess situational confidence for drug and alcohol abstention. Each of these measures has evidence of good reliability, internal consistency, and validity in adults (Annis & Graham, 1988; DiClemente, et al., 1994; Sklar et al., 1997). While lower self-efficacy to abstain from substances in certain contexts is associated with relapse, research has shown that this is a modifiable trait. For example, higher self-efficacy following treatment is associated with positive outcomes, including alcohol use moderation (Maisto et al., 1999). These measures can be used repeatedly throughout substance use treatment to monitor changes in self-efficacy regarding situations that pose a risk to relapse (Donovan, 2003).

Environmental Reinforcement Questionnaires

Two rating scales measure reinforcement received from the environment, the *Environmental Reward Observation Scale* (EROS; Armento & Hopko, 2007) and the *Reward Probability Index* (RPI; Carvalho et al., 2011). The EROS is a 10-item Likert scale that assesses self-observed environmental reward. The RPI, a 20-item Likert questionnaire, extended the EROS and includes two factors, environmental suppressors (the availability of rewarding opportunities within one's environment) and reward probability (ability to experience reward; Carvalho et al., 2011). The two scales were developed to measure response-contingent positive reinforcement (i.e., the increase in frequency of a behavior due to reinforcer presentation), a concept central to depression research and treatment (Boswell et al., 2017). Validity studies showed that scores on the RPI were strongly associated with daily diary reports of activity engagement and enjoyment among undergraduate students (Carvalho et al., 2011). The EROS and RPI have several strengths; i.e., they are very brief, possess sound psychometric properties, are useful for treatment planning, and have demonstrated associations with treatment response.

The EROS and RPI have primarily been used to examine individual differences in reward functioning among college students and as markers of changes in reward functioning following treatment for harmful substance use (Acuff et al., 2018b; Joyner et al., 2016; Meshesha et al., 2018). Among college students, the environmental suppressor subscale of the RPI, but not the reward probability subscale, predicts harmful alcohol use (Joyner et al., 2016) and explains variance in the relation between PTSD symptoms and harmful alcohol use (Acuff et al., 2018b; Luciano et al., 2019). Scores on both the environmental suppressor and reward probability subscales differentiated heavy drinkers who also reported polysubstance use from those who did not (Meshesha et al., 2018). The environmental suppressor subscale contains items related to resource availability and negative reinforcement, suggesting that it is likely capturing access to the intended constructs of reinforcement.

Clinical Utility of Contextual and Reinforcement Surveys

Definitions of substance use recovery are shifting from an exclusive focus on abstinence to identifying improvements in substance-related risks and harms and increasing general quality of life. Hence, assessment should identify contextual alternatives to substance use to target for intervention even if the client is not interested in changing his or her overall level of use. Contexts and reinforcing features that precede and maintain substance use are factors that can be assessed and monitored throughout treatment. Utilizing survey instruments like the ones summarized here highlight clients' experience of reinforcement that is related to both substance-involved and substance-free activities. This information can be used to identify deficits in alternative substance-free rewards and the contexts that increase the value of the substance-related reward, which can guide interventions to reduce substance use and promote behaviors incompatible with it, as described below (Epstein & McCrady, 2009; Marlatt & Donovan, 2005).

Research utilizing *reinforcement surveys* provide evidence that diminished substance-free reinforcement predicts naturalistic changes in substance use (Audrain-McGovern et al., 2010; Khoddam et al., 2018) and response to intervention (Dennhardt et al., 2015; Murphy et al., 2005). Similarly, changes in relative substance-related reinforcement during the month following an intervention predict changes in substance use over time (Dennhardt et al., 2015). Related findings led to the development of a behavioral economic supplement to brief alcohol interventions, known as the Substance-Free Activity Session (SFAS) that is designed to increase future orientation and engagement in constructive alternatives to substance use. Both an initial pilot study (Murphy et al., 2012a) and randomized controlled trials (Murphy et al. 2012b; Murphy et al., 2019) demonstrated that the addition of the behavioral economic supplement to a brief motivational intervention reduced substance use over 6- to 16-month follow-up intervals. The intervention was particularly effective, relative to control, for heavy drinkers with symptoms of depression or lower levels of substance-free reinforcement. This suggests that the supplement can be used to target students with a specific behavior pattern previously identified as a risk factor for substance use.

Similarly, increases in engagement in substance-free activities have been associated with increases in abstinence from drug use during a trial of contingency management for individuals receiving methadone who met criteria for cocaine use disorder (Rogers et al., 2008). This is also the case among trials focused on smoking cessation; e.g., smokers who increased substance-free reinforcement (assessed using the PES) during a smoking cessation trial were twice as likely to quit smoking at the end of treatment (Audrain-McGovern et al., 2009; Schnoll et al., 2016). Murphy and colleagues (2015) found that a measure of substance-related reinforcement relative to total reinforcement (reinforcement ratio) incrementally predicted post-intervention drinking following a brief intervention for college student drinkers. Drinkers with greater proportional activity participation and enjoyment related to substance use reported greater post-intervention drinking. Hence, reinforcement surveys can be used to inform personalized interventions based on levels of reward value as well as to monitor changes in reward during and after treatment.

Measures of *monetary spending on substances* can be used to evaluate treatment response and are predictive of positive treatment outcomes (Murphy et al., 2015; Worley et al., 2015). The ASDE index similarly predicts stability of recovery, particularly low-risk drinking outcomes, among middle-class adult heavy drinkers who attempted to quit harmful alcohol use without treatment (e.g., Tucker et al., 2006, 2009, 2016). Thus, assessing spending patterns prior and throughout attempts to stop harmful substance use can be used to monitor changes in substance use preference and evaluate recovery progress.

Time allocation measures also have great potential for clinical utility. These measures have been used as part of the SFAS intervention feedback aimed at shifting time allocation away from substance-related to substance-free activities. The time allocation data are displayed as a bar graph showing time spent in various categories to create discussion with a client about current activity engagement and its influence on choices to engage in substance use. This measure may also highlight areas of scarce engagement in specific categories of substance-free activities that are protective against substance use. For example, time spent in academic, athletic, religious, and service-related activities is associated with lower rates of substance use and binge drinking among college students (Fenzel, 2005; Meshesha et al., 2015; Vaughan et al., 2009; Wechsler et al., 1997). These assessments can be used to guide substance use treatment, facilitate increased engagement in substance-free activities, and monitor changes in value-driven behavior.

Identifying the antecedents to substance use using *general contextual surveys* can help both clinicians and clients better understand motives for use and what might trigger use that leads to negative consequences. Information gathered from these surveys can be used to isolate situations or contexts that increase the risk of use so they can be avoided and new coping skills can be developed and executed. These data can then be used to develop ways to manage high-risk situations, personalize interventions, and monitor treatment progress (Epstein & McCrady, 2009). Situational self-efficacy measures can similarly be used for treatment planning by identifying situations associated with high risk for relapse. Given that successful low-risk use of alcohol (moderation) is associated with higher self-efficacy following treatment (Maisto et al., 1999), assessing and monitoring confidence levels is another important dimension in tracking progress toward recovery.

The *RPI* and *EROS rating scales* have been used to examine changes in reward functioning following interventions such as behavioral activation for substance use and the Life Enhancement Treatment for Substance Use (LETS Act), a brief behavioral activation treatment delivered in six sessions over two weeks (Daughters et al., 2008, 2016; Magidson et al., 2011). However, the results are inconsistent. Although one study examining LETS Act found significant treatment effects on EROS scores (Daughters et al., 2008), results of another study were not significant (Magidson et al., 2011). Further, two studies using these measures to examine changes in reward functioning following behavioral activation were non-significant in both adults (MacPherson et al., 2010) and young adults (MacPherson et al., 2017). With these qualifications, these measures may be useful to establish baseline levels of reward functioning and guide treatment planning.

Finally, indices of alcohol demand as measured by *purchase tasks* show promise as proxy indicators of actual drinking behavior and therefore may be used to measure treatment progress and success. Alcohol demand predicts poor intervention response (MacKillop & Murphy, 2007), pharmacotherapy and brief motivational interventions can reduce demand, and the degree of reduction predicts subsequent changes in drinking (Bujarski et al., 2012; Murphy et al., 2015). The burgeoning literature on contextual manipulations of alcohol demand demonstrates a number of factors that may influence value in a discrete choice context, which can help clients and clinicians understand contextual risk levels and which contexts will be likely to result in increased or decreased drinking levels.

Conclusions and Recommendations

The research reviewed suggests that contextual and reinforcement measures provide novel information regarding an individual's strength of preference for substance use. Utilizing these measures provides data relevant to understanding and promoting recovery from substance use disorders that goes above and beyond assessing levels of substance use by measuring level of risk based on an overall pattern of behavioral allocation and obtained reinforcement (Murphy et al., 2015). This expanded scope of assessment is vitally important for expanding the recovery concept to include improvements in life-health functioning. The assessment approaches summarized here have sound measurement properties with a range of individuals who use a variety of substances and are firmly grounded in behavioral economic theory and research.

These measures can also be used to guide clinical practice. For clients whose substance use accounts for a large proportion of their total reinforcement compared to valued alternatives, a more intensive intervention such as contingency management or community reinforcement may be needed to increase substance-free sources of reinforcement (Daughters et al., 2018; Higgins et al., 2004; Murphy et al., 2019). For clients with present and future sources of substance-free reinforcement, less intensive brief interventions such as the SFAS are more suitable even if clients are currently engaging in high-risk levels of substance use. Response to treatment can also be assessed using these measures. Identifying any reallocation of behavior towards reinforcing activities other than substance use (e.g., career and educational pursuits, rewarding hobbies) is one way to document recovery in response to an intervention (Miller & Rollnick, 2012).

In summary, the behavioral economic measurement approach presented in this chapter has promise to continue to advance an expanded view of recovery as a dynamic process of behavior change in which improvements in biopsychosocial functioning and circumstances of living are fundamental. Focusing on substance use contexts, the behavioral economic factors that support continued substance use, and the availability of substance-free reinforcement should be an integral feature of substance-related assessment and interventions that are developed to promote recovery. Behavioral economic factors should be considered at least as vital in understanding and assessing recovery as substance use practices.

References

Acuff, S. F., Amlung, M. T., Dennhardt, A. A., MacKillop, J., & Murphy, J. G. (2020b). Experimental manipulations of behavioral economic demand for addictive commodities: A meta-analysis. *Addiction*, *115*(5), 817–831. https://doi.org/10.1111/add.14865

Acuff, S. F., Luciano, M. T., Soltis, K. E., Joyner, K. J., McDevitt-Murphy, M. E., & Murphy, J. G. (2018b). Access to environmental reward mediates the relation between posttraumatic stress symptoms and alcohol problems and craving. *Experimental and Clinical Psychopharmacology*, *25*(5), 412–421. https://doi.org/10.1037/pha0000181

Acuff, S. F., & Murphy, J. G. (2017). Further examination of the temporal stability of alcohol demand. *Behavioral Processes*, *141*(Part 1), 33–41. https://doi.org/10.1016/j.beproc.2017.03.020

Acuff, S. F., Soltis, K. E., Dennhardt, A. A., Borsari, B., Martens, M. P., & Murphy, J. G. (2017). Future so bright? Delay discounting and consideration of future consequences predict academic performance among college drinkers. *Experimental and Clinical Psychopharmacology*, *25*(5), 412–421. https://doi.org/10.1037/pha0000143

Acuff, S. F., Soltis, K. E., & Murphy, J. G. (2020a). Using demand curves to quantify the reinforcing value of social and solitary drinking. *Alcoholism: Clinical and Experimental Research*, *44*(7), 1497–1507. https://doi.org/10.1111/acer.14382

Ainslie, G., & Herrnstein, R. J. (1981). Preference reversal and delayed reinforcement. *Animal Learning & Behavior*, *9*(4), 476–482. https://doi.org/10.3758/BF03209777

Amlung, M. T., Acker, J. D., Stojek, M. K., Murphy, J. G., & MacKillop, J. (2012). Is talk "cheap"? An initial investigation of the equivalence of alcohol purchase task performance for hypothetical and actual rewards. *Alcoholism: Clinical and Experimental Research*, *36*(4), 716–724. https://doi.org/10.1111/j.1530-0277.2011.01656.x

Amlung, M. T., & MacKillop, J. (2015). Further evidence of close correspondence for alcohol demand decision making for hypothetical and incentivized rewards. *Behavioral Processes*, *113*, 187–191. https://doi.org/10.1016/j.beproc.2015.02.012

Andrabi, N., Khoddam, R., & Leventhal, A. M. (2017). Socioeconomic disparities in adolescent substance use: Role of enjoyable alternative substance-free activities. *Social Science & Medicine*, *176*, 175–182. https://doi.org/10.1016/j.socscimed.2016.12.032

Annis, H. M., & Graham, J. M. (1988). *Situational Confidence Questionnaire user's guide*. Addiction Research Foundation.

Annis, H. M., Graham, J., & Davis, C. (1987). *Inventory of Drinking Situations (IDS) user's guide*. Addiction Research Foundation.

Annis, H. M., Martin, G., & Graham, J. M. (1992). *Inventory of Drug-Taking Situations (IDTS): User's guide*. Addiction Research Foundation.

Armento, M. E. A., & Hopko, D. R. (2007). The environmental reward observation scale (EROS): Development, validity, and reliability. *Behavior Therapy*, *38*(2), 107–119. https://doi.org/10.1016/j.beth.2006.05.003

Audrain-McGovern, J. E., Rodriguez, D., Epstein, L. H., Rodgers, K., Cuevas, J., & Wileyto, E. P. (2009). Young adult smoking: What factors differentiate ex-smokers, smoking cessation treatment seekers, and nontreatment seekers? *Addictive Behaviors*, *34*(12), 1036–1041. https://doi.org/10.1016/j.addbeh.2009.06.012

Audrain-McGovern, J. E., Rodriguez, D., Rodgers, K., & Cuevas, J. (2010). Declining alternative reinforcers link depression to young adult smoking. *Addiction*, *106*(1), 178–187. https://doi.org/10.1111/j.1360-0443.2010.03113.x

Baum, W. M. & Rachlin, H. C. (1969). Choice as time allocation. *Journal of Experimental Annals of Behavior, 12,*861–874. https://doi.org/10.1901/jeab.1969.12-861

Benson, T. A., Little, C. S., Henslee, A. M., & Correia, C. J. (2009). Effects of reinforcer magnitude and alternative reinforcer delay on preference for alcohol during a multiple-choice procedure. *Drug and Alcohol Dependence*, *100*(1–2), 161–163. https://doi.org/10.1016/j.drugalcdep.2008.09.005

Berry, M. S., Sweeney, M. M., Morath, J., Odum, A. L., & Jordan, K. E. (2014). The nature of impulsivity: Visual exposure to natural environments decreases impulsive decision-making in a delay discounting task. *PloS one*, *9*(5), e97915. https://doi.org/10.1371/journal.pone.0097915

Berry, M. S., Repke, M. A., Nickerson, N. P., Conway, L. G., Odum, A. L., & Jordan, K. E. (2015). Making time for nature: Visual exposure to natural environments lengthens subjective time perception and reduces impulsivity. *PloS one*, *10*(11), e0141030. https://doi.org/10.1371/journal.pone.0141030

Bertholet, N., Murphy, J. G., Daeppen, J. B., Gmel, G., & Gaume, J. (2015). The alcohol purchase task in young men from the general population. *Drug and Alcohol Dependence*, *146*(1), 39–44. https://doi.org/10.1016/j.drugalcdep.2014.10.024

Bickel, W. K., Johnson, M. W., Koffarnus, M. N., MacKillop, J., & Murphy, J. G. (2014). The behavioral economics of substance use disorders: Reinforcement pathologies and their repair. *Annual Review of Clinical Psychology*, *10*, 641–677. https://doi.org/10.1146/annurev-clinpsy-032813-153724

Boswell, J. F., Iles, B. R., Gallagher, M. W., & Farchione, T. J. (2017). Behavioral activation strategies in cognitive-behavioral therapy for anxiety disorders. *Psychotherapy*, *54*(3), 231–236. https://doi.org/10.1037/pst0000119

Bujarski, S., MacKillop, J., & Ray, L. A. (2012). Understanding naltrexone mechanism of action and pharmacogenetics in Asian Americans via behavioral economics: A preliminary study. *Experimental and Clinical Psychopharmacology, 20*(3), 181–190. https://doi.org/10.1037/a0027379

Carvalho, J. P., Gawrysiak, M. J., Hellmuth, J. C., McNulty, J. K., Magidson, J. F., Lejuez, C. W., & Hopko, D. R. (2011). The reward probability index: Design and validation of a scale measuring access to environmental reward. *Behavior Therapy*, *42*(2), 249–262. https://doi.org/10.1016/j.beth.2010.05.004

Correia, C. J., & Carey, K. B. (1999). Applying behavioral theories of choice to substance use in a sample of psychiatric outpatients. *Psychology of Addictive Behaviors*, *13*(3), 207–212. https://doi.org/10.1037/0893-164X.13.3.207

Correia, C. J., Carey, K. B., & Borsari, B. (2002). Measuring substance-free and substance-related reinforcement in the natural environment. *Psychology of Addictive Behaviors*, *16*(1), 28–34. https://doi.org/10.1037//0893-164X.16.1.28

Correia, C. J., Simons, J. S., Carey, K. B., & Borsari, B. E. (1998). Predicting drug use: Application of behavioral theories of choice. *Addictive Behaviors*, *23*(5), 705–709. https://doi.org/10.1016/S0306–4603(98)00027-6

Daughters, S. B., Braun, A. R., Sargeant, M. N., Reynolds, E. K., Hopko, D. R., Blanco, C., & Lejuez, C. W. (2008). Effectiveness of a brief behavioral treatment for inner-city illicit drug users with elevated depressive symptoms: The life enhancement treatment for substance use (LETS Act!). *Journal of Clinical Psychiatry*, *8*, 1–8. https://doi.org/10.4088/jcp.v69n0116

Daughters, S. B., Magidson, J. F., Anand, D., Seitz-Brown, C. J., Chen, Y., & Baker, S. (2018) The effect of a behavioral activation treatment for substance use on post-treatment abstinence: A randomized controlled trial. *Addiction*, 113: 535–544. https://doi.org/10.1111/add.14049

Daughters, S. B., Magidson, J. F., Lejuez, C. W., & Chen, Y. (2016). LETS ACT: A behavioral activation treatment for substance use and depression. *Journal of Dual Diagnosis*, *9*(2/3), 74–84. https://doi.org/10.1108/ADD-02-2016-0006

Davison, M., & Baum, W. M. (2000). Choice in a variable environment: Every reinforcer counts. *Journal of the Experimental Analysis of Behavior*, *74*(1), 1–24. https://doi.org/10.1901/jeab.2000.74-1

(2003). Every reinforcer counts: Reinforcer magnitude and local preference. *Journal of the Experimental Analysis of Behavior*, *80*(1), 95–129. https://doi.org/10.1901/jeab.2003.80-95

Dennhardt, A. A., Yurasek, A. M., & Murphy, J. G. (2015). Change in delay discounting and substance reward value following a brief alcohol and drug use intervention. *Journal of the Experimental Analysis of Behavior*, *103*(1), 125–140. https://doi.org/10.1002/jeab.121

DiClemente, C. C., Carbonari, J. P., Mongomery, R. P. G., & Hughes, S. O. (1994). The Alcohol Abstinence Self-Efficacy Scale. *Journal of Studies on Alcohol*, *55*(2), 141–148. https://doi.org/10.15288/jsa.1994.55.141

Donovan, D. M. (2003). Assessments to aid in the treatment planning process. In J. P. Allen & V. B. Wilson (Eds.), *Assessing alcohol problems: A guide for clinicians and researchers* (2nd ed., pp. 125–188) (NIH Publication No. 03–3745). National Institute of Alcohol Abuse and Alcoholism.

(2013). Evidence-based assessment: Strategies and measures in addictive behaviors. In B. S. McCrady & E. E. Epstein (Eds.), *Addictions: A comprehensive guidebook* (2nd ed., pp. 311–351). Oxford University Press.

Epstein, E. E., & McCrady, B. S. (2009). *A cognitive-behavioral treatment program for overcoming alcohol problems: Therapist guide*. Oxford University Press. http://ezproxy.memphis.edu/login?url=http://search.ebscohost.com/login.aspx?direct=true&db=psyh&AN=2009-06101-000&site=ehost-live

Fenzel, L. M. (2005). Multivariate analyses of predictors of heavy episodic drinking and drinking-related problems among college students. *Journal of College Student Development*, *46*(2), 126–140. https://doi.org/10.1353/csd.2005.0013

Gilbert, L. J., Murphy, J. G., & Dennhardt, A. A. (2014). A behavioral economic analysis of the effect of next-day responsibilities on drinking. *Psychology of Addictive Behaviors*, *28*(4), 1253–1258. https://doi.org/10.1037/a0038369

Griffiths, R. R., Brady, J. V., & Bradford, L. D. (1979). Predicting the abuse liability of drugs with animal drug self-administration procedures: Psychomotor stimulants and hallucinogens. In T. Thompson & P. B. Dews (Eds.), *Advances in Behavioral Pharmacology* (vol. 2) (pp. 163–208). Academic Press.

Halkitis, P. N., Parsons, J. T., & Wilton, L. (2003). An exploratory study of contextual and situation factors related to methamphetamine use among gay and bisexual men in New York City. *Journal of Drug Issues, 33*,413–432. https://doi.org/10.1177/002204260303300207

Hallgren, K. A., Greenfield, B. L., & Ladd, B. O. (2016). Psychometric properties of the adolescent reinforcement survey schedule-alcohol use version with college student drinkers. *Substance Use and Misuse*, *51*(7), 812–822. https://doi.org/10.3109/10826084.2016.1155609

Herrnstein, R. J. (1970). On the law of effect. *Journal of Experimental Analysis of Behavior, 13,* (2), 243–266. https://doi.org/10.1901/jeab.1970.13-243

Higgins, S. T., Heil, S. H., & Lussier, J. P. (2004). Clinical implications of reinforcement as a determinant of substance use disorders. *Annual Review of Psychology, 55,* 431–461. https://doi.org/10.1146/annurev.psych.55.090902.142033

Holmes, G. R., Heckel, R. V., Chestnut, E., Harris, N., & Cautela, J. (1987). Factor analysis of the adolescent reinforcement survey schedule (ARSS) with college freshmen. *Journal of Clinical Psychology, 43*(4), 386–390. https://doi.org/10.1002/1097-4679(198707)43:4<386::AID-JCLP2270430408>3.0.CO;2-E

Holmes, G. R., Sakano, Y., Cautela, J., & Holmes, G. L. (1991). Comparison of factor-analyzed adolescent reinforcement survey schedule (ARSS) responses from Japanese and American adolescents. *Journal of Clinical Psychology, 47* (6), 749–755. https://doi.org/10.1002/1097-4679(199111)47:6<749::AID-JCLP2270470604>3.0.CO;2-G

Hursh, S. R. (1984). Behavioral economics. *Journal of the Experimental Analysis of Behavior, 42*(3), 435–452. https://doi.org/10.1901/jeab.1984.42-435

Johnson, M. W. & Bickel, W. K. (2006). Replacing relative reinforcing efficacy with behavioral economic demand curves. *Journal of the Experimental Analysis of Behavior, 85,*73–93. https://doi.org/10.1901/jeab.2006.102-04

Johnson, M. W., Bickel, W. K., & Baker, F. (2007). Moderate drug use and delay discounting: A comparison of heavy, light, and never smokers. *Experimental and Clinical Psychopharmacology, 15*(2), 187–194. https://doi.org/10.1037/1064-1297.15.2.187

Joyner, K. J., Meshesha, L. Z., Dennhardt, A. A., Borsari, B., Martens, M. P., & Murphy, J. G. (2019). High opportunity cost demand as an indicator of weekday drinking and distinctly severe alcohol problems: A behavioral economic analysis. *Alcoholism: Clinical and Experimental Research, 43*(12), 2607–2619. https://doi.org/10.1111/acer.14206

Joyner, K. J., Pickover, A. M., Soltis, K. E., Dennhardt, A. A., Martens, M. P., & Murphy, J. G. (2016). Deficits in access to reward are associated with college student alcohol use disorder. *Alcoholism: Clinical and Experimental Research, 40*(12), 2685–2691. https://doi.org/10.1111/acer.13255

Kelly, B. C., & Parsons, J. T. (2008). Predictors and comparisons of polydrug and non-polydrug cocaine use in club subcultures. *American Journal of Drug and Alcohol Abuse, 24,* 774–781. https://doi.org/10.1080/00952990802455451

Khoddam, R., Cho, J., Jackson, N. J., & Leventhal, A. M. (2018). Diminished alternative reinforcement as a mechanism linking conduct problems and substance use in adolescence: A longitudinal examination. *Addiction, 113*(6), 1139–1148. https://doi.org/10.1111/add.14160

Koffarnus, M. N., Jarmolowicz, D. P., Mueller, E. T., & Bickel, W. K. (2013). Changing delay discounting in the light of the competing neurobehavioral decision systems theory: A review. *Journal of the Experimental Analysis of Behavior, 99*(1), 32–57. https://doi.org/10.1002/jeab.2

Lau-Barraco, C., Linden-Carmichael, A. N., Braitman, A. L., & Stamates, A. L. (2016). Identifying patterns of situation antecedents to heavy drinking among college students. *Addiction Research and Theory, 24*(6), 431–440. https://doi.org/10.3109/16066359.2016.1153077

Lemley, S. M., Kaplan, B. A., Reed, D. D., Darden, A. C., & Jarmolowicz, D. P. (2016). Reinforcer pathologies: Predicting alcohol related problems in college drinking men and women. *Drug and Alcohol Dependence*, *167*, 57–66. https://doi.org/10.1016/j.drugalcdep.2016.07.025

Lewinsohn, P. M. (1974). A behavioral approach to depression. In R. J. Friedman & M. M. Katz (Eds.), The psychology of depression: Contemporary theory and research *(pp. 157–174).* John Wiley & Sons.

Lewinsohn, P. M., Sullivan, J. M., & Grosscup, Sally, J. (1980). Changing reinforcing events: An approach to the treatment of depression. *Psychotherapy: Theory, Research, & Practice*, *17*(3), 322–334. https://doi.org/10.1037/h0085929

Luciano, M. T., Acuff, S. F., McDevitt-Murphy, M. E., & Murphy, J. G. (2019). Behavioral economics and coping-related drinking motives in trauma exposed drinkers: Implications for the self-medication hypothesis. *Experimental and Clinical Psychopharmacology*, *28*(3), 265–270. https://doi.org/10.1037/pha0000318

MacKillop, J., Amlung, M. T., & Acker, J. D. (2010a). Further validation of an alcohol purchase task: Equivalence of versions for hypothetical and actual rewards. *Alcoholism: Clinical and Experimental Research*, *34*(6), 48A. https://doi.org/10.1111/j.1530-0277.2010.01210.x

MacKillop, J. & Murphy, J. G. (2007). A behavioral economic measure of demand for alcohol predicts brief intervention outcomes, *Drug and Alcohol Dependence, 89* (2–3), 227–233. https://psycnet.apa.org/doi/10.1016/j.drugalcdep.2007.01.002

MacKillop, J., O'Hagen, S., Lisman, S. A., Murphy, J. G., Ray, L. A., Tidey, J. W., McGeary, J. E., & Monti, P. M. (2010b). Behavioral economic analysis of cue-elicited craving for alcohol. *Addiction*, *105*(9), 1599–1607. https://doi.org/10.1111/j.1360-0443.2010.03004.x

MacPherson, L., Collado, A., Ninnemann, A., & Hoffman, E. (2017). Development of a behavioral activation-based intervention for cigarette-smoking young adults. *Cognitive and Behavioral Practice*, *24*(1), 101–114. https://doi.org/10.1016/j.cbpra.2016.03.004

MacPherson, L., Tull, M. T., Matusiewicz, A. K., Rodman, S., Strong, D. R., Kahler, C. W., Hopko, D. R., Zvolensky, M. J., Brown, R. A., & Lejuez, C. W. (2010). Randomized controlled trial of behavioral activation smoking cessation treatment for smokers with elevated depressive symptoms. *Journal of Consulting and Clinical Psychology*, *78*(1), 55–61. https://doi.org/10.1037/a0017939

MacPhillamy, D. J., & Lewinsohn, P. M. (1982). The pleasant events schedule: Studies on reliability, validity, and scale intercorrelation. *Journal of Consulting and Clinical Psychology*, *50*(3), 363–380. https://doi.org/10.1037/0022-006X.50.3.363

Magidson, J. F., Gorka, S. M., MacPherson, L., Hopko, D. R., Blanco, C., Lejuez, C. W., & Daughters, S. B. (2011). Examining the effect of the life enhancement treatment for substance use (LETS ACT) on residential substance abuse treatment retention. *Addictive Behaviors*, *36*(6), 615–623. https://doi.org/10.1016/j.addbeh.2011.01.016

Magidson, J. F., Robustelli, B. L., Seitz-Brown, C. J., & Whisman, M. A. (2016). Activity enjoyment, not frequency, is associated with alcohol-related problems and heavy episodic drinking. *Psychology of Addictive Behaviors*, *31*(1), 73–78. https://doi.org/10.1037/adb0000220

Maisto, S. A, Carey, K. B, & Bradizza, C. M. (1999). Social learning theory. In K. E. Leonard & H. T. Blaine (Eds.), *Psychological theories of drinking and alcoholism* (pp. 106–163). Guilford.

Marlatt, G. A. & Donovan, D., M. (Eds.). (2005). *Relapse prevention: Maintenance strategies in the treatment of addictive behaviors*. Guildford.

Marlatt, G. A. & Gordon, J. R. (Eds.) (1985). *Relapse prevention: Maintenance strategies in the treatment of addictive behaviors*. Guilford.

Mazur, J. E. (1987). An adjusting procedure for studying delayed reinforcement. In M. L. Commons, J. E. Mazur, J. A. Nevin, & H. Rachlin (Eds.), *Quantitative analyses of behavior (vol. 5). The effect of delay and of intervening events on reinforcement value* (pp. 55–73). Lawrence Erlbaum.

Meshesha, L. Z., Dennhardt, A. A., & Murphy, J. G. (2015). Polysubstance use is associated with deficits in substance-free reinforcement in college students. *Journal of Studies on Alcohol and Drugs*, *76*(1), 106–116. www.ncbi.nlm.nih.gov/pubmed/25486399

Meshesha, L. Z., Pickover, A. M., Teeters, J. B., & Murphy, J. G. (2017). A longitudinal behavioral economic analysis of non-medical prescription opioid use among college students. *The Psychological Record*, 241–251. https://doi.org/10.1007/s40732–017-0235-2

Meshesha, L. Z., Soltis, K. E., Wise, E. A., Rohsenow, D. J., Witkiewitz, K., & Murphy, J. G. (2020). Pilot trial investigating a brief behavioral economic intervention as an adjunctive treatment for alcohol use disorder. *Journal of Substance Abuse Treatment*, *113*, 108002. https://doi.org/10.1016/j.jsat.2020.108002

Meshesha, L. Z., Utzelmann, B., Dennhardt, A. A., & Murphy, J. G. (2018). A behavioral economic analysis of marijuana and other drug use among heavy drinking young adults. *Translational Issues in Psychological Science*, *4*(1), 65–75. https://search.proquest.com/docview/2019667186?accountid=14568%0Ahttp://rj9jj8rc3u.search.serialssolutions.com?ctx_ver=Z39.88-2004&ctx_enc=info:ofi/enc:UTF-8&rfr_id=info:sid/ProQ%3Apsycinfo&rft_val_fmt=info:ofi/fmt:kev:mtx:journal&rft.genre=article&rft.jt

Miller, W. R., & Rollnick, S. (2012). *Motivational interviewing: Helping people change* (3rd ed). Guilford.

Morris, V., Amlung, M. T., Kaplan, B. A., Reed, D. D., Petker, T., & MacKillop, J. (2017). Using crowdsourcing to examine behavioral economic measures of alcohol value and proportionate alcohol reinforcement. *Experimental and Clinical Psychopharmacology*, *25*(4), 314–321. https://doi.org/10.1037/pha0000130

Moskal, D., Maisto, S. A., De Vita, M., & Ditre, J. W. (2018). Effects of experimental pain induction on alcohol urge, intention to consume alcohol, and alcohol demand. *Experimental and Clinical Psychopharmacology*, *26*(1), 65–76. https://doi.org/10.1037/pha0000170

Murphy, J. G., Barnett, N. P., Goldstein, A. L., & Colby, S. M. (2007). Gender moderates the relationship between substance-free activity enjoyment and alcohol use. *Psychology of Addictive Behaviors*, *21*(2), 261–265. https://doi.org/10.1037/0893-164X.21.2.261

Murphy, J. G., Correia, C. J., Colby, S. M., & Vuchinich, R. E. (2005). Using behavioral theories of choice to predict drinking outcomes following a brief intervention.

Experimental and Clinical Psychopharmacology, 13(2), 93–101. https://doi.org/10.1037/1064-1297.13.2.93

Murphy, J. G., Dennhardt, A. A., Martens, M. P., Borsari, B., Witkiewitz, K., & Meshesha, L. Z. (2019). A randomized clinical trial evaluating the efficacy of a brief alcohol intervention supplemented with a substance-free activity session or relaxation training. *Journal of Consulting and Clinical Psychology, 87*(7), 657–669. https://doi.org/10.1037/ccp0000412

Murphy, J. G., Dennhardt, A. A., Martens, M. P., Yurasek, A. M., Skidmore, J. R., MacKillop, J., & McDevitt-Murphy, M. E. (2015). Behavioral economic predictors of brief alcohol intervention outcomes. *Journal of Consulting and Clinical Psychology, 83*(6), 1033–1043. https://doi.org/10.1038/nbt.3121.ChIP-nexus

Murphy, J. G., Dennhardt, A. A., Skidmore, J. R., Borsari, B. E., Barnett, N. P., Colby, S. M., & Martens, M. P. (2012b). A randomized controlled trial of a behavioral economic supplement to brief motivational interventions for college drinking. *Journal of Consulting and Clinical Psychology, 80*(5), 876–886. https://doi.org/10.1037/a0028763

Murphy, J. G., & MacKillop, J. (2006). Relative reinforcing efficacy of alcohol among college student drinkers. *Experimental and Clinical Psychopharmacology, 14*(2), 219–227. https://doi.org/10.1037/1064-1297.14.2.219

Murphy, J. G., MacKillop, J., Skidmore, J. R., & Pederson, A. A. (2009). Reliability and validity of a demand curve measure of alcohol reinforcement. *Experimental and Clinical Psychopharmacology, 17*(6), 396–404. https://doi.org/10.1037/a0017684

Murphy, J. G., Skidmore, J. R., Dennhardt, A. A., Martens, M. P., Borsari, B., Barnett, N. P., & Colby, S. M. (2012a). A behavioral economic supplement to brief motivational interventions for college drinking. *Addiction Research & Theory, 20*(6), 456–465. https://doi.org/10.3109/16066359.2012.665965.A

Owens, M. M., Ray, L. A., & MacKillop, J. (2015). Behavioral economic analysis of stress effects on acute motivation for alcohol. *Journal of the Experimental Analysis of Behavior, 103*(1), 77–86. https://doi.org/10.1002/jeab.114

Palamar, J. J., Mukherjee, P. P., & Halkitis, P. N. (2008). A longitudinal investigation of powder cocaine use among club-drug using gay and bisexual men. *Journal of Studies on Alcohol and Drugs, 69*(6), 806–813. https://doi.org/10.15288/jsad.2008.69.806

Reed, D. D., Niileksela, C. R., & Kaplan, B. A. (2013). Behavioral economics: A tutorial for behavior analysts in practice. *Behavior Analysis in Practice, 6*(1), 34–54. https://doi.org/10.1007/BF03391790

Rogers, R. E., Higgins, S. T., Silverman, K., Thomas, C. S., Badger, G. J., Bigelow, G., & Stitzer, M. (2008). Abstinence-contingent reinforcement and engagement in non-drug-related activities among illicit drug abusers. *Psychology of Addictive Behaviors, 22*(4), 544–550. https://doi.org/10.1037/0893-164X.22.4.544

Samo, J. A., Tucker, J. A., & Vuchinich, R. E. (1989). Agreement between self-monitoring, recall, and collateral observation measures of alcohol consumption in older adults. *Behavioral Assessment, 11*(4), 391–409.

Schneider, W. (1973). Reinforcer effectiveness as a function of reinforcer rate and magnitude: A comparison of concurrent performances. *Journal of the*

Experimental Analysis of Behavior, *20*(3), 461–471. https://doi.org/10.1901/jeab.1973.20-461

Schnoll, R. A., Hitsman, B., Blazekovic, S., Veluz-Wilkins, A., Wileyto, E. P., Leone, F. T., & Audrain-McGovern, J. E. (2016). Longitudinal changes in smoking abstinence symptoms and alternative reinforcers predict long-term smoking cessation outcomes. *Drug and Alcohol Dependence*, *165*, 245–252. https://doi.org/10.1016/j.drugalcdep.2016.06.017

Skidmore, J. R., Murphy, J. G., & Martens, M. P. (2014). Behavioral economic measures of alcohol reward value as problem severity indicators in college students. *Experimental and Clinical Psychopharmacology*, *22*(3), 198–210. https://doi.org/10.1016/j.pestbp.2011.02.012.Investigations

Sklar, S. M., Annis, H. M. & Turner, N. E. (1997). Development and validation of the drug-taking questionnaire: A measure of coping self-efficacy. *Addictive Behaviors, 22*(5), 655–670. https://doi.org/10.1016/S0306–4603(97)00006-3

Sobell, L. C., & Sobell, M. B. (1992). Timeline Follow-Back. In R. Z. Litten & J. P. Allen (Eds.), *Measuring alcohol consumption*. Springer. https://doi.org/10.1007/978-1-4612-0357-5_3

Spelman, P. J., & Simons, J. S. (2018). Effects of sexual arousal and alcohol cues on acute motivation for alcohol. *Archives of Sexual Behavior, 0123456789*. https://doi.org/10.1007/s10508–018-1195-6

Stein, J. S., Tegge, A. N., Turner, J. K., & Bickel, W. K. (2017). Episodic future thinking reduces delay discounting and cigarette demand: An investigation of the good-subject effect. *Journal of Behavioral Medicine, 42* (2), 269–276. https://doi.org/10.1007/s10865–017-9908-1

Thaler, R. H., & Sunstein, C. R. (2008). *Nudge: Improving decisions about health, wealth, and happiness.* Yale University Press.

Tucker, J. A., Chandler, S. D., & Cheong, J. (2017). Role of choice biases and choice architecture in behavioral economic strategies to reduce addictive behaviors. In N. Heather & G. Segal (Eds.), *Addiction and choice: Rethinking the relationship* (pp. 346–364). Oxford University Press.

Tucker, J. A., Cheong, J., Chandler, S. D., Lambert, B. H., Kwok, H., & Pietrzak, B. (2016). Behavioral economic indicators of drinking problem severity and initial outcomes among problem drinkers attempting natural recovery: A cross-sectional naturalistic study. *Addiction*, 111: 1956–1965. https://doi.org/10.1111/add.13492

Tucker, J. A., Foushee, H. R., Black, B. C., & Roth, D. L. (2007). Agreement between prospective interactive voice response self-monitoring and structured retrospective reports of drinking and contextual variables during natural resolution attempts. *Journal of Studies on Alcohol and Drugs*, *68*(4), 538–542. https://doi.org/10.15288/jsad.2007.68.538

Tucker, J. A., Roth, D. L., Vignolo, M. J., & Westfall, A. O. (2009). A behavioral economic reward index predicts drinking resolutions: Moderation re-visited and compared with other outcomes. *Journal of Consulting and Clinical Psychology, 31*(9), 1713–1723. https://doi.org/10.1109/TMI.2012.2196707.Separate

Tucker, J. A., Vuchinich, R. E., Black, B. C., & Rippens, P. D. (2006). Significance of a behavioral economic index of reward value in predicting drinking problem resolution. *Journal of Consulting and Clinical Psychology, 74*(2), 317–326. https://doi.org/10.1037/0022-006X.74.2.317

Tucker, J. A., Vuchinich, R. E., Harris, C. V., Gavornik, M. G., & Rudd, E. J. (1991). Agreement between subject and collateral verbal reports of alcohol consumption in older adults. *Journal of Studies on Alcohol, 52*(2), 148–155. https://doi.org/10.15288/jsa.1991.52.148

Tucker, J. A., Vuchinich, R. E., & Rippens, P. D. (2002). Predicting natural resolution of alcohol-related problems: A prospective behavioral economic analysis. *Experimental and Clinical Psychopharmacology, 10*, 248–257. https://doi.org/10.1037/1064-1297.10.3.248

Turner, N. E., Annis, H. M., & Sklar, S. M. (1997). Measurement of antecedents to drug and alcohol use: Psychometric properties of the Inventory of Drug-taking Situations (IDTS). *Behavior Research and Therapy, 35,* 465–483. https://doi.org/10.1016/S0005–7967(96)00119-2

Victorio-Estrada, A. & Mucha, R. F. (1997). The inventory of drinking situations (IDS) in current drinkers with different degrees of alcohol problems. *Addictive Behaviors, 22*, 557–565. https://doi.org/10.1016/S0306–4603(96)00061-5

Vaughan, E. L., Corbin, W. R., & Fromme, K. (2009). Academic and social motives and drinking behavior. *Psychology of Addictive Behaviors, 23*(4), 564–576. https://doi.org/10.1037/a0017331

Vuchinich, R. E., & Heather, N. (Eds.) (2003). *Choice, behavioural economics, and addiction*. Elsevier.

Vuchinich, R. E., & Tucker, J. A. (1988). Contributions from behavioral theories of choice to an analysis of alcohol abuse. *Journal of Abnormal Psychology, 97*(2), 181–195. https://doi.org/10.1037/0021-843X.97.2.181

(1996). Alcoholic relapse, life events, and behavioral theories of choice: A prospective analysis. *Experimental and Clinical Psychopharmacology, 4*(1), 19–28. https://doi.org/10.1037/1064-1297.4.1.19

Waldrop, A. E., Back, S. E., Verduin, M. L., & Brady, K. T. (2007). Triggers for cocaine and alcohol use in the presence and absence of posttraumatic stress disorder. *Addictive Behaviors, 32*,634-9. https://doi.org/10.1016/j.addbeh.2006.06.001

Wechsler, H., Davenport, A. E., Dowdall, G. W., Grossman, S. J., & Zanakos, S. I. (1997). Binge drinking, tobacco, and illicit drug use and involvement in college athletics: A survey of students at 140 American colleges. *Journal of the American College Health Association, 45*(5), 195–200. https://doi.org/10.1080/07448481.1997.9936884

Worley, M. J., Shoptaw, S. J., Bickel, W. K., & Ling, W. (2015). Using behavioral economics to predict opioid use during prescription opioid dependence treatment. *Drug and Alcohol Dependence, 148*, 62–68. https://doi.org/10.1016/j.drugalcdep.2014.12.018.Using

Young, J. S. (1981). Discrete-trial choice in pigeons: Effects of reinforcer magnitude. *Journal of the Experimental Analysis of Behavior, 35*(1), 23–29. https://doi.org/10.1016/j.bbr.2014.03.044

PART III

Macro Level: Creating Environments, Resources, Incentives, and Policies to Promote Harm Reduction and Recovery

16 Recovery Communities

Resources and Settings

David Best, Charlotte Hargreaves, Philip Hodgson, and David Patton

Recovery Communities: Resources and Settings

Recovery is characterized as a unique and personalized process and one that is embedded in a relational context both at the individual and at the societal level. Social group membership, social networks, and social identity have all been reported as central to the process of recovery, and this network of relationships is also embedded in societal processes and structures (Best et al., 2016). This chapter will define recovery as an intrinsically social process (cf. Tucker & Witkiewitz, Chapter 1 this volume) and considers the accrual of recovery capital as its underlying mechanism. Within this model, the personal resources needed to sustain a recovery journey build in a dynamic and interactive way based on the social and community resources the person is able to access and his or her ability to transcend exclusion and stigma, in an ongoing journey of personal growth and social and societal belonging.

How Has Recovery Been Defined and What Are Its Characteristics?

According to two of the most frequently cited consensus group definitions of recovery (Betty Ford Institute Consensus Group, 2007: UK Drug Policy Commission, 2008), recovery can be characterized as consisting of three component parts – sobriety, historically but not uniformly defined as abstinence; global health and well-being; and citizenship and active participation in community life. The Betty Ford definition goes on to describe recovery as a process that typically lasts for around five years until "stable recovery" is achieved, based on the research findings of recovery pathways by Dennis et al. (2014).

A key research question that emanates from recovery studies explores the proportion of people that recover from substance use disorders (SUD). A review for the United States (US) Substance Abuse and Mental Health Services Administration (SAMHSA) by Sheedy and Whitter (2009) concluded that of all those who experience a lifetime SUD, 58 percent will achieve stable recovery, although there was marked variability in rates among the studies included in the review. Similarly, in a review of 415 studies, White (2012) concluded that the overall recovery rate is just over 50 percent. More recently, Kelly and colleagues (2017) asked the prevalence question in a different way assessing what proportion of the US adult population defined themselves as being "recovered" or "in recovery." The overall reported rate, from a survey of 39,809 adults, was 9.1 percent, indicating that just under one in ten of the US population would regard themselves as being in recovery. At the time of writing, this survey has not been replicated in any other countries.

Another issue in defining recovery concerns its time course. Dennis et al. (2007) examined the relationship between abstinence duration and other recovery outcomes related to health and well-being and found that mental health problems increased through years one to three of abstinence and then diminished, while physical health problems appeared to increase. The authors also reported that it typically took over three years for significant improvements in financial status to occur, in spite of employment starting much earlier and criminal offending largely being eliminated in the first year of recovery. The authors were keen to caution that, even among those who maintained abstinence for five years, about 14 percent subsequently returned to substance use on more than one occasion ("relapse"), suggesting that recovery is not a journey that is "completed." Rather, it should be considered as an ongoing and dynamic change process. Nonetheless, as discussed next, such prevalence and proportions alone do not adequately address the question of who will recover, and when or why.

Quantifying Recovery Pathways: Recovery Capital as a System of Measurement and Planning

This section addresses the question of pathways to recovery including candidate mechanisms that predict recovery change and the emergence of the metric "recovery capital," which has been operationalized to quantify recovery growth and well-being (Cano et al., 2017). The concept of "negative recovery capital" is introduced to examine factors that can act as a barrier to effective recovery progress. Early empirical evidence about recovery pathways and mechanisms was provided by Moos (2007). His review of the evidence on the psychological mechanisms underpinning recovery concluded that there were two fundamental interpersonal processes – social learning (in which role models provide an example of how to live recovery) and social control (through which group members will learn and conform to the group's norms). In addition, opportunities for social learning by observing and imitating the recovery behaviors of more experienced peers in recovery promote the two changes – first, the development of coping skills, and second, the development of and engagement in rewarding alternative activities other than substance use (e.g., school and work, physical activity), which can promote recovery and protect against relapse (Bickel & Vuchinich, 2000). Over time, positive attitudes, beliefs, and expectations that support sustained recovery come to dominate the individual's value system.

The intrinsically social component of the majority of recovery pathways is further illustrated by the work of Litt and colleagues (2009). In this randomized controlled trial, people who completed residential detoxification from alcohol were randomly allocated to either "treatment as usual" (which was standard aftercare) or to a "network support" condition that involved developing a relationship with at least one non-drinking peer. Compared to standard aftercare, those who added at least one non-drinking member to their social network showed a 27 percent increase at 12 months post-treatment in the likelihood of treatment success (defined as being without alcohol 90 percent of the time).

In an analysis of the COMBINE Study data (Longabaugh et al., 2010) following up on earlier examination of social network effects (Longabaugh et al., 1993), the authors found that greater opposition to a person's drinking from within their social network predicted more days without alcohol use both during and after treatment, and fewer heavy drinking days after treatment. In addition, less frequent drinking within the person's social network predicted more days without alcohol use during and after treatment. The role of social norms was also a key feature of Best et al.'s (2008) United Kingdom study of recovery pathways, in which sustained recovery was associated with moving away from drug-using or drinking networks and actively engaging in social networks supportive of recovery. Thus, changes in social networks and identities are associated both with the initiation of recovery and with managing and sustaining the ongoing recovery journey.

Social Capital and Recovery Capital

The previous section introduced some of the evidence about social factors in recovery, highlighting that creating bonds and networks of people in recovery and with others who do not use substances are critical components of many individuals' recovery journeys, as is the process of leaving behind social groups that use substances and personal identities that were associated with active use patterns. To incorporate this component within a coherent model of recovery, the concept of recovery capital and its origins in the concept of social capital are described next.

Bourdieu (1985) argued that social networks are a valuable asset and that social interaction, a sense of belonging, and the relationships of trust and tolerance that are subsequently developed are key resources, particularly in communities where there is a lack of financial capital and a resulting limitation in access to community resources. In the United States, Putnam (2000) described social capital as a resource that individuals can draw upon, as well as a commitment to the group. As such, reciprocity is central to Putnam's conceptualization of social capital. He differentiated between "bonding" capital (the strength of links within established groups) and "bridging" capital which referred to the links and associations between groups. Putnam argued that individuals from marginalized communities can have strong bonds in their social networks but still have little access to community resources if there are not bridges to more groups that are engaged effectively with community assets and resources.

The history of social capital writing is central to our understanding of the emerging concept of recovery capital, which we define as the set of "resources and capacities that enable growth and human flourishing." We use this working definition of recovery capital for the remainder of this chapter. It fits with the broader characterization of recovery in this book as a dynamic process of behavior change. The assumption here is that recovery capital is a key marker of recovery progress and well-being and will increase or diminish in reasonably predictable ways in response to social and societal activities and forces. This assumption hinges on White and Cloud's (2008) assertion that long-term recovery pathways are better predicted on the basis of building strengths rather than managing or attempting to reduce deficits.

The term recovery capital was originally coined by Cloud and Granfield (2008) as "the sum total of one's resources that can be brought to bear on the initiation and maintenance of substance misuse cessation" (Cloud & Granfield, 2008, p. 1972). Cloud and Granfield (2008) argued that recovery capital applies not only to assets and strengths, but they also discussed the concept of "negative recovery capital" for factors that constitute barriers to recovery change. Cloud and Granfield identified four such barriers, suggesting that recovery is more difficult for those with histories of mental health problems, histories of involvement with the criminal justice system, for people who are older and, more controversially, for women. Within the model outlined in this chapter, it is also important to recognize that recovery is a dynamic concept that will change over time and is bidirectional, meaning that it is just as likely to go down as it is to go up if an individual experiences adversity and the removal or inability to access desired goods or resources.

The other key advance precipitated by the introduction of the recovery capital concept was the promise of quantification and the development of a metric. While there have been a number of ways of characterizing recovery capital, Best and Laudet (2010) argued that there are three primary domains to recovery capital:

a. Personal recovery capital, which refers to those qualities and capabilities a person acquires in the course of their recovery journey, including resilience, coping skills, communication skills, self-esteem, and self-efficacy.
b. Social recovery capital, which refers to the relationships a person has and, crucially, as Putnam (2000) argued, to the strength of their commitment to those relationships and networks.
c. Community recovery capital, which refers to the resources in the community that the person can access, such as educational courses, safe and secure accommodation, and meaningful employment opportunities. Community recovery capital also includes recovery-specific resources in the community, like mutual help groups, visible recovery champions, and recovery-oriented treatment services.

As Best (2019) argued, these components of recovery capital do not accrue consistently or evenly, and there are grounds for suggesting that the transition to recovery as a self-determined state (Dennis et al., 2014) is, for many, about utilizing social and community capital as scaffolding around the individual to afford them the opportunity to grow core personal attributes and skills necessary to support sustainable recovery pathways.

Two research studies illustrate how this can be achieved. The first is the Glasgow Recovery Study (Best et al., 2011) in which 202 individuals in recovery from alcohol and heroin dependence were assessed in terms of well-being and quality of life. There were two central predictors of well-being in recovery – how much time participants had spent with other people in recovery and how much time people spent in meaningful activities (defined as average hours in a week spent on childcare, volunteering, community group activities, education, and employment). In other words, spending time with people who acted as social learning role models and engaging in meaningful activities were associated in greater well-being and quality of life.

A similar relationship was found in a later study of recovery residences in Florida (Cano et al., 2017). Based in eight recovery residences that were members of the Florida Association of Recovery Residences, structured equation modeling showed that longer duration of stay was associated with lower barriers to recovery and less unmet needs, thus generating higher levels of well-being. However, there was also a second path to well-being that was "strengths-based." For those who used their time in residence to engage in more positive and meaningful activities, there was growth in personal and social recovery capital that was associated with positive changes in overall well-being. The authors concluded that while treatment duration confers a beneficial effect, it is the active engagement in meaningful activities that generates recovery well-being.

The above study utilized an emerging metric for recovery capital, the REC-CAP (Cano et al., 2017), which included an earlier scale, the Assessment of Recovery Capital (Groshkova et al., 2012). The aim of these measures, which have acceptable psychometric properties, was to assess the resources that individuals have and, in the case of the REC-CAP, to utilize the scores derived on the scale to inform recovery care planning. What is most important about the measures is that they are based on strengths and predicated on the assumption that strengths build further strengths. Moreover, the use of a "positive" model of measurement in itself contributes to an emerging sense of self-esteem and self-efficacy in study participants, and that it is part of a relational approach in which recovery capital presumably grows through relationships with both the recovery community and the local, lived community. The scale provides an immediate score profile in an accessible form when completed online that the client and their recovery mentor, referred to within this approach as a "recovery navigator," can use to plan further recovery actions. The impact this has on personal identity is discussed in the following section.

Social Identity and the Role of Group Belonging in Recovery Change

Since the early work of Biernacki (1986), identity change has been recognized as a central part of addiction recovery, and Biernacki asserted that the transition to recovery required "new identities, perspectives, and social world involvements" (Biernacki, 1986, p. 141). McIntosh and McKeganey (2000, 2002) collected the recovery narratives of 70 individuals with previous SUD in Glasgow, Scotland, and concluded that SUD may result in "identities [that] have been seriously damaged" (McIntosh & McKeganey, 2002, p. 152). They concluded that for recovery to happen, the individual required the restoration of identity. This has been challenged, however, by subsequent work that suggested that identity is a much more complex issue. For example, Radcliffe (2011) used motherhood as an example of a positive identity that could assist in overcoming the addiction identity and enable an initiation of recovery endeavors.

The early focus on personal identity has gradually transitioned over time into an increased research focus on identity that is embedded in group membership and in the sense of belonging that emerges from recovery identity (Best et al., 2016). The switch to a social lens for understanding identity dates back to the work of Tajfel and Turner on Social Identity Theory and Self-Categorization Theory, respectively (Tajfel & Turner, 1979; Turner et al., 1987). The model emphasizes the importance of group belonging on identity and in particular how membership in a group involves adherence to the norms and rules of the group and the internalization of its values. The more important the group is to the person, the more salient will its rules and values be across multiple life domains.

In terms of health and stigmatization, this was brought to particular prominence by work on "the social cure" (Jetten et al., 2012). This refers to the health benefits that are associated with active group memberships and their potentially protective effects against adverse life experiences and, in particular, the importance of group membership and group support in times of key life transitions. This perspective has been adapted to support understanding of addiction recovery processes in the Social Identity Model of Recovery (SIMOR; Best et al., 2016), which asserts that individuals' "identification with a recovery group will shape their understanding of substance-related events (e.g., an offer to go to the pub with friends) and their response to it (rejection on the grounds that it would put their recovery at risk). Thus, group memberships exert influence on individuals through the transmission of social norms which are internalized, and shape subsequent attitudes and behavior" (Best et al., 2016, p. 9). What SIMOR outlines is a model that frames recovery as a process of social identity change in which a person's most salient identity shifts from being defined by membership in a group whose norms and values revolve around substance use to being defined by membership in a group whose norms and values encourage recovery.

The SIMOR model, which focuses specifically on the process of change in social networks and the resulting social identities, is based on a growing body of research evidence. Dingle et al. (2015) assessed retention and treatment outcomes among residents of a Therapeutic Community in Queensland, Australia and showed that longer retention was associated with the growth of a recovery identity as well as with the diminution of a SUD identity, and that this transition was associated with better treatment outcomes. Similarly, Beckwith et al. (2015)

undertook research in the same Therapeutic Community and showed that the extent of change from a dominant SUD identity to a dominant recovery identity was associated with positive outcomes in this population.

This model has been examined in considerably more depth in the Social Networks and Recovery Study (SONAR; Best et al., 2016). The study was a longitudinal cohort study that followed 307 individuals entering one of five Therapeutic Community (TC) services in three states in Eastern Australia from admission to six months (around the time of planned discharge) and then at 12 months after admission, when all participants should have returned to the community. Haslam et al. (2019) interviewed participants about about their individual- and group-based social relationships prior to treatment entry, their social identification with the TC and as "a user" and a person "in recovery," and their current recovery capital and quality of life. A key finding was group identities (for instance, to families, mutual help groups, and friendship groups) reported by participants prior to TC admission predicted the extent of their engagement with the treatment service they attended. Individual identities did not predict outcomes. Furthermore, a mediation analysis indicated that TC identification was the mechanism through which social group memberships prior to TC admission protected quality of life in the early phases of treatment.

Collectively, this research shows the importance of transitioning from social group membership in groups committed to substance use and the related lifestyle and to the consequent engagement in pro-social groups. The mechanism that underpins this transition is about identification and the complex inter-play between membership in a group and the adoption and internalization of its beliefs, values, and norms. Thus, being part of a social group that uses substances is not simply about "peer pressure" to use, but also about a shared set of assumptions and values around the merits of substance use and the resultant lifestyle. Conversely, immersion in recovery groups is about a different set of social norms and beliefs and a different set of expectations around membership that extend beyond sobriety and involve decisions about the merits and drawbacks of substance use and sobriety (Moos, 2007).

There is one further aspect of this process that links the concepts of social identification with two types of recovery capital – social and community. This concerns access to community resources among people in groups that use substances and are marginalized and excluded compared to groups of individuals in recovery who are embedded in multiple pro-social networks. Jetten et al. (2015), in the context of studying homelessness, initially observed that all groups were not equal in terms of the merits and benefits of membership. Membership in marginalized groups, like individuals who are homeless and those with SUD, does not afford the same psychological benefits (e.g., to self-esteem, self-efficacy, and so on) or practical benefits as does membership in pro-social groups engaged in meaningful activities that are consistent with conventional norms and values. The link to personal and social capital is that engagement in a recovery group acts as a form of linking and bridging capital (Putnam, 2000) to community resources that would otherwise be denied the individual. This includes not only practical assistance but informational resources about job opportunities, available college courses, and access to housing. However, this is a dynamic process that is bi-directional, and changes in access to social and community capital can generate reductions as well as increases in social capital.

Connectedness Hope Identity Meaning and Empowerment (CHIME) and the Role of Social Networks

While much has been written about definitions of recovery and recovery stages and processes, there is much less evidence on what can be done by others to support recovery pathways and processes. Much of the evidence that does exist has focused on peer processes and mutual help groups (White, 2009; Humphreys & Lembke, 2013), whereas relatively little attention has been given to what support services (statutory services and non-governmental organizations as well as peer-based) should do to support the individual and the group in their recovery journey.

A systematic review of the mental health recovery literature by Leamy et al. (2011) concluded that there were five essential elements in recovery supportive programmes – Connectedness, Hope, Identity, Meaning, and Empowerment (CHIME). The evidence was based on 97 papers that reviewed 87 distinct studies and supported the authors' conclusion that these are "essential elements" in an effective recovery program relating to recovery processes. What is crucial about this model is that it outlines what external agencies and groups can do to support an individual in their recovery journey, and thus switches the focus to the conditions or facilitators of individual and group recovery.

Best (2019) translated this model to the addiction recovery area and suggested that there is a clear order to the model. As in the acronym, Connection is the starting point with the social contagion of recovery effectively initiating a social contagion of Hope, and so the catalyst for the process is fundamentally social and interpersonal. Visible and successful role models create the belief that recovery is possible, and generate the energy, conviction, and focus to allow individuals to overcome barriers and exclusions – including lethargy, fear, and self-doubt – to taking meaningful action. The first two stages are connection and hope, but what they then trigger is a virtuous circle of meaningful activities (Meaning), growth in self-esteem and self-efficacy (Empowerment), and changes in both self-perceptions and group membership and belonging (Identity). It is at this point that the cyclical and ongoing nature of CHIME continues to promote and enhance recovery change, although that does not mean that recovery is linear or that positive growth is inexorable.

Overall, this integrative model of recovery capital, social contagion, and social identity emphasizes that recovery is a change process and one that is firmly embedded in social and societal triggers and sustained by group involvement.

Public policy, public attitudes, and community connections are all important contextual drivers for recovery (in both positive and negative directions). Access to visible recovery champions and community resources are essential contextual facilitators of addiction recovery.

The "contagion" component of the model also draws heavily on the work of Christakis and Fowler (2010) and the principles of social epidemiology. Specifically, if recovery is both visible and attractive in its presentation, then it is likely that it will spread more rapidly through social networks both as a behavioral phenomenon among individuals with addiction histories and also as a socially desirable and acceptable aspiration within communities. This in turn should open more doors and create further pathways that increase the opportunities for sustainable recovery growth and change. These are the ideas that have generated the "Recovery Cities" (i.e., Inclusive Cities) movement (Best & Colman, 2019), promoting community inclusiveness based on the principles of the recovery movement and designed to continue to support effective recovery pathways. The Recovery Cities/Inclusive Cities initiative involved three cities initially – Doncaster in the UK, Ghent in Belgium, and Gothenburg in Sweden. In all three cities, the aim was to mobilize community resources through a recruited cohort of "community connectors" to challenge exclusion and create pathways to community resources for people who misuse substances and then to other marginalized and stigmatized groups. The initiative has now extended to a number of other cities in Europe and New Zealand, and is building a community model for supporting and enhancing personal journeys to well-being.

Conclusions and Recommendations

The evidence presented here challenges the dominant tendency historically to view addiction as a disease (White & Cloud, 2008). The disease model has oftentimes been critiqued for having the effect of overly individualizing, pathologizing, and dehumanizing the person and the perceived problem (Pienaar & Dilkes-Frayne, 2017), while at the same time individualizing the responsibility for resolution. Individuals have differentiated capacities and resources to overcome addiction (Cloud & Granfield, 2008). The same set of factors can and do affect individuals differently depending on their personal, situational, and social contexts, as well as their resources. However, this differentiated capacity is also deeply affected by factors, forces, and structures that operate at the meso and macro levels.

Therefore, the processes and forces operating in individuals' recovery journey are nuanced, interactive, and dynamic and are not always within the control or responsibility of the individual. To simply individualize and ascribe responsibility to the person in recovery for their lack of "success" does little to acknowledge the existence of the social inequalities and dire social realities, levels of exclusion, and stigma faced by certain populations within the recovery population (Cloud & Granfield, 2008). There will be some individuals who can recover in stigmatizing and hostile settings if they have enough personal and social recovery capital. For most, however, it will be the ability to access community resources, (houses, jobs, meaningful activities, and recovery support groups) as well as personalized and individualized relationships, that will be prerequisites for sustainable change. This is why CHIME offers a model for how recovery-oriented services should deploy their resources and assess their impact and effectiveness.

Some have argued that substance use has become a normalized activity (Aldridge et al., 2011; Parker et al., 1998), whilst Lloyd (2010) has highlighted that those who experience drug and alcohol problems are one of the most stigmatized groups. The forces of exclusion and stigma manifest in different guises that can block or impede continuing routes out of addiction. O'Gorman (2016, p. 253) usefully questioned "why the use of similar drugs and similar drug using behaviors by different social groups is differentially accommodated and accepted by mainstream society?" This highlights the relative as well as differentiated nature of acceptability and accommodation of harmful drug use and related behaviors.

As recovery is centered around relationships embedded in societal processes and structures, the Recovery Cities initiative is one example of attempting to change societal responses in order to address structural barriers to effective group engagement. Individuals in recovery need both "the will and the ways" on their journey (Burnett & Maruna, 2004). It is acknowledged that this transition at the meso and macro levels is not simple, quick, or easy. Therefore, it requires mapping existing assets in the community that promote belonging and inclusion, provide meaningful activities, act as social connection points, build awareness of existing strengths, and offer a vision for the future. These processes highlight the powerful impact that environments and organizations can have in promoting recovery. Supporting and promoting recovery at a policy level will require increased resources for community infra-structures and crucially for (primarily peer-based) pathways to community resources, including housing, education, training, and leisure activities.

Building on this further to create inclusive cities that promote participation and inclusion whilst challenging stigmatization and exclusion is key (Best & Colman, 2019). This is predicated on the idea that individual recovery journeys have the ability to generate further community recovery capital and to increase the visibility and accessibility of recovery. The Recovery Cities/Inclusive Cities model is based on the assumption that there is a generative dynamism between individual transformation and collective recovery potential, although this model has not yet been evaluated. Operating from this framework requires us to rethink and redefine our understanding of the operation of recovery in a way that transcends the personal to incorporate the social, societal, and community forces that are essential to promoting growth and human flourishing. Through building inclusive and recovery-oriented systems and communities, we are suggesting a form of "giving back" that is transformative in placing the values of recovery at the heart of communities and, in doing so, promotes a broad base of community connections and active participation as fundamental for growth and well-being at a collective level.

Acknowledgments

We would like to thank all of the colleagues, friends, and people in recovery who have supported our work in this area.

References

Aldridge, J., Measham, F. & Parker, H. (2011) *Illegal leisure revisited: Changing patterns of alcohol and drug use in adolescents and young adults.* Routledge.

Beckwith, M., Best, D., Lubman, D., Dingle, G. & Perryman C. (2015). Predictors of flexibility in social identity among people entering a therapeutic community for substance abuse. *Alcoholism Treatment Quarterly, 33*(1), 93–104. https://doi.org/10.1080/07347324.2015.982465

Best, D. (2019). *Pathways to desistance and recovery: The role of the social contagion of hope.* Policy Press.

Best, D., Beckwith, M., Haslam, C., Haslam, S. A., Jetten, J., Mawson, E., & Lubman, D. I. (2016). Overcoming alcohol and other drug addiction as a process of social identity transition: The social identity model of recovery (SIMOR). *Addiction Research & Theory, 24*(2), 111–123. https://doi.org/10.3109/16066359.2015.1075980

Best, D. & Colman, C. (2019). Desistance and recovery special issue – introduction and overview, *Addiction Research and Theory, 27*(1), 55–64. https://doi.org/10.1080/16066359.2018.1535059

Best, D., Ghufran, S., Day, E., Ray, R. & Loaring, J. (2008). Breaking the habit: A retrospective analysis of desistance factors among formerly problematic heroin users. *Drug and Alcohol Review, 27*(6), 619–624. https://doi.org/10.1080/09595230802392808

Best, D., Gow, J., Taylor, A., Knox, A. & White, W. (2011). Recovery from heroin or alcohol dependence: A qualitative account of the recovery experience in Glasgow. *Journal of Drug Issues, 41*(3), 359–378. https://doi.org/10.1177/002204261104100303

Best, D., Haslam, C., Staiger, P., Dingle, G., Savic, M., Bathish, R., Mackenzie, J., Beckwith, M., & Lubman, D. I. (2016). Social networks and recovery (SONAR): Characteristics of a longitudinal outcome study in five therapeutic communities in Australia. *Therapeutic Communities: International Journal of Therapeutic Communities, 37*(3), 131–139. https://doi.org/10.1108/TC-04-2016-0012

Best, D. & Laudet, A. (2010). *The potential of recovery capital.* RSA.

Betty Ford Institute Consensus Group (2007). What is recovery? A working definition from the Betty Ford Institute. *Journal of Substance Abuse Treatment, 33*(3), 221–8. https://doi.org/10.1016/j.jsat.2007.06.001

Bickel, W. K., & Vuchinich, R. E. (2000). *Reframing health behavior change with behavioral economics*. Lawrence Erlbaum.

Biernacki, P. (1986). *Pathways from heroin addiction: Recovery without treatment*. Temple University Press.

Bourdieu, P. (1985). The forms of capital. In J. G. Richardson (Ed.), *Handbook of theory and research for the sociology of education* (pp. 241–258). Greenwood.

Burnett, R., & Maruna, S. (2004). So "prison works," does it? The criminal careers of 130 men released from prison under Home Secretary, Michael Howard. *Journal of Criminal Justice, 43*(4): 390–404. https://doi.org/ 10.1111/j.1468-2311.2004.00337.x

Cano, I., Best, D., Edwards, M. & Lehman, J. (2017). Recovery capital pathways: Mapping the components of recovery well-being. *Drug and Alcohol Dependence*, 181, 11–19. https://doi.org/10.1016/j.drugalcdep.2017.09.002

Christakis, N., & Fowler, J. (2010). *Connected: The amazing power of social networks and how they shape our lives*. Harper Press.

Cloud, W., & Granfield, R. (2009). Conceptualizing recovery capital: Expansion of a theoretical construct. *Substance Use and Misuse, 43*(12–13), 1971–1986. https://doi.org/10.1080/10826080802289762

Dennis, M., Foss, M. & Scott, C. (2007). An eight-year perspective on the relationship between the duration of abstinence and other aspects of recovery. *Evaluation Review, 31*(6), 585–612. https://doi.org/10.1177/0193841X07307771

Dennis, M., Scott, C., & Laudet, A. (2014). Beyond bricks and mortars: Recent research on substance abuse disorder recovery management. *Current Psychiatry Report, 16*(4), 442. https://doi.org/doi: 10.1007/s11920-014-0442-3

Dingle, G., Stark, C., Cruwys, T. & Best, D. (2015). Breaking good: Breaking ties with social groups may be good for recovery from substance misuse. *British Journal of Social Psychology, 54*(2), 236–254. https://doi.org/10.1111/bjso.12081

Granfield, R. & Cloud, W. (2001). Social context and "natural recovery": The role of social capital in the resolution of drug-associated problems. *Substance Use &Misuse, 36*(11), 1543–1570. https://doi.org/ 10.1081/ja-100106963

Groshkova, T., Best, D., & White, W. (2012). The assessment of recovery capital: Properties and psychometrics of a measure of addiction recovery strengths. *Drug and Alcohol Review, 32*(2), 187–194. https://doi.org/10.1111/j.1465-3362.2012.00489.x

Haslam, C., Best, D., Dingle, G., Staiger, G., Savic, M., Bathish, R., Mackenzie, J., Beckwith, M., Kelly, A. & Lubman, D. (2019). Social group membership before treatment for substance dependence predicts early identification and engagement with treatment communities. *Addiction Research and Theory, 27*(5), 363–372. https://doi.org/10.1080/16066359.2018/1537393

Humphreys, K., & Lembke, A. (2013). Recovery-oriented policy and care systems in the UK and USA. *Drug and Alcohol Review, 33*(1), 13–18. https://doi.org/10.1111/dar.12092

Jetten, J., Branscombe, N., Haslam, S., Haslam, C., Cruwys, T., Jones, J., & Zhang, A. (2015). Having a lot of a good thing: Multiple important group memberships as a source of self-esteem. *PLoS One*, 10(5), e0131035. https://doi.org/0.1371/journal.pone.0124609

Jetten, J., Haslam, C., & Haslam, S. A. (Eds.) (2012). *The social cure: Identity, health, and well-being*. Psychology Press.

Kelly, J., Bergman, B., Hoeppner, B., Vilsaint, C., & White, W. (2017). Prevalence and pathways of recovery from drug and alcohol problems in the United States population: Implications for practice, research, and policy. *Drug and Alcohol Dependence*, *181*, 162–169. https://doi.org/10.1016/j.drugalcdep.2017.09.028

Leamy, M., Bird, V., Le Boutillier, C., Williams, J., & Slade, M. (2011). A conceptual framework for personal recovery in mental health: Systematic review and narrative synthesis. *British Journal of Psychiatry, 199*(6), 445–452. https://doi.org/ 10.1192/bjp.bp.110.083733

Litt, M. D., Kadden, R. M., Kabela-Cormier, E., & Petry, N. (2007). Changing network support for drinking: Initial findings from the Network Support Project. *Journal of Consulting and Clinical Psychology*, *75*(4), 542–55. https://doi.org/10.1037/0022-006X.75.4.542

Lloyd, C. (2010). *Sinning and sinned against: The stigmatization of problem drug users*. The UK Drug Policy Commission.

Longabaugh, R., Beattie, M., Noel, N., Stout, R., & Malloy P. (1993). The effect of social investment on treatment outcome. *Journal of Studies on Alcohol*, *54*(4), 465–478. https://doi.org/10.15288/jsa.1993.54.465

Longabaugh, R., Wirtz, P. W., Zywiak, W. H., & O'Malley, S. S. (2010). Network support as a prognostic indicator of drinking outcomes: The COMBINE study. *Journal of Studies on Alcohol and Drugs*, *71*(6), 837–846. https://doi.org/10.15288/jsad.2010.71.837

McIntosh, J. & McKeganey, N. (2000). Addicts' narratives of recovery from drug use: Constructing a non-addict identity. *Social Science & Medicine*, *50*(10), 1501–1510. https://doi.org/10.1016/s0277–9536(99)00409-8

Moos, R. H. (2007). Theory-based active ingredients of effective treatments for substance use disorders. *Drug and Alcohol Dependence*, *88*(2–3): 109–121. https://doi.org/10.1016/j.drugalcdep.2006.10.010.

O'Gorman, A (2016). Chillin', buzzin', getting mangled, and coming down: Doing differentiated normalization in risk environments. *Drugs: Education, Prevention and Policy*, *23*(3), 247–254.

Parker, H., Aldridge, J., & Measham, F. (1998) *Illegal leisure: The normalization of adolescent recreational drug use*. Routledge.

Pienaar, K., & Dilkes-Frayne, E (2017). Telling different stories, making new realities: The ontological politics of "addiction" biographies, *International Journal of Drug Policy, 44,* 145–154. http://dx.doi.org/10.1016/j.drugpo.2017.05.011

Putnam, R. D. (2000). *Bowling alone: The collapse and revival of American community*. Simon & Schuster.

Radcliffe, P. (2011). Motherhood, pregnancy, and the negotiation of identity: The moral career of drug treatment. *Social Science & Medicine*, *72*(6), 984–991. https://doi.org/10.1016/j.socscimed.2011.01.017

Sheedy, C. & Whitter, M. (2009) *Guiding principles and elements of recovery-oriented systems of care: What do we know from the research?* (HHS Publication No. (SMA) 09-4439). Substance Abuse, and Mental Health Services

Administration. www.naadac.org/assets/2416/sheedyckwhitterm2009_guiding_principles_and_elements.pdf

Tajfel, H., & Turner, J. C. (1979). An integrative theory of intergroup conflict. In W. G. Austin & S. Worchel (Eds.), *The social psychology of intergroup relations* (pp. 33–47). Brooks/Cole.

Turner, J., Hogg, M., Oakes, P., Reicher, S., & Wetherell, MS. (1987). *Rediscovering the social group: A self-categorization theory*. Blackwell.

UK Drug Policy Commission (2008). *The UK drug policy commission recovery consensus group: A vision of recovery*. UK Drug Policy Commission.

White, W. (2012). *Recovery/remission from substance use disorders: An analysis of reported outcomes in 415 scientific reports*. Philadelphia Department of Behavioral Health and Intellectual Disability Services and the Great Lakes Addiction Technology Transfer Center.

(2009). *Peer-based addiction recovery support: History, theory, practice, and scientific evaluation*. Great Lakes Addiction Technology Transfer Center and Philadelphia Department of Behavioral Health and Mental Retardation Services.

White, W., & Cloud, W. (2008). Recovery capital: A primer for addictions professionals. *Counselor, 9*(5), 22–27.

17 Disparities in Alcohol Treatment Access in Rural Areas

Opportunities for Change

Claire Snell-Rood, Kara Bensley, and
Laura Schmidt

Disparities in Alcohol Treatment Access in Rural Areas: Opportunities for Change

Rural communities within the United States (US) are under-represented in research on alcohol use and also possess fewer resources for treatment. There is considerable diversity – racially, ethnically, culturally, economically, and geographically – across communities that fall within the conceptual group known as "rural" (Showalter, 2020), with dozens of definitions of "rural" in use by the US government and researchers that present complications in comparing and classifying studies (Dixon & Chartier, 2016). While this chapter describes studies of national and regional samples, it is important to stay cognizant of the fact that "rural" is a lived experience that varies community by community. Despite such variation, people living in rural areas face a common set of barriers to accessing alcohol treatment services (Ali et al., 2020; Bensley et al., 2019; Davis et al., 2016; Edmonds et al., 2020), including higher rates of persistent poverty, limited behavioral health personnel, limited resources for health departments, and fewer public health policies overall (Harris et al., 2016). Socially, rural communities are characterized by high social integration which means that individuals have a deep knowledge of their fellow community members. This can make it more challenging to pursue care for an alcohol problem due to challenges in maintaining confidentiality (Gordon et al, 2011; Saunders et al., 2019).

This chapter engages with epidemiological definitions of alcohol use based on the presence or absence of AUD as these predominate the research. However, while the epidemiological literature holds the potential to understand differences in and across communities, it can inadvertently construct people as individuals apart from the social worlds in which they live. This focus on the individual, together with the tendency to pathologize people seen as "problem drinkers," can lead to portrayals of "isolated, passive, and de-contextualized individuals" rather than "as active agents, immersed in a complex social structure, relating to other actors in their social group" (Hunt & Barker, 2001). In considering this interdisciplinary literature, an anthropological orientation is applied toward treatment and recovery that prioritizes how alcohol use is defined within communities, often in diverse ways (Hunt & Barker, 2001).

Patterns of Alcohol Use in Rural Communities

In the 1990s, health services researchers Booth and Fortney led the first large-scale studies to understand patterns of drinking among rural people in the United States. They conducted a four-wave longitudinal study of "at-risk" drinkers across the US South, comparing urban and rural populations. They found that rural people at-risk for AUD were sicker overall and had more symptoms over time, but also were more likely to use services to address their alcohol use than urban people (Booth et al., 2000). Booth's later work with Tyrone Borders used the National Epidemiologic Survey on Alcohol and Related Conditions (NESARC) to compare alcohol use by rurality. The 2001–2002 NESARC data revealed more variation in alcohol use by region than absolute differences between rural, suburban, and urban residents. Alcohol abstinence was more common among people living in the rural Northeast, Midwest, and South than among those living in suburban areas. The odds of drinking more than weekly, and of having AUD, were greater among rural and urban people living in the Midwest than in other regions (Borders & Booth, 2007). People in rural areas were more likely to abstain from alcohol use than their urban counterparts. However, among those who drank, those in rural areas drank at a similar or even higher consumption level relative to those in urban areas. Rural residents drank more per occasion (Dixon & Chartier, 2016), were more likely to experience heavy episodic drinking, and were more likely to drink frequently than those living in urban areas (Borders & Booth, 2007).

More recent studies have attempted to compare alcohol use patterns among different ethnic communities in rural areas. This work suggests that social conditions are more influential in determining the outcomes of alcohol use compared to ethnic status (Ponicki et al., 2018). While these analyses do not highlight meaningful differences between African Americans and indigenous people living in rural areas, they underline the intersectional disadvantage of not being white plus living in a rural area as it relates to poverty and age (Ponicki et al., 2018).

Other studies have drawn attention to the challenges inherent in attempts to capture drinking patterns in rural sub-populations using quantitative methods. Early epidemiological research on alcohol use among rural American Indians/Alaska Natives has long found higher prevalence of AUD compared to nearly all other ethnic groups. Yet later studies found that early studies over-estimated alcohol use and under-counted abstinence due to limited sampling and thus failed to capture the immense diversity between and within indigenous communities (Beals et al., 2009). People living on rural American Indian/Alaska Native reservations have commented that studies reliant on treatment facility data overestimate AUD prevalence and are an inaccurate guide for estimating drinking in the community (Lee et al., 2018). Moreover, in communities that have experienced dispossession and impoverishment for generations, limitations in housing could increase the visibility of problem drinking, thus increasing the perceived prevalence of AUD (Beals et al., 2009).

Research on alcohol use in rural settings illuminates the role that the social determinants of health play in alcohol problems, including poverty, structural racism, and other social dislocations. Growing societal wealth is typically accompanied by increased alcohol consumption. Yet it is people living in poverty who are disproportionately affected by alcohol use, even though alcohol abstinence may be more common and patterns of alcohol consumption are not significantly different compared to people not living at poverty level (Mulia et al, 2009; Schmidt et al., 2010). Socioeconomic inequities put people at risk for AUD via community environments that facilitate high exposures to alcohol and myriad sources of stress. At the same time, inequities exacerbate the consequences of having an AUD by deepening the negative social effects (e.g., criminalization, loss of secure jobs) and increasing barriers to recovery (e.g., lower quality healthcare options, treatment costs) (Mulia et al, 2009; Schmidt et al., 2010).

Recent research has charted a rise in "deaths of despair" among white, non-Hispanic, middle aged, especially rural, people (Case & Deaton, 2015). Situating the declining mortality in this group in the current social-economic context, economists Case and Deaton argued that the decline of stable, high-quality jobs for white, non-college educated people – particularly in rural areas – and subsequent downward mobility leads to "despair" that is evident through a rise in deaths from alcohol-induced cirrhosis, poisonings from alcohol and other drug overdose, and suicide. The deaths produce declines in social support in sparsely populated rural communities, compounding despair, thus limiting the capacity of families and communities to recover. Most research on "deaths of despair" has highlighted opioids as the key substance even though rural deaths from alcohol grew between 2000 and 2018, among both men and women (Spencer et al., 2020).

"Deaths of despair" scholarship has brought substance use among rural whites to the fore, in part because it portended political shifts among rural whites that shaped Donald Trump's 2016 election as president (Goldman et al., 2019). This narrative may, however, minimize the persistently deep health inequities affecting rural people of color that often is obscured in national datasets. Research along the Texas-Mexico border, for instance, links AUD and binge drinking in rural *colonia* settlements to the boom and bust cycles driven by the passage of 1994 North Atlantic Free Trade Agreement and a subsequent regional recession impacting maquiladora factories and communities throughout the area. Amid economic challenges, these rural communities lacked an older generation to support families through the stress, and strong community institutions like churches and city government were absent (Spence & Wallisch, 2007).

Qualitative studies conducted among rural youth highlight how substance use is a reaction to the dismal economic prospects of their communities (Boyd et al., 2009; Gordon et al., 2011; Willging et al., 2014). Feminist approaches to substance use draw attention to the social institutions and gendered power relationships that shape alcohol use (Travis, 2019). Research on rural Black women in the South reveals how alcohol use responds to a paucity of social opportunities, violence, and persistent marginalization resulting in "self-alienation" (Boyd & Mackey, 2000; Boyd et al., 2009).

More recent accounts focus on alcohol use alongside other substances that are more heavily criminalized, illuminating the emotional fallout of historic poverty, domestic colonialism, and dispossession that influence substance use in Appalachia, rural American Indian reservations and Pueblos in the West, and northern New Mexico (Buer, 2020; Garcia, 2010; Radin et al., 2015; Lee et al., 2018). These studies directly confront the structural violence and inward-directed personal violence that lead to and sustain alcohol and substance use. Attention to alcohol use has receded to the background as researchers focus on opioids and methamphetamines, and shifting drug markets have changed patterns of substance use and related premature deaths.

Increasingly, research on rural alcohol use acknowledges its impact on community life (Radin et al., 2015). In such contexts, families form the most critical sites of caring for people with substance use, even as alcohol use is understood to restrict family members' ability to care for one another (Garcia, 2010). Yet multiple accounts of alcohol use in rural families reveal the tension between consuming alcohol to belong in relationships and acknowledging its destructive effects (Novins et al., 2012). Family members note tensions between not "turning your back on your family," and the potential for "enabling" or denying alcohol problems (Radin et al., 2015).

The criminalization of drinking and drug use becomes a tool through which local officials identify rural community members as "unfit" parents, mandating their participation in (often punitive) treatment and removing their children (Buer, 2020; Garcia, 2010). While alcohol is not criminalized to the same extent as other substances, some research indicates that alcohol-related incarceration is more common than treatment (Feldstein et al., 2006). This is especially the case for rural American Indians living on reservations, where alcohol laws are stricter and residents endure persistent healthcare shortages. This criminalization of AUD can result in a loss of eligibility for tribal employment and subsequent loss of family income, impacting multiple people within the community (Lee et al., 2018).

The past 20 years have seen a gradual shift in rural alcohol research from rural-urban comparisons to an explicit engagement with the inequities that lead to alcohol consumption and increase its harms. This shift necessarily confronts the ethnic and racial diversity that characterizes rural communities across the United States (Lee & Sharp, 2017) and is responsive to calls for research to be driven by community-based, participatory approaches. This expands opportunities for theorizing about rural alcohol use (with Lee et al., 2018 as a model) to follow the explosion of theoretical work on rural disparities in opioid use and treatment in the wake of the US opioid epidemic.

Increasing Alcohol Treatment Availability in Rural Communities

Rural treatment researchers have argued that limited treatment capacity severely limits the ability of rural people to adequately sustain treatment engagement and to choose a program that meets their specific needs (Booth et al., 2000). The immense barriers that rural people face to receiving treatment likely contribute to the increased severity of their AUD (Booth et al., 2000). A US federal "parity" law in 2008 sought to bring care for AUD and other behavioral health problems into the mainstream of the US medical care system by requiring parity in coverage. The impact of the federal parity law, however, was mostly felt in states that had already implemented parity laws on their own and did not systematically vary by the degree of rurality across states (Mulia et al., 2019). Then, in 2010, the US Affordable Care Act (ACA) dramatically expanded Medicaid, mandated employers to offer insurance, created health insurance exchanges with subsidies for low-income people, and included other reforms that expanded coverage (Barry & Huskamp, 2011). State governors, however, were allowed to turn down expansions in Medicaid, which disproportionately affected rural populations, leading to a growing sense of white, rural resentment (Mulligan & Castañeda, 2017). Current efforts by the Republican party to repeal the ACA could significantly worsen access to care in rural areas and accelerate "deaths of despair" (Friedmann et al., 2017).

Perhaps the most important shift in rural access to care has been a push to offer AUD treatment in primary care settings over the past two decades (Young et al., 2018). Increasingly, alcohol treatment has been guided by a public health orientation focused on expanding access to treatment to a broader group of people and creating a continuum of care to connect a fragmented treatment landscape (Babor et al., 2007). Primary care-based treatment for substance use problems has been enabled by new clinical interventions and policy developments. While stand-alone specialty treatment previously predominated among treatment options, now pharmacotherapy and "medication-assisted treatments" (MAT) for AUD are available (Bensley et al., 2019; Edmonds et al., 2020). In addition, effective brief screening tools have been developed that are suitable for primary care engagement, and brief psychosocial interventions have been developed that can be delivered in primary care settings. One such innovation was the Screening, Brief Intervention, and Referral to Treatment (SBIRT) tool, a stepped care intervention that uses screening to identify level of need and assigns patients to a brief intervention, a longer multi-session treatment to be delivered in primary care settings, or referral to intensive specialist treatment (Babor et al., 2007). Comparative studies of brief alcohol interventions and referral to treatment in real-world settings have shown lasting benefits, and additional "booster" sessions can increase reductions in alcohol use (Gryczynski et al., 2011).

MAT and SBIRT are more feasible interventions to implement in low-resource rural settings than the traditional behavioral, psychotherapy, and 12 Step-oriented treatments. Locating rural AUD treatment capacity in primary care settings bypasses the persistent rural shortages in specialty providers across all fields of behavioral health (Lambert et al., 1999). New funding streams created by the ACA have supported the shift from specialty treatment settings to primary care settings. The ACA included substantial investments in federally qualified health centers (FQHCs), now one of the predominant types of primary care organizations in rural settings. FQHCs have proven well positioned to expand options for AUD treatment. Policies that grant FQHCs access to special drug pricing have enabled them to offer pharmacotherapy that might otherwise not have been possible, resulting in a quality of care comparable to specialty care (Substance Abuse and Mental Health Services Administration & Office of the Surgeon General, 2016). States that did not expand Medicaid – and are more likely to have higher rural and small-town populations – instead tended to provide more support for treatment interventions in criminal justice settings (McCarty, 2019).

Despite the changes associated with the ACA, national studies continue to show that rural people are less likely to receive evidence-based AUD treatments than urban people (Edmonds et al., 2020). Rural people experiencing intersectional disadvantages experience additional barriers, including women, American Indians, and those living in the most remote areas. Women with substance use disorders (including AUD) who live in rural counties have 90 percent lower odds of obtaining treatment than similar women in urban settings. This is primarily due to the challenges of finding transportation, a lack of treatment options, and long program waitlists (Ali et al., 2020). In isolated and American Indian reservation areas, many people seeking alcohol treatment are challenged by primary care access and therefore are significantly less likely to receive treatment (Davis et al., 2016). AUD medications are still used less in rural settings (Bensley et al., 2019; Edmonds et al., 2020). There is an appalling dearth of research on MAT delivery for AUD across rural primary care sites, especially in states that did not expand Medicaid. While screening for harmful substance use now occurs for almost three-quarters of rural patients, less than half receive follow-up care, with an even lower proportions (13.6 percent) receiving follow-up in small and isolated rural settings (Chan et al., 2016).

Barriers to Expanding AUD Treatment in Rural Communities

Researchers bemoan the fact that effective implementation strategies to increase AUD treatment access have not yet been identified (Williams et al., 2019). The particular challenges of implementing AUD treatments in rural settings, particularly through primary care, are discussed next.

Screening

Increased screening in primary care settings is seen as a critical strategy for identifying rural people in need of treatment, and many studies underscore the challenges of reaching some groups. Providers and patients across the age spectrum agree that computer-based screening would enable patients to overcome fears of stigma, thus allowing for a fuller disclosure of alcohol use (Saunders et al., 2019; Gordon et al., 2011). Yet less research has explored how screening in rural communities can address culturally variable thresholds of drinking that are perceived to constitute a problem in need of treatment and ascertain whether such thresholds need to be higher in rural areas (e.g., Broffman et al., 2017; Radin et al., 2015). Additional considerations pertain to the ethics of screening vulnerable populations (e.g., African American women facing violence) for whom identifying alcohol use may be intertwined with uncovering sensitive domestic circumstances (Boyd et al., 2009) that expose patients' personal challenges within tight-knit rural communities.

Training

Historically, there has been limited funding for behavioral health training for rural providers (Pullen & Oser, 2014). Recent public health efforts to respond to the opioid crisis have resulted in a number of system-level initiatives to build ongoing training and support for addiction treatment among rural providers (e.g., Hub & Spoke, ECHO), although the focus has been on opioid treatment, not AUD treatment (Komaromy et al., 2016). This infrastructure has not translated into increased confidence among rural providers in offering AUD treatment. Although AUD pharmacotherapy is technically feasible for primary care settings, many rural providers feel unsure about offering it, lack the support staff to facilitate medication management, and remain convinced of the need for oversight from specialty addictions providers (Saunders et al., 2019; Young et al., 2018). Rural primary care teams may consequently feel that they lack the training to provide these treatments, and their patients perceive this discomfort, making it more challenging to raise concerns (Saunders et al., 2019).

Encounters with Providers and Patients

Several studies noted how challenges in establishing relationships between rural providers and patients can obstruct the trust necessary to address sensitive issues involving alcohol use (Gordon et al., 2011; Saunders et al., 2019). Some studies of rural people who drink or are at-risk for AUD suggest that patients fear that their privacy will be breached in primary care settings (Gordon et al., 2011; Radin et al., 2015). Less acknowledged are the ways that bias and racism shape rural primary care interactions around treatment. One study of rural New Mexico highlighted providers' cultural stereotypes about Latinos; some providers viewed families as responsible for socializing their children about alcohol and suggested that a "culture of poverty" could be passed along generationally, affecting alcohol use in offspring (Quintero et al., 2007). Training must encourage providers to acknowledge how racism can influence their interpretation of patients' substance use and encourage respect for community strengths as resources for recovery (Quintero et al., 2007).

Continuum of Care

SBIRT is a stepped care model with referral to treatment as the highest level of care, yet numerous studies underscore the challenges of establishing a continuum of care for alcohol treatment in rural settings. Rural dwellers often have to leave the community for in-patient intensive treatment, detoxification facilities, and sober housing (Lee et al., 2018; Radin et al., 2015). Rural treatment centers deliver fewer wrap-around services and fewer specialty treatment options tailored to specific populations (Edmond et al., 2015). The need to travel to distant cities to receive specialty care can make it challenging for rural patients' family members to provide support, due to limitations on transportation and other resources (Lee et al., 2018). The lack of referral options puts the onus on rural primary care providers to offer all levels of follow-up care even when they feel they are insufficiently trained to do so (Gordon et al., 2011; Young et al., 2018). Without the complete network of needed providers, rural patients may face breaks in their care (Pullen & Oser, 2014), struggle to maintain recovery after discharge (Radin et al., 2015), or experience harsh alternatives like jail when there is no detoxification facility available (Lee et al., 2018). Researchers have recommended offering coordinating councils between counties to comprehensively link resources across jurisdictions (Browne et al., 2016).

Telemedicine

Telemedicine has long been imagined as a strategy to overcome provider shortages, hesitancy about confidentiality in provider interactions, and the transportation barriers that keep rural people from engaging in AUD treatment (Davis et al., 2016; Pullen & Oser, 2014). Telemedicine could facilitate a continuum of care by connecting primary care providers to specialty providers when acute care is needed and connecting providers to hard-to-reach populations. Telemedicine technology could further enable rural practices to efficiently use their personnel, increasing the time available to see patients remotely by obviating the need for providers to commute between clinics (Browne et al., 2016). Remote providers of telemedicine services may remove the fear of confidentiality breaches, thereby offering the potential to explore sensitive issues that may be related to alcohol use (Marsch & Dallery, 2012).

Nevertheless, telemedicine is less available for AUD treatment than many other forms of care, particularly because of regulations that have mandated in-person care to dispense AUD medications (Huskamp et al., 2018). In 2020, loosened federal restrictions on telemedicine enabled a vast expansion to limit the spread of COVID-19. However, rural primary care providers lack standard protocols for identifying which patients can benefit from telemedicine and strategies for initiating relationships with new patients remotely (e.g., Shore et al., 2018). Many people living in rural areas lack the broadband internet connectivity required to engage in telemedicine care (Browne et al., 2016). Increased access to broadband internet is essential to prevent the current expansion of telehealth from deepening disparities in access to care.

Lessons from Efforts to Expand Primary Care Opioid Use Disorder (OUD) Treatment

As rural communities have struggled to address rising rates of OUD since 2000, public health professionals have invested significantly in training and technical support to primary care providers to offer medication for OUD in primary care settings. Some primary care providers have argued that such efforts have made substance use screening more of a priority (Saunders et al., 2019). Evidence suggests that attention to opioid use has eclipsed awareness of other substance use in rural areas, particularly among policymakers (Woodruff & Roberts, 2019). Efforts to expand AUD treatment capacity in primary care could build upon the inter-organizational relationships and technical assistance provided for OUD treatment (Cole et al., 2019; Department of Health and Human Services, Health Resources, and Services Administration, 2018). The scale of research on rural primary care capacity for AUD treatment (screening, brief interventions, and pharmacotherapy) is dwarfed by that on OUD treatment, and there is comparatively little understanding of what will be needed to expand AUD treatment in rural areas.

Alcohol Treatment in the Community

In rural settings, which typically are already beset with healthcare disparities, it is imperative that interventions centrally address the socioeconomic context (e.g., Schmidt et al., 2010), building on the tight social networks in rural communities to facilitate social support-driven intervention strategies (Booth et al., 2000). Rural American Indian communities in particular have been leaders in developing community-driven alcohol treatment and prevention strategies (Brave Heart et al., 2011; Kelley et al., 2018; Lee et al., 2018; Radin et al., 2015). Some promising possibilities to respond to alcohol problems in rural communities are highlighted below.

Treatment through Carceral Systems

Alcohol treatment systems are deeply intertwined with criminal justice and social service systems (Weisner & Schmidt, 2001). People in rural areas on probation, those charged for crimes, and particularly for a DUI, are more likely to receive alcohol treatment (Booth et al., 2000). Mechanisms such as "drug courts" that can mandate treatment for offenders as an alternative to incarceration have become more common across the United States, but not in many rural areas. While treatment mandates can successfully link individuals to treatment, they do not automatically result in successful treatment outcomes because personal motivations often make more of a difference (Broffman et al., 2017). While the use of jails has declined in urban areas over the past ten years, rural jail populations have grown (Kang-Brown & Subramanian, 2017). Programs for diversion (from jail or prison to treatment) have become common in urban areas, but much less so in rural areas (Kang-Brown & Subramanian, 2017). Until trends in rural incarceration change, primary care providers located in jails should be trained to offer pharmacotherapy and brief interventions.

Policy Interventions to Prevent AUD

Policy interventions that limit access to alcohol through taxation, bans, and by regulating alcohol sales have been shown to be extremely effective in reducing alcohol consumption and, therefore, AUD rates at the population level (Babor, 2018). Such interventions may use community leaders to mobilize awareness of the consequences of community-level alcohol use and generate strategies to confront the selective marketing of alcohol, such as limiting the location of alcohol sales through zoning and enforcing statutes on public drunkenness. US-based research has shown the salutary impact of stronger alcohol policies in controlling dangerous alcohol use like binge drinking, youth drinking, and in curbing cirrhosis, but there is a need for more in-depth research explorations of rural jurisdictions, which have distinct patterns of policy implementation (e.g., Showalter, 2020). Research on rural health departments shows that their limited resources hamper their capacity for new policy development (Harris et al., 2016).

Studies exploring the regulation of alcohol on rural tribal lands found that policies punishing alcohol users (e.g., for DUIs) are more commonly enforced than those punishing vendors (e.g., sales restrictions) (Lee et al., 2018). Some tribal communities are reluctant to enforce regulations on alcohol bootleggers because of the impact this has on relationships within close-knit communities (Lee et al., 2018). Some rural counties in the United States have employed alcohol prohibition policies that limit the sale or even possession of alcohol. But evidence indicates that these policies have often led to increased drinking in neighboring counties and drinking-driving (Keyes, 2017), substitution of illicit drugs for alcohol, and decreased local tax revenues (Keyes, 2017; Lee et al., 2018). Ensuring that some community spaces and events remain free of alcohol can be important both for shifting community norms about drinking and restricting access to minors (Kelley et al., 2018; Palombi et al., 2019). Given their diversity, rural communities must generate their own decisions using local data (Lee et al., 2018).

Peer Approaches and Self-Help Groups

Alcoholics Anonymous (AA) is the most commonly used peer approach for AUD, but may be best used to extend clinical treatment rather than substitute for it (Weisner & Schmidt, 2001). Research has not systematically examined the delivery of AA in rural areas and evaluated its outcomes, although some evidence indicates that rural people face substantially higher barriers to engaging in AA. The barriers are familiar ones: long distances to reach groups, a shortage of groups offered, challenges to anonymity in small communities, and a lack of options for tailored support (such as single-gender, sexual, and gender minorities) (Browne et al., 2016). For rural women in particular, especially women of color experiencing violence and racism, AA's core tenets of surrender and powerlessness may seem oppressive (Boyd et al., 2005).

Other peer models may respond to the unique challenges of rural populations (Boyd et al., 2005). While community health workers or *promotoras* are not widely used in substance use treatment, they may be appropriate for linking low-income and underinsured rural communities to alcohol treatment by addressing key logistical barriers (Spence & Wallisch, 2007). Some rural community evidence suggests that building a new peer network is key for recovery, especially when it links people with shared cultural practices or experiences of marginalization (Palombi et al., 2019; Willging et al., 2018). Peer interventions may also focus on the self-advocacy of rural marginalized people within existing treatment systems where their needs are often misunderstood or ignored, such as those who are LGBTQ (Willging et al., 2018).

As with other health personnel in rural areas, retention is a key challenge to sustaining peer-driven interventions (Boyd et al., 2005); this can be addressed through building career ladders and improved pay. Moreover, peers may not share all aspects of lived experience; for instance, gender and sexual minorities in rural communities face challenges to overcoming their own feelings of stigma (Willging et al., 2018). Optimally, peer interventions should bolster, not substitute for, rural behavioral health systems that anchor continua of care (Willging et al., 2018).

Addressing Historic Oppression

A large body of research centering on rural American Indian communities stresses the need for community leadership in culturally tailoring or prioritizing prevention messages (Kelley et al., 2018). In rural American Indian/Alaska Native communities where alcohol use has emerged from historical trauma, interventions should centrally address grief and employ culturally specific sources of healing, such as sweat lodges (Brave Heart et al., 2011; Lee et al., 2018). Locating treatment within community rather than in healthcare settings can increase their cultural relevance and distance care from conventional clinical hierarchies (Radin et al., 2015; Willging et al., 2018). Interventions that have been centered on American Indian culture are efficacious for alcohol cessation, particularly when they integrate traditional spirituality and practices (Torres Stone et al., 2006). There is limited attention, however, to implementation strategies for scaling up funding and appropriate personnel, as well as community partnerships that identify the culturally specific forms of resilience and histories of marginalization that treatment efforts must address.

Economic Inequality

Rural alcohol use and problems are linked to the socioeconomic contexts of rural communities where opportunities for economic advancement and social mobility may be dim (Broffman et al., 2017). Rural programs must thus address employment insecurity and educational limitations (Quintero et al., 2007), including rural childcare disparities that limit women's employment. However, by and large, there are limited strategies for integrating economic opportunities into alcohol interventions for rural communities. Research on the next generation of policy interventions must examine the mechanisms that can have the greatest impact on rural alcohol use, AUD treatment, and recovery.

Conclusions and Recommendations

Increasingly, research demonstrates the historic challenges and inequities that shape how alcohol is used across diverse rural communities. Passage of the ACA has expanded access to treatment, and effective new AUD treatment strategies hold promise for rural access, including MAT and SBIRT. In particular, strategies for delivering alcohol treatment through primary care providers holds dramatic potential for making care accessible to people living in rural areas. But significant changes need to be made to expand training, create acceptable screening tools for rural populations, adjust patient-provider interactions to privacy concerns, and increase the capacity for telemedicine in ways that repair considerable tears and gaps in the continuum of care. Investing in community-based interventions is necessary to address the root causes of rural alcohol disparities. Newly developed peer and culturally grounded interventions can mitigate the longstanding inaccessibility and deficiencies of clinically-based AUD treatment in rural communities. Despite some advances in recent years, there is a paucity of evidence on policy and economic interventions that can be effective in rural areas to address alcohol problems and the unique elements of rural environments.

Acknowledgments

This work was supported by US National Institute on Drug Abuse award R21 DA046051 and UL1 TR001872 from the US National Center for Advancing Translational Sciences.

References

Ali, M. M., Nye, E., & West, K. (2020). Substance use disorder treatment, perceived seed for treatment, and barriers to treatment among parenting women with substance use disorder in US rural counties. *The Journal of Rural Health*. https://doi.org/10.1111/jrh.12488

Babor, T. F. (2018). Effective policy measures to reduce alcohol-related harm: An update of the book, "Alcohol: No ordinary commodity." *Alcoholism: Clinical and Experimental Research, 42,*85A. https://doi.org/10.1111/j.1360-0443.2010.02945.x

Babor, T. F., McRee, B. G., Kassebaum, P. A., Grimaldi, P. L., Ahmed, K., & Bray, J. (2007). Screening, brief intervention, and referral to treatment (SBIRT): Toward a public health approach to the management of substance abuse. *Substance Abuse, 28*(3), 7–30. https://doi.org/10.1300/J465v28n03_03

Barry, C. L. & Huskamp, H. A. (2011). Moving beyond parity—mental health and addiction care under the ACA. *The New England Journal of Medicine, 365* (11), 973. https://doi.org/10.1056/NEJMp1108649

Beals, J., Belcourt-Dittloff, A., Freedenthal, S., Kaufman, C., Mitchell, C., Whitesell, N., Albright, K., Beauvais, F., Belcourt, G., Duran, B., Fleming, C., Floersch, N., Foley, K., Jervis, L., Kipp, B. J., Mail, P., Manson, S., May, P., Mohatt, G., & Walters, K. (2009). Reflections on a proposed theory of reservation-dwelling American Indian alcohol use: Comment on Spillane and Smith (2007). *Psychological Bulletin, 135*(2), 339–343. https://doi.org/10.1037/a0014819

Bensley, K. M., Fortney, J., Chan, G., Dombrowski, J. C., Ornelas, I., Rubinsky, A. D., Lapham, G. T., Glass, J. E., & Williams, E. C. (2019). Differences in receipt of alcohol-related care across rurality among VA patients living with HIV with unhealthy alcohol use. *Journal of Rural Health, 35*(3), 341–353. https://doi.org/10.1111/jrh.12345

Booth, B. M., Kirchner, J., Fortney, J., Ross, R., & Rost, K. (2000). Rural at-risk drinkers: Correlates and one-year use of alcoholism treatment services. *Journal of Studies on Alcohol, 61*(2), 267–277. https://doi.org/10.15288/jsa.2000.61.267

Borders, T. F., & Booth, B. M. (2007). Rural, suburban, and urban variations in alcohol consumption in the United States: Findings from the national epidemiologic survey on alcohol and related conditions. *Journal of Rural Health, 23*(4), 314–321. https://doi.org/10.1111/j.1748-0361.2007.00109.x

Boyd, M. R., Berger, K. C., Baliko, B., & Tavakoli, A. (2009). Predictors of alcohol and drug problems in rural African American women. *Issues in Mental Health Nursing, 30*(6), 383–391. https://doi.org/10.1080/01612840802509478

Boyd, M. R., & Mackey, M. C. (2000). Alienation from self and others: The psychosocial problem of rural alcoholic women. *Archives of Psychiatric Nursing, 14*(3), 134–141. https://doi.org/10.1053/py.2000.6383

Boyd, M. R., Moneyham, L., Murdaugh, C., Phillips, K. D., Tavakoli, A., Jackwon, K., Jackson, N., & Vyavaharkar, M. (2005). A peer-based substance abuse intervention for HIV+ rural women: A pilot study. *Archives of Psychiatric Nursing, 19*(1), 10–17. https://doi.org/10.1016/j.apnu.2004.11.002

Brave Heart, M. Y. H., Chase, J., Elkins, J., & Altschul, D. B. (2011). Historical trauma among indigenous peoples of the Americas: Concepts, research, and clinical considerations. *Journal of Psychoactive Drugs*, *43*(4), 282–290. https://doi.org/10.1080/02791072.2011.628913

Broffman, L., Spurlock, M., Dulacki, K., Campbell, A., Rodriguez, F., Wright, B., McConnell, K. J., Warne, D., & Davis, M. M. (2017). Understanding treatment gaps for mental health, alcohol, and drug use in South Dakota: A qualitative study of rural perspectives. *Journal of Rural Health, 33*(1), 71–81. https://doi.org/10.1111/jrh.12167

Browne, T., Priester, M. A., Clone, S., Iachini, A., DeHart, D., & Hock, R. (2016). Barriers and facilitators to substance use treatment in the rural south: A qualitative study. *The Journal of Rural Health, 32*(1), 92–101. https://doi.org/10.1111/jrh.12129

Buer, L. (2020). *RX Appalachia: Stories of treatment and survival in rural Kentucky*. Haymarket Books.

Case, A., & Deaton, A. (2015). Rising morbidity and mortality in midlife among white non-Hispanic Americans in the 21st century. *Proceedings of the National Academy of Sciences of the United States of America, 112*(49), 15078–15083. https://doi.org/10.1073/pnas.1518393112

Chan, Y. F., Lu, S. E., Howe, B., Tieben, H., Hoeft, T., & Unützer, J. (2016). Screening and follow-up monitoring for substance use in primary care: An exploration of rural–urban variations. *Journal of General Internal Medicine, 31*(2), 215–222. https://doi.org/10.1007/s11606–015-3488-y

Davis, M. M., Spurlock, M., Dulacki, K., Meath, T., Li, H. F. G., McCarty, D., Warne, D., Wright, B., & McConnell, K. J. (2016). Disparities in alcohol, drug use, and mental health condition prevalence and access to care in rural, isolated, and reservation areas: Findings from the South Dakota health survey. *Journal of Rural Health, 32*(3). https://doi.org/10.1111/jrh.12157

Department of Health and Human Services, Health Resources, and Services Administration (2018). *HRSA's home visiting program: Supporting families impacted by opioid use and neonatal abstinence syndrome*. US Department of Health and Human Services. https://mchb.hrsa.gov/sites/default/files/mchb/MaternalChildHealthInitiatives/HomeVisiting/MIECHV-Opioid-NAS-Resource.pdf

Dixon, M. A., & Chartier, K. G. (2016). Alcohol use patterns among urban and rural residents: Demographic and social influences. *Alcohol Research: Current Reviews*, *38*(1), 69–77. www.ncbi.nlm.nih.gov/pmc/articles/PMC4872615/

Edmond, M. B., Aletraris, L., & Roman, P. M. (2015). Rural substance use treatment centers in the United States: An assessment of treatment quality by location. *American Journal of Drug and Alcohol Abuse, 41*(5), 449–457. https://doi.org/10.3109/00952990.2015.1059842

Edmonds, A. T., Bensley, K. M., Hawkins, E. J., & Williams, E. C. (2020). Geographic differences in receipt of addictions treatment in a national sample of patients with alcohol use disorders from the US Veterans Health Administration. *Substance Abuse*. https://doi.org/10.1080/08897077.2020.1803176

Feldstein, S. W., Venner, K. L., & May, P. A. (2006). American Indian/Alaska Native alcohol-related incarceration and treatment. *American Indian and Alaska Native*

Mental Health Research (Online), 13(3), 1–22. https://doi.org/10.5820/aian.1303.2006.1

Friedmann, P. D., Andrews, C. M., & Humphreys, K. (2017). How ACA repeal would worsen the opioid epidemic. *New England Journal of Medicine, 376*(10), e16. https://doi.org/10.1056/NEJMp1700834

Garcia, A. (2010). *The pastoral clinic: Addiction and dispossession along the Rio Grande*. University of California Press.

Goldman, L., Lim, M. P., Chen, Q., Jin, P., Muennig, P., & Vagelos, A. (2019). Independent relationship of changes in death rates with changes in US presidential voting. *Journal of General Internal Medicine, 34*(3), 363–371. https://doi.org/10.1007/s11606–018-4568-6

Gordon, A. J., Ettaro, L., Rodriguez, K. L., Mocik, J., & Clark, D. B. (2011). Provider, patient, and family perspectives of adolescent alcohol use and treatment in rural settings. *Journal of Rural Health, 27*(1), 81–90. https://doi.org/10.1111/j.1748-0361.2010.00321.x

Gryczynski, J., Mitchell, S. G., Peterson, T. R., Gonzales, A., Moseley, A., & Schwartz, R. P. (2011). The relationship between services delivered and substance use outcomes in New Mexico's screening, brief intervention, referral and treatment (SBIRT) initiative. *Drug and Alcohol Dependence, 118*(2–3), 152–157. https://doi.org/10.1016/j.drugalcdep.2011.03.012

Harris, J. K., Beatty, K., Leider, J.P., Knudson, A., Anderson, B. L., & Meit, M. (2016). The double disparity facing rural local health departments. *Annual Review of Public Health, 37*(1), 167–84. https://doi.org/10.1146/annurev-publhealth-031914-122755

Hunt, G., & Barker, J. C. (2001). Socio-cultural anthropology and alcohol and drug research: Towards a unified theory. *Social Science and Medicine, 53*(2), 165–188. https://doi.org/10.1016/S0277–9536(00)00329-4

Huskamp, H. A., Busch, A. B., Souza, J., Uscher-Pines, L., Rose, S., Wilcock, A., Landon, B. E., & Mehrotra, A. (2018). How is telemedicine being used in opioid and other substance use disorder treatment? *Health Affairs, 37*(12), 1940–1947. https://doi.org/10.1377/hlthaff.2018.05134

Kang-Brown, J., & Subramanian, R. (2017). *Out of sight: The growth of jails in rural America*. Vera Institute on Justice.

Kelley, A., Fatupaito, B., & Witzel, M. (2018). Is culturally based prevention effective? Results from a 3-year tribal substance use prevention program. *Evaluation and Program Planning, 71*, 28–35. https://doi.org/10.1016/j.evalprogplan.2018.07.001

Keyes, S. (2017). *Alcohol prohibition in America is not over yet*. Pacific Standard. https://psmag.com/news/gin-and-tonic-hold-the-gin

Komaromy, M., Duhigg, D., Metcalf, A., Carlson, C., Kalishman, S., Hayes, L., Burke, T., Thornton, K., & Arora, S. (2016). Project ECHO (Extension for Community Healthcare Outcomes): A new model for educating primary care providers about treatment of substance use disorders. *Substance Abuse, 37*(1), 20–24. https://doi.org/10.1080/08897077.2015.1129388

Lambert, D., Agger, M., & Hartley, D. (1999). Service use of rural and urban Medicaid beneficiaries suffering from depression: The role of supply. *Journal of Rural Health, 15*(3), 344–355. https://doi.org/10.1111/j.1748-0361.1999.tb00756.x

Lee, B. A., & Sharp, G. (2017). Ethnoracial diversity across the rural-urban continuum. *Annals of the American Academy of Political and Social Science*, 672(1), 26–45. https://doi.org/10.1177%2F0002716217708560

Lee, J. P., Pagano, A., Moore, R. S., Tilsen, N., Henderson, J. A., Shell, A. I., Davids, S., LeBeaux, L., & Gruenewald, P. (2018). Impacts of alcohol availability on tribal lands where alcohol is prohibited: A community-partnered qualitative investigation. *International Journal of Drug Policy, 54*, 77–86. https://doi.org/10.1016/j.drugpo.2018.01.010

Marsch, L. A., & Dallery, J. (2012). Advances in the psychosocial treatment of addiction: The role of technology in the delivery of evidence-based psychosocial treatment. *Psychiatric Clinics of North America*. https://doi.org/10.1016/j.psc.2012.03.009

McCarty, D. (2019). A changing landscape for treatment of alcohol and drug use disorders. *American Journal of Public Health, 35*(2), 481–493. https://doi.org/10.2105/AJPH.2019.305080

Mulia, N., Lui, C. K., Ye, Y., Subbaraman, M. S., Kerr, W. C. & Greenfield, T. K. (2019). US alcohol treatment admissions after the Mental Health Parity and Addiction Equity Act: Do state parity laws and race/ethnicity make a difference? *Journal of Substance Abuse Treatment, 106*, 113–121. https://doi.org/10.1016/j.jsat.2019.08.008

Mulia, N., Ye, Y., Greenfield, T. K. & Zemore, S. E. (2009). Disparities in alcohol-related problems among White, Black, and Hispanic Americans. *Alcoholism: Clinical and Experimental Research, 33*(4), 654–662. https://doi.org/10.1111/j.1530-0277.2008.00880.x

Mulligan, J. M., & Castañeda, H. eds. (2017). *Unequal coverage: The experience of health care reform in the United States*. New York University Press. www.jstor.org/stable/j.ctt1pwtbzp

Novins, D. K., Spicer, P., Fickenscher, A., & Pescosolido, B. (2012). Pathways to care: Narratives of American Indian adolescents entering substance abuse treatment. *Social Science and Medicine, 74*(12), 2037–2045. https://doi.org/10.1016/j.socscimed.2012.02.004

Palombi, L., Hawthorne, A. N., Irish, A., Becher, E., & Bowen, E. (2019). "One out of ten ain't going to make it": An analysis of recovery capital in the rural upper midwest. *Journal of Drug Issues, 49*(4), 680–702. https://doi.org/10.1177/0022042619859309

Ponicki, W. R., Henderson, J. A., Gaidus, A., Gruenewald, P. J., Lee, J. P., Moore, R. S., Davids, S., & Tilsen, N. (2018). Spatial epidemiology of alcohol- and drug-related health problems among Northern Plains American Indians: Nebraska and South Dakota, 2007 to 2012. *Alcoholism: Clinical and Experimental Research, 42*(3), 578–588. https://doi.org/10.1111/acer.13580

Pullen, E., & Oser, C. (2014). Barriers to substance abuse treatment in rural and urban communities: Counselor perspectives. *Substance Use & Misuse, 49*(7), 891–901. https://doi.org/10.3109/10826084.2014.891615

Quintero, G. A., Lilliott, E., & Willging, C. (2007). Substance abuse treatment provider views of "culture": Implications for behavioral health care in rural settings. *Qualitative Health Research, 17*(9), 1256–1267. https://doi.org/10.1177/1049732307307757

Radin, S. M., Kutz, S. H., Marr, J. L., Vendiola, D., Vendiola, M., Wilbur, B., Thomas, L. R., & Donovan, D. M. (2015). Community perspectives on drug/alcohol use, concerns, needs, and resources in four Washington state tribal communities. *Journal of Ethnicity in Substance Abuse, 14*(1), 29–58. https://doi.org/10.1080/15332640.2014.947459

Saunders, E. C., Moore, S. K., Gardner, T., Farkas, S., Marsch, L. A., McLeman, B., Meier, A., Nesin, N., Rotrosen, J., Walsh, O., & McNeely, J. (2019). Screening for substance use in rural primary care: A qualitative study of providers and patients. *Journal of General Internal Medicine*, *34*(12), 2824–2832. https://doi.org/10.1007/s11606–019-05232-y

Schmidt, L. A., Makelia, P., Rehm, J., & Room, R. (2010). Alcohol: Equity and social determinants. In E. Blas & A. S. Kurup (Eds.), *Equity, social determinants, and public health programs* (pp. 11–30). World Health Organization.

Shore, J. H., Yellowlees, P., Caudill, R., Johnston, B., Turvey, C., Mishkind, M., Krupinski, E., Myers, K., Shore, P., Kaftarian, E., & Hilty, D. (2018). Best practices in videoconferencing-based tele mental health April 2018. *Telemedicine and E-Health, 24*(11), 827–832. https://doi.org/10.1089/tmj.2018.0237

Showalter, D. (2020). Steps toward a theory of place effects on drug use: Risk, marginality, and opportunity in small and remote California towns. *International Journal of Drug Policy, 85.*https://doi.org/10.1016/j.drugpo.2019.102629

Spence, R. T., & Wallisch, L. S. (2007). Alcohol and drug use in rural *colonias* and adjacent urban areas of the Texas border. *Journal of Rural Health, 23*(Suppl.), 55–60. https://doi.org/10.1111/j.1748-0361.2007.00124.x

Spencer, M. R., Curtin, S. C., & Hedegaard, H. (2020). *Rates of alcohol-induced deaths among adults aged 25 and over in urban and rural areas: United States, 2000–2018.* (NCHS Data Brief, No 383). US Department of Health and Human Services. www.cdc.gov/nchs/products/databriefs/db383.htm

Substance Abuse and Mental Health Services Administration & Office of the Surgeon General (2016). *Facing addiction in America: The surgeon general's report on alcohol, drugs, and health.* US Department of Health and Human Services. www.ncbi.nlm.nih.gov/books/NBK424848/

Torres Stone, R. A., Whitbeck, L. B., Chen, X., Johnson, K., & Olson, D. M. (2006). Traditional practices, traditional spirituality, and alcohol cessation among American Indians. *Journal of Studies on Alcohol, 67*(2), 236–244. https://doi.org/10.15288/jsa.2006.67.236

Travis, T. (2019). Toward a feminist history of the drug-using woman—and her recovery. *Feminist Studies, 45*(1), 209–233. https://doi.org/10.15767/feministstudies.45.1.0209

Weisner, C., & Schmidt, L. A. (2001). Rethinking access to alcohol treatment. In M. Galanter (ed.), *Recent developments in alcoholism — services research in the era of managed care, 15*, 107–136. New York: Kluwer Academic Publishers.

Willging, C. E., Harkness, A., Israel, T., Ley, D., Hokanson, P. S., DeMaria, C., Joplin, A., & Smiley, V. (2018). A mixed-method assessment of a pilot peer advocate intervention for rural gender and sexual minorities. *Community Mental Health Journal, 54*(4), 395–409. https://doi.org/10.1007/s10597–017-0168-x

Willging, C. E., Quintero, G. A., & Lilliott, E. A. (2014). Hitting the wall: Youth perspectives on boredom, trouble, and drug use dynamics in rural New Mexico. *Youth and Society, 46*(1), 3–29. https://doi.org/10.1177/0044118X11423231

Williams, E. C., Matson, T. E., & Harris, A. H. S. (2019). Strategies to increase implementation of pharmacotherapy for alcohol use disorders: A structured review of care delivery and implementation interventions. *Addiction Science & Clinical Practice, 14*(6). https://doi.org/10.1186/s13722–019-0134-8

Woodruff, K., & Roberts, S. C. M. (2019). "Alcohol during pregnancy? Nobody does that anymore": State legislators' use of evidence in making policy on alcohol use in pregnancy. *Journal of Studies on Alcohol and Drugs, 80*(3), 380–388. https://doi.org/10.15288/jsad.2019.80.380

Young, J. P., Achtmeyer, C. E., Bensley, K. M., Hawkins, E. J., & Williams, E. C. (2018). Differences in perceptions of and practices regarding treatment of alcohol use disorders among VA primary care providers in urban and rural clinics. *The Journal of Rural Health, 34*(4), 359–68. https://doi.org/10.1111/jrh.12293

18 Recovery, Communities, and the Organized Recovery Movement

Robert D. Ashford

Recovery, Communities, and the Organized Recovery Movement

Substance use, misuse, and disorders have been a continuous point of scientific, political, and community discourse in the United States, ranging as far back as the Puritanical leaders of the Massachusetts Bay Colony in the 1600s (Influence and Cotton Mather) and their focus on the moral implications of intoxicant use (Barrows & Room, 1991). While the conversation about the impact and importance of substance use continues in the modern era, it has decidedly evolved past moral relativism, with substance use disorders (SUD) now accurately depicted not as moral failings, but as a medical condition requiring treatment and support across a continuum of care (Jellinek, 1960; Leshner, 1997). However, as it concerns recovery, and perhaps even the accepted etiology of SUD, the roots of past historical understanding are not so easily forgotten.

In the United States, the fusion of medical science and psychology began to shape definitions of chronic inebriation as a biological and psychological problem in the early 1900s. William James and Carl Jung introduced "moral psychology" (Finlay, 2000) into the scientific discourse, almost as a treatise between the moral prohibitionists of the growing temperance movement and the medical and psychological sciences. It is no wonder that traditional recovery processes, achieved through mutual aid, still hold the middle line between a "spiritual malady" and the disease model of SUD (Kurtz, 2002). Mutual aid is very much a reflection of the intersection of forces that have historically shaped the American view of SUD and recovery (White, 1998). This paradigm of mutual aid recovery, with community-based groups such as Alcoholics Anonymous (AA), is still dominant in the United States and elsewhere (Donovan et al., 2013; see Tonigan Chapter 6). However, concurrent with our growing understanding of SUD, so too has our understanding of recovery grown, and the manifestations of that knowledge within the community have continued to evolve in recent decades.

Over the past 20 years there has been a surge of empirical knowledge about SUD and recovery from SUD. Recent trends have established recovery as the keystone in organizing paradigms related to systems of care, research endeavors, public policy, and the social organizing of communities with a shared identity and lived experience – i.e., the recovery community (Brown & Ashford, 2019). It is important to note that such shared identities and lived experience extend past a personal identity as "in recovery" and include those directly and indirectly affected, such as family members and loved ones, friends, allies, etc. It is this collective community of individuals across a spectrum of shared experiences and identities who have, and continue to, organize themselves into the recovery community. These developments have resulted in a shift in the foundational understanding of the recovery phenomenon, the creation of new recovery support mechanisms and institutions, and in many cases, ushered in new levels of public and private support for individuals who have SUD or are living in recovery (i.e., those actively engaged and identifying as within the recovery process). It is this last point – the increasing support of the public and private sectors of society for those with SUD or who are living in recovery – that has likely supported the emerging organized recovery community more than anything else.

Conceptualizing Recovery

Recovery, best viewed not only as a process but as a shared identity amongst individuals and collective communities, is useful as an organizing construct for research (Brown & Ashford, 2019), policy (Laudet & Humphreys, 2013), and for community and social mobilization (White, 2005). Recent efforts to define recovery have been numerous, with the most recent and salient perhaps being from the Recovery Science Research Collaborative (RSRC) that defined recovery as "an individualized, intentional, dynamic, and relational process involving sustained efforts to improve wellness" (p. 183; Ashford et al., 2019a). This definition views recovery as both dynamic (i.e., ever changing) and relational (i.e., involving connections and community). The framework has served as a galvanizing call to action within community settings and given rise to community-based participatory research efforts (Ashford et al., 2019a), organized policy advocacy agendas through the New Recovery Advocacy Movement (N-RAM; White, 2007), and community-based direct services such as recovery community organizations (Ashford et al., 2019b). Recovery and community are thus inexorably linked, with advances for the benefit of individuals in recovery and living with SUD being directly associated with the evolution of organized recovery within, by, and for the community itself.

Creations of and for the Recovery Community

As mentioned, recovery and its relationship to the community serve an identity in which individuals and community stakeholders can organize around socially or politically, which has led to the development of central elements of the organized recovery community. These include direct services and direct service models (e.g., recovery-oriented systems of care and recovery support services), academic inquiry concerning the recovery process and outcomes (e.g., recovery science), and recovery-informed policy and advocacy. Each of these elements has a synergistic effect with individual recovery outcomes and also contributes to further support and grow of the size and impact of the organized recovery community itself.

Recovery-Oriented Systems of Care

The recovery-oriented systems of care (ROSC) model and framework was designed and largely influenced by the efforts of the recovery community to support geographic communities in the coordination of services supporting recovery from SUD (Davidson & White, 2007; DiClemente et al., 2016; White, 2009). Davidson and White (2007) described the guiding principles of ROSC as: (1) recovery looks different for different individuals; (2) interventions and resources should be matched to where an individual is in their recovery process; (3) recovery is a process along a continuum; and (4) peer support, family support and involvement, and spirituality are important components of the recovery process.

A key feature of ROSC is the recognition that recovery support often relates to non-SUD specific domains that support attainment of social capital (Davidson & White, 2007). SUD is a complex disorder that often affects social spheres in negative and corrosive ways that degrade overall function and social support relationships during the time a person is using substances (Cadet et al., 2014). Co-occurrence of mental health disorders, combined with social and environmental barriers (lack of employment, social support, transportation, access to care, etc.), often present formidable obstacles to sustaining recovery. As such, recovery is a continuous process punctuated by benchmarks of social capital restructuring and goal attainment, such as education, stable housing, and recovery-affirmative activities and relationships (Muller et al., 2016).

The development of the ROSC model and the practical implementation of the model provide the assertive linkages between recovery support services and resources within and surrounding a geographic, identity, or social community. In doing so, the ROSC model helps to ensure that an individual's perception of the benefits of services offered and/or rendered is positive, along with serving to bring a community closer together through intentional linkage and collaboration. In this way, the ROSC model has not only helped to improve direct service delivery efforts for individuals seeking or in recovery from SUD, but also has fostered increased formal organizing of the recovery community within itself and in relation to the tertiary supports (housing programs, vocational and employment supports, etc.), which are part of the organized recovery community as allied services.

Recovery Support Services

Recovery support services are a diverse array of direct and indirect services, delivered most frequently via peer channels, that are concerned with promoting improved long-term recovery outcomes (Kaplan, 2008; Sheedy & Whitter, 2009; White, 2009). Recovery support services may be categorized into the domains of education, employment, housing, and social/peer support aimed at improving the functioning and wellness of individuals (Kaplan, 2008).

Education

Increased educational opportunity supports those in the recovery process by improving self-esteem and self-efficacy and by increasing long-term gainful employment opportunities. The most widely available educational recovery support services are collegiate recovery programs and recovery high schools. Over 200 of these programs are available in the United States (Ashford et al., 2018). In addition to focusing on educational support, collegiate recovery programs and recovery high schools often contain many other elements of recovery support services, such as peer services, housing, vocational services, and advocacy (Laudet et al., 2014).

Employment

Employment recovery support services are focused on both increasing the vocational and technical skills of individuals and finding gainful employment opportunities for them during the recovery process (White et al., 2012). Services that help individuals craft resumes and cover letters, fill out job applications, practice interviewing skills, or secure interview attire are all employment recovery support services. These services and resources exist for a variety of individuals in need in the general population, and the subset of services that are recovery-informed may pay special attention to SUD history and current status, criminal records, recovery stigma, and recovery disclosure status. Further, they may be delivered by individuals currently in the recovery process themselves.

Peer Services

Peer recovery support services – sometimes referred to as recovery coaching or mentoring – are peer-delivered support services that focus on the individual navigation of the recovery process (White, 2009). Peer recovery support services should not be confused with mutual aid recovery services (e.g., 12 Step groups), as peer recovery support services differ in several ways. Perhaps most importantly, peer recovery support services are delivered through formal and specialized roles by individuals with personal experience of the recovery process (i.e., lived recovery experience) (White, 2009). Similar to membership in the organized recovery community, lived experience is not simply identifying as in recovery or having a past SUD, but any involvement within the larger recovery process; meaning, individuals of many types may also be peers just as they may consider themselves part of the recovery community. Peer recovery support services may exist as a service within a physical recovery support service location, such as within a recovery community organization or a recovery residence, but also may be delivered as part of medical treatment (Laudet & Humphreys, 2013).

Recovery Housing

Housing, as a recovery support service, provides supportive living arrangements, such as substance-free and safe living environments for individuals in recovery. Many models of recovery housing exist within the United States, including Oxford Houses^{TM}, recovery residences that are not associated with clinical services or programs, and clinically supported recovery residences (Polcin, 2001, 2010). Additionally, for individuals in sustained recovery (e.g., greater than one year), "housing first" resources that allow for the securing of safe and affordable housing may also be considered a recovery support service (Tsemberis et al., 2012). Housing first programs that do not impose strict abstinence or other behavior change requirements are also critically important for those pursuing non-abstinent recovery pathways (see Collins et al., Chapter 12).

Recovery Community Organizations

Recovery community organizations serve as community-based entities that support the individual recovery process through a variety of mechanisms (Ashford et al., 2019a; White, 2009). These can include (1) offering a physical space (e.g., recovery community center) for recovery related activities and service delivery; (2) engaging in and organizing advocacy efforts at the local, state, and federal level meant to improve policy and increase availability of recovery resources and services; (3) offering recovery support services, often as peer recovery support services, meant to enhance the recovery process; and (4) educating the local community on SUD and the recovery process. Recovery community organizations can be standalone entities or exist within faith-based communities, tribal communities, or educational communities (Taylor, 2009; see Best et al., Chapter 16).

Mutual Aid Organizations

Different from peer recovery support services, mutual aid organizations (e.g., 12 Step groups like Alcoholics Anonymous) are both a recovery pathway and a community-based recovery support service (see Tonigan et al., Chapter 6). Mutual aid organizations are informal, decentralized, and autonomous, and are the most widely available recovery support service in the United States (Donovan et al., 2013). As a public service, mutual aid organizations offer key elements of recovery support that are free, local, and widely available to anyone (Kelly, 2017).

Recovery Science

Diversifying and separating the study of recovery from the more general study of SUD is perhaps the most important academic advance for the organized recovery community in the twenty-first century. The critical ontological shift has occurred at a timely moment in the development of the recovery movement, wherein both the scientific pursuit of understanding recovery and an organized populace of persons in recovery are seeking to make positive changes in the way society addresses SUD and promotes long-term recovery. Public health officials have worked to develop solutions as the opioid-driven overdose crisis continues across communities, social classes, and geographic regions, and as the death toll mounts (Christie et al., 2017). Much of this public policy response has been reactive and aimed at public health outcomes, such as mortality reduction. Often lost in this response is the pursuit of sustainable, long-term solutions that support an individual with SUD to reconstitute their lives in comprehensive and meaningful ways. Policy focus has been primarily in the realm of prescription drug controls (Kirschner, et al., 2014; Kolodny et al., 2015), as well as in the prevention of death and crime related to opioid use disorders (OUD; Mathis et al., 2018; Volkow, 2014). In addition to immediate concerns with opioids, the larger SUD situation in the United States remains even more complex and broader in scope than concerns about opioids alone (Substance Abuse and Mental Health Service Administration [SAMHSA], 2017). As unfortunate as the current opioid crisis has been, the substantial scientific efforts that have emerged from renewed interest in the broader SUD field have paved the way for recovery science to emerge as a unique field of academic investigation.

Recovery science is founded upon the pioneering work of recovery-oriented systems of care (White, 2008); the development of recovery capital frameworks and theory (Cloud & Granfield, 2008; Laudet & White, 2008), which were adapted from theories of social capital (Bourdieu, 1986; Granfield & Cloud, 2001); and identity models of recovery, including personal identities (Biernacki, 1986; McIntosh & McKeganey, 2000) and social identities (Best et al., 2016; Frings & Albery, 2014). As recovery science has begun to mature, comprehensive theories such as the recovery-informed theory (Brown & Ashford, 2019) have been put forth to serve as a framework for studying recovery in ways that center on the experiences of the recovery community as a form of epistemology – i.e., as a conjoining between science and organized recovery community values.

While recovery science will undoubtedly continue to evolve in the next several decades, its creation has already contributed tangible outputs, such as a body of work on peer-based recovery support services, recovery ready communities, collegiate recovery programs and recovery high schools, recovery housing, and digital recovery support services (Ashford et al., 2019b, 2020; White et al., 2012). As an extension of the organized recovery community – one in which scientists are increasingly members of the community and may or may not be in recovery themselves – the new science of recovery is likely to continue advancing and leading the recovery paradigm in which the recovery community itself is centered.

Recovery-Informed Advocacy and Policy

Though recovery community organizations often use advocacy as a means of education and policy change as part of their recovery support service models

(Ashford et al., 2019c), stand-alone advocacy organizations that engage in advocacy work without a direct service component also exist within the organized recovery community. Advocacy organizations serve two primary functions focusing on the education of the community and positive policy change that can support the recovery process and further promote and promulgate the efforts and goals of the organized recovery community. The presence of advocacy organizations within a community can support the creation of new recovery support services, change discriminatory public policy, and increase funding of institutional and community service systems (White, 2007).

Within the recovery community, advocacy and policy are often two sides of the same coin. Advocacy efforts are used to help create and enact recovery-informed policy, whether through direct political advocacy (e.g., meeting with policy makers) or through indirect political advocacy (e.g., educating and mobilizing community members to advocate on the behalf of the organized recovery community). Community mobilization advocacy efforts are often informed by national advocacy organizations, such as Faces and Voices of Recovery (https://facesandvoicesofrecovery.org/), a consequence of the formalization of the recovery community through its growth and presence in the past two decades (White, 2007).

In the last decade alone, the organized recovery community has advanced several important recovery-informed policies, including the state level Good Samaritan legislation that protects individuals who assist persons experiencing opiate overdose from legal consequences (Zadoretzky et al., 2017), as well as increasing the availability of naloxone to reverse opioid overdoses to family and other social network members of opiate users who are not medical personnel or frontline responders (Humphreys, 2015). Federally, policies such as the Mental Health Parity and Addiction Equity Act (Beronio et al., 2014), the Comprehensive Addiction and Recovery Act (Kennedy-Stewart, 2016), the Twenty-First Century Cures Act (Jones et al., 2019), and the SUPPORT Act (Substance Use-Disorder Prevention that Promotes Opioid Recovery and Treatment for Patients and Communities Act, 2018) have all benefited from the momentum and contributions of the organized recovery community.

Conclusions and Recommendations

Understanding of SUD and recovery has dramatically shifted over the last two decades, with the most prominent evolution being increased recognition of recovery as an organizing paradigm for individuals and communities. Recovery, by definition, is antithetical to active SUD. Recovery from SUD enjoys a necessary relational aspect, be it individual or familial relationships, or likely most important, community relationships. The advancement of recovery science is shaping the understanding of recovery and is amassing an evidence base to support long-term improvements in the human condition by ameliorating the heavy burden of SUD on individuals, their social networks, and the population at large. Despite the challenges faced within the United States, enormous progress has been made in the adaptive responses and strides that individuals and communities have achieved in order to address SUD. Moving forward, the evidence base on recovery will be informed by the restoration of families, the reconstituting of lives, the social organizing of the community, and the empowerment of new healthy ways of living and being for individuals. The work and growth of recovery is intimately connected with the work and growth of the community, and when one progresses, the other naturally does too.

References

Ashford, R. D., Bergman, B. G., Kelly, J. F., & Curtis, B. (2020). Systematic review: Digital recovery support services used to support substance use disorder recovery. *Human Behavior and Emerging Technologies*, *2*(1), 18–32. https://doi.org/10.1002/hbe2.148

Ashford, R. D., Brown, A., Brown, T., Callis, J., Cleveland, H. H., Eisenhart, E., Groover, H., Hayes, N., Johnston, T., Kimball, T., Manteuffel, B., McDaniel, J., Montgomery, L., Phillips, S., Polacek, M., Statman, M., & Whitney, J. (2019a). Defining and operationalizing the phenomena of recovery: A working definition from the recovery science research collaborative. *Addiction Research & Theory*, 27(3), 179–188. https://doi.org/10.1080/16066359.2018.1515352

Ashford, R. D., Brown, A. M., Canode, B., McDaniel, J., & Curtis, B. (2019c). A mixed-methods exploration of the role and impact of stigma and advocacy on substance use disorder recovery. *Alcoholism Treatment Quarterly*, *37*(4), 462–480. https://doi.org/10.1080/07347324.2019.1585216

Ashford, R. D., Brown, A. M., Eisenhart, E., Thompson-Heller, A., & Curtis, B. (2018). What we know about students in recovery: Meta-synthesis of collegiate recovery programs, 2000-2017. *Addiction Research & Theory*, *26*(5), 405–413. https://doi.org/10.1080/16066359.2018.1425399

Ashford, R. D., Brown, A. M., Ryding, R., & Curtis, B. (2019b). Building recovery ready communities: The recovery ready ecosystem model and community framework. *Addiction Research & Theory*, *28* (1), 1–11. https://doi.org/10.1080/16066359.2019.1571191

Barrows, S., & Room, R. (1991). *Drinking: Behavior and belief in modern history.* University of California Press.

Beronio, K., Glied, S., & Frank, R. (2014). How the affordable care act and mental health parity and addiction equity act greatly expand coverage of behavioral health care. *The Journal of Behavioral Health Services & Research*, *41*(4), 410–428. https://doi.org/10.1007/s11414–014-9412-0

Best, D., Beckwith, M., Haslam, C., Haslam, A., Jetten, J., Mawson, E., & Lubman, D. (2016). Overcoming alcohol and other drug addiction as a process of social identity transition: The social identity model of recovery (SIMOR). *Addiction Research and Theory*, *24*(2), 111–123. https://doi.org/10.3109/16066359.2015.1075980

Biernacki, P. (1986). *Pathways from heroin addiction: Recovery without treatment.* Temple University Press.

Bourdieu, P. (1986). The forms of capital. In Richardson, J. (Ed.), *Handbook of theory and research for the sociology of education.* (pp. 241–258). Greenwood.

Brown, A. M., & Ashford, R. D. (2019). Recovery-informed theory: Situating the subjective in the science of substance use disorder recovery. *Journal of Recovery Science, 1*(3), 1–15. https://doi.org/10.31886/jors.13.2019.38

Cadet, J. L., Bisagno, V. & Milroy, C. M. (2014). Neuropathology of substance use disorders. *Acta Neuropathologica, 127*(91), 91–107. https://doi.org/10.1007/s00401–013-1221-7

Christie, C., Baker, C., Cooper, R., Kennedy, C. P. J., Madras, B., & Bondi, F. A. G. P. (2017). *The President's commission on combating drug addiction and the opioid crisis.* US Government Printing Office.

Cloud, W., & Granfield, R. (2008). Conceptualizing recovery capital: Expansion of a theoretical construct. *Substance Use & Misuse, 43*(12–13), 1971–1986. https://doi.org/10.1080/10826080802289762

Davidson, L., & White, W. (2007). The concept of recovery as an organizing principle for integrating mental health and addiction services. *The Journal of Behavioral Health Services & Research, 34*(2), 109–120. https://doi.org/10.1007/s11414–007-9053-7

DiClemente, C. C., Norwood, A. E. Q., Gregory, W. H., Travaglini, L., Graydon, M. M., & Corno, C. M. (2016). Consumer-centered, collaborative, and comprehensive care: The core essentials of recovery-oriented system of care. *Journal of Addictions Nursing, 27*(2), 94–100. https://doi.org/10.1097/JAN.0000000000000120

Donovan, D. M., Ingalsbe, M. H., Benbow, J., & Daley, D. C., 2013. 12 Step interventions and mutual support programs for substance use disorders: An overview. *Social Work in Public Health, 28*(0), 313–332. http://doi.org/10.1080/19371918.2013.774663

Finlay, S. W. (2000). Influence of Carl Jung and William James on the origin of Alcoholics Anonymous. *Review of General Psychology, 4*(1), 3–12. https://doi.org/10.1037/1089-2680.4.1.3

Frings, D., & Albery, I. (2014). The social identity model of cessation maintenance: Formulation and initial evidence. *Addictive Behaviors, 44*, 35–42. https://doi.org/10.1016/j.addbeh.2014.10.023

Granfield, R., & Cloud, W. (2001). Social context and "natural recovery": The role of social capital in the resolution of drug-associated problems. *Substance Use & Misuse, 36*(11), 1543–1570. https://doi.org/10.1081/ja-100106963

Humphreys, K., 2015. An overdose antidote goes mainstream. *Health Affairs, 34*(10), 1624–1627. https://doi.org/10.1377/hlthaff.2015.0934

Jellinek, E. M. (1960). *The disease concept of alcoholism.* Hillhouse Press.

Jones, M. R., Novitch, M. B., Sarrafpour, S., Ehrhardt, K. P., Scott, B. B., Orhurhu, V., Viswanath, O., Kaye, A. D., Gill, J., & Simopoulos, T. T. (2019). Government legislation in response to the opioid epidemic. *Current Pain and Headache Reports, 23*(6), 40. https://doi.org/10.1007/s11916–019-0781-1

Kaplan, L. (2008). *The role of recovery support services in recovery-oriented systems of care.* DHHS publication no. (SMA) 08-4315. Substance Abuse and Mental Health Services Administration.

Kelly, J. F. (2017). Is Alcoholics Anonymous religious, spiritual, neither? Findings from 25 years of mechanisms of behavior change research. *Addiction, 112*(6), 929–936. https://doi.org/10.1111/add.13590

Kennedy-Stewart, S. (2016). So what's all this talk of the CARA bill? *MedSurg Nursing, 25*(6), S16.

Kirschner, N., Ginsburg, J., & Sulmasy, L. S. (2014). Prescription drug abuse: Executive summary of a policy position paper from the American College of Physicians. *Annals of Internal Medicine, 160*(3), 198–200. https://doi.org/10.7326/M13–2209

Kolodny, A., Courtwright, D. T., Hwang, C. S., Kreiner, P., Eadie, J. L., Clark, T. W., & Alexander, G. C. (2015). The prescription opioid and heroin crisis: A public health approach to an epidemic of addiction. *Annual Review of Public Health, 36*, 559–574. https://doi.org/10.1146/annurev-publhealth-031914-122957

Kurtz, E. (2002). Alcoholics Anonymous and the disease concept of alcoholism. *Alcoholism Treatment Quarterly, 20*(3/4), 5–39. https://doi.org/10.1300/J020v20n03_02

Laudet, A., Harris, K, Kimball, T., Winters, K. C., & Moberg, P. (2014). Collegiate recovery communities programs: What do we know and what do we need to know? *Journal of Social Work Practice in the Addictions, 14*(1), 84–100. https://doi.org/10.1080/1533256X.2014.872015

Laudet, A. B., & Humphreys, K. (2013). Promoting recovery in an evolving policy context: What do we know and what do we need to know about recovery support services? *Journal of Substance Abuse Treatment, 45*(1), 126–133. https://doi.org/10.1016/j.jsat.2013.01.009

Laudet, A. B., & White, W. L. (2008). Recovery capital as prospective predictor of sustained recovery, life satisfaction, and stress among former poly-substance users. *Substance Use & Misuse, 43*(1), 27–54. https://doi.org/10.1080/10826080701681473

Leshner, A. I. (1997). Addiction is a brain disease, and it matters. *Science, 278*(5335), 45–47. https://doi.org/10.1126/science.278.5335.45

Mathis, S. M., Hagemeier, N., Hagaman, A., Dreyzehner, J., & Pack, R. P. (2018). A dissemination and implementation science approach to the epidemic of opioid use disorder in the United States. *Current HIV/AIDS Reports, 15*(5), 359–370. https://doi.org/10.1007/s11904–018-0409-9

McIntosh, J., & McKeganey, N. (2000). Addicts' narratives of recovery from drug use: Constructing a non-addict identity. *Social Science & Medicine, 50*(10), 1501–1510. https://doi.org/10.1016/s0277–9536(99)00409-8

Muller, A. E., Skurtveit, S., & Clausen, T. (2016). Many correlates of poor quality of life among substance users entering treatment are not addiction-specific. *Health and Quality of Life outcomes, 14*(1), 39. https://doi.org/10.1186/s12955–016-0439-1

Polcin, D. L. (2001). Sober living houses: Potential roles in substance abuse services and suggestions for research. *Substance Use & Misuse, 36*(3), 301–311. https://doi.org/10.1081/ja-100102627

Polcin, D. L., Korcha, R. A., Bond, J., & Galloway, G. (2010). Sober living houses for alcohol and drug dependence: 18-month outcomes. *Journal of Substance Abuse Treatment, 38*(4), 356–365. https://doi.org/10.1016/j.jsat.2010.02.003

Sheedy, C. K., & Whitter, M. (2009). *Guiding principles and elements of recovery oriented systems of care: What do we know from the research?* HHS publication no. (SMA) 09-4439. Substance Abuse and Mental Health Services Administration.

Substance Abuse and Mental Health Services Administration. (2017). *Key substance use and mental health indicators in the United States: Results from the 2016 national survey on drug use and health* (HHS Publication No. SMA 17-5044, NSDUH Series H-52). Substance Abuse and Mental Health Services Administration.

Substance Use Disorder Prevention that Promotes Opioid Recovery and Treatment for Patients and Communities Act, Public Law 115-271, Stat. 3894, (2018). www.govinfo.gov/content/pkg/PLAW-115publ271/html/PLAW-115publ271.htm

Taylor, P. (2009). *Recovery community organizations.* In G. L. Fisher & N. A. Roget (Eds.), *Encyclopedia of substance abuse prevention, treatment, & recovery* (pp. 765–765). SAGE Publications Ltd. https://doi.org/10.4135/9781412964500.n263

Tsemberis, S., Kent, D., & Respress, C. (2012). Housing stability and recovery among chronically homeless persons with co-occurring disorders in Washington, DC. *American Journal of Public Health, 102*(1), 13–6. https://doi.org/10.2105/AJPH.2011.300320

Volkow, N. D., Frieden, T. R., Hyde, P. S., & Cha, S. S. (2014). Medication assisted therapies—tackling the opioid-overdose epidemic. *New England Journal of Medicine, 370*(22), 2063–2066. https://doi.org/10.1056/NEJMp1402780

White, W. L. (1998). *Slaying the dragon: The history of addiction treatment and recovery in America.* Chestnut Health Systems/Lighthouse Institute Bloomington, IL.

(2005). Recovery: Its history and renaissance as an organizing construct concerning alcohol and other drug problems. *Alcoholism Treatment Quarterly, 23*(1), 3–15. https://doi.org/10.1300/J020v23n01_02

(2007). The new recovery advocacy movement in America. *Addiction, 102*(5), 696–703. https://doi.org/10.1111/j.1360-0443.2007.01808.x

(2009). The mobilization of community resources to support long-term addiction recovery. *Journal of Substance Abuse Treatment, 36*(2), 146–158. https://doi.org/10.1016/j.jsat.2008.10.006

White, W. L., Kelly, J. F., & Roth, J. D. (2012). New addiction-recovery support institutions: Mobilizing support beyond professional addiction treatment and recovery mutual aid. *Journal of Groups in Addiction & Recovery, 7*(2–4), 297–317. https://doi.org/10.1080/1556035X.2012.705719

Zadoretzky, C., McKnight, C., Bramson, H., Des Jarlais, D., Phillips, M., Hammer, M., & Cala, M. E. (2017). The New York 911 Good Samaritan law and opioid overdose prevention among people who inject drugs. *World Medical & Health Policy, 9*, 318–340. https://doi.org/10.1002/wmh3.234

19 Alcohol Control Policy and Regulations to Promote Recovery from Alcohol Use Disorder

William C. Kerr and Meenakshi S. Subbaraman

Alcohol Control Policy and Regulations to Promote Recovery from Alcohol Use Disorder

This chapter discusses key areas of the alcohol policy literature from the perspective of effects on those with alcohol use disorders (AUD) and in recovery from AUD. These groups are always relevant to policy effectiveness, but much of the focus of policies is on preventing heavy drinking, new cases of AUD, and reducing drinking consequences. Thus, the current review will be from a different perspective, and some policies may be more important or effective for these purposes. For example, driving under the influence (DUI) and 24/7 alcohol monitoring policies may be more important for initiating recovery from AUD, while reducing outlet density and banning advertising may be more important for maintaining recovery. Most evidence of policy effectiveness is more general, often at the population level, but those with AUD contribute substantially to alcohol sales, heavy drinking, and most alcohol-related mortality and morbidity, so there is a strong relevant research base. Still, significant need remains for studies focused on AUD and maintaining recovery, recognizing the substantial measurement and sampling issues that such studies face.

Pricing Policies

Taxes are viewed as one of the most effective policies for reducing alcohol–related harm, and considerable evidence supports this view (Cook, 2007). Studies have found that price increases for alcoholic beverages lead to reduced alcohol consumption and binge drinking (defined as five or more drinks on an occasion for men or four or more drinks for women), both in the general population and in high-risk populations, including heavy drinkers, youth, and young adults (Nelson et al., 2013). Tax and price increases also have been shown to reduce the adverse consequences of alcohol consumption and AUD, including drinking and driving, traffic crashes, alcohol-involved crimes, alcohol-related mortality, and risky sexual behavior and its consequences (Xu & Chaloupka, 2011). A review by the Centers for Disease Control and Prevention (CDC) found strong evidence that raising alcohol excise taxes is an effective strategy for reducing excessive alcohol consumption and related harms (Elder et al., 2010). Similarly, an international team found taxation to be a key recommended effective policy for reducing alcohol-related harms that is backed by strong empirical evidence (Babor et al., 2010). Further, the heaviest drinkers bear a substantial share of the tax burden, along with those with higher incomes (Naimi et al., 2016). Drinkers who exceed United States (US) low-risk drinking guidelines ($<$ 14 drinks per week for men and $<$ 7 drinks per week for women) would pay an estimated 72 percent of a hypothetical tax increase on all alcoholic beverage types. The cost of alcohol is most relevant to those who buy the most, such that high taxes and prices may lead quickly to personal financial problems, reduce consumption through disposable income constraints, and potentially encourage quitting and discourage re-starting through the high financial cost of frequent heavy drinking.

Taxes of Different Types

Taxes in the United States are mostly beverage-type-specific on the basis of beverage volume; for example, $2.00 per gallon of wine. The federal spirits tax is applied directly on the ethanol volume and some states apply *ad valorem* taxes on all beverage types, adding a percentage of the sale price like a general sales tax. Beer, wine, and spirits are nearly always taxed at different rates, with the highest rates on spirits. There is some attention to alcohol content by volume (percent ABV) with higher rates for wine over 14 percent ABV for example, but US states pay much less attention to this than other countries. US tax rates are also not indexed to inflation, as is done in some countries to maintain the real value of the tax. US alcohol taxes have declined substantially in real value and relative to average incomes since the 1950s (Kerr et al., 2013). Taxes imposed directly on the alcohol unit, such as a standard drink or gallon of ethanol, that increase with the product's percent ABV and are adjusted to inflation would be the most appropriate for preventing heavy drinking, AUD, and alcohol-related harms. No US taxes have all of these features.

Tax pass-through refers to the degree to which taxes and tax changes are ultimately paid by the consumer and depends on the market power of producers, wholesalers, retailers, and consumers. In a competitive market, less than the full amount of the tax would be passed through to consumers. Some studies have found producers use a tax increase as an opportunity to raise prices more than the amount of the tax increase (Kenkel, 2005; Shrestha & Markowitz, 2016; Young & Bielinska-Kwapisz, 2002). However, it is difficult to know how the tax impacts prices over time, as future price increases may also be affected. A US study comparing prices across states found that the tax pass-through rate was closer to a full pass-through of the tax to consumers (Siegel et al., 2013). Similar to some results for cigarettes, a study in the United Kingdom (UK) found that tax pass-through rates depend on product price and quality level. The cheapest beer and spirits had tax pass-through rates of approximately 85 percent of the tax, while more expensive products had pass through rates greater than the tax amount (Ally et al., 2014). This suggests that taxes are not completely passed through to the consumer on the cheapest products, which are disproportionally favored by heavy drinkers (Black et al., 2010; Kerr & Greenfield, 2007; Wall et al., 2017).

Other Pricing Policies

Minimum unit pricing (MUP), minimum markups, price posting, and price floors are non-tax pricing policies utilized in the United States and other countries aimed at avoiding predatory pricing. MUP has been adopted in several countries in recent years and is aimed at increasing the price of the lowest cost products targeting heavy drinkers, many of whom have AUD. MUP policies establish an overall or beverage-specific minimum retail price for a unit of alcohol, such as the US standard drink. This typically increases the prices of the lowest cost alcohol products and also appears to shift the prices of other products upward to maintain price differences with higher quality brands to some extent. Substantial evidence from Canada has established the effectiveness of these polices in reducing alcohol consumption (Stockwell et al., 2012), alcohol-attributable morbidity (Zhao & Stockwell, 2016, 2017), and alcohol-attributable mortality (Zhao et al., 2013).

Market Structure Policies Affecting Prices

Market structure policies that affect prices include: the three-tier system separating (1) alcohol production, (2) wholesaling, and (3) retailing; government control of alcohol wholesaling and retailing; restriction on store types allowed to sell each beverage type; and restrictions on delivery. The three-tier system was designed to prevent vertical integration based on the pre-Prohibition era experiences with "tied-houses" (bars that are owned or controlled by alcohol producers). These included price competition and marketing schemes, such as free lunches with alcohol purchase, that are facilitated by producers controlling distribution and consumer on- and off-premise sales. Current examples include large volume discounts on cases or other larger quantities of beer, wine, and spirits used as loss leader products (which are sold below costs to induce customers into the store) in supermarkets in the UK and Australia, where supermarkets have a large share of off-premise sales and can buy directly from producers. Government control also prevents such activities and allows strong policies around pricing.

Evidence of Tax Effectiveness

Beer, wine, spirits, and total alcohol (all alcoholic beverages combined) assessed using surveys and per capita alcohol sales consistently show a negative price elasticity of demand, meaning that higher prices lead consumers to reduce their consumption. In a meta-analysis, the mean price elasticity estimate was -0.5, meaning that a 10 percent increase in prices would result in a 5 percent reduction in consumption (Wagenaar et al., 2009). All types of beverages were found to be responsive to price changes, with spirits being the most responsive and beer the least. More recently, the Maryland 3 percent ad valorem tax increase was associated with a 3.8 percent decline in alcohol sales, suggesting that taxes can have a greater impact in some cases (Esser et al., 2016).

Major reviews have shown significant effects of alcohol taxes and prices on alcohol-related disease, injury, and traffic crashes (Wagenaar et al., 2010), and have confirmed the effectiveness of alcohol taxes and prices in reducing drinking, heavy drinking, and alcohol-related mortality (Guide to Community Preventive Services, 2013). Several studies have evaluated changes in alcohol-attributable mortality across increases in tax rates utilizing time-series methods that control for trends in rates prior to the tax change. A study of New York state taxes found that alcohol-related mortality declined by 7.0 percent after a 1990 tax increase on spirits and beer (Delcher et al., 2012). A Florida study found alcohol-attributable mortality to be reduced by 2.2 percent for each 10 percent increase in tax rates (Maldonado-Molina & Wagenaar, 2010). A study of two tax increases in Alaska found substantial and significant reductions in alcohol-attributable mortality rates to be associated with each tax increase (Wagenaar et al., 2009). Regarding specific mortality types, an analysis of spirits taxes found a substantial and significant inverse association with mortality from liver cirrhosis (Ponicki & Gruenewald, 2006).

The responsiveness of alcohol-related mortality outcomes and traffic crashes to tax rates strongly suggests that individuals with AUD are influenced by taxes. Supporting this, surveys show that drinkers with symptoms of AUD are responsive to price changes (S. Farrell et al., 2003) and that taxes reduce both adult and youth binge drinking (Xuan et al., 2013). However, a recent US study did not find significant protective effects of state-level taxes on the odds of past-year AUD in subgroups defined by gender and race/ethnicity (Subbaraman et al., 2020). Thus, while taxes could mitigate alcohol-related harms among those with AUD, they might not prevent AUD from occurring.

Alcohol Availability Policies

Availability policies restrict the places and times of alcohol sales and include regulations such as licensed vs. government monopolies on sales; restrictions on the number, types, and location of alcohol outlets; and limits on hours and/or days of sale. These policies can differ by beverage type (e.g., beer vs. spirits) and are often correlated; e.g., government control of retail alcohol sales usually coincides with fewer alcohol outlets or more limited sales hours compared to states with privatized or open market alcohol sales.

In general, evidence supports the effectiveness of government-controlled retail monopolies, limits on the number and types of outlets, and limits on hours and days of sale for reducing heavy alcohol consumption (Babor et al., 2010) and alcohol-related problems (Gruenewald, 2011). For example, in the United States, states with government control of spirits retail sales have fewer spirits outlets and earlier outlet closing hours, as well as lower per capita consumption of spirits, compared to states without government control (National Alcohol Beverage

Control Association (NABCA), 2011). Similarly, simulation studies of alcohol policies in Sweden show that re-instating its government monopoly on beer sales would result in decreases in beer retail outlets, beer consumption, hospital admissions for alcohol-related harms, and motor vehicle crashes (Holder et al., 2007; Norström et al., 2010; Stockwell et al., 2018). Thus, government control of both spirits and beer retail sales and its related restrictions on outlet density and sales hours may be relevant for those in recovery or who are attempting to reduce heavy drinking and its related consequences.

Restricting the kinds of stores (e.g., grocery stores, gas stations) that sell alcohol could also be valuable for those in recovery, as allowing alcohol in grocery, drug, and department stores inherently makes alcohol more visible, and individuals in recovery from AUD are often vulnerable to alcohol-related cues (Witteman et al., 2015). Related to alcohol visibility, a survey of Washington residents after its privatization of liquor sales in 2012 found that past-year abstainers were dissatisfied with having liquor available in grocery stores as opposed to having liquor sales restricted to government stores (Subbaraman & Kerr, 2016). Individuals in recovery might similarly find alcohol availability at grocery stores or other places where they need to shop dissatisfying or even triggering, and therefore may prefer stronger restrictions on the kinds of stores that are allowed to sell alcohol.

Supporting the idea that limiting the types and number of alcohol outlets can aid those with AUD, a review of outlet density-limiting laws found that reducing alcohol outlet density can reduce excessive alcohol consumption and related harms (Campbell et al., 2009). Similarly, a study in British Columbia found that rapid growth in private liquor store density led to an increase in both per capita consumption and alcohol-related mortality, particularly from chronic causes such as AUD and alcoholic liver disease (Stockwell et al., 2011).

Several reviews have also concluded that restricting hours of sales and bar closing times are effective strategies for reducing excessive drinking and related harms (Hahn et al., 2010), though most studies have focused on outcomes such as emergency room visits, police calls (Room, 2004), and violent assaults (Rossow & Norström, 2012) rather than heavy drinking or AUD specifically. Still, studies of bar closing times and late night patrons show a strong relationship between participants' expected home time and predicted Blood Alcohol Content (percent BAC) at that time. For example, a study in the UK showed that the average percent BAC among patrons intending to leave at midnight was 0.09 percent compared to 0.21 percent BAC among those intending to leave at or after 4 a.m. (Deacon et al., 2010). Thus, restricting bar closing times could reduce contexts and opportunities for binge drinking and may be especially important for individuals in recovery from AUD who are particularly susceptible to binge drinking.

Under a similar hypothesis that people with high propensities for risky drinking may be more prone to harmful consumption if alcohol is highly visible and available, a Swiss study examined whether more liberal alcohol policies intensified the effects of individual-level factors on heavy drinking among Swiss men (Foster et al., 2015). An analysis of interactions between alcohol policy strength and within-person variables of sensation-seeking, antisocial personality disorder, and attention-deficit hyperactivity disorder indicated stronger alcohol laws protected against heavy alcohol use, though this protective effect was lost in individuals with high levels of sensation-seeking or an antisocial personality disorder (Foster et al., 2015). A similar study of the same Swiss cohort also found that more control policies per jurisdiction were related to reduced probabilities of heavy episodic drinking, weekend heavy volume drinking, and AUD, though effects weakened at the heavy end of the drinking spectrum (Foster et al., 2019). The authors concluded that stricter alcohol policy environments were associated with a shift towards lighter drinking. Though these findings may be more relevant for AUD prevention efforts rather than recovery efforts per se, they show that availability restrictions can interact with individual-level factors to protect individuals who are particularly vulnerable to persistent AUD.

Alcohol Delivery Services

In recent years, home delivery of alcohol has increased substantially. Delivery from licensed retail stores by staff of those stores has long been available in many states. Partnerships with online ordering platforms has increased their use. Direct shipping through third parties such as UPS and FedEx have also increased as most states now allow this from wineries, and some states allow deliveries from in-state retailers and, in a few, even out-of-state retailers. The internet has also facilitated a substantial increase in unlicensed direct shipping, which is difficult to control. Such deliveries are more convenient than going to a store in some cases, but can also be less convenient in many cases where the delivery time is uncertain and an adult signature is required. Delivery fees are also common, especially on smaller orders, increasing the cost of these services. As this market develops, the potential for low cost rapid delivery presents the greatest potential for adversely affecting those in recovery through increasing the ease of access to alcohol products.

COVID-19 and Alcohol Availability

When this chapter was prepared, the COVID-19 pandemic had directly impacted the contexts in which people drink all over the world. Although the pandemic should be curtailed or resolved at an uncertain future date, the current context highlights the impact of such widespread contextual changes on drinking and possible policy-related avenues to mitigate the effects. The onset of the pandemic resulted in rapid mitigation measures involving the closing of bars and restaurants, continued enforcement of distancing, and consequent shifts to drinking at home. Furthermore, and particularly relevant to individuals with a history of alcohol-related problems and/or AUD, the shift from on-premise (e.g., bars and restaurants) to off-premise (e.g., buying alcohol at a liquor or grocery store to drink at home) consumption might coincide with a shift in alcohol-related consequences. For example, while drunk-driving should decline due to less travelling to and from drinking locations, violence may increase due to its positive relationship with drinking off-premise (e.g., at home) (Rehm et al., 2020; Trangenstein et al., 2018a, 2018b). Potential increases in domestic and other violence were cited as the main rationale for temporary bans on alcohol in some jurisdictions, e.g., in Northern France (Rehm et al., 2020).

In response to COVID-19, India banned both on- and off-premise alcohol sales nationwide without exception in March 2020. This total non-availability of alcohol resulted in individuals with severe AUD going into withdrawal, and in extreme cases reported suicides resulted from frustrations of not having access to alcohol (Nadkarni et al., 2020). After "a small wave of suicides attributed to alcohol withdrawal" (p. 105) occurred in Kerala, India, state authorities directed citizens with alcohol withdrawal symptoms to approach doctors at government hospitals for alcohol "passes" (Varma, 2020). For individuals in recovery, the consequences of total prohibition and lockdown are both biological (e.g., forced withdrawal) and psychosocial (e.g., isolation increases the risk of relapse among those attempting to recover, access to recovery services is limited) (Nadkarni et al., 2020).

In Australia, the UK, and the United States, governments have allowed off-premise alcohol outlets to remain open as "essential" services, whereas on-premise drinking locations such as bars and restaurants have been forced to close. Forced isolation combined with access to purchasing alcohol may exacerbate social and health harms associated with home drinking (Reynolds & Wilkinson, 2020). The pandemic's context is a "perfect storm" for exacerbating substance use problems because access to valued non-drinking activities has been seriously curtailed, which shifts preference in favor of drinking (Acuff et al., 2020); reflecting this shift, alcohol sales in both the US and UK have increased substantially as of March 2020 (Nadkarni et al., 2020). Further, the stress imposed by COVID-19 is probably causing some to drink as a coping mechanism. For those in recovery, access to support could also affect drinking outcomes. For example, a study of high-risk drinkers in England found that the prevalence of high-risk drinking had increased since the COVID-19 lockdown despite increased attempts at reduced consumption, perhaps because evidence-based support like in-person therapy had decreased without compensatory increase in use of remote support (Jackson et al., 2021).

Marketing and Advertising Policies

Marketing policies include bans and/or content restrictions on advertising alcohol on television, on the radio, in print, outdoors, in public places, and on the Internet. Like availability policies, marketing and advertising policies may differ by beverage type and are often primarily aimed at reducing underage drinking. In the United States, the enforcement of marketing and advertising policies relies on self-regulation by the alcohol industry, which does not have particularly vested interests in protecting vulnerable populations like minors or individuals in recovery from AUD (Noel et al., 2017).

A recent meta-review of alcohol control interventions from 2006–2017 concluded that restricting alcohol advertising was "possibly beneficial" in reducing heavy drinking based on evidence from both systematic reviews and experimental studies (Siegfried & Parry, 2019). However, the literature regarding the effectiveness of marketing restrictions on reduced heavy drinking is dominated by studies of students and younger adults (Esser & Jernigan, 2018). A systematic review and meta-analysis of experimental studies of the immediate effects of alcohol marketing and media portrayals on consumption concluded that viewing alcohol advertisements (but not alcohol portrayals, e.g., of a TV character drinking) may increase immediate alcohol consumption (Stautz et al., 2016). Yet again, this study only included young adult students, and the additional amounts consumed (0.14–0.94 standard drinks for females, 0.22–1.52 standard drinks for males) might be considered negligible for those in AUD recovery or with a history of heavy drinking. Still, a household survey of South African drinkers found that perceptions of alcohol availability, exposure to alcohol promotions and advertising through SMS/text messaging, and free offers when buying alcohol all increased heavy drinking, and that exposure to alcohol advertising in magazines and newspapers increased symptoms of alcohol problems (Williams et al., 2019). Thus, alcohol advertising can increase negative alcohol-related consequences among drinkers.

Alcohol marketing and advertising policies can negatively affect individuals in AUD recovery or those who are trying to reduce drinking because exposure to alcohol ads can trigger cravings to drink (Guillou-Landréat et al., 2020). Results from a functional magnetic resonance imaging (fMRI) study indicated that advertising of alcohol (or cannabis) use activated the brain's reward circuit, suggesting that reducing marketing exposure would reduce brain exposure to reward cues that motivate substance use (de Sousa Fernandes Perna et al., 2017). An ongoing study in France is examining the influence of alcohol marketing on drinkers with AUD who are seeking treatment to assess the impact of marketing on vulnerable drinkers. If found to increase drinking, the results will put pressure on public authorities to initiate preventive measures specifically related to marketing to individuals with AUD (Guillou-Landréat et al., 2020). Since alcohol advertisements were initially authorized in France in 1993, exposure to alcohol marketing has grown to an "omnipresence in the daily environment of the citizens: posters in the street, promotions, competitions in shops, in the press, on the internet (official sites and social networks), radio, and also in films and series, etc." (Guillou-Landréat et al., 2020, p. 7). In response to this "omnipresence," a primary aim of the French study is the development of counter-marketing messages specifically targeting individuals with AUD (Guillou-Landréat et al., 2020).

Appeals made in advertisements are often designed to reflect or even shape cultural norms (Albers-Miller & Gelb, 1996). Alcohol advertisements inherently encourage drinking and promote positive norms around a drinking lifestyle (T. Farrell & Gordeon, 2012). However, a relatively new wave of movements like "Sober Curious" (Warrington, 2018), campaigns for "Dry January" (and "Dry July" and "Sober September"), as well as revived marketing of products like "mocktails" and "booze-free beer," all promote an abstinence-based lifestyle, and may reflect a cultural shift in drinking norms (Splitter, 2020). For example, registrations for Dry January in the UK increased 15-fold over four years, and Dry January participants reported reduced harmful drinking and enhanced capacity to refuse alcohol (de Visser et al., 2017). A follow-up study of the UK sample concluded that Dry January appears to attract heavier drinkers who are concerned about their alcohol intake, and that successful completion of Dry January was associated with both short- and longer-term benefits to well-being for participants wanting to reduce consumption (de Visser & Piper, 2020). Thus, social marketing of abstinence-based challenges can help people change harmful drinking patterns (de Visser & Nicholls, 2020) and may be a useful tool to counter alcohol industry marketing and aid individuals in recovery.

Driving Under the Influence (DUI) Policies

Except for Utah, all US states currently have laws establishing a blood alcohol content of 0.08 milligrams per deciliter (0.08 BAC) as per se intoxication in relation to driving a motor vehicle with varying criminal penalties for those found driving with a BAC exceeding this limit. Utah has a per se limit of 0.05 BAC. The implementation of 0.08 BAC in US states from previous limits of 0.10 BAC or higher has significantly reduced alcohol-related traffic crashes and fatalities (Voas & Fell, 2011). Policies targeting impaired driving include these per se BAC limits, enforcement measures (such as road blocks and penalties for exceeding limits, like immediate jailing and car impounding), mandated alcohol education, license revocation, monetary fines, and ignition interlocks. These polices help discourage heavy drinking outside the home. Many individuals with AUD and those in recovery have had one or more DUI incidents, and these incidents are an opportunity for brief intervention and treatment that is often mandated.

Trends in DUI in the United States from roadside surveys conducted in 1996 and 2007 show that while reductions have been achieved, driving while intoxicated remains dangerously prevalent. In 2007, 12.4 percent of nighttime drivers had a positive BAC, 4.4 percent were above 0.05 BAC, and 2.2 percent were above 0.08 BAC. These percentages were reduced from 16.7 percent, 7.4 percent, and 4.1 percent, respectively, in 1996 (Kelley-Baker et al., 2013). Virtually all drivers are impaired with regard to driving performance at 0.05 BAC, and the risk of being involved in a crash increases significantly at 0.05 BAC (Fell & Voas, 2013). The majority of drinkers are significantly impaired in their ability to operate a motor vehicle at 0.05 BAC or above, including heavy drinkers. The risk of death in a single vehicle crash for BAC levels between 0.05 and 0.079 BAC is seven times higher compared to no alcohol consumption. Relative risk of any crash is elevated (1.38) at 0.05 BAC and rises to 2.69 at 0.08 BAC (Voas & Fell, 2011).

Most European countries such as the UK, Germany, Spain, Italy, and Denmark set per se limits at 0.05 BAC. Other countries such as Japan, Russia, and Poland have limits of 0.03 BAC, and still others such as Sweden, Norway, and Ukraine have limits of 0.02 BAC. Studies of countries implementing 0.05 BAC illegal per se limits have supported its effectiveness in reducing accident and other alcohol-related harms in the Netherlands, France, Austria, Australia, Japan, and Sweden (Fell & Voas, 2009). For example, an evaluation of Japan's 0.05 BAC law in 1972 along with other complementary measures found that there were immediate and sustained reductions in alcohol-related accidents, as well as driving while intoxicated arrests, resulting over time in very low levels of both (Deshapriya & Iwase, 1998).

Certainty and celerity are key elements of effective deterrence. Individuals who choose to drive drunk tend to have a strong present orientation leading to heavy discounting of future penalties, even if severe (Nagin & Pogarsky, 2001). A recent US study found that drinking drivers are relatively knowledgeable about the laws in their state. They were, however, less likely to plan events involving drinking, such as selecting a designated driver in advance, and were more impulsive. The study also found evidence of hyperbolic discounting among drinking drivers confirming the present orientation of this group (Sloan et al., 2014). So, immediate and certain penalties such as license revocation, car seizure, and arrest of impaired drivers will be more effective than delayed consequences. New penalties for impaired driving and speeding offences implemented in 2010 in British Columbia, Canada, included significant fines, potential vehicle impoundment, and increasing penalties for repeat offenses for those exceeding 0.05 BAC. More immediate penalties for exceeding 0.08 BAC and increased penalties for speeding and street racing were also implemented. An evaluation of the new penalties found a 21 percent reduction in fatal crashes and a 52 percent reduction in alcohol-related fatal crashes, suggesting that the alcohol and driving penalty changes were the major cause of these dramatic results (Brubacher et al., 2014).

Ignition interlocks are devices installed on motor vehicles to prevent individuals from driving with a positive BAC level. The devices are installed on the vehicles of individuals convicted of impaired driving. Drivers blow into the device to measure their BAC level, and the vehicle cannot start if a set minimal level, such 0.02 BAC, is exceeded. Research has shown that ignition interlocks significantly reduce re-arrest rates for alcohol-impaired driving (Elder et al., 2011). In addition, mandatory ignition interlock laws for all impaired driving offenders reduce alcohol-involved fatal crashes, and interlocks on all vehicles could prevent 85 percent of crash fatalities from drinking drivers (Carter et al.,

2015). The use of ignition interlocks for offenders may be an under-utilized tool. In 2013, only 21 percent of people arrested for alcohol-impaired driving had interlocks installed. The number of installed devices varies greatly across states, partially due to policy differences. Although mandatory laws increase the likelihood of requiring ignition interlock devices, additional measures are needed to ensure the devices are actually installed in their vehicles by addressing cost barriers to installation and increasing penalties for those who drive without a license (Elder et al., 2011). States could also turn to alternative policies, such as transdermal alcohol sensor monitoring devices for those who opt out of ignition interlock programs. This could provide greater incentives to have an ignition interlock installed (Elder et al., 2011).

Court-Ordered Alcohol Monitoring

For DUI and other alcohol-related offences such as domestic violence, individuals can be ordered by the court to not drink. Compliance is monitored through twice-a-day testing with breathalyzer at a police station or through wearing a transdermal alcohol sensor device. These devices continuously measure blood alcohol content through the skin and will alert authorities if alcohol consumption is detected (Bond et al., 2014). These measures have been shown to reduce DUI and domestic violence arrests (Kilmer et al., 2013).

Conclusions and Recommendations

Policies that could reduce AUD and promote recovery include taxation, pricing policies such as minimum unit pricing (MUP), controls on alcohol availability such as government-run stores, limits on the types of stores selling alcoholic beverages, outlet density limits and hours of sale restrictions, marketing and advertising restrictions, and DUI policies. The United States has low and poorly structured taxes compared to many developed countries, making this a priority area for improvement. Increasing alcoholic beverage tax rates, changing the basis of taxation to alcohol instead of beverage volume, indexing rates to inflation, and addressing the lowest cost products with MUPs are suggested. Marketing and advertising policies could also be strengthened to reduce exposure to alcohol messaging for those in recovery. DUI policies could be strengthened with further adoption of the 0.05 BAC per se limit and wider use of ignition interlocks for offenders. Strengths of the current US policies and regulations include the mandated three-tier system preventing vertical integration and associated pricing and marketing schemes, government control of wholesale and retail operations for spirits and wine in some states, and local control over alcohol outlet numbers and locations.

Alcohol policies shape the alcohol market and other aspects of the environment promoting and constraining alcohol use and the behaviors of drinkers and those in recovery. Support for strengthening weaker alcohol control policies such as taxation and maintaining stronger polices such as government control and the three-tier system are needed to promote recovery as well as to reduce heavy drinking and prevent AUD.

References

Acuff, S. F., Tucker, J. A., & Murphy, J. G. (2020). Behavioral economics of substance use: Understanding and reducing harmful use during the COVID-19 pandemic. *Experimental and Clinical Psychopharmacology*. Advance online publication. https://doi.org/10.1037/pha0000431

Albers-Miller, N. D., & Gelb, B. D. (1996). Business advertising appeals as a mirror of cultural dimensions: A study of eleven countries. *Journal of Advertising, 25*(4), 57–70. https://doi.org/10.1080/00913367.1996.10673512

Ally, A. K., Meng, Y., Chakraborty, R., Dobson, P. W., Seaton, J. S., Holmes, J., Angus, C., Guo, Y., Hill-McManus, D., Brennen, A., & Meier, P. S. (2014). Alcohol tax pass-through across the product and price range: Do retailers treat cheap alcohol differently? *Addiction, 109*(12), 1994–2002. https://doi.org/10.1111/add.12590

Babor, T., Caetano, R., Casswell, S., Edwards, G., Giesbrecht, N., Graham, K., Grube, J. S., Hill, L., Holder, H., Homel, R., Livingston, M., Osterberg, E., Rehm, J., Room, R., & Rossow, I. (2010). *Alcohol: No ordinary commodity: Research and public policy* (2nd ed.). Oxford University Press.

Ballard, J. (2016). What is Dry January? *British Journal of General Practice, 66*(642), 32. https://doi.org/10.3399/bjgp16X683173

(2019). One in five Americans is participating in Dry January. *YouGov*. https://today.yougov.com/topics/health/articles-reports/2019/01/11/dry-january-2019

Black, H., Gill, J., & Chick, J. (2010). The price of a drink: Levels of consumption and price paid per unit of alcohol by Edinburgh's ill drinkers with a comparison to wider alcohol sales in Scotland. *Addiction, 106*(4), 729–736. https://doi.org/10.1111/j.1360-0443.2010.03225.x

Bond, J. C., Greenfield, T. K., Patterson, D., & Kerr, W. C. (2014). Adjustments for drink size and ethanol content: New results from a self-report diary and transdermal sensor validation study. *Alcoholism: Clinical and Experimental Research 38* (12), 3060–3067. https://doi.org/10.1111/acer.12589

Brubacher, J. R., Chan, H., Brasher, P., Erdelyi, S., Desapriya, E., Asbridge, M., Purssell, R., Macdonald, S., Schuurman, N., & Pike, I. (2014). Reduction in fatalities, ambulance calls, and hospital admissions for road trauma after implementation of new traffic laws. *American Journal of Public Health, 104*(10), e89–e97. https://doi.org/10.2105/AJPH.2014.302068

Campbell, C. A., Hahn, R. A., Elder, R., Brewer, R., Chattopadhyay, S., Fielding, J., Naimi, T. S., Toomey, T., Lawrence, B., & Middleton, J. C. (2009). The effectiveness of limiting alcohol outlet density as a means of reducing excessive alcohol consumption and alcohol-related harms. *American Journal of Preventive Medicine, 37*(6), 556–569. https://doi.org/10.1016/j.amepre.2009.09.028

Carter, P. M., Flannagan, C. A. C., Bingham, C. R., Cunningham, R. M., & Rupp, J. D. (2015). Modeling the injury prevention impact of mandatory alcohol ignition interlock installation in all new US vehicles. *American Journal of Public Health, 105*(5), 1028–1035. https://doi.org/10.2105/AJPH.2014.302445

Chaudhuri, S., & Maloney, J. (2019). As Americans drink less alcohol, booze makers look beyond the barrel: Brewers and liquor companies seek nonalcoholic alternatives as beer volumes fall and growth in wine, spirits slow. *The Wall Street Journal.* www.wsj.com/articles/americans-are-drinking-less-alcohol-11547733600#:~:text=Americans%27%20consumption%20of%20ethanol,%20or,according%20to%20research%20firm%20Bernstein

Cook, P. J. (2007). *Paying the tab: The costs and benefits of alcohol control.* Princeton University Press.

De Sousa Fernandes Perna, E. B., Theunissen, E. L., Kuypers, K. P. C., Evers, E. A., Stiers, P., Toennes, S. W., Witteman, J., van Dalen, W., & Ramaekers, J. G. (2017). Brain reactivity to alcohol and cannabis marketing during sobriety and intoxication. *Addiction Biology, 22*(3), 823–832. https://doi.org/10.1111/adb.12351

De Visser, R. O., & Nicholls, J. (2020). Temporary abstinence during Dry January: Predictors of success; impacts on well-being and self-efficacy. *Psychology and Health*, 35(11), 1293–1305. https://doi.org/10.1080/08870446.2020.1743840

De Visser, R. O., & Piper, R. (2020). Short- and longer-term benefits of temporary alcohol abstinence during "Dry January" are not also observed among adult drinkers in the general population: Prospective cohort study. *Alcohol and Alcoholism, 55*(4), 433–438. https://doi.org/10.1093/alcalc/agaa025

De Visser, R. O., Robinson, E., Smith, T., Cass, G., & Walmsley, M. (2017). The growth of "Dry January": Promoting participation and the benefits of participation. *European Journal of Public Health, 27*(5), 929–931. https://doi.org/10.1093/eurpub/ckx124

Deacon, L., Morleo, M., Hannon, K. L., Cook, P. A., Tocque, K., Perkins, C., & Bellis, M. A. (2010). *Alcohol consumption: Segmentation series report 2.* Center for Public Health, Liverpool. John Moores University. Archived by WebCite® at www.webcitation.org/6RJLlXfGS

Delcher, C., Maldonado-Molina, M. M., & Wagenaar, A. C. (2012). Effects of alcohol taxes on alcohol-related disease mortality in New York state from 1969 to 2006. *Addictive Behaviors, 37*(7), 783–789. https://doi.org/10.1016/j.addbeh.2012.02.019

Deshapriya, E. B. R., & Iwase, N. (1998). Impact of the 1970 legal BAC 0.05 mg percent limit legislation on drunk-driver-involved traffic fatalities, accidents, and DWI in Japan. *Substance Use and Misuse, 33*(14), 2757–2788. https://doi.org/10.1080/17457300701440634

Dry July Foundation (2020). *Donate to a Dry July participant or team: Help us improve the comfort and well-being of people affected by cancer.* www.dryjuly.com/

Elder, R. W., Lawrence, B., Ferguson, A., Naimi, T. S., Brewer, R. D., Chattopadhyay, S. K., Toomey, T. L., & Fielding, J. E. (2010). The effectiveness of tax policy interventions for reducing excessive alcohol consumptions and related harms. *American Journal of Preventive Medicine, 38*(2), 217–229. https://doi.org/10.1016/j.amepre.2009.11.005

Elder, R. W., Voas, R., Beirness, D., Shults, R. A., Sleet, D. A., Nichols, J. L., & Compton, R. (2011). Effectiveness of ignition interlocks for preventing alcohol-impaired driving and alcohol-related crashes: A community guide systematic review. *American Journal of Preventive Medicine, 40*(3), 362–376. https://doi.org/10.1016/j.amepre.2010.11.012

Esser, M. B., & Jernigan, D. H. (2018). Policy approaches for regulating alcohol marketing in a global context: A public health perspective. *Annual Review of Public Health, 39*(1), 385–401. https://doi.org/10.1146/annurev-publhealth-040617-014711

Farrell, S., Manning, W. G., & Finch, M. D. (2003). Alcohol dependence and the price of alcoholic beverages. *Journal of Health Economics, 22*(1), 117–147. https://doi.org/10.1016/s0167–6296(02)00099-1

Farrell, T., & Gordeon, R. (2012). Critical social marketing: Investigating alcohol marketing in the developing world. *Journal of Social Marketing, 2*(2), 138–156. https://doi.org/10.1108/20426761211243973

Fell, J. C., & Voas, R. B. (2009). Reducing illegal blood alcohol limits for driving: Effects on traffic safety. In J. C. Verster, S. R. Pandi-Perumal, J. G. Ramaekers, & J. J. de Gier (Eds.), *Drugs, driving and traffic safety* (pp. 415–437). Birkhäuser Basel.

(2013). The effectiveness of a 0.05 blood alcohol concentration (BAC) limit for driving in the United States. *Addiction and Recovery, 109*(6), 869–874.

Foster, S., Gmel, G., & Mohler-Kuo, M. (2019). Light and heavy drinking in jurisdictions with different alcohol policy environments. *International Journal of Drug Policy, 65*, 86–96 https://doi.org/10.1016/j.drugpo.2019.01.014.

Foster, S., Held, L., Estevez, N., Gmel, G., & Mohler-Kuo, M. (2015). Liberal alcohol legislation: Does it amplify the effects among Swiss men of person-related risk factors on heavy alcohol use? *Addiction, 110*(11), 1746–1756. https://doi.org/10.1111/add.13032

Gruenewald, P. J. (2011). Regulating availability: How access to alcohol affects drinking and problems in youth and adults. *Alcohol Research and Health, 34*(2), 248–256.

Guide to Community Preventive Services (2013). *Preventing excessive alcohol consumption: Increasing alcohol taxes.* Archived by WebCite® at www.webcitation.org/6RPQ9FmIY

Guillou-Landréat, M., Dany, A., Yves Le Reste, J., Le Goff, D., Benyamina, A., Grall-Bronnec, M., & Gallopel-Morvan, K. (2020). Impact of alcohol marketing on drinkers with alcohol use disorders seeking treatment: A mixed-method study protocol. *BMC Public Health, 20*, 467. https://doi.org/10.1186/s12889–020-08543-6

Hahn, R. A., Kuzara, J. L., Elder, E., Brewer, R., Chattopadhyay, S., Fielding, J., Naimi, T. S., Toomey, T., J Middleton, J. C., & Lawrence, B. (2010). Effectiveness of policies restricting hours of alcohol sales in preventing excessive alcohol consumption and related harms. *American Journal of Preventive Medicine, 39*(6), 590–604. https://doi.org/10.1016/j.amepre.2010.09.016

Holder, H., Agardh, E., Högberg, P., Miller, T., Norström, T., Österberg, E., & Stockwell, T. (2007). *If retail alcohol sales in Sweden were privatized, what would be the potential consequences?* Swedish National Institute of Public Health. Archived by WebCite® at www.webcitation.org/6tQvTDPrl

Holland, K. (2018). A "Sober September" may be just what you need for a healthy fall season. *Healthline*. www.healthline.com/health-news/what-are-health-benefits-of-a-sober-september#:~:text=Sober%20September%20is%20one%20such,a%20chance%20to%20dry%20out

Jackson, S. E., Garnett, C., Shahab, L., Oldham, M., & Brown J. (2021). Association of the Covid-19 lockdown with smoking, drinking, and attempts to quit in England: an analysis of 2019–2020 data. *Addiction, 116*(5), 1233–1244. https://doi.org/10.1111/add.15295

Kelley-Baker, T., Lacey, J. H., Voas, R. B., Romano, E., Yao, J., & Berning, A. (2013). Drinking and driving in the United States: Comparing results from the 2007 and 1996 National Roadside Surveys. *Traffic Injury Prevention, 14*(2), 117–126. https://doi.org/10.1080/15389588.2012.697229

Kenkel, D. S. (2005). Are alcohol tax hikes fully passed through to prices? Evidence from Alaska. *The American Economic Review, 95*(2), 273–277. https://doi.org/10.1257/000282805774670284

Kerr, W. C., & Greenfield, T. K. (2007). Distribution of alcohol consumption and expenditures and the impact of improved measurement on coverage of alcohol sales in the 2000 National Alcohol Survey. *Alcoholism: Clinical and Experimental Research, 31*(10), 1714–1722. https://doi.org/10.1111/j.1530-0277.2007.00467.x

Kerr, W. C., Patterson, D., Greenfield, T. K., Jones, A. S., McGeary, K. A., Terza, J. V., & Ruhm, C. J. (2013). US alcohol affordability and real tax rates, 1950–2011. *American Journal of Preventive Medicine, 44*(5), 459–464. https://doi.org/10.1016/j.amepre.2013.01.007

Kilmer, B., Nicosia, N., Heaton, P., & Midgette, G. (2013). Efficacy of frequent monitoring with swift, certain, and modest sanctions for violations: Insights from South Dakota's 24/7 sobriety project. *American Journal of Public Health, 103*(1), e37–e43. https://doi.org/10.2105/AJPH.2012.300989

Maldonado-Molina, M .M., & Wagenaar, A. C. (2010). Effects of alcohol taxes on alcohol-related mortality in Florida: Time-series analyses from 1969 to 2004. *Alcoholism: Clinical and Experimental Research, 34*(11), 1915–1921. https://doi.org/10.1111/j.1530-0277.2010.01280.x

Nadkarni, A., Kapoor, A., & Pathare, S. (2020). COVID-19 and forced alcohol abstinence in India: The dilemmas around ethics and rights. *International Journal of Law and Psychiatry*, 101579. https://doi.org/10.1016/j.ijlp.2020.101579

Nagin, D. S., & Pogarsky, G. (2001). Integrating celerity, impulsivity, and extra-legal sanction threats into a model of general deterrence: Theory and evidence. *Criminology, 39*(4), 865–892. https://doi.org/10.1111/j.1745-9125.2001.tb00943.x

Naimi, T. S., Daley, J. I., Xuan, Z., Blanchette, J. G., Chaloupka, F. J., & Jernigan, D.H. (2016). Who would pay for state alcohol tax increases in the United States? *Preventing Chronic Disease, 13*, 150450. https://doi.org/10.5888/pcd13.150450

National Alcohol Beverage Control Association (NABCA) (2011). *The effects of privatization of alcohol control systems* (3rd ed.). Prepared by the Alcohol Research Group.

Nelson, T. F., Xuan, Z., Babor, T. F., Brewer, R. D., Chaloupka, F. J., Gruenewald, P. J., Holder, H., Klitzner, M., Mosher, J. F., Ramirez, R. L., Reynolds, R., Toomey, T. L., Churchill, V., & Naimi, T. S. (2013). Efficacy and the strength of evidence of US alcohol control policies. *American Journal of Preventive Medicine, 45*(1), 19–28. https://doi.org/10.1016/j.amepre.2013.03.008

Noel, J. K., Babor, T. F., & Robaina, K. (2017). Industry self-regulation of alcohol marketing: A systematic review of content and exposure research. *Addiction, 112*(S1), 28–50. https://doi.org/10.1111/add.13410

Norström, T., Miller, T., Holder, H., Österberg, E., Ramstedt, M., Rossow, I., & Stockwell, T. (2010). Potential consequences of replacing a retail alcohol monopoly with a private license system: Results from Sweden. *Addiction, 105*(12), 2113–2119. https://doi.org/10.1111/j.1360-0443.2010.03091.x

Ponicki, W. R., & Gruenewald, P. J. (2006). The impact of alcohol taxation on liver cirrhosis mortality. *Journal of Studies on Alcohol, 67*(6), 934–938. https://doi.org/10.15288/jsa.2006.67.934

Rehm, J., Kilian, C., Ferreira-Borges, C., Jernigan, D., Monteiro, M., Parry, C. D. H., Sanchez, A. M., & Manthey, J. (2020). Alcohol use in times of the COVID 19: Implications for monitoring and policy. *Drug and Alcohol Review, 39*(4), 301–304. https://doi.org/10.1111/dar.13074

Reynolds, J., & Wilkinson, C. (2020). Accessibility of "essential" alcohol in the time of COVID-19: Casting light on the blind spots of licensing? *Drug and Alcohol Review, 39*(4), 305–308. https://doi.org/10.1111/dar.13076

Room, R. (2004). Effects of alcohol controls: Nordic research traditions. *Drug and Alcohol Review, 23*(1), 43–53. https://doi.org/10.1080/09595230410001645547

Rossow, I., & Norström, T. (2012). The impact of small changes in bar closing hours on violence: The Norwegian experience from 18 cities. *Addiction, 107*(3), 530–537. https://doi.org/10.1111/j.1360-0443.2011.03643.x

Shrestha, V., & Markowitz, S. (2016). The pass-through of beer taxes to prices: Evidence from state and federal tax changes. *Economic Inquiry, 54*(4), 1946–1962. https://doi.org/10.1111/ecin.12343

Siegel, M., Grundman, J., DeJong, W., Naimi, T.S., King III, C., Albers, A. B., Williams, R. S., & Jernigan, D. H. (2013). State-specific liquor excise taxes and retail prices in eight US states, 2012. *Substance Abuse, 34*(4), 415–421. https://doi.org/10.1080/08897077.2013.792314

Siegfried, N., & Parry, C. (2019). Do alcohol control policies work? An umbrella review and quality assessment of systematic reviews of alcohol control interventions (2006-2017). *PLOS One, 14*(4), e0214865. https://doi.org/10.1371/journal.pone.0214865

Sloan, F. A., Eldred, L. M., & Xu, Y. (2014). The behavioral economics of drunk driving. *Journal of Health Economics, 35*, 64–81. https://doi.org/10.1016/j.jhealeco.2014.01.005

Splitter, J. (2020). How to make a "beer-like beverage" without the booze. *Forbes.* www.forbes.com/sites/forbes-personal-shopper/2020/07/01/best-gas-grills/#15c6d8c15ff6

Stautz, K., Brown, K. G., King, S. E., Shemilt, I., & Marteau, T. M. (2016). Immediate effects of alcohol marketing communications and media portrayals on consumption and cognition: A systematic review and meta-analysis of experimental studies. *BMC Public Health, 16*, 465. https://doi.org/10.1186/s12889-016-3116-8

Stockwell, T., Sherk, A., Norström, T., Angus, C., Ramstedt, M., Andréasson, S., Chikritzhs, T., Gripenberg, J. Holder, H. Holmes, J. & Mäkelä, P. (2018). Estimating the public health impact of disbanding a government alcohol monopoly: Application of new methods to the case of Sweden. *BMC Public Health, 18*(1400), https://doi.org/10.1186/s12889-018-6312-x

Stockwell, T., Zhao, J., Giesbrecht, N., Macdonald, S., Thomas, G., & Wettlaufer, A. (2012). The raising of minimum alcohol prices in Saskatchewan, Canada: Impacts on consumption and implications for public health. *American Journal of Public Health, 102*(12), e103–e110. https://ajph.aphapublications.org/doi/full/10.2105/AJPH.2012.301094

Stockwell, T., Zhao, J., Macdonald, S., Vallance, K., Gruenewald, P., Ponicki, W., Holder, H., & Treno, A. (2011). Impact on alcohol-related mortality of a rapid rise in the density of private liquor outlets in British Columbia: A local area multi-level analysis. *Addiction, 106*(4), 768–776. https://doi.org/10.1111/j.1360-0443.2010.03331.x

Subbaraman, M. S., & Kerr, W. C. (2016). Opinions on the privatization of distilled-spirits in Washington State: Did voters change their minds? *Journal of Studies on Alcohol and Drugs, 77*(4), 568–576. https://doi.org/10.15288/jsad.2016.77.568

Subbaraman, M. S., Mulia, N., Kerr, W. C., Patterson, D., Karriker-Jaffe, K. J., & Greenfield, T. K. (2020). Relationships between US state alcohol policies and alcohol outcomes: Differences by gender and race/ethnicity. *Addiction, 115*(7), 1285–1294. https://doi.org/10.1111/add.14937

Trangenstein, P. J., Curriero, F. C., Jennings, J. M., Webster, D., Latkin, C., Eck, R., & Jernigan, D. H. (2018a, November 10–14). *Outlet type, access to alcohol, and violent crime.* American Public Health Association Annual Meeting and Expo. San Diego, CA.

Trangenstein, P. J., Curriero, F. C., Webster, D., Jennings, J. M., Latkin, C., Eck, R., & Jernigan, D. H. (2018b). Outlet type, access to alcohol, and violent crime. *Alcoholism: Clinical and Experimental Research, 42*(11), 2234–2245. https://doi.org/10.1111/acer.13880

Varma, R. P. (2020). Alcohol withdrawal management during the Covid-19 lockdown in Kerala. *Indian Journal of Medical Ethics, V*(2), 105–106. https://doi.org/10.20529/IJME.2020.042

Voas, R. B., & Fell, J. C. (2011). Preventing impaired driving opportunities and problems. *Alcohol Research and Health, 34*(2), 225–235.

Wagenaar, A. C., Maldonado-Molina, M. M., & Wagenaar, B. H. (2009). Effects of alcohol tax increases on alcohol-related disease mortality in Alaska: Time-series analyses from 1976 to 2004. *American Journal of Public Health, 99*(9), 1464–1470. https://doi.org/10.2105/AJPH.2007.131326

Wagenaar, A. C., Salois, M. J., & Komro, K. A. (2009). Effects of beverage alcohol price and tax levels on drinking: A meta-analysis of 1003 estimates from 112 studies. *Addiction, 104*(2), 179–190. https://doi.org/10.1111/j.1360-0443.2008.02438.x

Wagenaar, A. C., Tobler, A. L., & Komro, K. A. (2010). Effects of alcohol tax and price policies on morbidity and mortality: A systematic review. *American Journal of Public Health, 100*(11), 2270–2278. https://doi.org/10.2105/AJPH.2009.186007

Wall, M., Casswell, S., & Yeh, L.-C. (2017). Purchases by heavier drinking young people concentrated in lower priced beverages: Implications for policy. *Drug and Alcohol Review, 36*(3), 352–358. https://doi.org/10.1111/dar.12495

Warrington, R. (2018). *Sober curious: The blissful sleep, greater focus, deep connection, and limitless presence awaiting us all on the other side of alcohol.* HarperCollins.

Williams, P. P., Morojele, N., Londani, M., Burnhams, N. H., & Parry, C. D. H. (2019). Alcohol advertising, affordability and availability, and the effect on adult heavy drinking and symptoms of alcohol problems: international alcohol control study (South Africa). *Substance Use and Misuse, 54*(11), 1751–1762. https://doi.org/10.1080/10826084.2019.1609987

Witteman, J., Post, H., Tarvainen, M., de Bruijn, A., De Sousa Fernandes Perna, E., Ramaekers, J. G., & Wiers, R. W. (2015). Cue reactivity and its relation to craving and relapse in alcohol dependence: A combined laboratory and field study. *Psychopharmacology, 232*(20), 3685–3696. https://doi.org/10.1007/s00213-015-4027-6

Xu, X., & Chaloupka, F. J. (2011). The effects of prices on alcohol use and its consequences. *Alcohol Research and Health, 34*(2), 236–245.

Xuan, Z., Nelson, T. F., Heeren, T., Blanchette, J., Nelson, D. E., Gruenewald, P., & Naimi, T. S. (2013). Tax policy, adult binge drinking, and youth alcohol consumption in the United States. *Alcoholism: Clinical and Experimental Research, 37*(10), 1713–1719. https://doi.org/10.1111/acer.12152

Young, D. J., & Bielinska-Kwapisz, A. (2002). Alcohol taxes and beverage prices. *National Tax Journal, 55*(1), 57–73. https://doi.org/dx.doi.org/10.17310/ntj.2002.1.04

Zhao, J., & Stockwell, T. (2017). The impacts of minimum alcohol pricing on alcohol attributable morbidity in regions of British Colombia, Canada, with low, medium, and high mean family income. *Addiction, 112*(11), 1942–1951. https://doi.org/10.1111/add.13902

Zhao, J., Stockwell, T., Martin, G., Macdonald, S., Vallance, K., Treno, A., Ponicki, W. R., Tu, A., & Buxton, J. (2013). The relationship between minimum alcohol prices, outlet densities, and alcohol-attributable deaths in British Columbia, 2002–09. *Addiction, 108*(6), 1059–1069. https://doi.org/10.1111/add.12139

20 Causal Inference Approaches to Studying Recovery from Alcohol Use Disorder

Douglas Steinley

Causal Inference Approaches to Studying Recovery from Alcohol Use Disorder

In recent years, the health, behavioral, and social sciences have undertaken a certain degree of soul-searching due to the so-called "replication crisis." Simply put, several effects – sometimes even highly publicized effects – have failed to be replicated by independent researchers (or even sometimes the same research group). Several reasons have been proposed for this, including but not limited to misunderstanding statistics and *p*-values, using sample sizes that are too small, lack of theoretical underpinnings, exploratory data analysis, and many more (see Tackett & Miller 2019). Likely, it is a confluence of many factors. However, in this chapter, two drivers will be highlighted that may be more to blame than others: exploratory data analysis and lack of theory that have led to such difficulties in replicating results and subsequently establishing causality between a cause and an effect.

Historically, the gold standard for determining causality in the field of statistics has been experimental manipulation through randomization. Perhaps apocryphally, Fisher (1935) famously developed this method to test whether an individual could tell whether tea or milk was added to a cup of tea first by creating four glasses of tea where the tea was added prior to the milk and four glasses where the milk was added before the tea and then randomly permuted their order and presented them for tasting (Salsburg, 2001). Fisher called randomization the "reasoned basis for inference" in experiments; consequently, he demonstrated that treatment effects could be estimated based on distributions that are created from the randomization process itself. Almost miraculously, no assumptions are required and the randomization process accounts for all covariates (both measured and unmeasured). The notion of randomization revolutionized the early field of statistics, leading to substantial gains in both theory and application throughout the twentieth century. In the health and behavioral sciences, the most likely place to first encounter randomization is in the discussion of simple experimental designs that are often analyzed with a *t*-test or a one-way analysis of variance. The general idea is that a treatment effect is hypothesized and participants are randomly assigned to one of two groups, either the treatment group or the control group. After this random assignment, the treatment is administered to the treatment group (but not the control group) and then subsequent differences between the groups are analyzed on an outcome of interest. Due to the randomization, and given adequate sample size, it is then assumed that any observed differences must be due to the treatment – such differences are often termed treatment effects.

Unfortunately, researchers often find themselves in a position where conducting a true experiment is not feasible for a variety of reasons (cost, ethics, resources, etc.) and can attempt to turn to approximations of the gold standard. In other words, what types of studies can be designed that are as close as possible to a true experiment – even though a randomization protocol cannot be implemented. This chapter discusses a variety of these quasi-experimental designs, including regression discontinuity, differences-in-differences, and interrupted time series. Most of the data collected with these designs can be analyzed in the framework of the general linear model; consequently, a brief review of regression is provided to provide a common ground to understand the rationale underlying each of these quasi-experimental designs. Structural equation modeling (SEM) and causal graphical modeling can also help disentangle causal effects in a system, and these methodologies undoubtedly have much to contribute to the discussion. However, they are excluded from this chapter because the associated assumptions and technical expertise necessary for implementation and interpretation preclude their sufficient discussion in this chapter format and because the data collected in the psychological sciences often fall short of supporting causal statements from such complex, multivariable models.

Beyond the focus on quasi-experimental designs, there has been an explosion of the development of statistical methods for causal inference among observational data (see Rosenbaum, 2002, 2010; Rubin, 2006). However, as Shadish et al. (2002) noted, these advanced statistical methodologies are not a knight in shining armor that can save poor study design. In fact, without well-planned study design, no amount of statistic machinery will reveal a causal structure between variables.

Randomized Experiments

As mentioned above, in the course of developing statistical methods for agricultural advances, Fisher (1925, 1926, 1935) concretely established the rationale for linking causal inference to the act of randomization of experimental units to treatment. Shadish et al. (2002) noted one of the main advantages of randomization is that all possible confounding variables are unlikely to be correlated with the condition (either treatment or control) to which an experimental unit is assigned. For instance, imagine a study investigating whether there is a causal relationship between alcohol use and depression. In this instance, depression would be the outcome, and alcohol use would be the predictor. Randomly assigning people to the alcohol use condition allows separation of all the variation in depression that is due to the treatment condition from variation that is due to all other factors (e.g., all other sources of depression). This notion of randomization can be utilized in several experimental designs (see Lash et al., 2021; Maxwell et al., 2017; Shadish et al., 2002). Using a taxonomy similar to Shadish et al. (2002), some common designs that are used to infer causality are described next.

Treatment vs. Control

The most basic experimental design is to have two groups, where experimental units are randomly assigned to the treatment group and the control group (usually with equal probability). After random assignment, the two groups are compared on some outcome of interest. A natural variant on this design is when the experimental units are randomly assigned to two treatment groups, where one of the treatment groups is considered to be the best available current treatment and the other is a new, competitor treatment. Alternatively, it is easy to imagine experimental units being randomly assigned to multiple treatments or the control.

Factorial Designs

When two or more independent variables (called "factors," hence the name of the design) have at least two levels each, then a factorial design can be used. There are numerous factorial designs. The most common is likely the fully-crossed factorial design where all experimental units (ideally an equal number) are assigned to each combination of factor levels across all of the factors. Two advantages of these designs are that the same power as other designs can be achieved with fewer experimental units and the interaction between factors (e.g., independent treatment variables) can be tested. Although the fully-crossed factorial design is often recommended, it is possible to have fractional-factorial designs (e.g., experimental units are not assigned to all cross-classifications), nested factor designs (e.g., not all levels of one factor are crossed with each other), Latin square designs, and split-plot/strip-plot designs, to mention a few.

Designs with Pre-Test and Longitudinal Designs

All of the above designs can also be used with a pre-test, where the pre-test ideally measures the outcome of interest prior to the intervention being tested. The randomization can be conducted prior to pre-test (most common) or after the pre-test has been administered to all experimental units. Designs with a pre-test/post-test component tend to increase the power to detect group differences. Longitudinal designs are basically an extension of the pre-test/post-test designs. Instead of only measuring the outcome once prior to the treatment and once after the treatment, the variable of interest can be measured several times before and several times after the treatment. It is most common to measure it more times after the intervention than before the intervention. Again, experimental units are randomly assigned to groups that receive different interventions.

The cross-over design is a type of longitudinal design where experimental units are randomly assigned to treatment groups. After the treatment occurs, the individuals receive a post-test and then receive the other treatment followed by another post-test. As a process, it would look like: Randomization ➔ Treatment 1 ➔ Post-test ➔ Treatment 2 ➔ Post-test. Naturally, there would be a second group that had the structure: Randomization ➔ Treatment 2 ➔ Post-test ➔ Treatment 1 ➔ Post-test. As with all of these designs, it can be made more complex in multiple fashions, such as inserting a pre-test between the randomization and the first treatment phase or more than two treatments can be used. The crossover design is a special case of the more general Latin square design (Fisher & Yates, 1953).

Multiple Regression

Maxwell et al. (2017) explicated the data analysis of the above mentioned designs (among many more) in the traditional analysis of variance framework. However, it is well-known that equivalent analyses can be conducted within the general linear modeling framework. For instance, consider the basic design of investigating the effect of treatment vs. control on an outcome variable. This can be represented by the following equation

$$Y_{ij} = \mu + \tau_i + \varepsilon_{ij},$$

where Y_{ij} is the outcome for the *jth* observation in the *ith* treatment, μ is the overall mean, τ_i is the treatment effect of the *ith* group, and ε_{ij} is the residual for the *jth* observation in the *ith* treatment. This can be easily rewritten as the standard regression equation

$$Y = \mathbf{X}\beta + \mathbf{e}$$

where Y is the vector of outcomes, **X** is the design matrix with g columns (e.g., a column of ones that represents the intercept, or the overall mean, and g-1 dummy coded variables, where g is the number of treatment groups). In the simple example with only a treatment group and a control group, β is the estimate for the treatment effect.

Similarly, an observational study that does not have a randomization component can be represented in the same format, with additional covariates, **Z**

$$Y = \mathbf{X}\beta_x + \mathbf{Z}\beta_z + \mathbf{e}.$$

Often, covariates are included in the model to "control" for existing variables whose effects could not be accounted for by the randomization process. Furthermore, in observational studies, no assumption is made about the relationship between the covariates (**Z**) and the predictor of interest (**X**), and they can be expected to have some non-zero correlation. Consequently, the relationship between **X** and *Y* is then confounded by the covariates **Z**, making the pure treatment effect (e.g., between **X** and *Y*) difficult to tease apart from the effect of the covariates (e.g., between **Z** and *Y*) since the covariates and the treatment are correlated – not to mention, all of the covariates that are not included in the model. In contrast, the randomization of experimental units to groups makes all covariates included in the model, as well as those not included in the model, independent of the predictor variable (e.g., group membership). It is important to note that covariates could be included in the experimental model as well, resulting in the traditional Analysis of Covariance (ANCOVA) model. For ANCOVA to be successful, three assumption are generally assumed to hold: (1) the dependent variable is linearly related to the covariate, (2) groups (e.g., treatments) have the same slope – in other words, there is not an interaction between the treatment variable and the covariate, and (3) the covariate is unaffected by differences among the means of the groups

Since the model formulation for experimental designs and observational studies can be equivalently represented (e.g., above as a general linear model), it becomes clear that the causality is not related to the statistical estimation of the model. In fact, in this example, causality is related to the randomization of experimental units to groups. In the absence of this randomization, causality is very difficult to establish. Nevertheless, as discussed next, there are a handful of quasi-experimental designs that can be applied in observational studies that can approximate the process of randomization.

Quasi-Experimental Designs

Two quasi-experimental designs that can come close to approximating causality are regression discontinuity and interrupted time series. Additionally, propensity scores – an analytic approach often assumed to uncover causality – is discussed.

Regression Discontinuity

The observational design that is closest to a randomized experiment is the regression discontinuity design. At its heart, the regression discontinuity is a pre-test/post-test design. Experimental units are assigned to groups based on a predetermined cutoff value of a variable (termed the "forcing" variable) that is collected prior to intervention. The entire notion of a cutoff value is an advantage for regression discontinuity designs as it allows the treatment to be provided to the experimental units who are in most need (whether the treatment group is above or below the cutoff). After the cutoff value on the forcing variable has been determined and the experimental units have been assigned to the treatment or control group, comparisons on the outcome variable can be made. A simple example could be where the forcing variable are scores on the Alcohol Use Disorders Identification Test (AUDIT; Saunders et al. 1993) administered to all college freshmen, the cutoff criterion could be eight, the "treatment" could be a prevention program for the subset of freshmen who scored above an eight, and then the outcome could be college GPA, with the goal to determine if receiving the prevention program had an effect on the subsequent college GPA. It has been well-documented that this type of design is the optimal quasi-experimental design and approaches the interval validity exhibited by a randomized experiment, albeit less efficiently.

However, for this to be the case, several assumptions must be met. First, there must be strict adherence to the cutoff criterion. That is, in this simple study example, if someone has an AUDIT score of eight or above, they must receive and attend the prevention program. Likewise, if they have a score less than eight, they cannot receive the prevention program. Deviations away from strict adherence will weaken subsequent causal claims.

Second, the more narrow the comparison around the cutoff, the stronger the causal claim. For instance, in this example, drawing from classical test theory, it could be assumed that each expressed measurement of AUDIT is really a combination of the true score plus error score, and any group of individuals around the cutoff are basically being drawn from the same portion of the distribution. In this example, some subjects who scored a nine on the AUDIT might have a true score of seven, and, conversely, some subjects who scored a seven on the AUDIT might have a true score of nine. In reality, there is some degree of randomness on who "lands" slightly above and slightly below the cutoff. If we compared participants with a seven on the AUDIT with participants with an eight on the AUDIT, where the latter received the prevention program and the former did not, confounding variables can be safely assumed to be equivalent between the two groups. However, as the window around the cutoff grows, the assumption of equivalence of confounding variables between the two groups becomes less tenable.

Figure 20.1 provides a hypothetical example of the regression discontinuity design. The general assumption is that, absent of the treatment, the linear trend would stay the same. Additionally, it is assumed that there is not a spurious discontinuity that coincides with the cutoff point by happenstance (generally, this is not too much of a concern). The treatment effect is the difference between the end of the line on the left side of the cutoff and the beginning of the line on the right side of the cutoff.

To highlight the issue around a narrow bandwidth, consider Figure 20.2, where there is no treatment effect. Two possible bandwidths are illustrated: (1) a bandwidth containing only the observations between the two dotted vertical lines and (2) considering all observations on each side of the cutoff. For the first bandwidth, the conclusion would be that there is no treatment effect as there is no discontinuity between the two lines. However, if all observations on each side of the cutoff were considered, the means of both sides would correspond to the

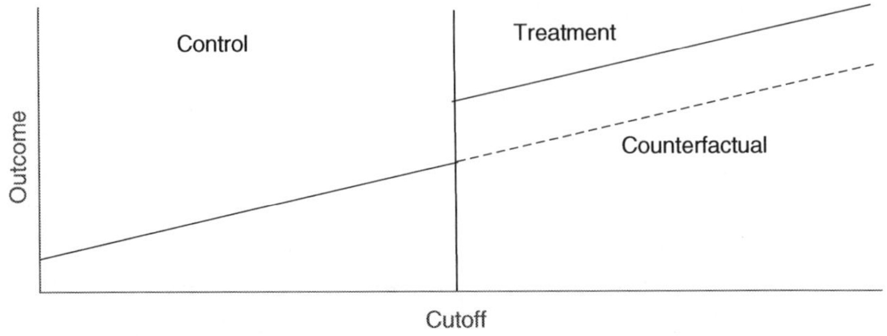

Figure 20.1 *Regression discontinuity example.*

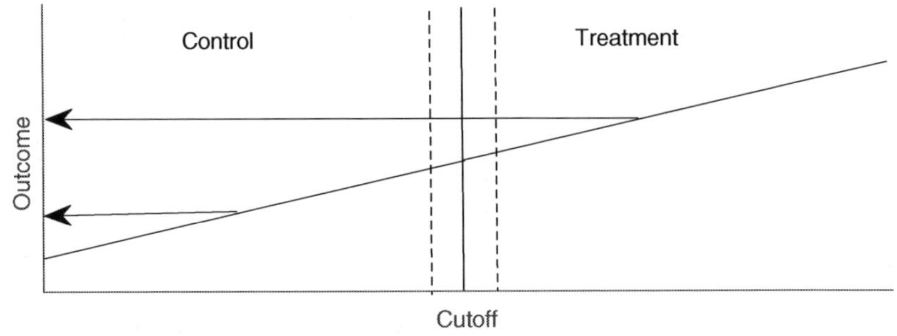

Figure 20.2 *Effect of bandwidth around a cutoff.*

arrows that are projected onto the y-axis. In this case, there is a much greater difference between the treatment and control, leading to the erroneous conclusion that there is a treatment effect.

Similar mistaken conclusions can occur if the wrong functional form is fit to the data, such as fitting a linear model when the true relationship is curvilinear. As such, it is recommended to fit a higher-order polynomial to the data than what is expected; generally, fit a polynomial that is an order or two higher than what is observed when visually inspecting the relationship between the forcing variable and the outcome. Much like fitting a higher order polynomial, it is recommended to fit a model with as many covariates, polynomial terms, and interactions as necessary. In fact, it is better to have an over-identified model, capture the correct functional form of the model, and risk inefficiency in the estimate of the treatment effect than it is to have an under-identified model and risk bias in the estimate of the treatment effect (Lee et al., 2016). Beyond strict adherence to the cutoff and modeling the correct functional form, it is necessary to have a large sample size, ensure that all observations are drawn from the same population, and ensure that those who receive the treatment receive the same amount for the same duration of time (see Linden et al., 2006).

In terms of applying this methodology to alcohol use disorder and associated research, regression discontinuity designs were recommended by Hester and

Miller (1988) more than 30 years ago. As an example, consider the study by Flam-Zalcman et al. (2013), who used a regression discontinuity design to determine if increased treatment is beneficial for individuals with more serious alcohol problems; in other words, should the amount of treatment be correlated with the degree of severity of problems? The variable collected prior to the treatment and used as the forcing variable was based on scale scores extracted from the Research Institute on Addictions Self-Inventory (Mann et al., 2009). Participants who exceeded the cutoff score received a 16-hour intervention, whereas those who did not received an 8-hour intervention. Flam-Zalcman et al. (2013) found that participants who received the longer intervention showed significant reductions in the days of alcohol use at the cutoff score, which determined the individuals who received the treatment. This highlights a benefit of the regression discontinuity design in that participants who have the highest scale scores are those who receive the treatment.

Interrupted Time Series

Another quasi-experimental design that is considered to provide strong insight into causality is the interrupted time series design. The basic premise of this design is that the dependent variable is measured at numerous time points (much like a regular time series) and, at some point in time, an intervention (e.g., an interruption) occurs. Much like the regression discontinuity design, a break in the time series is tested – whether that is a change in level, trend, slope, etc. Any change at the point of the intervention is attributed as a causal effect due to the intervention.

Naturally, there are threats to validity surrounding such a design. Namely, other "events" could occur around the same time and could cause the same effect – this is similar to the threat of an ancillary change occurring at exactly the cutoff in the regression discontinuity design. There are safeguards that can be used to help provide confidence that the causal effects are due to the intervention. First, shrink the width of the measurement intervals in the time series design. Second, add a non-equivalent dependent variable that is hypothesized will not be affected by the intervention. Third, add a control group time series that is not affected by the intervention. Fourth, ensure that the manner in which the outcome is measured stays constant across the entire time series (especially when the intervention occurs).

While there has been a call for greater use of interrupted time series designs in intervention research (Biglan et al., 2000), alcohol research has only seen occasional use of these designs. For example, Humphreys et al. (2013) evaluated the effect of lifting regulatory restrictions on the times at which alcohol could be sold on measures of community violence, as measured by police records of violence, robbery, and total crime before and after the regulatory restrictions were lifted. Results indicated no effect on the overall level of violence, although the pattern of violence did shift to be later in the evenings. A renewed call for an increase in time series analyses in addiction research was recently provided by Beard et al. (2019). Although speculative, it seems plausible that some of the lack of use of these methods is due to the increased statistical complexities of collecting and modeling time series data (Shadish et al., 2002), with the primary issue being the presence of autocorrelation among the error terms. In the context of terror management theory, Stein et al. (2011) showed that modeling the 9/11 terrorist attacks "intervention" as a breakpoint (e.g., similar to a knot in a regression spline) in a piecewise linear model resulted in the same conclusions as an interrupted time series using an Autoregressive Integrated Moving Average (ARIMA) model. In both analyses, results indicated that there was an increase in federal sentencing in morally charged crimes, as compared to amoral crimes, from before to after the 9/11 terrorist attacks.

When compared to regression discontinuity, interrupted time series differs in the following ways: (1) it operates in the time domain rather than as a cutoff on a continuous variable, (2) it is much easier to do retrospectively (generally, regression discontinuity has to establish the cutoff score prospectively), (3) it is sensitive to competing interventions, and (4) it is sensitive to changes in the population. Both designs must rule out competing interventions, and both designs can test for changes in level (e.g., intercept) and trend (e.g., slope).

Propensity Scores

In an observational study, individuals self-select into participating in the "treatment" or the "control" condition. As in the other designs discussed, it is common to include several covariates in the model with the non-randomized treatment variable. Unsurprisingly, these covariates will be correlated with the non-randomized treatment variable, and the problems discussed within observational studies will rear their ugly heads. The aim of propensity scores is to recognize this correlation and create a "match" on the covariates (often called instrumental variables) between the individuals who self-selected into the treatment and those who self-selected into the control. After matching, the matched individuals will not be significantly different on the covariates. This process is basically extracting a portion of the multivariate covariate space where the covariates are uncorrelated with the non-randomized control. Propensity score analysis has been used more extensively in alcohol research than the quasi-experimental designs discussed earlier. For example, Magura et al. (2014) used propensity score matching to estimate the effect of Alcoholics Anonymous on drinking outcomes, and Vocht et al. (2016) used propensity score matching to estimate the effects of alcohol policies in case series and quasi-case control designs.

The assumption is then that the propensity score creates a group of participants that are nearly equivalent to what would be found in a randomized experiment, using the following logic: first, if experimental units are randomized to groups, then measured and unmeasured covariates are uncorrelated with the group membership (this was shown by Fisher, 1935). Second and conversely, if group membership is uncorrelated with measured covariates, then the experimental units are as good as randomized. Clearly, from classical logic this is very close to the logical fallacy of affirming the consequent (specifically, if "A" is true, then "B" is true, when "B" is true, therefore "A" is true). Original developers of the propensity score system recognized this and provided a suite of tests to help determine how close the propensity score matching process approximates balanced covariates and, by extension, randomization. Nonetheless, there is a problem that can never be addressed – randomization balances all the covariates, both measured and unmeasured. Propensity score matching on measured covariates can never verify that the matched groups are also balanced on the unmeasured covariates. This almost always will not be true in that it is possible to imagine an infinite number of unmeasured covariates that could be related to both the outcome and the group membership. In fact, when discussing instrumental variables, Hernan and Robins (2006, p. 360) stated, "Can you guarantee that the results from your observational study are unaffected by unmeasured confounding? The only answer an epidemiologist can provide is 'no'."

Beyond the issue of omitted variables complicating the inference of causality, the model relating the covariates to group membership to generate the propensity scores needs to be sound and make good predictions; otherwise, the matching will basically be worthless. Unfortunately, the covariate model cannot be too good because there will not be anyone left to match as the distribution of the propensity scores will not overlap between the "treatment" and the "control" group. In other words, creating perfect predictions will result in no overlap in the propensity to be in the treatment group versus the propensity to be in the control group. Basically, this involves trying to thread the model building needle where the relationship between the covariates and the treatment variable is good, but not too good. The goal is to fit a mediocre model.

While such a mediocre model might seem to be the ticket to finding a suitable set of observations on which to match in order to approximate a randomized experiment, it likely is not. The risk is that researchers using propensity scores are misleading themselves into thinking they have revealed a slice of the observational space that mirrors an experiment. Unfortunately, as propensity score models are compared to randomized experiments, they are commonly found not to agree in their conclusions (see Atkins & Aldea, 2018; Mnatzaganian et al., 2015). Somewhat ironically, Loux (2015) and Xu and Kalbfleisch (2012) showed that propensity score matching performs well in highlighting the causal relationship when propensity score matching is combined with randomized clinical trials, illustrating that one of the key components to a sound study design is randomization.

In addition to this overview of propensity score matching, it should be noted that there are myriad ways to both estimate the propensity scores, match the observations, and estimate the final treatment effect. Having so many options opens up propensity scores to be selectively chosen to obtain the desired result. As such, it is recommended that every propensity score analysis also use a sensitivity analysis to determine the degree to which the final estimated treatment effect is due to specific decisions made by the researcher. Such an analysis, often termed a multiverse analysis (see Irvin et al. 2020 for an example), recommends making all possible combinations of subjective decisions (all matching methods, propensity score estimation, etc.) to generate a distribution of treatment effects. Ideally, the observed treatment effect will fall in the middle of the distribution of treatment effects, indicating that the results are not driven by the subjective decisions of the researcher.

Given the questionable utility in uncovering causal effects, propensity score analysis can also be thought of as a way to conduct data reduction in a high-dimensional covariate space. When many covariates are present, the propensity score can serve as a way to represent all of them as a single value computed from a linear combination. However, much like principal components analysis or factor analysis, not all information will be captured in this singular dimension. Furthermore, as the number of variables increases, the number of observations required due to the increase in dimensionality will increase exponentially (see Steinley, 2006).

Psychometric Network Modeling

As mentioned in the introduction, causal graphical modeling can be used to attempt tease causal information out of complicated models, such as structural equation modeling (SEM). While there is not space to discuss this type of modeling in detail, it would be a disservice not to mention a type of modeling that has taken the clinical psychology field – especially areas concerned with diagnoses – by storm over the last five years: psychometric network modeling. The general notion of this type of modeling is laudable and follows a medical model; namely, symptoms cause symptoms and are agents in a broader causal system (Borsboom, 2008). A tacit goal is to supplant (or perhaps supplement) latent variable modeling, which posits that symptoms arise from an unobserved, common cause. Indeed, much work has been done in developing networks of mental disorders (see Fried et al., 2017, for an example) that seek to point to underlying causal mechanisms.

That being said, the vast majority of the methods that are used to estimate these networks are based on association/correlation: (1) association networks (Epskamp et al., 2012), which often have zero-order correlations between items; (2) concentration networks (van Borkulo et al., 2014), which are usually based on partial correlations; (3) directed acyclic graphs (Scutari, 2010), in which the presence of one symptom is likely to suggest the presence of another symptom; and (4) relative importance networks (Gromping, 2015), which are based on the proportion of variance one symptoms in another symptom after controlling for all other symptoms. Of these, concentration networks seem to be the most prevalent, which represent the partial correlations through Gaussian graphical models

(GGM) for continuous data (Epskamp & Fried, 2018) and the Ising model for binary data (Brusco et al., 2019).

Often, the GGM is estimated with the inverse of the covariance matrix (also referred to as the concentration matrix – hence the name "concentration network"), and the Ising model is estimated with a series of logistic regressions. The elements of the concentration matrix can be used to compute the parameter estimates in a standard linear regression model; consequently, both the GGM and the Ising model are basically just a series of regressions (one for each symptom). As such, there should be no expectation that causality can be inferred from these methods. Rather, unless an appropriate design is utilized, these methods should be viewed as exploratory.

Software

To estimate these models, there are several software packages available. For instance, there are numerous software packages available for estimating experimental designs and traditional general linear models, such as SAS, SPSS, and Mplus. However, as more specialized quasi-experimental designs (regression discontinuity, interrupted time series, propensity scores, instrumental variables, etc.) are utilized, the free software package R is a good place to turn to. Specifically, the following packages are quite useful: **rdd** (regression discontinuity designs); **changepoint** (interrupted time series analysis); **Matching, MatchIT, twang** (propensity score analysis); **pcalg** (causal inference using graphical models); **experiment** (experimental design specifically for clinical trials); and **qgraph** (psychometric network visualization and graphical model estimation).

Conclusions and Recommendations

Much like the famous real estate saying, often attributed to Lord Harold Samuel, "There are three things that matter in property: *location, location, location*," we can say that there are three things that matter in causal inference: *design, design, design*. In fact, Rubin (2001, 2007, 2008) argued that the design and analysis of observational studies should mirror that of randomized trials and suggests propensity scores can be used at the data collection phase – before outcome data are collected – to match the treatment and controls on a wide array of covariates to ensure that the data are properly balanced prior to analyzing the data. No amount of statistical wizardry or advanced computational methods can result in scientific alchemy and magically create causal relationships in the absence of a well-conceived research design rooted in theory pertinent to the research area being studied.

While linear regression and other forms of the general linear model have revolutionized the analysis of data across many fields by providing both a cognitive framework for conceptualizing relationships and expressing magnitudes of effects, it is questionable whether its widespread deployment has done more harm than good. Every regression model comes with parameter estimates and associated statistical tests, on which numerous statistical inferences within a single research study are based. Unfortunately, these statistical inferences are often mistaken for clues to causal inference (even outright for causal inference itself), when most of the time it is little better than exploratory data analysis. The desire to infer causality increases as the linear regression model becomes more complex; for example, the morass of directional arrows in a structural equation model practically cries out for a causal interpretation. These methods are merely layering a patina of causality over complicated methods for representing correlations between variables. Pearl (2009, 2017), under the guise of the "structural causal model," established methods to highlight the effects of interventions and counterfactuals that move well beyond just interpreting parameters from a statistical analysis. In fact, Pearl (2009) offered the following principle: "One cannot substantiate causal claims from associations alone, even at the population level – behind every causal conclusion there must lie some causal assumption that is not testable in observational studies" (p. 99).

Combining this weakness of associative methods (such as the general linear model) with the need for the data collection of observational studies to mirror randomized control trials as closely as possible provides a strong argument that the social and behavioral sciences have many foundational deficiencies to shore up with respect to supporting causal statements. The wide array of experimental designs discussed at the beginning of this chapter can provide a template for data collection and study design (even if it is an observational study) to help the study hew as closely as possible to an experiment. Beyond aiding in supporting advances toward causal statements, such careful approaches are likely to result in stronger theory building and greater replication. As Heinlein famously said in *The Moon is a Harsh Mistress,* "There ain't no such thing as a free lunch." In this case, there is no causality without appropriate design and theory, and it is critically important to consider these issues in order to advance research on a multidimensional view of recovery from alcohol use disorder.

References

Atkins, B. Z., & Aldea, G. S. (2018). The paradox between randomized controlled trials and propensity score-matched real-world data: Moving dissonance to dialog? *The Journal of Thoracic and Cardiovascular Surgery, 156*(3), 1026–1027. https://doi.org/10.1016/j.jtcvs.2018.06.003

Beard, E., Marsden, J., Brown, J., Tombor, I., Stapleton, J., Michie, S., & West, R. (2019). Understanding and using time series analyses in addiction research. *Addiction, 114*(10), 1866–1884. https://doi.org/10.1111/add.14643

Biglan, A., Ary, D., & Wagenaar, A. C. (2000). The value of interrupted time-series experiments for community intervention research. *Prevention Science, 1*(1), 31–49. https://doi.org/10.1023/a:1010024016308

Borsboom, D. (2008). Psychometric perspectives on diagnostic systems. *Journal of Clinical Psychology, 64*(9), 108–109. https://doi.org/10.1002/jclp.20503

Brusco, M. J., Steinley, D., Hoffman, M., Davis-Stober, C., & Wasserman, S. W. (2019). On Ising models and algorithms for the construction of symptom networks in psychopathological research. *Psychological Methods, 24*(6), 735–753. https://doi.org/10.1037/met0000207

Epskamp, S., Cramer, A. O., Waldorp, L. J., Schmittmann, V. D., & Borsboom, D. (2012). *Qgraph:* Network visualizations of relationships in psychometric data. *Journal of Statistical Software, 48*(4), 1–18. https://doi.org/10.18637/jss.v048.i04

Epskamp, S., & Fried, E. I. (2018). A tutorial on regularized partial correlation networks. *Psychological Methods, 23*(4), 617–634. https://doi.org/10.1037/met0000167

Fisher, R. A. (1925). *Statistical methods for research workers*. Oliver & Boyd.

(1926). The arrangement of field experiments. *Journal of the Ministry of Agriculture of Great Britain, 33,* 505–513.

(1935). *The design of experiments*. Oliver & Boyd.

Fisher, R. A., & Yates, F. (1953). *Statistical tables for biological, agricultural, and medical research* (4th ed.). Oliver & Boyd.

Flam-Zalcman, R., Mann, R. E., Studoto, G., Nochajski, T. H., Rush, B. R., Koski-Jannes, A., Wickens, C. M., Thomas, R. K., & Rehm, J. (2013). Evidence from regression-discontinuity analyses for beneficial effects of a criterion-based increase in alcohol treatment. *International Journal of Methods in Psychiatry Research, 22*(1), 59–70. https://doi.org/10.1002/mpr.1374

Fried, E. I., van Borkulo, C. D., Cramer, A. O., Boschloo, L., Schoevers, R. A., & Borsboom, D. (2017). Mental disorders as networks of problems: A review of recent insights. *Social Psychiatry and Psychiatric Epidemiology, 52*(1), 1–10. https://doi.org/10.1007/s00127–016-1319-z

Gromping, U. (2015). Variable importance in regression models. *WIREs Computational Statistics, 7*(2), 137–152. https://doi.org/10.1002/wics.1346

Hernan, M. A., & Robins, J. M. (2006). Instruments for causal inference: An epidemiologists dream? *Epidemiology, 17*(4), 360–372. https://doi.org/10.1097/01.ede.0000222409.00878.37

Hester, R. K., & Miller, W. R. (1988). Empirical guidelines for optimal client-treatment matching. *NIDA Research Monograph, 77,* 27–38.

Humphreys, D. K., Eisner, M. P.., & Wieber, D. J. (2013). Evaluating the impact of flexible alcohol trading hours on violence: An interrupted time series analysis. *PLoS One, 8*(2), e55581. https://doi.org/10.1371/journal.pone.0055581

Irvin, K. M., Bell, D. J., Steinley, D., & Bartholow, B. (2020). The thrill of victory: Savoring positive affect, psychophysiological reward processing, and symptoms of depression. *Emotion*. Advance online publication. https://doi.org/10.1037/emo0000914

Lash, T. L., VanderWeele, T. J., Haneuse, S., & Rothman, K. J. (2021). *Modern epidemiology* (4th ed.). Wolters Kluwer.

Lee, M.-J. (2016). *Matching, regression discontinuity, differences in differences, and beyond.* Oxford University Press.

Linden, A. Adams, J. L., & Roberts, N. (2006). Evaluating disease management programme effectiveness: An introduction to the regression discontinuity design. *Journal of Evaluation in Clinical Practice, 12*(2), 124–131. https://doi.org/10.1111/j.1365-2753.2005.00573.x

Loux, T. M. (2015). Randomization, matching, and propensity scores in the design and analysis of experimental studies with measured baseline covariates. *Statistics in Medicine, 34*(4), 558–570. https://doi.org/10.1002/sim.6361

Magura, S., McKean, J., Kosten, S., & Tonigan, J. S. (2014). A novel application of propensity score matching to estimate Alcoholics Anonymous' effects on drinking outcomes. *Drug and Alcohol Dependence, 129*(1–2), 54–59. https://doi.org/10.1016/j.drugalcdep.2012.09.011

Mann, R. E., Stoduto, G., Flam-Zalcman, R., Nochajski, T. H., Hall, L., Dill, P., & Wells-Parker, E. (2009). Examining factors in the research institute on addictions self inventory (RIASI): Associations with alcohol use and problems at assessment and follow-up. *International Journal of Environmental Research and Public Health, 6*(11), 2898–2918. https://doi.org/10.3390/ijerph6112898

Maxwell, S. E., Delaney, H. D., & Kelley, K. (2017). *Designing experiments and analyzing data: A model comparison perspective.* Routledge.

Mnatzaganian, G., Davidson, D. C., Hiller, J. E., & Ryan, P. (2015). Propensity score matching and randomization. *Journal of Clinical Epidemiology, 68*(7), 760–768. https://doi.org/10.1016/j.jclinepi.2015.01.002

Pearl, J. (2009). Causal inference in statistics: An overview. *Statistics Surveys, 3,* 96–146. https://doi.org/10.1214/09-SS057

(2017). A linear "microscope" for interventions and counterfactuals. *Journal of Causal Inference, 5*(1), 1–15. https://doi.org/10.1515/jci-2017-0003

Rosenbaum, P.R. (2002). *Observational studies* (2nd ed.). Springer-Verlag.

(2010). *Design of observational studies.* Springer-Verlag.

Rubin, D. B. (2001). Estimating the causal effects of smoking. *Statistics in Medicine, 20* (9-10), 1395–1414. https://doi.org/10.1002/sim.677

(2006). *Matched sampling for causal effects.* Cambridge University Press.

(2007). The design versus the analysis of observational studies for causal effects: Parallels with the design of randomized trials. *Statistics in Medicine, 26*(1), 20–30. https://doi.org/10.1002/sim.2739

(2008). For objective causal inference, design trumps analysis. *The Annals of Applied Statistics, 2*(3), 808–840. https://doi.org/10.1214/08-AOAS187

Salsburg, D. (2001). *The lady tasting tea: How statistics revolutionized science in the twentieth century.* Henry Holt & Co.

Saunders, J. B., Aasland, O. G., Babor, T. F., de la Fuente, J. R., & Grant, M. (1993). Development of the alcohol use disorders identification test (AUDIT): WHO collaborative project on early detection of persons with harmful alcohol consumption–II. *Addiction, 88*(6), 791–804. https://doi.org/10.1111/j.1360-0443.1993.tb02093.x

Scutari, M. (2010). Learning Bayesian networks with the bnlearn R package. *Journal of Statistical Software, 35*(3), 1–22. https://doi.org/10.18637/jss.v035.i03

Shadish, W. R., Cook, T. D., & Campbell, D. T. (2002). *Experimental and quasi-experimental designs for generalized causal inference*. Wadsworth.

Stein, J. H., Steinley, D., & Cropanzano, R. (2011). How and why terrorism corrupts the consistency of organizational justice. *Journal of Organizational Behavior, 32* (7), 984–1007. https://doi.org/10.1002/job.729

Steinley, D. (2006). Curse of dimensionality. In N. J. Salkind (Ed.), *Encyclopedia of Measurement and Statistics* (pp. 209–211). Sage.

Tackett, J. L., & Miller, J. D. (2019). Introduction to the special section on increasing replicability, transparency, and openness in clinical psychology. *Journal of Abnormal Psychology, 128*(6), 487–492. https://doi.org/10.1037/abn0000455

van Borkulo, C. D., Borsboom, D., Epskamp, S., Blanken, T. F., Boschloo, L., Schoevers, R. A., & Waldrop, L. J. (2014). A new method for constructing networks from binary data. *Scientific Reports, 4,* 5918. https://doi.org/10.1038/srep05918

Vocht, F. de., Campbell, R., Brennan, A., Mooney, J., Angus, C., & Hickman, M. (2016). Propensity score matching for selection of local areas as controls for evaluation of effects of alcohol policies in case series and quasi case-control designs. *Public Health, 132,* 40–49. https://doi.org/10.1016/j.puhe.2015.10.033

Xu, Z., & Kalbfleisch, J. D. (2012). Propensity score matching in randomized clinical trials. *Biometrics, 66*(3), 813–823. https://doi.org/10.1111/j.1541-0420.2009.01364.x

21 Building on Collaborative Research to Co-Design *SURE Recovery*, a Mobile Application for People with Experience of Alcohol and Other Drug Problems

Alice Bowen, Melanie Getty, Casandra Hogan, Paul Lennon, Elle Long, John Strang, and Joanne Neale

Building on Collaborative Research to Co-Design SURE Recovery, a Mobile Application for People with Experience of Alcohol and Other Drug Problems

Mobile health (mHealth) applications (apps) allow people to monitor and share information about their health via a smartphone, tablet, or wearable device. Their use is becoming increasingly common amongst clinical and non-clinical populations, including people who use substances. In this chapter, we explain how we extended an existing program of collaborative research to co-design one of the first addiction recovery apps.

Collaborative Research and Co-Design

Defining Collaborative Research

"Collaborative research" refers to research that is carried out "with" or "by" members of the population being studied, rather than "to," "about" or "for" them (Jennings et al., 2018; Involve, 2019). The terms that describe this concept vary and are often used interchangeably. The most appropriate terminology will depend on the situation, but includes "community-based participatory research," "service user involvement in research," "patient and public involvement in research," "peer involvement in research," and "community involvement in research" (Neale et al., 2017; Trivedi & Wykes, 2002).

In this chapter, we refer to "peer researchers" or "members of our Service User Research Group (SURG)" when referring to people with lived experience of addiction treatment who worked as partners on our team when developing the app. We use the terms "community members," "people who use substances," "service users," and "people in recovery" when describing people with lived experience of addiction who participated in interviews and workshops during the development process or who provided general advice and feedback.

The Benefits of Collaborative Research

Collaborative research requires team members to treat each other as equal partners and to trust and respect each other throughout the research process (Neale et al., 2017; Trivedi & Wykes, 2002). University researchers must value the opinions of peer researchers and also be willing to change their views in response to their suggestions and feedback (Neale et al., 2017). Collaborative research requires both effort and resources, but the benefits are increasingly being documented (Ashcroft et al., 2016; Brett et al., 2014; Ennis & Wykes, 2013; Neale et al., 2017; Staley, 2017).

A recent editorial published in the journal *Addiction* highlighted utilitarian, ethical, epistemological, and consequentialist reasons for conducting studies in collaboration with people who use substances (Neale et al., 2017). From a utilitarian perspective, research funders often require collaboration as part of study applications; from an ethical perspective, people have a right to be involved in research that might affect them; from an epistemological perspective, people who use substances have better knowledge and understanding about their own health status, circumstances, support needs, and goals than researchers; and from a consequentialist perspective, involving community members from the outset of a study can increase the quality and impact of research (e.g., by preventing researchers from making unrealistic assessments, by forcing researchers to explain their work clearly, and by adding credibility to study findings) (Neale et al., 2017).

Our Collaborative Research Program

University researchers from our team had previously collaborated with members of a Service User Research Group (SURG) linked to a peer mentoring service in South London, UK, to complete a program of research that resulted in the development of two validated Patient Reported Outcome Measures (or PROMs) (Neale et al., 2016, 2018). PROMs are self-completion questionnaires that focus on health status and health-related quality of life from the perspective of the patient, client, or service user. They attempt to capture those health indicators that are meaningful to the particular population for whom the measure is intended, rather than indicators that are deemed important by clinicians and researchers (Dawson, 2008).

Our first collaborative study led to the development of a PROM for recovery from alcohol and other drug problems. The team worked with community members to ensure that the measure developed only included questions that were clear, relevant, and easily interpretable (Neale & Strang, 2015; Neale et al., 2015). The published validated PROM – named the Substance Use Recovery

Evaluator (SURE) – comprises 21 questions that assess five recovery domains: (1) substance use, (2) self-care, (3) relationships, (4) material resources, and (5) outlook on life (Neale et al., 2016). Our second study generated the Substance Use Sleep Scale (SUSS) (Neale et al., 2018). Its development was guided by previous research that had found that service users repeatedly identified sleep as a crucial but overlooked problem in treatment and recovery from a substance use disorder (Nettleton et al., 2011). SUSS has 23 questions that assess two components of sleep: (1) mind and body sleep problems and (2) substance-related sleep problems (Neale et al., 2018).

Although SURE and SUSS were designed for pen and paper completion, community members expressed a desire to complete them on their mobile phones and tablet computers so that they could record and refer back to their scores. Some also explained that they wanted personalized feedback. Accordingly, the university researchers and SURG members decided to co-design and build an app. To achieve this, funding was secured from a variety of not-for-profit sources, and a new partnership was established with Mindwave Ventures, a company with expertise in the co-design of digital products.

From Collaborative Research to Co-Design

The principles of co-design mirror those of collaborative research, but the terms refer to developing new products, services, or interventions, such as apps. Co-design involves "end users" throughout the design process as active partners (Islind et al., 2019), providing people whose lives might be affected by a problem with a voice in its solution (Kensing & Greenbaum, 2012; Visser et al., 2005). Evidence suggests that the inclusion of end-users in the early stages of the design process leads to better outcomes and more benefits compared with ideas developed by designers alone (Trischler et al., 2018).

Co-Designing a Recovery App

In order to co-design our new recovery app, we followed a framework widely used in the design industry known as the Double Diamond design process (The Design Council, 2015). This has four distinct phases that are repeated in iterative cycles: (1) discover, (2) define, (3) develop, and (4) deliver. Our methods are described below and summarized in Table 21.1.

Phase 1: Discover

During the discovery phase, the team conducted two sets of semi-structured interviews and two workshops with paid volunteers who were all currently attending community addiction services. The interviews and workshops were led by Mindwave Ventures in order to provide them with a better understanding

Table 21.1. *Timeframe, activity, and participants for each key phase of app development*

	Timeframe	Activity	Participants
PHASE 1: DISCOVER	November 2018	One-hour, semi-structured interviews focusing on experiences of recovery conducted by MW	Five people at a peer support service
	November 2018	Ninety-minute workshop focusing on mobile phone and app use, conducted by MW and a KCL researcher	Ten people at a community day program
	December 2018	One-hour, semi-structured interviews focusing on experiences of recovery, conducted by MW	Four people at a community support service
	February 2019	Forty-minute visual identity workshop conducted by MW to establish the types of apps that were visually appealing and a name for the app	Nine people at a peer support service
PHASE 2: DEFINE	January 2019	*Discovery Report* outlining findings from Phase 1	MW
	January 2019	MoSCoW exercise to prioritize key features for inclusion in the app	MW, KCL, and SURG
	January–February 2019	Preliminary flowchart including key features, app navigation, and research questions	KCL and review by SURG
PHASE 3: DEVELOP	January 2019	Creation of app prototype and initial designs	MW
	January 2019	Testing, review, and feedback of prototype and designs	KCL and SURG
	February 2019	Further iterations of designs and prototype based on ongoing feedback	MW, KCL, and SURG
	February 2019	Two one-hour workshops to check findings from Phase 1 and gather feedback on the app design, conducted by MW and KCL	People at a residential rehabilitation service
	February 2019	Digital prototype testing and feedback to MW	People at a residential rehabilitation service
	February 2019	Final designs and sign-off	MW, KCL, and SURG
	February–March 2019	Development of app content	KCL and SURG
	March–May 2019	Ethics application for data collection via the app	KCL
	April–August 2019	Test versions of the app released and reviewed using Test Flight	MW, KCL, and SURG

Table 21.1. (*cont.*)

	Timeframe	Activity	Participants
PHASE 4: DELIVER	September 2019	Near final versions of the app shared at conferences and amended based on feedback	KCL, SURG, and conference attendees
	September 2019	Final version of the app agreed	MW, KCL, and SURG
	September 2019	App submitted to Apple and Google Play Stores	MW
	September 2019	App accepted by Google Play	Google Play
	October 2019	App accepted by Apple	Apple
	October 2019	"Soft" launch and sharing with SURG, researchers, and KCL clinicians	KCL and SURG
	October 2019	Official launch	KCL and SURG
	October 2019–present	Dissemination by email and presentations at organizations working in the addictions field	KCL and SURG
	November 2019	Press release	KCL
	October 2019–December 2019	Creation of Facebook, Twitter, and YouTube channels and content	KCL and SURG
COVID-19	March 2020	Increased use of social media for dissemination	KCL and SURG
	April 2020	Discussions with the UK Recovery Champion, PHE, and NHS England regarding use of the app to communicate and learn from people in recovery	KCL and SURG
	March 2020	Ethics amendment to collect Covid-19 data	KCL
	April 2020	Development of a framework and content for the temporary Covid-19 feature	MW, KCL, and SURG
	April 2020	Development of the Covid-19 feature	MW
	April 2020	Submission of the updated app to Google Play and Apple App stores	MW
	April 2020	Acceptance of the new Covid-19 feature by Google Play	Google Play
	April 2020	Acceptance of the new Covid-19 feature by Apple app store	Apple
	April–May 2020	Dissemination of the new Covid-19 feature online	KCL, SURG, PHE, and the UK Recovery Champion

Note. KCL: King's College London; MW: Mindwave Ventures; MoSCoW: "Must-have," "Should-have," "Could-have," and "Will not have at this time"; PHE: Public Health England; SURG: Service User Research Group members of recovery, insights into the population's use of mobile technology and apps, and ideas on what a recovery app might look like and include.

The interviews and first workshop focused on participants' personal recovery journeys and use of technology and apps. In the second "visual identity" workshop, participants were shown images of various apps and websites and asked to place a green sticker on any image that appealed to them and a red sticker on those that did not. The images with most green and red stickers were then discussed, and key descriptions of the visual elements that people liked and disliked were recorded. Participants next completed a word association exercise in which they suggested words that described what a recovery app should do, identified other associated words, used all the words to create several potential app names, and finally voted for their favorite.

Phase 2: Define

Members of the Mindwave Ventures team summarized findings from phase one in a *Discovery Report*, which identified challenges that people encountered during recovery ("pain points") and potential app features that might address those pain points. The report also outlined a range of "personas" that reflected potential users of the app and helped the design team understand the target audience.

Team members from Mindwave Ventures, King's College London, and SURG next completed a MoSCoW ("Must-have," "Should-have," "Could-have," and "Will not have at this time") prioritization exercise (Hatton, 2008). This technique enables teams to establish key elements of a product, whilst being mindful of timeframe and budget. To this end, each potential app feature was allocated a number of days for development and a total number of days was assigned to the project according to the budget. Team members then jointly discussed each feature and placed them in one of the MoSCoW categories, thus informing decisions about the features to include.

At this point, the university researchers developed a preliminary flow chart that outlined where each feature might be positioned within the app, navigation between features, the kinds of research questions that might be asked within the app, and where and how frequently those questions would appear. Members of SURG reviewed and advised on the flowchart at every stage.

Phase 3: Develop

At the start of the develop phase, a designer from Mindwave Ventures created a prototype of the app on a laptop. This included a site map and initial designs based on findings from the visual identity workshop and the flowchart developed by the rest of the team. The prototype and designs were shared with members of the research team and SURG who reviewed them and offered comments. Further iterations were then developed by Mindwave Ventures.

Two workshops were subsequently held at a residential treatment service in order to check the findings from the discovery phase and to gather feedback on the initial designs. Participants in this workshop were also invited to test the digital prototype of the app on a laptop and those who agreed were asked to "think aloud" as they worked their way through the app. The aim of these testing sessions was to establish whether the prototype was user-friendly and simple to navigate. Mindwave Ventures then provided final designs that were agreed upon and signed off on by members of the wider team.

Over the following weeks, additional content for the app was developed, produced, reviewed, and agreed on collaboratively by members of the university research team and SURG, other community members, and other university colleagues with a clinical background. This content included text for each page of the app, a privacy statement, terms of service, research questions, naloxone information, external information sources for signposting within the app, artwork, and individualized feedback for SURE and SUSS. Ethical approval with respect to the analyses of data collected within the app was also obtained from King's College London's Research Ethics Committee.

Next, over a period of four months, Mindwave Ventures released approximately weekly test versions of the app to the rest of the team on Test Flight (an online service for over-the-air installation and testing of mobile applications). Researchers and members of SURG reviewed and provided feedback on each version.

Phase 4: Deliver

Near final versions of the app were shared at conferences and amended once again to include feedback. Once a final version (Figure 21.1) had been approved by the whole team, Mindwave Ventures submitted it to Google Play and the Apple app store. The app was immediately accepted by Google Play and was ready to download within 24 hours. In contrast, the app was rejected by Apple because the name of the app (*SURE Recovery*) did not match the name of the app developer account (Mindwave Ventures). A new app developer account was therefore established for *SURE Recovery*, and the app was accepted by Apple seven weeks later.

As soon as the app was published, team members completed a "soft" launch. This involved sharing it with all members of SURG, research colleagues and clinicians at King's College London, and others who had offered advice and feedback during the development process. People were encouraged to download the app, inform the researchers of any bugs, and provide any general comments (although the team did not plan to undertake any significant changes at this point). As no bugs were identified, we progressed to an official launch in October 2019.

Once officially launched, the team began disseminating the app by emailing organizations working in the addictions field with a short summary of the app

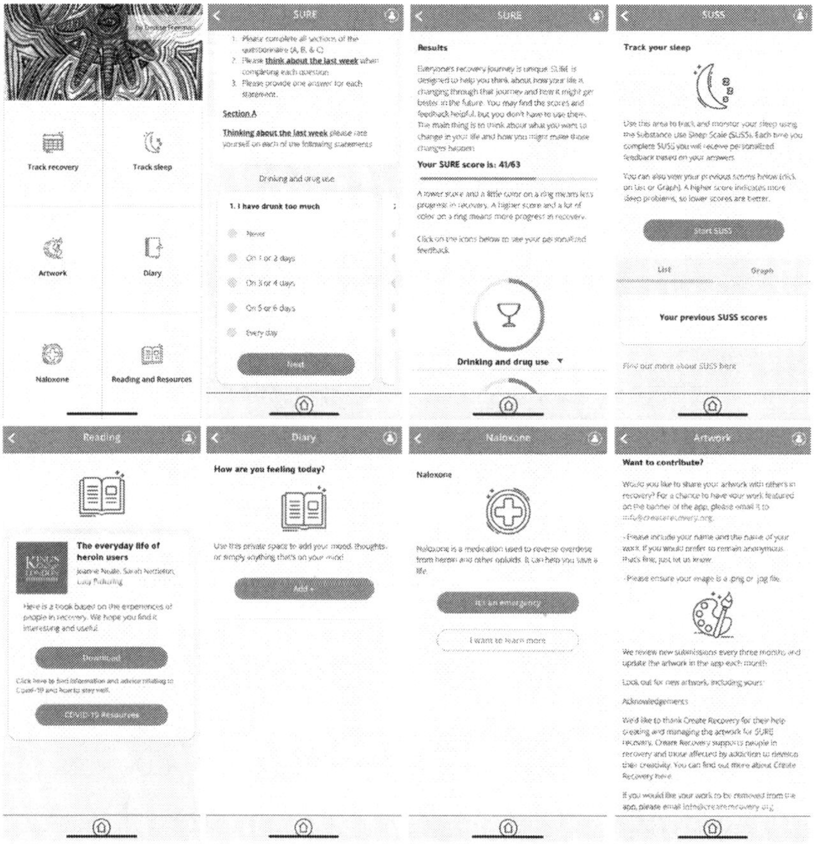

Figure 21.1 *Screenshots from the final version of the app launched in the Apple app store and Google Play.*

and a link to a university webpage that described its functionality and development in more detail. We also shared the app with peer-led organizations and mutual-aid groups. In addition, we contacted news outlets for the sector, issued a press release, and created *SURE Recovery* Twitter and Facebook accounts. These efforts were combined with presentations at addiction services and conferences. Over time, the team expanded their dissemination activities with regular postings on social media and plans to initiate a network of *SURE Recovery* champions who would support others in using the app.

Effects of Covid-19

At the end of March 2020, six months after launching the app, the UK went into lockdown in response to Covid-19. In-person dissemination activities could not continue, and so we adapted our dissemination strategy to accomplish more online. This involved increasing the use of Twitter and Facebook and creating a *SURE Recovery* Instagram account and YouTube channel. Members of the research team and SURG then prepared several short promotional videos and continued to contact people who might be interested in the app via email and video chat. Throughout lockdown, two members of the research team and two members of SURG also held regular Skype meetings to share ideas and make decisions.

During April 2020, discussions with the UK Recovery Champion, Public Health England (PHE), and NHS England soon indicated that the app offered an opportunity to communicate with and learn about the experiences of people in recovery during the pandemic. The team therefore decided to develop an additional temporary Covid-19 feature that included links to information about the pandemic and a space where people could submit their experiences and any impact of Covid-19 on their lives. The overall framework and content were decided by members of the research team and SURG, Mindwave Ventures developed the new feature within 10 days, and NHS England provided financial support for the build. After updating the app on the App Store and Google Play, the team continued to promote the app via email and social media. PHE and NHS England also disseminated the app to their contacts and regional networks.

Lessons Learned during the Co-Design Process

Knowledge and insights gained from the co-design process are described below, including our retrospective reflections on what we learned at each stage.

Phase 1: Discovery

Participant Experiences of Recovery

Participants in the interviews and workshops reported that personal experiences of recovery were diverse: "The same type of recovery doesn't necessarily work for everyone." Equally, people valued different types of formal and informal support, but did not always find the same support helpful. For example, one participant stated, "I didn't go down the routes of AA [Alcoholics Anonymous] or rehab. I had explored [those] options many times in the past and it just made me worse." In contrast, another identified AA as playing a large and positive part in their recovery.

Participants also identified common activities that had helped them with their recovery. These included making connections with others, sharing their stories and experiences with others, meeting others in a similar situation, keeping busy and distracted, supporting others, and receiving support from peers: "Supportive networks are key. If you're not in that, then it is very difficult to stay in recovery." Additionally, participants often noted that keeping a log of their recovery, to which they could refer back, was valuable (e.g., writing a diary, tracking their mood, or keeping a gratitude list).

Conversely, participants identified many common problems. These included cravings, boredom, isolation, stress, managing new responsibilities, financial difficulties, living with past behaviors, needing to avoid certain people and places, and poor sleep: "If you can't sleep, you're in trouble." Furthermore, finding and accessing services were identified as a challenge, particularly when first thinking about recovery, and this was exacerbated by the lack of readily available information on support sources: "It takes a long time to find out what is going on, who to see, how to seek help." In response, participants generally agreed that having advice and tips about the types of support available would be very useful: "Advice and knowledge of what is available where – that would be amazing."

Participant Use of Technology and Apps

All participants had a smart phone and used apps, and most felt that other people using substances or in recovery would have similar access to mobile technology. Features of existing apps that participants particularly liked included the simplicity and ease of finding information, clear layout, and tracker features (e.g., for mood, anger, or anxiety). Additionally, participants welcomed the idea of having some way of connecting with others within the app, receiving inspirational quotations, and sharing artwork. In contrast, they disliked apps that they perceived as being "busy" or "crowded" with too much text, and those that contained "too much information" or advertisements that looked "technical."

Participants suggested several names for the app, including, "Recovery Mate," "One Day at a Time," "Toolkit," "Freedom," "Recovery Tracker," "Connect," and "Wellness Journey." These generated mixed opinions within the workshop, particularly regarding the appropriateness of certain terms and whether the word "recovery" would deter some people from using the app. Following discussion, participants agreed on the name *SURE Recovery* because they felt that it clearly described the content of the app, made them feel positive, and linked well to the SURE measure.

Team Reflections

In practice, the discovery phase focused predominantly on personal experiences of addiction and recovery, rather than on technology and apps. This was valuable for members of the Mindwave Ventures design team who were new to the addictions field. However, other team members had been living or studying recovery for several years and, with hindsight, could have informed Mindwave Ventures about key features of addiction without the need for new data collection. Furthermore, some information collected during the discovery phase was sensitive, and the research team wished they had known more about the topics to be covered so that they could have given participants notice that so many personal questions would be asked.

These various difficulties seemed to have arisen because members of the Mindwave Ventures team and the research team did not communicate adequately before the discovery stage started. Additional initial discussion by Mindwave Ventures and the research team about the content and format of the interviews and workshops might have improved participants' experiences, whilst reducing unnecessary data collection and project resources.

Phase 2: Define

Deciding on Features

Following the workshops and interviews, members of the Mindwave Ventures team concluded that the app might usefully include: (1) information, recommendations, and advice; (2) a directory of services; (3) help in finding people or groups to meet; (4) a sense of community; (5) sharing of personal stories, experiences, and advice; (6) artwork; (7) coping strategies/resources; (8) options for helping others/volunteering; (9) different types of support; (10) tracking (progress, mood, or problems); (11) a way to be reminded of the app; (12) encouragement and motivation; and (13) sleep tracking.

All of these suggestions could not be accommodated within the project budget and timeframe, so the MoSCoW method previously outlined was used to narrow the options to six more concrete and viable features. These were: (1) a recovery tracker that would allow people to monitor their recovery via SURE and receive personalized feedback and a score that could be viewed on a graph; (2) a sleep tracker that would enable people to monitor their sleep via SUSS and also produce personalized feedback, a score, and a graph; (3) information concerning the use of naloxone in the event of an opioid overdose and further overdose resources; (4) reading material, including a free downloadable book based on the lived experiences of people in recovery; (5) a diary offering a private space for people to record their thoughts and feelings; and (6) an artwork feature through which people could submit their own artwork for potential display in the banner on the home screen of the app. A set of research questions covering basic demographic, substance use, and treatment-related topics were also deemed to be within scope, plan, and budget.

Team Reflections

One feature that was not included in the final design of the app, despite being highly valued by people in recovery, was a social feature where app users could "chat" and share experiences, stories, and advice. This exclusion was particularly difficult, but the team concluded that it would need constant monitoring to ensure that all information or personal stories shared would be safe, not have any ethical issues, and be compliant with data protection regulations. Professional input, beyond the resources available, would also likely be needed to guarantee that anyone posting to the feature would be supported if they experienced a crisis.

Developing the research questions and flowchart for the app was, meanwhile, more complicated than the team had anticipated and resulted in a number of false starts. Eventually, three statisticians from King's College London were consulted in order to ensure that the data generated from the research questions would be suitable for analysis. On the advice of one of these statisticians, the team also stopped trying to set out the flow chart in a Word document and swapped to the diagram builder program, yEd (www.yworks.com/products/yed), which made the process clearer and more manageable.

Phase 3: Develop

Developing the App

The click through prototype of the app produced by Mindwave was particularly helpful in enabling others to envisage how the app might work and what it could look like. It additionally allowed Mindwave Ventures to check that they had correctly understood and incorporated findings from the earlier phases. Data from the two workshops conducted in the initial Develop phase supported findings from the later Discovery phase with respect to participants' experiences of recovery, challenges encountered, and support needed.

When participants reviewed the four possible designs for the app, they preferred simple, clear designs that used bright colors on a light background, as they said this looked positive. They did not like designs that were "overly simple," with little color or text, as they felt these were boring and unappealing. Workshop participants reported that they wanted an app that enabled them to connect with others and provided non-judgemental advice and information on where to get help. They also said they would be disinclined to use an app if it was not easy to use, felt judgemental, or did not "look nice." When asked how they might find out about the app, participants referred to various possibilities, including via drug treatment services and word of mouth; none said that they would search directly on Google Play or the Apple app store.

Participants who tested the app prototype on the laptop described it as "clean-looking," "simple," and "easy to use." They noted that the app would be "a good distraction" from substance use and useful in "setting goals." They particularly liked the way the app allowed them to track their recovery over time and hoped that the feedback would be encouraging if they were not doing well. Participants also suggested several changes. For example, most did not recognize, or know how to use, the "burger menu" used in the prototype. Instead they wanted a "home button" that was subsequently incorporated instead.

The content for the app, which was initially written by the university researchers, was also changed significantly based on feedback from SURG members, people in recovery, and clinical colleagues. For example, the scope of the naloxone feature was extended to include a video and validated scale, the Opioid Overdose Attitude Scale (OOAS) (Williams et al., 2013). In addition, modifications were made to the app text, particularly to the SURE and SUSS personalized feedback, to ensure that the language was non-judgemental and supportive throughout. Such changes meant that the budget for development (originally 66,400 GBP) had to be increased on several occasions (final sum 77,600 GBP without the Covid-19 feature).

Early test versions of the app also had multiple glitches in the build structure that required repeated cycles of changes and testing by the whole team. Furthermore, once the content and structure had been "brought to life," some of the research team's ideas about navigation did not work as expected and had to be amended. Although these changes often seemed simple to the research team, they usually required significant work on the underlying functionality of the app by Mindwave Ventures. This meant that the timeline for developing the app was constantly being extended (from 6 to 12 months), and a total of 31 versions of the app were tested before the final version was ready for dissemination.

Securing ethical approval to analyze the research questions within the app was also more complex than had been expected. The ethical approval application was different from that of a standard research project because there was no study protocol, no pre-specified research questions, and no data analysis plan (since we did not yet know what data would be generated). This resulted in the team having to respond to multiple questions and clarifications raised by the ethics committee.

Lastly, finding a successful mechanism and format for exporting the research data from the app ready for analyses proved challenging. The initial output format developed by Mindwave Ventures did not meet the needs of the research team and, when reviewed by statisticians, was deemed unusable. The research team therefore spent a long time explaining in detail the type of output needed in ways that the app developers might understand. Once the developers understood, they in turn had to undertake a significant amount of extra work reformatting the app's content management system.

Team Reflections

During this phase of the work, research team members again felt that unnecessary time was spent asking workshop participants about their personal experiences of recovery. Nonetheless, they recognized that it was important to talk with different groups of people from residential and community settings to maximize the range of opinions and feedback received. Indeed, participants in the phase three residential workshop made some very helpful observations that subsequently shaped the design and usability of the app.

As the app content was developed, the benefits of having a diverse team of researchers, people in recovery, and clinicians became very apparent. People in recovery and clinicians gave crucial feedback on the text used within the app, whilst the statisticians gave vital advice on how to design the flow of the research questions and format the data output. Having peer researchers and strong connections to people with lived experience were also invaluable as they helped test, and provided feedback on, each iteration.

As none of the research team had any prior experience with app development, it was difficult for them to imagine how the app features and research questions would link together. Using Test Flight increased their understanding and was relatively easy to use, although testing repeated versions of the app was very time-consuming. The embedded research questions also challenged the ethical approval process, and team members had to find new ways of explaining the data and their origins when interacting with the research ethics committee.

Again, earlier communication between the research team and Mindwave Ventures might have led to fewer setbacks during this phase. One particular issue was that members of each team assumed that members of the other would use the same language and have similar knowledge and understanding. For example, the Mindwave Ventures team presumed that the research team would understand the processes and intricacies of developing an app, whilst the research team presumed the developer would understand how data should be formatted for analysis. That said, the complexity and novelty of the project meant that some delays and additional costs were probably unavoidable, and the team was fortunate in having some flexibility with respect to their budget and deadlines.

Phase 4: Deliver

Finalizing the App

The final testing was essential in identifying several small bugs that had been previously overlooked and also led to significant changes to the graphs in both the recovery and sleep features. The graphs had been designed to allow app users to view their SURE and SUSS scores over the course of a week, but feedback suggested that they were not very functional. Several people noted that they would be better if they incorporated a weekly, monthly, and yearly view, so that people using the app could visually track and monitor their scores over longer periods. Mindwave Ventures was therefore invited to provide a quotation to redevelop the graph features. The design was agreed, and two new versions were built before final sign off by the wider team.

Launching the App

Our initial dissemination plan comprised a list of organizations to be contacted and a number of discrete tasks (presentations, press release, setting up social media) to be completed. Although we generated a slow and steady increase in app downloads, it soon became apparent that we were reaching people "working" in the addictions field, rather than people who might actually use the app. We therefore increased our use of social media to connect with more community members, identified new contacts and people to visit, sought advice on dissemination from key professionals and community players in the sector, and started to read about and research app promotion.

During this phase, we also discovered that people had interests in using the app in ways that we had not anticipated. For example, some treatment providers said they would like to use the data generated by the app to monitor their clients;

some service users thought that it would be helpful to share their scores and feedback from the app with supportive drug workers or family and friends; and some researchers suggested that the app could offer a way of recruiting out-of-treatment populations to studies. In addition, conversations with the UK Recovery Champion highlighted how questions within the app could potentially offer a way of gathering rapid feedback from community members on national treatment and policy issues.

At the time of writing (August 2020), the app had been downloaded 619 times from Google Play and 631 times from the Apple app store. In total, 543 users had consented to allowing their data to be used for research, and 90 had responded to the Covid-19 question. Between April and August, we saw a slow and steady increase in the numbers of people using the app and returning to complete SURE (Neale et al., 2016), SUSS (Neale et al., 2018), OOAS (Williams et al., 2013), and the research questions. Users were based in a number of countries, although mostly from the UK. In addition, the team was being contacted by both service providers and service user forums requesting further information and suggestions on how to use the app to support their clients, patients, and peers.

Team Reflections

The repetitive process of testing, followed by the "soft" launch amongst close colleagues, delayed the app's main launch and dissemination. Nonetheless, our cautious approach likely explains why there have been no bugs reported to-date. The process of getting the app published by the Apple app store, meanwhile, proved very stressful for the whole team. Although Mindwave Ventures had been prepared for a delay, nobody was expecting Apple's changes in requirements that set the launch date back by seven weeks. This did, however, have one unanticipated benefit, as it brought the team very close together with a shared common goal in the final development stages. The research team appreciated how much Mindwave Ventures had invested in the app and how hard they were working to solve the app store problem. In turn, Mindwave Ventures could see that other members of the team trusted and valued their knowledge and expertise in navigating a way through the Apple bureaucracy.

Initial downloads and use of the app were not as high as had been hoped and generated some disappointment. Nonetheless, the team recognized that prolonged engagement with mHealth apps is notoriously low (Krebs & Duncan, 2015; Serrano et al., 2017; Szinay et al., 2020) and their target population might not always have ready access to mobile devices, IT skills, or data packages (Milward et al., 2015). Accordingly, the team focused on the fact that the app would not be suitable for everyone and that the goal should be to maximize uptake amongst as many people as possible. Furthermore, dissemination should be seen as a creative, evolving, and ongoing endeavor, rather than a one-off event or time-limited phase. Unexpectedly, the advent of Covid-19 seemed to increase downloads and engagement, probably because more people than usual were connecting with, and searching for, resources online.

As the team started to consider new and innovative ways of disseminating *SURE Recovery*, their attention turned to the implementation science literature. The underlying philosophy behind the app and its content had always been collaboration and co-design, but the team began to realize that they also needed strategies, and ideally a framework, to help them optimize the app's reach, adoption, and embeddedness amongst users. Efforts to identify such a framework specific to mHealth apps failed. Nonetheless, we found a refined compilation of implementation strategies from the Expert Recommendations for Implementing Change (ERIC) project to be very helpful (Powell et al., 2015). This reinforced some of the approaches we had already used (e.g., conducting outreach visits, building coalitions and partnerships, networking and attending educational meetings) and provided ideas for other initiatives (e.g., identifying new funding streams, developing and distributing educational materials, identifying and preparing champions, informing local opinion leaders, and exploring train-the-trainer strategies).

In particular, the practice of "reexamining the implementation" (that is, continuously adjusting practices and the planned implementation strategy; Powell et al., 2015) is likely to be useful going forward as the team deliberates the pros and cons of enabling service providers to use the app to monitor their clients; encouraging clients to share their scores and feedback with trusted others; permitting researchers to use the app for study recruitment; and allowing national bodies and organizations to adopt the app for collating anonymized service user feedback on treatment and policy decisions. These all appear to be interesting innovations and opportunities. However, decisions about repurposing the app for any new activities will only be made with the involvement of peer researchers and people with lived experience in order to maintain the open collaboration that has guided the project so far.

Conclusions and Recommendations

Multiple partners, with different areas of expertise, worked collaboratively to develop the *SURE Recovery* app. It is interesting to note that when inefficiencies and miscommunications occurred in the development process, these tended to be between the researchers and the app developers rather than between the researchers and team members with lived experience of addiction. We suspect that is because the researchers and members of SURG had already worked together for several years and had established trusting relationships and effective systems of working. In contrast, new relationships had to be forged with the app developer, and differences in language and knowledge had to be worked through in order to build a cohesive team with a common goal. As argued in our Introduction, undertaking collaborative research requires effort and resources. Our experiences show how this is not exclusive to research teams working with community members and is likely to apply to all collaborations when partners have different backgrounds and expertise.

In terms of the specific benefits of collaboration with people who use substances in developing *SURE Recovery* (Neale et al., 2016), we believe that the app is more useful for, and acceptable to, the community for which it was built because of all the input and guidance from SURG and other community members. For example, our collaborative approach has helped ensure that the app content is useful, the language is appropriate and accessible, the design is appealing, the usability is good, and the app runs without glitches or system crashes. Crucially, having people with personal experience of harmful substance use and recovery as part of the team and available to help with dissemination activities has generated a level of trust in *SURE Recovery* that could never have been achieved by researchers or app developers alone. To date, the app has been positively received, but it is still early days, and its real value will become apparent from download and usage figures going forward.

The version of *SURE Recovery* currently in use could undoubtedly be improved, and we are now starting to undertake further research to enhance its utility. This will combine analyses of quantitative data from the app's content management system with new qualitative data from interviews conducted with users of the app. Findings should help us better understand who is using the app; their patterns of engagement; who is finding it most useful and why; which features users like, dislike, and would wish to see improved; any positive or negative outcomes of using the app; and the types of changes to the app that users would find acceptable or unacceptable. Our hope is to then secure further funding to update the app in line with the research findings.

Based on our collaborative app development experience and reflecting upon the strengths and weaknesses of our approach, we end with five simple recommendations for others working on similar apps. First, we cannot overemphasize how important it is to have team members with diverse experiences and expertise, including people who are part of the community for whom the app is being developed. This helps to ensure that the needs and wishes of the target audience and end user are always central. Second, regular and open communication between the various parties throughout the project is essential, but particularly during the early stages when all team members need to understand each other's' terminology and knowledge base and work to ensure that they share the same project aim and goals. Third, developing the app in phases and iterative cycles enables feedback from the various partners to be incorporated as work progresses and allows lessons to be learned before it is too late. Fourth, given the complexities and inevitable uncertainties of app development, all parties need to build flexibility into both the budget and timetable to allow for mistakes, changes in direction, and unforeseen costs. Fifth, having a carefully considered short-, medium-, and longer-term dissemination strategy that involves community members and is informed by the implementation science literature should help raise awareness and facilitate uptake of the app once it is launched.

Acknowledgments

The authors would like to acknowledge the following organizations for providing financial support in developing the app: Action on Addiction, the Alexander Moseley Charitable Trust, the Mackie Foundation, the NIHR Maudsley Biomedical Research Centre, and NHS England. They would also like to thank everyone who provided insights and feedback into the design and content of *SURE Recovery*, including all members of SURG, the Aurora Project, Create Recovery, Mindwave Ventures, and colleagues at King's College London and the South London and Maudsley NHS Foundation Trust. Joanne Neale is part-funded by, and John Strang is supported by, the NIHR Maudsley Biomedical Research Center. John Strang's declarations are available at: www.kcl.ac.uk/ioppn/depts/addictions/people/hod.aspx.

SURE Recovery is free to download from Google Play and the App Store.

References

Ashcroft, J., Wykes, T., Taylor, J., Crowther, A., & Szmukler, G. (2016). Impact on the individual: What do patients and carers gain, lose, and expect from being involved in research? *Journal of Mental Health, 25*(1), 28–35. https://doi.org/10.3109/09638237.2015.1101424

Brett, J., Staniszewska, S., Mockford, C., Herron-Marx, S., Hughes, J., Tysall, C., & Suleman, R. (2014). Mapping the impact of patient and public involvement on health and social care research: A systematic review. *Health Expectations, 17* (5), 637–650. https://doi.org/10.1111/j.1369-7625.2012.00795.x

Dawson, J. (2008). Measuring health status. In J. Neale (Ed.), *Research methods for health and social care* (pp. 181–194). London: Palgrave Macmillan.

Ennis, L., & Wykes, T. (2013). Impact of patient involvement in mental health research: longitudinal study. *British Journal of Psychiatry, 203*(5), 381–386. https://doi.org/10.1192/bjp.bp.112.119818

Hatton, S. (2008). Choosing the right prioritization method. In *19th Australian Conference on Software Engineering (aswec 2008)* (pp. 517–526). IEEE. https://doi.org/10.1109/ASWEC.2008.4483241

Involve (2019). *National standards for public involvement in research.* www.invo.org.uk/wp-content/uploads/2019/02/71110_A4_Public_Involvement_Standards_v4_WEB.pdf

Islind, A. S., Lindroth, T., Lundin, J., & Steineck, G. (2019). Co-designing a digital platform with boundary objects: Bringing together heterogeneous users in healthcare. *Health and Technology, 9*, 425–438. https://doi.org/10.1007/s12553-019-00332-5

Jennings, H., Slade, M., Bates, P., Munday, E., & Toney, R. (2018). Best practice framework for patient and public involvement (PPI) in collaborative data analysis of qualitative mental health research: Methodology development and refinement. *BMC Psychiatry*, *18*(1), 213. https://doi.org/10.1186/s12888–018-1794-8

Kensing, F., & Greenbaum, J. (2012). Heritage: Having a say. In J. Simonsen & T. Robertson (Eds.), *Routledge International Handbook of Participatory Design* (pp. 21–36). Routledge. www.forskningsdatabasen.dk/da/catalog/2444729034

Krebs, P., & Duncan, D. T. (2015). Health app use among US mobile phone owners: A national survey. *JMIR MHealth and UHealth*, *3*(4), e101. https://doi.org/10.2196/mhealth.4924

Milward, J., Day, E., Wadsworth, E., Strang, J., & Lynskey, M. (2015). Mobile phone ownership, usage, and readiness to use by patients in drug treatment. *Drug and Alcohol Dependence*, *146*(1), 111–115. https://doi.org/10.1016/j.drugalcdep.2014.11.001

Neale, J., Bouteloup, A., Getty, M., Hogan, C., Lennon, P., Mc Cusker, M., & Strang, J. (2017). Why we should conduct research in collaboration with people who use alcohol and other drugs. *Addiction*, *112*(12), 2084–2085. https://doi.org/10.1111/add.14015

Neale, J., & Strang, J. (2015). Philosophical ruminations on measurement: Methodological orientations of patient reported outcome measures (PROMS). *Journal of Mental Health*, *24*(3), 123–125. https://doi.org/10.3109/09638237.2015.1036978

Neale, J., Tompkins, C., Wheeler, C., Finch, E., Marsden, J., Mitcheson, L., Rose, D., Wykes, T., & Strang, J. (2015). "You're all going to hate the word 'recovery' by the end of this": Service users' views of measuring addiction recovery. *Drugs: Education, Prevention and Policy*, *22*(1), 26–34. https://doi.org/10.3109/09687637.2014.947564

Neale, J., Vitoratou, S., Finch, E., Lennon, P., Mitcheson, L., Panebianco, D., Rose, D., Strang, J., Wykes, T., & Marsden, J. (2016). Development and validation of "SURE": A patient reported outcome measure (PROM) for recovery from drug and alcohol dependence. *Drug and Alcohol Dependence*, *165*, 159–167. https://doi.org/10.1016/j.drugalcdep.2016.06.006

Neale, J., Vitoratou, S., Lennon, P., Meadows, R., Nettleton, S., Panebianco, D., Strang, J., & Marsden, J. (2018). Development and early validation of a patient-reported outcome measure to assess sleep amongst people experiencing problems with alcohol or other drugs. *Sleep*, *41*(4), 1–14. https://doi.org/https://dx.doi.org/10.1093/sleep/zsy013

Nettleton, S., Neale, J., & Pickering, L. (2011). Techniques and transitions: A sociological analysis of sleeping practices amongst recovering heroin users. *Social Science and Medicine*, *72*(8), 1367–1373. https://doi.org/10.1016/j.socscimed.2011.02.040

Powell, B. J., Waltz, T. J., Chinman, M. J., Damschroder, L. J., Smith, J. L., Matthieu, M. M., Proctor, E. K., & Kirchner, J. A. E. (2015). A refined compilation of implementation strategies: Results from the expert recommendations for implementing change (ERIC) project. *Implementation Science*, *10*(1), 21. https://doi.org/10.1186/s13012–015-0209-1

Serrano, K. J., Coa, K. I., Yu, M., Wolff-Hughes, D. L., & Atienza, A. A. (2017). Characterizing user engagement with health app data: A data mining approach.

Translational Behavioral Medicine, *7*(2), 277–285. https://doi.org/10.1007/s13142–017-0508-y

Staley, K. (2017). Changing what researchers "think and do": Is this how involvement impacts on research? *Research for All*, *1*(1), 158–167. https://doi.org/10.18546/RFA.01.1.13

Szinay, D., Jones, A., Chadborn, T., Brown, J., & Naughton, F. (2020, May 29). Influences on the uptake of and engagement with health and well-being smartphone apps: Systematic review. *Journal of Medical Internet Research*. NLM (Medline). https://doi.org/10.2196/17572

The Design Council (2007). *Eleven lessons: Managing design in eleven global companies*. www.designcouncil.org.uk

(2015). *Design methods for developing services*. www.designcouncil.org.uk/sites/default/files/asset/document/DesignCouncil_Design%20methods%20for%20developing%20services.pdf

Trischler, J., Pervan, S. J., Kelly, S. J., & Scott, D. R. (2018). The value of co-design. *Journal of Service Research*, *21*(1), 75–100. https://doi.org/10.1177/1094670517714060

Trivedi, P., & Wykes, T. (2002). From passive subjects to equal partners: Qualitative review of user involvement in research. *The British Journal of Psychiatry: The Journal of Mental Science*, *181*, 468–472. www.ncbi.nlm.nih.gov/pubmed/12456515

Visser, F. S., Stappers, P. J., & Remko, V. D. L. (2005). Context mapping: Experiences from practice. *Co-Design: International Journal of CoCreation in Design and the Arts*, *1*(2). Taylor and Francis. https://cpb-us-w2.wpmucdn.com/u.osu.edu/dist/1/8276/files/2015/02/Contextmapping_SleeswijkVisseretal_05–10ugkj1.pdf

Williams, A. V., Strang, J., & Marsden, J. (2013). Development of opioid overdose knowledge (OOKS) and attitudes (OOAS) scales for take-home naloxone training evaluation. *Drug and Alcohol Dependence*, *132*(1–2), 383–386. https://doi.org/10.1016/j.drugalcdep.2013.02.007

22 Economic Methods Used to Evaluate Recovery Programs for Alcohol Use Disorder

Brady P. Horn

Economic Methods Used to Evaluate Recovery Programs for Alcohol Use Disorder

It is not uncommon for people to wonder why economic analysis of alcohol use disorder (AUD) interventions, or really any intervention designed to improved health, is necessary. Moreover, economics can be characterized as a cold discipline, which distills the complex impact of many different types of treatment that improve human lives into monetary decisions or cost-effectiveness ratios. In contrast to its reputation as the "dismal" science, the purpose of economics is actually to maximize human welfare and/or create the greatest possible amount of benefit to society. A fundamental assumption of economic models is that resources (e.g., tax revenues) are limited. Because there are many valuable social programs, or more generally valuable "public goods" to put money, time, and effort into, difficult decisions must be made about which programs or treatment modalities to pursue. Economic analysis is designed to consider tradeoffs, or the relative value of potential programs and/or uses of our time and resources, in order to create the greatest possible amount of benefit to society.

To relate these ideas of budget constraints and maximizing human welfare to AUD interventions, consider a simple hypothetical situation where the government has only $10 million available and is considering two potential treatment modalities: (1) a more costly but relatively more efficacious intervention, such as an intensive outpatient intervention or (2) a less costly and less intensive intervention with lower treatment efficacy, perhaps such as a screening and brief intervention in emergency departments. Considering efficacy alone, or assuming money is not an issue, the government should choose the more efficacious, more expensive intensive outpatient treatment modality. However, if budgets are limited, then tradeoffs must be considered – notably that because the brief intervention is less costly and amenable to wider dissemination and adoption, it could be used to reach substantially more people. Thus, depending on relative efficacy and the difference in the number of individuals that could receive treatment, a brief intervention could potentially cause a bigger overall impact on population health than an intensive outpatient intervention. The goal of economic analysis is to provide an analytical framework to think about these tradeoffs.

Beyond improvements in health, there are also considerable societal benefits associated with AUD treatment. AUD treatment has been found to have many benefits to society, including increased labor market participation and productivity of employees while at work, reduced healthcare utilization, and reduced crime. Economic models can be designed to estimate the impact of AUD treatment on these outcomes. If an AUD recovery program is found to produce societal benefits that outweigh its costs, it can provide compelling evidence to policy makers that the program should be implemented and/or that usage of the recovery program could be expanded. The fact that Alcoholics Anonymous has been found to produce comparable treatment outcomes with 45 percent lower treatment costs is one possible explanation for its widespread usage and support among policy makers (Humphreys & Moos, 1996). The objective of this chapter is to describe the economic costs and benefits associated with alcohol consumption and the economic models used to evaluate AUD interventions and/or recovery programs.

The Economic Costs and Benefits of Alcohol Consumption

The negative consequences of alcohol consumption are substantial. Studies that evaluate the total societal costs associated with an illness or condition are known as burden of illness or cost of illness studies. A number of these studies have attempted to evaluate the overall economic costs associated with AUD. Sacks et al. (2015) estimated the annual economic cost of excess alcohol consumption in the United States to be about $249 billion, or approximately 1.5 percent of the country's gross domestic product (GDP), an economic measure of the size of an economy. For reference, the economic burden of HIV in the United States has been estimated to be $36.4 billion (Hutchinson et al., 2006), and the economic burden of cancer in the United States has been estimated to be $80.2 billion (American Cancer Society, 2020). Similar results have been estimated in numerous other countries. The annual economic burden of alcohol in India has been estimated to be 1.45 percent of GDP (Jyani et al., 2019) and the burden of alcohol dependence in Europe has been estimated to be as high as 0.095 percent of GDP (Laramée et al., 2013). Overall, the worldwide burden of alcohol is estimated to be as much as $650 billion, or 2.0 percent of global GDP (Baumberg, 2006).

This substantial burden of alcohol on society stems from a combination of individual health outcomes and societal outcomes. Alcohol has been linked with liver disease (Becker et al., 1996) and cancer (Boffetta & Hashibe, 2006), and high levels of alcohol consumption have been linked to lower life expectancy (Wood et al., 2018). Up to six percent of deaths worldwide are related to alcohol consumption (Bardach et al., 2019). Alcohol has been shown to be associated with reduced employment and poor workplace performance (Mullahy & Sindelar, 1996; Pidd et al., 2006). Also, while there is a complicated relationship between alcohol and crime, a large proportion of crimes are committed when an individual has been drinking (Dingwall, 2013; Greenfeld, 1998).

Although the substantial costs associated with alcohol are clear, there are also societal benefits associated with alcohol. People's enjoyment of alcohol is real, if hard to quantify. Also, alcohol is big business. For instance, in California the wine industry employs more than 700,000 Americans and generates over $100 billion in economic activity (Wine Institute, 2020). Thus, social programs designed to mitigate the burden of alcohol must be evaluated through a complex lens.

Economic Methods Used to Evaluate AUD Recovery Programs

To guide policy makers, clinicians, program administrators, and the general public on the tradeoffs associated with AUD recovery programs, a number of economic methodologies have been developed, including cost, cost-effective, cost-utility, burden of illness, and benefit-cost models. French (2000) and Bray and Zarkin (2006) reviewed these methods in further detail. The reason that a number of economic methodologies exist is that economic studies serve diverse audiences with a range of different perspectives. Policy makers are particularly interested in the societal impact of an intervention. Benefit-cost models are designed to assess the overall societal impact of AUD recovery programs. Clinicians may be primarily interested in comparing different types of programs in order to maximize health benefit (e.g., maximizing the number of successful recovery outcomes). Cost-effectiveness models are particularly well suited to answer these questions. Also, healthcare and jail-system administrators and managers of businesses may have budget constraints and/or profit motives that may be important drivers of their decisions to incorporate AUD recovery programming into their protocols. The next several sections describe the three most common methodologies used to evaluate AUD interventions and/or recovery programs: cost, benefit-cost, and cost-effectiveness models.

Cost Analysis

The first step in evaluating an intervention/recovery program from an economic perspective is evaluating the costs associated with providing the program. Standalone cost analyses can be important in understanding the feasibility of implementing an AUD recovery program. For instance, policy makers or program administrators may simply want to know, if they were to implement a recovery program, how much it would cost. Also, understanding how much a program costs is an important reference point with which to compare the benefits of the program.

When generating cost estimates, there is an important distinction between accounting costs and economic costs. Accounting costs are the actual costs incurred by the program (e.g., rent, wages paid to staff, and amount paid for supplies and materials). Economic costs equal accounting costs plus other "opportunity" costs that may not directly be paid for by the program. For instance, sometimes labor, materials, or space may be donated to a recovery program. These are not accounting costs, as the program does not explicitly pay for them; however, they are economic costs because, if the recovery program did not exist, these resources could be used productively elsewhere. Also, economic costs include the cost of participant time.

Which type of cost estimates (accounting or economic) to use depends on the perspective of the analysis. Analysis designed to understand the incentives and/or behavior of program administrators should evaluate the program from the perspective of the provider (usually limited to accounting costs). Analysis designed to inform policy should evaluate economic costs. Also, economic costs provide a more realistic approximation of the cost of replicating a recovery program elsewhere.

To estimate the cost of AUD and other substance-related treatments, a couple of standardized costing procedures have been developed. While it is not essential to use a standardized costing procedure, these procedures provide a comprehensive and standardized way to collect cost data. Also, it is easier to compare cost estimates for different types of treatment programs if the same cost program is used. One standardized instrument is the Drug Abuse Treatment Cost Analysis Program (DATCAP), a program developed by French et al. (1997). This instrument has been widely used to calculate the economic costs of over 100 substance use disorder treatment programs (French et al., 2008). Another program that has been developed is the Substance Abuse Services Cost Analysis Program (SASCAP) (Zarkin et al., 2004). The benefit of the SASCAP is that it is relatively quicker and easier to implement and is easier to estimate costs at the individual component service level (Bray & Zarkin, 2006).

To generate cost estimates, program administrators (or research staff for a clinical trial) are interviewed, and additional information can be obtained from financial statements, budgets, and/or fiscal reports of a program. This is usually an iterative process that begins with semi-structured meetings with program administrators who explain the treatment protocol and general details about the program. Program administrators or research staff provide financial documents, which can be used to determine a number of cost components. After financial statements are reviewed, additional meetings are held with program administrators to review, validate, and clarify cost estimates obtained from financial records.

Cost categories to be considered include screening, equipment, labor, administrative, laboratory, information technology (IT), start-up, and space costs. Depending on the type of intervention, some of these cost categories may not be relevant. Screening costs are explicitly noted because they are easily missed and can be a considerable cost component (Barbosa et al., 2016; Horn et al., 2017; Kunz Jr et al., 2004; Zarkin et al., 2003). Equipment, laboratory, and labor costs are relatively straightforward to estimate. Equipment should be depreciated over time, with the length of time depending on how long each piece of equipment is expected to last. Sometimes prices or the value of equipment and materials change over time. When necessary, it is appropriate to use replacement costs rather than the price paid by the program; also, it may be necessary to adjust for inflation. Labor is typically the most expensive cost component. The cost of labor is usually estimated by determining the number of hours worked for each general work category (e.g., clinical psychologist, AUD counselor) and multiplying the number of hours worked in each category by either the regional median wage rate for that category or the self-reported hourly wage (plus benefits).

Start-up costs can be a complicated cost component to incorporate because they may involve high, one-time, initial costs. Including these costs at the beginning of a project's life could produce an artificially high cost estimate compared with what is expected once the program has been running for some time. However, not including these costs may create cost estimates that are too low. Barbosa et al. (2018) provided a framework to estimate start-up costs. Also, a distinction can be made between fixed costs and quasi-fixed costs (Bray et al., 2015). To address the complicated long-run impact of start-up costs, it may make sense to provide robustness estimates that exclude start-up costs. Additionally, average start-up costs can be extrapolated using a stepwise cost structure analysis (Horn et al., 2018).

If a program uses rented or financed space and uses the space full time, then rent or mortgage payments can serve as a good approximation for space costs. However, some programs do not directly pay for their space (e.g., programs implemented as part of a larger hospital system) or may not pay market rates (e.g., property that was donated or provided at a discount). Under these circumstances it is common to obtain the square footage of space and approximate square footage costs using comparable property values or hourly rental rates.

When evaluating costs for a clinical trial, there are a number of additional considerations (Polsky & Glick, 2009). A treatment implemented for the first time may be more time consuming, and some costing elements may be different in a clinical trial than when implemented in clinical practice (e.g., a research assistant's time rather than a substance use disorder counselor's time). Grant activities not associated with the intervention (e.g., implementing survey questions) are generally not included in cost analysis. Finally, while it may be difficult to quantify using clinical data, AUD treatment programs as well as other types of treatment programs may exhibit economies of scale, meaning that the average cost of treatment decreases as the annual number of patients treated increases (Barbosa et al., 2016; Horn et al., 2016, 2018; Yilmaz et al., 2018).

Benefit-Cost Analysis

The method used to evaluate the overall economic impact of an AUD treatment interaction from a societal perspective is benefit-cost analysis (interchangeably termed cost-benefit analysis). The objective of benefit-cost analysis is to quantify all the societal benefits of an intervention and contrast them with the intervention's costs. If the benefits of the program are found to outweigh its costs, this provides evidence that the program benefits society. However, just because a program's benefits are larger than its costs does not necessarily mean a program will be adopted. There are many valuable societal programs and projects, and budgets are limited. Benefit-cost analysis allows social programs to be evaluated across treatment modalities or even societal projects. For instance, the benefits and costs of an AUD recovery program could be compared with the benefits and costs of building a bridge or constructing a professional sporting stadium. Theoretically, this allows policy makers to spend money in a way that maximizes the societal benefits that can be generated within government budget allocations.

Several papers have found AUD interventions to have benefits that considerably outweigh their costs. For instance, Fleming et al. (2000) and Mundt et al. (2005) found that, compared to a no-treatment comparison group in which participants received a general health booklet, brief physician advice for problem drinkers resulted in societal benefits that were considerably higher than the societal cost of treatment. Note that because the goal of benefit-cost analysis is to determine the overall societal benefits of an intervention, it is ideal to have a comparison group that did not receive any treatment. Many clinical trials are designed to compare an advanced treatment strategy with a treatment-as-usual comparison group. While benefit-cost analysis can be applied to this type of study design, the resulting economic analysis will not capture the overall societal impact of the program; instead, it will capture the benefits using one treatment modality compared with another. Many times, cost-effective analysis, described in the next section, is used to compare two (or more) different types of interventions. Also, for studies with quasi-experimental designs, propensity score or entropy matching techniques can be used to create a comparison group that is similar in terms of pre-treatment characteristics (e.g., age, gender, race, employment, substance use, and/or criminal histories) (Barbosa et al., 2015; Hainmueller, 2012; Horn et al., 2020).

While AUD is linked with a myriad of economic outcomes, the outcome domains evaluated in economic evaluations are usually individual health, criminal activity, labor market participation, and healthcare utilization. To elicit information about these outcome domains, data can be obtained from either administrative datasets (e.g., insurance claims data and administrative crime datasets) or self-reported survey data. More comprehensive data can usually be collected via surveys. The specific survey questions that should be asked depend on context. Fleming et al. (2000) provides a good template. Also, the Economic Form 90 can be used to capture patient-level cost and outcome data (Bray et al., 2007; Tonigan et al., 1997).

At this stage, a researcher needs to beware of double counting. Double counting is a common error in all types of benefit-cost analysis, which involves counting the same benefit multiple times. For instance, when evaluating the economic impact of an AUD recovery program, it is tempting to use outcome domains such as the psychic benefit, or increased happiness, that friends and family might receive from an individual abstaining or drinking in a healthier way. However, counting the increased "happiness" that others receive from the direct recipients increase in "happiness" is an example of the circular extra-counting process that benefit-cost analysis tries to avoid. Although, note that direct benefits to family members, such as reductions in domestic abuse, can and should be included.

Once the impact of a recovery program has been estimated, outcomes must be monetized. This involves multiplying the estimated impact of the recovery program for each economic outcome by its corresponding societal value. These values, known as unit cost estimates, are usually obtained from the literature. Everything else equals, the more recent the unit cost estimate, the better. Also note that all unit costs will need to be adjusted for inflation and reflect a base year. Recent unit cost estimates for different types of crime have been generated by McCollister et al. (2017). However, these estimates do not include the expected costs for drinking and driving. Although a recent source for the expected cost of drinking and driving does not appear to be available, Barbosa et al. (2015) used a combination of data from Miller (1996) and the Fatality Analysis Reporting System (FARS) from the National Highway Traffic Safety Administration. Also, a large impact of AUD interventions has been found for labor market participation. Typically, this outcome is measured by calculating changes in a patient's self-reported number of hours worked and then monetizing this outcome by the patient's average hourly wage. Median wage rates can usually be obtained from the Bureau of Labor Statistics.

To construct a benefit-cost ratio, all monetized outcome variables are summed and then divided by estimated societal costs. Also, a net benefit approach can be utilized (Bray & Zarkin, 2006). Note that societal costs of a recovery program include participant time costs. Also, to accurately compare benefits of a recovery program with its costs, outcomes must be adjusted for inflation. Inflation is a natural part of an economy, where the price of goods and services gets more expensive over time, and thus the value of money decreases over time. Because the costs of an AUD recovery program are immediate and the benefits deferred, the future stream of benefits derived from an AUD program must be adjusted for inflation. Consumer Price Index data obtained from the Bureau of Labor Statistics supply a standard measure of inflation.

To test the significance of individual economic outcomes, some papers have used standard *t*-tests or one-way analysis of variance. However, economic outcomes often suffer from skewness or kurtosis. To mitigate the non-normality associated with these outcomes, a number of non-parametric tests can be used, including a Mann-Whitney (or Wilcoxon rank-sum) test, a Kolmogorov-Smirnov test, or a Kruskall-Wallis test (Polsky & Glick, 2009). To test the significance of benefit-cost ratios, it is common to use non-parametric bootstrapping. Finally, it is also important to determine the sensitivity of estimated results to model assumptions and imputed parameters. It is common to calculate sensitivity analysis by estimating separate models that both increase and decrease the value of imputed parameters. Also, probability distributions can be used, and worst- and best-case scenarios can be calculated.

Cost-Effective Analysis

The most common method used to evaluate AUD interventions is cost-effective analysis. As the name suggests, this method compares the tradeoff between the differences in effectiveness of two or more treatment modalities and the differences in cost between the two interventions. For instance, Zarkin et al. (2008) studied the cost-effectiveness of three different outpatient treatments for AUD: (1) medical management with placebo, (2) medical management plus naltrexone, and (3) medical management plus combined naltrexone and acamprosate therapy. To estimate the cost-effectiveness of one treatment modality compared with another, it is common to use incremental cost-effectiveness ratios (ICER), which can be represented by the following ratio: $(C_j - C_i)/(E_j - E_i)$. In this equation C_j indicates the cost of intervention j, C_i indicates the cost of intervention i, E_j indicates the clinical effect of intervention j (e.g., average number of weekly drinks, days abstinent, avoided heavy drinking outcomes) and E_i indicates the clinical effect of intervention i. Thus, this equation is simply the ratio of the difference in the average costs of the two interventions to the difference in average treatment effects. Again, non-parametric tests (e.g., Kruskal-Wallis) and bootstrapping methods are usually used for significance testing.

Also, for cost-effective analysis, an important distinction concerns what constitutes the economic costs in the numerator. For baseline models, it is common to use treatment costs (i.e., cost estimates generated by the DATCAP or SASCAP instruments); however, it is also not uncommon to estimate models that include societal costs, such as health, social services, criminal justice, and productivity losses (Barbosa et al., 2015; Barrett et al., 2006). Note that this is different from benefit-cost analysis, where changes in these types of societal outcomes were considered "benefits." However, the same monetizing methods can be used.

When comparing two different recovery programs, there are two notable relationships between cost and effectiveness. First, one recovery program could be both more effective and less costly than another recovery program. In this case, the first is said to *economically dominate* the second, and it is obvious which recovery program is preferred. Second, one recovery program could be more effective but also more costly than another. In this case, an incremental cost-effectiveness ratio is presented, and the acceptable tradeoff between recovery outcomes and costs is left up to program administrators or policy makers.

Interested readers can learn more about interpreting cost-effectiveness from Bala and Zarkin (2002). For a cost-effectiveness example, Zarkin et al. (2008) estimated that a medical management plus naltrexone therapy intervention modality costed approximately $262 more per patient than medical management plus a placebo, but it also had a nine percentage point increase in the proportion of patients who avoided heavy drinking. Thus, to obtain a patient who avoided heavy drinking using medical management plus naltrexone therapy compared with medical management alone, we estimate that it would cost $262 divided by 0.09 or approximately $2,911.

Like benefit-cost analysis, the final step of cost-effective analysis is to calculate sensitivity analysis. This can involve varying modeling assumptions and imputed cost parameters. Also, it is common to estimate cost-effectiveness acceptability curves. As mentioned earlier, which recovery program should be adopted depends on how much program administrators or policy makers "value" recovery outcomes. Cost-effectiveness acceptability curves plot the probability that a recovery program is cost-effective across different levels of willingness to pay for the health outcome of interest.

Conclusions and Recommendations

Economic analysis can be an important tool used to consider tradeoffs associated with AUD recovery interventions and can help guide policy decisions to allocate resources in the most effective way possible. However, there are many different types of study designs and data sources that can be used to evaluate the economic impact of AUD interventions, and numerous different types of economic questions and perspectives are important in understanding the economics of interventions. This chapter outlines the three most common types of economic methods used to evaluate AUD interventions: cost, cost-effective, and benefit-cost analysis.

There is a substantial literature evaluating the economic impact of interventions for substance use disorders, and, while still relatively sparse, a subset of studies evaluated the economic impact of AUD interventions. Notably, this research has shown a valuable impact of brief interventions for alcohol in emergency departments (Barbosa et al., 2015; Barrett et al., 2006; Kunz Jr et al., 2004). However, the economic impact of the broader range of available professional treatment and other services to support AUD recovery has not been well researched. For example, as previously mentioned, Humphreys and Moos (1996) found that Alcoholics Anonymous produced similar drinking outcomes at much lower costs than an outpatient comparison group, but there are many relatively unknown economic aspects of Alcoholics Anonymous, other mutual help groups, and alcohol services associated with the criminal justice system. Yet, not considered in this prior work are the societal costs associated with mutual help groups such as the opportunity cost of attending meetings and the space used for holding meetings. It is also difficult to quantify the considerable societal benefit associated with AUD intervention services and mutual help groups, such as Alcoholics Anonymous, including decreased crime and increased labor market participation.

Finally, while it is commonplace to narrowly define alcohol treatment success as abstinence, there appear to be substantial economic benefits associated with reductions in drinking that fall short of abstinence (Magnus et al., 2012). Also, there are many pathways to AUD recovery, treatment-assisted recovery is only one pathway to change, and the majority of people with AUD will eventually recover on their own without receiving treatment (see Tucker, Chapter 9 this volume). The economic costs and benefits of alternative pathways are largely unknown, including in relation to treatment-assisted change. Broader market interventions such as alcohol taxation and policies designed to reduce alcohol outlet densities (e.g., more restrictive liquor license laws) could reduce alcohol consumption and potentially nudge individuals toward recovery (see Kerr & Subbaraman, Chapter 19 this volume). These topics deserve empirical inquiry and will help inform the relative costs and benefits of alcohol interventions across the spectrum of services and support rational decisions about relative resource allocation to different segments of the spectrum of AUD and the population in need.

References

American Cancer Society (2020, October 30). *Economic impact of cancer.* www.cancer.org/cancer/cancer-basics/economic-impact-of-cancer.html

Bala, M. V., & Zarkin, G. A. (2002). Application of cost-effectiveness analysis to multiple products: A practical guide. *American Journal of Managed Care, 8* (3), 211–220. PMID: 11915971

Barbosa, C., Cowell, A., Bray, J., & Aldridge, A. (2015). The cost-effectiveness of alcohol screening, brief intervention, and referral to treatment (SBIRT) in emergency and outpatient medical settings. *Journal of Substance Abuse Treatment, 53*, 1–8. https://doi.org/10.1016/j.jsat.2015.01.003

Barbosa, C., Cowell, A. J., Landwehr, J., Dowd, W., & Bray, J. W. (2016). Cost of screening, brief intervention, and referral to treatment in health care settings. *Journal of Substance Abuse Treatment, 60*, 54–61. https://doi.org/10.1016/j.jsat.2015.06.005

Barbosa, C., Wedehase, B., Dunlap, L., Mitchell, S. G., Dusek, K., Schwartz, R. P., Gryzcynski, J., Kirk, A. S., Oros, M., & Hosler, C. (2018). Start-up costs of SBIRT implementation for adolescents in urban US federally qualified health centers. *Journal of Studies on Alcohol and Drugs, 79*(3), 447–454. https://doi.org/10.15288/jsad.2018.79.447

Bardach, A. E., Alcaraz, A. O., Ciapponi, A., Garay, O. U., Riviere, A. P., Palacios, A., Cremonte, M., & Augustovski, F. (2019). Alcohol consumption's attributable disease burden and cost-effectiveness of targeted public health interventions:

A systematic review of mathematical models. *BMC Public Health, 19*(1), 1378. https://doi.org/10.1186/s12889–019-7771-4

Barrett, B., Byford, S., Crawford, M. J., Patton, R., Drummond, C., Henry, J. A., & Touquet, R. (2006). Cost-effectiveness of screening and referral to an alcohol health worker in alcohol misusing patients attending an accident and emergency department: A decision-making approach. *Drug and Alcohol Dependence, 81* (1), 47–54. https://doi.org/10.1016/j.drugalcdep.2005.05.015

Baumberg, B. (2006). The global economic burden of alcohol: A review and some suggestions. *Drug and Alcohol Review, 25*(6), 537–551. https://doi.org/10.1080/09595230600944479

Becker, U., Deis, A., Sorensen, T. I., Gronbaek, M., Borch-Johnsen, K., Muller, C. F., Schnohr, P., & Jensen, G. (1996). Prediction of risk of liver disease by alcohol intake, sex, and age: A prospective population study. *Hepatology, 23*(5), 1025–1029. https://doi.org/10.1002/hep.510230513

Boffetta, P., & Hashibe, M. (2006). Alcohol and cancer. *The Lancet Oncology, 7*(2), 149–156. https://doi.org/10.1016/s1470–2045(06)70577-0

Bray, J. W., & Zarkin, G. A. (2006). Economic evaluation of alcoholism treatment. *Alcohol Research & Health, 29*(1), 27–33.

Bray, J. W., Zarkin, G. A., Miller, W. R., Mitra, D., Kivlahan, D. R., Martin, D. J., Couper, D. J., & Cisler, R. A. (2007). Measuring economic outcomes of alcohol treatment using the Economic Form 90. *Journal of Studies on Alcohol and Drugs, 68*(2), 248–255. https://doi.org/10.15288/jsad.2007.68.248

Caliendo, M., & Kopeinig, S. (2008). Some practical guidance for the implementation of propensity score matching. *Journal of Economic Surveys, 22*(1), 31–72. https://doi.org/10.1111/j.1467-6419.2007.00527.x

Dingwall, G. (2013). *Alcohol and crime*. Routledge.

Fleming, M. F., Mundt, M. P., French, M. T., Manwell, L. B., Stauffacher, E. A., & Barry, K. L. (2000). Benefit-cost analysis of brief physician advice with problem drinkers in primary care settings. *Medical Care, 38*(1), 7–18. https://doi.org/10.1097/00005650-200001000-00003

French, M. T. (2000). Economic evaluation of alcohol treatment services. *Evaluation and Program Planning, 23*(1), 27–39.

French, M. T., Dunlap, L. J., Zarkin, G. A., McGeary, K. A., & McLellan, A. T. (1997). A structured instrument for estimating the economic cost of drug abuse treatment: The drug abuse treatment cost analysis program (DATCAP). *Journal of Substance Abuse Treatment, 14*(5), 445–455. https://doi.org/10.1016/s0740–5472(97)00132-3

French, M. T., Popovici, I., & Tapsell, L. (2008). The economic costs of substance abuse treatment: Updated estimates and cost bands for program assessment and reimbursement. *Journal of Substance Abuse Treatment, 35*(4), 462–469. https://doi.org/10.1016/j.jsat.2007.12.008

Greenfeld, L. A. (1998). *Alcohol and crime: An analysis of national data on the prevalence of alcohol involvement in crime*. US Department of Justice, Office of Justice Programs, Bureau of Justice Statistics.

Hainmueller, J. (2012). Entropy balancing for causal effects: A multivariate reweighting method to produce balanced samples in observational studies. *Political Analysis*, 20(1), 25–46. https://doi.org/https://doi.org/10.1093/pan/mpr025

Horn, B. P., Barragan, G. N., Fore, C., & Bonham, C. A. (2016). A cost comparison of travel models and behavioral telemedicine for rural, Native American populations in New Mexico. *Journal of Telemedicine and Telecare*, *22*(1), 47–55. https://doi.org/10.1177/1357633X15587171.

Horn, B. P., Crandall, C., Forcehimes, A., French, M. T., & Bogenschutz, M. (2017). Benefit-cost analysis of SBIRT interventions for substance using patients in emergency departments. *Journal of Substance Abuse Treatment*, *79*, 6–11. https://doi.org/10.1016/j.jsat.2017.05.003

Horn, B. P., Li, X., Mamun, S., McCrady, B., & French, M. T. (2018). The economic costs of jail-based methadone maintenance treatment. *American Journal of Drug and Alcohol Abuse*, *44*(6), 611–618. https://doi.org/10.1080/00952990.2018.1491048

Horn, B. P., Li, X., McCrady, B., Guerin, P., & French, M. T. (2020). Cost-effectiveness analysis of a large jail-based methadone maintenance treatment continuation program in New Mexico. *Journal of Substance Abuse Treatment*, *115*, [108042]. https://doi.org/10.1016/j.jsat.2020.108042

Humphreys, K., & Moos, R. H. (1996). Reduced substance-abuse-related health care costs among voluntary participants in Alcoholics Anonymous. *Psychiatric Services*, *47*(7), 709–713. https://doi.org/10.1176/ps.47.7.709

Hutchinson, A. B., Farnham, P. G., Dean, H. D., Ekwueme, D. U., Del Rio, C., Kamimoto, L., & Kellerman, S. E. (2006). The economic burden of HIV in the United States in the era of highly active antiretroviral therapy: Evidence of continuing racial and ethnic differences. *JAIDS Journal of Acquired Immune Deficiency Syndromes*, *43*(4), 451–457. https://doi.org/10.1097/01.qai.0000243090.32866.4e

Jyani, G., Prinja, S., Ambekar, A., Bahuguna, P., & Kumar, R. (2019). Health impact and economic burden of alcohol consumption in India. *International Journal of Drug Policy*, *69*, 34–42. https://doi.org/10.1016/j.drugpo.2019.04.005.

Kunz, Jr., F. M., French, M. T., & Bazargan-Hejazi, S. (2004). Cost-effectiveness analysis of a brief intervention delivered to problem drinkers presenting at an inner-city hospital emergency department. *Journal of Studies on Alcohol*, *65*(3), 363–370. https://doi.org/10.15288/jsa.2004.65.363

Laramée, P., Kusel, J., Leonard, S., Aubin, H.-J., François, C., & Daeppen, J.-B. (2013). The economic burden of alcohol dependence in Europe. *Alcohol and Alcoholism*, *48*(3), 259–269. https://doi.org/10.1093/alcalc/agt004

Magnus, A., Cadilhac, D., Sheppard, L., Cumming, T., Pearce, D., & Carter, R. (2012). The economic gains of achieving reduced alcohol consumption targets for Australia. *American Journal of Public Health*, *102*(7), 1313–1319. https://doi.org/10.2105/AJPH.2011.300453

McCollister, K., Yang, X., Sayed, B., French, M. T., Leff, J. A., & Schackman, B. R. (2017). Monetary conversion factors for economic evaluations of substance use disorders. *Journal of Substance Abuse Treatment*, *81*, 25–34. https://doi.org/10.1016/j

Miller, T. R. (1996). *Victim costs and consequences: A new look*. US Department of Justice, Office of Justice Programs, National Institute of Justice.

Mullahy, J., & Sindelar, J. (1996). Employment, unemployment, and problem drinking. *Journal of Health Economics*, *15*(4), 409–434. https://doi.org/10.1016/s0167–6296(96)00489-4

Mundt, M. P., French, M. T., Roebuck, M. C., Manwell, L. B., & Barry, K. L. (2005). Brief physician advice for problem drinking among older adults: An economic analysis of costs and benefits. *Journal of Studies on Alcohol*, *66*(3), 389–394. https://doi.org/10.15288/jsa.2005.66.389

Pidd, K. J., Berry, J. G., Roche, A. M., & Harrison, J. E. (2006). Estimating the cost of alcohol-related absenteeism in the Australian workforce: The importance of consumption patterns. *Medical Journal of Australia*, *185*(11–12), 637–641. https://doi.org/10.5694/j.1326-5377.2006.tb00738.x

Polsky, D., & Glick, H. (2009). Costing and cost analysis in randomized controlled trials: Caveat emptor. *Pharmacoeconomics*, *27*(3), 179–188. https://doi.org/10.2165/00019053-200927030-00001

Sacks, J. J., Gonzales, K. R., Bouchery, E. E., Tomedi, L. E., & Brewer, R. D. (2015). 2010 national and state costs of excessive alcohol consumption. *American Journal of Preventive Medicine*, *49*(5), e73–e79. https://doi.org/10.1016/j.amepre.2015.05.031

Tonigan, J. S., Miller, W. R., & Brown, J. M. (1997). The reliability of Form 90: An instrument for assessing alcohol treatment outcome. *Journal of Studies on Alcohol*, *58*(4), 358–364. https://psycnet.apa.org/doi/10.15288/jsa.1997.58.358

Wine Institute (2020, October 10). *Economic impact of California wine*. http://wine-economy.com

Wood, A. M., Kaptoge, S., Butterworth, A. S., Willeit, P., Warnakula, S., Bolton, T., Paige, E., Paul, D. S., Sweeting, M., . . . & Danesh, J. (2018). Risk thresholds for alcohol consumption: Combined analysis of individual-participant data for 599 912 current drinkers in 83 prospective studies. *The Lancet*, *391*(10129), 1513–1523. https://doi.org/10.1016/S0140–6736(18)30134-X

Yilmaz, S. K., Horn, B. P., Fore, C., & Bonham, C. A. (2018). An economic cost analysis of an expanding, multi-state behavioral telehealth intervention. *Journal of Telemedicine and Telecare*, *25*(6), 353–364. https://doi.org/10.1177/1357633X18774181

Zarkin, G. A., Bray, J. W., Aldridge, A., Mitra, D., Mills, M. J., Couper, D. J., & Cisler, R. A. (2008). Cost and cost-effectiveness of the COMBINE study in alcohol-dependent patients. *Archives of General Psychiatry*, *65*(10), 1214–1221. https://psycnet.apa.org/doi/10.1001/archpsyc.65.10.1214

Zarkin, G. A., Bray, J. W., Davis, K. L., Babor, T. F., & Higgins-Biddle, J. C. (2003). The costs of screening and brief intervention for risky alcohol use. *Journal of Studies on Alcohol*, *64*(6), 849–857. https://doi.org/10.15288/jsad.2012.73.911

Zarkin, G. A., Dunlap, L. J., & Homsi, G. (2004). The substance abuse services cost analysis program (SASCAP): A new method for estimating drug treatment services costs. *Evaluation and Program Planning*, *27*(1), 35–43. https://doi.org/10.1016/j.evalprogplan.2003.09.002

Conclusions and Future Directions

23 Dynamic Pathways to Recovery from Alcohol Use Disorder

Advancing the Scientific Agenda and Policy Priorities

Katie Witkiewitz and Jalie A. Tucker

Dynamic Pathways to Recovery from Alcohol Use Disorder: Advancing the Scientific Agenda and Policy Priorities

As noted in the Preface and described in chapters throughout this book, consensus has emerged that recovery from alcohol use disorder (AUD) encompasses improvements in health, functioning, and well-being, and abstinence may not be required to achieve improved functioning and quality of life. This expanded view of recovery is slowly being accepted in a variety of circles, including among alcohol researchers, service providers, policy-makers, mutual help groups, and persons with AUD. The United States has lagged behind many countries with respect to harm reduction policies and support for harm reduction services. Yet, at the time of finalizing this book, the people of the United States had recently elected Joseph R. Biden, Jr. as the 46th President, and President Biden has indicated support for a harm reduction agenda. Given these changes, we believe that the alcohol field is at a critical turning point for understanding and supporting the expanded definition of AUD recovery described in Chapter 1 and in chapters throughout this volume. The broader research, treatment, community, and policy landscape has started to consider extending definitions of recovery to include alternative pathways. Correspondingly, new research, assessment, analysis, and community engagement methods will be essential and critical to capturing nuanced changes in functioning and the multilevel influences that support heterogeneous recovery pathways. In this final chapter, we discuss each major section of the book with a specific focus on identifying research opportunities and limitations, novel developments, and innovative future directions. We conclude with a statement of hope and aspiration for the field.

The socio-ecological model of influences on AUD recovery guided the organization of the book with chapters presenting recovery research that ranged from micro to meso to macro level approaches, coupled with methodologies for studying the different levels of analysis. When developing the book prospectus and charting the course for the book, we were interested in including authors and voices with varied expertise and who were at various career stages. We took active roles as editors and provided extensive feedback to help authors consider a range of research, practice, and policy perspectives, often with a focus toward future directions and limitations in our understanding. We endeavored to push beyond the dominant micro-level perspective of individuals as change agents and to consider the broader ways in which environments can shape individual change and how policies can shape environments that support or hinder recovery. We sought to bring together harm reduction, behavioral, economic, and public health approaches to understanding and promoting recovery and to present methodological advances that may stimulate novel research questions and approaches for studying dynamic pathways to recovery at the micro, meso, and macro levels. Throughout the book, we were mindful of the needs and concerns of the diverse stakeholders in the alcohol field, ranging from researchers, service providers, policy makers, and, vitally important, persons with lived experience of AUD, their families and social networks, and those who are consumers of alcohol-focused services.

Micro-Level: The Individual as Change Agent

The focus on individual-level factors in the book's first section is consistent with much prior research on AUD and AUD recovery, including biopsychosocial processes of change during recovery (Witkiewitz & Maisto, Chapter 2), self-regulation strategies (Roos et al., Chapter 3), neuropsychological and biological influences on drinking behavior change (Bates et al., Chapter 4), lifespan developmental perspectives on recovery mechanisms (Lee et al., Chapter 5), and mutual help approaches and mechanisms of change (Tonigan, Chapter 6). Two methodological chapters focused on novel quantitative models for examining longitudinal data that can be used to study AUD recovery processes and outcomes at the individual level, including time-varying effect modeling (Linden-Carmichael et al., Chapter 7) and latent variable mixture modeling (Cheong et al., Chapter 8).

The chapters in the micro-level section identified several shortcomings in our understanding and suggested many future research directions. Despite decades of research on AUD relapse, Witkiewitz and Maisto highlighted the relative dearth of studies that examined processes of recovery at the individual level over time, and Roos and colleagues highlighted the lack of studies examining self-regulation during recovery. Most studies relied on individuals recruited from treatment programs and/or Alcoholics Anonymous (AA) members, who comprise highly selective samples in relation to the larger population of persons who engage in harmful alcohol use and/or fulfill AUD diagnostic criteria. The vast majority of these individuals never attend mutual support groups or receive formal alcohol treatment, and only a limited number of studies have been conducted with this untreated population segment. Thus, we know relatively little about individual level risk and protective factors that might support "natural" recovery from AUD, even though a raft of epidemiological research indicates it is the dominant pathway to recovery in the population. Further, the fact that AA is strictly abstinence-based – as are most treatment programs – has limited investigation of individual- and treatment-level factors that might support non-abstinent recovery pathways, even though these outcomes occur regardless of the intervention "program theory" and drinking goals.

The chapter by Roos and colleagues discussed the understudied concept of self-regulation and also identified areas that deserve further inquiry, including a greater focus on measurement of momentary contextual events and processes that might support recovery and more research on mindfulness- and acceptance-based treatments for supporting self-regulation and recovery pathways. Compared to conventional treatment approaches, mindfulness- and acceptance-based treatments are far less focused on specific behaviors (e.g., drinking or not drinking, amount of consumption) and much more focused on the whole person and their experience of the world, which is consistent with core tenets of dynamic and multidimensional recovery pathways. For example, in mindfulness-based relapse prevention the amount a person drinks is rarely (if ever) discussed, and treatment is far more focused on direct momentary experiences, including cultivating awareness during nourishing experiences and decreasing reactivity during depleting experiences (Witkiewitz et al., 2019a).

Bates and colleagues contributed a very broad and digestible overview of the neuropsychological, neurocognitive, and neurophysiological impairments that are commonly studied among individuals with AUD, while Lee and colleagues offered an overview of a lifespan developmental approach to AUD recovery with a specific focus on etiological models of AUD. Gaining a better understanding of the biological underpinnings of AUD that may attenuate recovery pathways and how recovery is experienced over the life course are both critically important for advancing research and treatment of dynamic AUD recovery pathways. Despite decades of research on the brain and neurodevelopmental processes in AUD progression, we still know very little about how individuals with AUD may recover. A common but myopic focus on the absence of disorder and total abstinence from alcohol has provided scant new knowledge about how individuals who develop risky drinking behaviors and AUD may return to a state of better health and functioning. The brain disease model of AUD in particular has failed to provide new insights into recovery, and it is unclear whether the study of brain development over time will further understanding of how recovery may manifest across the lifespan or as the disorder evolves (Heather et al., 2018).

Throughout the past century, AA has played a major role in dictating recovery definitions, recovery services, and supporting millions of people in recovery from AUD. Several meta-analytic reviews found participation in AA to be associated with increased abstinence and improved functioning. Most studies focused on AA engagement (e.g., attending meetings, having a sponsor) and attainment of abstinence, with fewer focusing on broader definitions of recovery and "sobriety," which is a central concept and vital aspiration in AA that goes beyond abstinence. As expressed by Tonigan, sobriety and recovery involve "enhanced well-being, awareness of serenity, an absence of economic insecurity, and a positive change in attitude and outlook on life." This definition is quite consistent with the broadened evidence-based definition of recovery described throughout this book, although the pathway AA embraces to achieve it is narrow and singular. More research is needed on mutual help alternatives to AA, including SMART Recovery, Women for Sobriety, and LifeRing. Many people are interested in alternative options, particularly options that are less focused on abstinence as the only acceptable goal. These other mutual help programs may be as effective as AA for those who self-select into them, and they may have more potential to support a life worth living, particularly among individuals who do not want to adhere to an abstinence recovery pathway.

The methodological chapters in the micro level section provide a clear and succinct overview of novel approaches to studying individual change processes over time, which may facilitate a more nuanced understanding of recovery as a dynamic process of change. Linden-Carmichael and colleagues provided an introduction to time-varying effect modeling, which is useful for studying the timing of dynamic changes in predictors and outcomes over time, without requiring specific functional forms of change (e.g., nonlinear change). Time-varying effect modeling may be particularly well suited to studying how changes in substance use and other functional outcomes may co-occur and dynamically interact across time. The chapter by Cheong and colleagues provided an overview of latent variable mixture modeling approaches to studying AUD recovery. Mixture models offer a useful tool for parsing heterogeneity in predictors and/or outcomes, as well as heterogeneity in trajectories of change over time. The chapters illustrated the use of these methods in research evaluating a continuing care intervention (Linden-Carmichael et al.) and research on natural recovery processes, as well as profiles of recovery up to 10 years following AUD treatment (Cheong et al.). Both methods may be useful tools for assessing dynamic recovery pathways, particularly those pathways that are not solely defined by levels of drinking and assess diverse recovery pathways characterized by improvements in both health and functioning.

Meso-Level: Understanding and Promoting Individual Behavior Change within Natural Environments

The book's second section focused on the role of the surrounding natural environment in individual behavior change, specifically contextual influences on beneficial change in alcohol-related and alcohol-free behavior patterns (Chapters 9–15). An overarching and empirically supported organizing principle is that alcohol and other drug use can be reduced by enriching the environment with rewarding alternatives to use. Murphy and colleagues (Chapter 10) discussed behavioral interventions ranging from very brief interventions to intensive alcohol treatment programs that focus on incentivizing behavior change and/or enriching the natural environment to provide rewarding alternatives to drinking. The interventions aim explicitly to expand and increase personally meaningful and/or enjoyable activities that can take the place of harmful alcohol use and thus contrast with many conventional treatments that emphasize reductions in substance use, including abstinence, without much concern with improving other areas of functioning. Evidence primarily using young adult samples indicated that these interventions can increase treatment adherence, engagement, and outcomes. Additional work is needed to address implementation challenges and methods for broadening the reach of these treatments to individuals in the untreated segment of the population with alcohol problems and those who live in rural and disadvantaged communities.

The core of the interventions discussed by Murphy and colleagues are based on behavioral principles, including behavioral economics. This approach is expanded in Chapter 9 by Tucker, who discussed the patterns, contexts, and behavioral economics of natural recovery from AUD. Tucker summarized a research program that spans over two decades, called Alcohol Recovery in Community (Project ARC), which followed individuals prospectively who self-identified as having recently resolved an alcohol problem on their own (i.e., “natural recovery”). Recovery status and outcomes were verified using objective measures of drinking practices, problems, and monetary allocation to activities and commodities available in the natural environment. Results highlighted how specific spending patterns (i.e., economic behaviors) were more or less favorable in supporting recovery. A key finding was that the spending patterns of persons who achieved stable non-abstinent recoveries differed from those who abstained or relapsed, who were more similar. Economic resources and expenditures may provide useful measures for characterizing recovery contexts and a common metric to assess relative preference for drinking compared to healthy alternatives. Project ARC findings underscore the importance of expanding the scope of assessment in line with a broadened definition of recovery and considering the role of surrounding life contexts.

Building on the theme of life context, Jarnecke and colleauges (Chapter 11) contributed a rich overview of research on family and social processes in AUD and recovery. Although the role of family and social environments on AUD and recovery are variable across individuals, there is a robust literture indicating the potential for close others to support, sustain, or impede heterogeneous and dynamic recovery pathways. The chapter also reviews interventions, programs, and approaches that have successfully integrated family and social support during the recovery process. More research is needed on the dynamics of family and social contexts in supporting recovery using an expanded definition of recovery, as well as on family and social factors that may be relevant among individuals from diverse cultural backgrounds and among those with a variety of recovery goals.

Drawing on a diverse community advisory board and years of coalition building and community engaged scholarship, the chapter by Collins et al. (Chapter 12) described a program of community-based harm reduction approaches for AUD that argues for taking a serious harm reduction approach to supporting AUD recovery. The chapter reviewed the relevant evidence and offered a compelling narrative about how their research team focused on recovery while embedded in and collaborating with the community being served by AUD harm reduction services. The chapter concluded with a call for more funding to support non-abstinence-based recovery services, including non-abstinence-based housing for those experiencing homelessness; community-based recovery services that offer harm reduction options; and greater focus on community building and engagement in meaningful activities.

The meso section included three chapters that describe an innovative range of assessment tools and quantitative methods to assess AUD recovery among individuals in context, including the application of mobile technologies to understand and improve recovery outcomes (Pearson et al., Chapter 13), quantitative methods for measuring and modeling social network data in studies of recovery in social context (Hallgren, Chapter 14), and measures assessing substance use contexts and substance-free reinforcement (Yurasek et al., Chapter 15). Mobile technologies are critical for assessing environmental and social contexts of recovery in near real time and could be expanded to provide interventions to support recovery in the moment. Mobile technology could also be used to assess social networks, which may further inform understanding of how recovery unfolds dynamically within complex social structures and processes. Using mobile technology would also be very useful in measuring substance-free reinforcement and meaningful engagement within substance-free contexts. The field of AUD recovery has traditionally relied on the measurement of drinking practices, but a range of tools like mobile technologies could be used to study the expanded definition of recovery. Assessing improvements in health and functioning during recovery is a vital next step for the field. Assessments in near real-time that capture social network and contextual effects will advance this objective and can be aggregated over varying temporal intervals to investigate contextual factors surrounding inflection points, transitions, and periods of stability during recovery attempts.

Macro-Level: Creating Environments, Resources, Incentives, and Policies to Promote Harm Reduction and Recovery

The book's final section focuses on understanding features of the broader macro environment that influence drinking and AUD recovery to inform the creation of environments, resources, incentives, and policies to promote harm reduction and recovery. Recovery communities, recovery identity, and "recovery capital" are important resources that can support an individual with AUD on a recovery pathway characterized by personal growth and societal belonging (Best et al., Chapter 16). A community-oriented recovery system is also essential to support a strengths-based approach to supporting recovery.

Whereas the chapter by Best and colleagues focused on recovery communities and cities, the chapter by Snell-Rood and colleagues (Chapter 17) focused on recovery at the community level in rural settings, highlighting the isolation and barriers to recovery that can exist in historically disadvantaged rural communities. The chapter covered trends in alcohol use and AUD in rural communities and discussed privacy and access concerns that are significant challenges to supporting interventions for AUD and AUD recovery among people living in rural areas. Increased access to AUD treatment and recovery services in primary care and greater capacity for telehealth care services (requiring corresponding increases in infrastructure for widespread broadband access) are offered as a few of the potential solutions to this longstanding problem. For example, New Mexico, a predominantly rural state where many chapter authors live and work, has the highest rate of alcohol-related mortality in the United States, yet treatment services are non-existent in many rural areas. Such gaps in rural care underscore the need for future research, treatment, and policy that invests in rural communities and supports community-based interventions that are culturally tailored and accessible.

The focus on recovery communities is expanded in the chapter by Ashford (Chapter 18), who covers broader goals for a recovery movement involving individuals, communities, and policies that seeks to increase access to evidence-based recovery services. Ashford outlined a case for building a recovery movement that supports long-term changes in how we treat, study, legislate, and empower individuals with AUD to connect within communities and develop a life worth living. Ashford's chapter covered the many barriers to successful recovery faced by individuals with AUD, including incarceration, family separation, and implicit and explicit biases that prevent securing basic support for living (e.g., housing, employment); and he offered recommendations for how specific policies and the advancement of recovery science may ameliorate decades of stigmatization towards individuals with AUD. Harm reduction and health promotion approaches to prevention, intervention, and policies are crucial to support well-being and engagement in meaningful activities during recovery.

The focus on policy is given fuller coverage in the chapter by Kerr and Subbaraman (Chapter 19) on alcohol control policy and regulations to promote AUD recovery. The task for Kerr and Subbaraman was not easy given that most policy-related research has focused on harmful alcohol use (e.g., driving while intoxicated, adolescent binge drinking) and trying to curb excessive alcohol use among those with severe AUD. Yet, much of this prior research may hold clues for policies that could potentially promote AUD recovery, including taxation, pricing policies, alcohol availability controls, outlet density limits, hours of sale restrictions, and marketing and advertising restrictions. As noted by the authors, alcohol policies shape the environmental availability and behavior of individuals who drink alcohol. Promoting and supporting alcohol control and taxation policies that favor reduced alcohol consumption and less social acceptability and availability of alcohol could potentially shape AUD recovery in ways that are similar to how tobacco control and taxation have changed the landscape of tobacco acceptability and smoking cessation outcomes.

The methodology chapters in the macro section take a broad view of how causal inference approaches can be used to address issues involved in studying recovery processes in the absence of experimental designs (Steinley, Chapter 20); how communities can be engaged in developing, designing, and implementing a mobile recovery program using a smartphone app (SURE; Bowen et al, Chapter 21); and how economic methods can be used to evaluate and promote cost-effective AUD recovery programs, with emphasis on diverse economic outcomes and policy considerations (Horn, Chapter 22). Future directions for the SURE application involve dissemination issues, including supporting service providers in using the app with their clients, receiving feedback from providers and clients on features to enhance the app experience, promoting research with the app, and allowing organizations to implement the app as part of policy initiatives. In his concluding comments, Horn noted that there are substantial economic benefits associated with drinking reductions, but the economic costs and benefits of recovery pathways that are not focused on abstinence are largely unknown. The notion that recovery could be defined by functioning, well-being, and quality of life indicators opens up new possibilities for market interventions and economic analyses of recovery pathways. As a group, these methodological chapters contribute to advancing understanding of how communities, natural environments, economic factors, and policies can be studied and expanded to extend the reach of recovery services and understand the role of economic factors in a broadened approach to defining and promoting recovery.

Conclusions and Recommendations

As noted in the Preface, this book is intended to advance our understanding and inspire new empirical work on AUD recovery. The chapters in the volume span multiple levels of analysis – from individuals to contexts to communities to policies – and provide a broader lens for considering domains of assessment and methodological tools that are fundamental to understanding and promoting an expanded definition of recovery. We endeavored to challenge the assumption that sustained abstinence was a necessary and sufficient condition for AUD recovery and underscored the strong empirical basis for a broadened definition of recovery that focuses on improvements in valued areas of living, functioning, and well-being. Further, we brought together experts in the field to identify and discuss new empirical research that is needed; what theories, treatments, and policies need to be reconsidered or adapted; and how this collective body of work can make a difference in helping individuals and communities.

Several shared challenges for the alcohol field were revealed across multiple chapters. First, we must address more effectively what the early psychotherapy evaluation field referred to as the "criterion problem" with respect to what outcomes are important to measure (Lambert, 2013). Much like early studies of psychodynamic psychotherapy effectiveness that focused on a simple dichotomous outcome of "cured" or not, the alcohol field has focused for far too long on a simple dichotomous outcome of abstinent or not. Decades ago the psychotherapy field expanded the domains of outcome assessment to provide a more nuanced picture of client changes in diagnostic symptoms and functioning in important life areas as viewed by the client and therapist. The alcohol field has made some progress in this direction, but there is much more to be done. On the one hand, we now have excellent measures of drinking practices, even though we often reduce them to a handful of outcome categories (e.g., number of abstinent and heavy drinking days). On the other hand, we have only begun to characterize drinking patterns over time, which exhibit considerable heterogeneity, including during recovery attempts. Exciting recent work has started to examine variability in the temporal patterning of alcohol use and corresponding levels of relative risk for poor outcomes, including but not limited to health risks. For example, research suggests intermittent binge drinking with intervening abstinent days carries relatively greater health risks than stable levels of daily drinking (e.g., Gronbach, 2009). Research that investigates risks associated with drinking patterns rather than single day or weekly thresholds and separates quantity/frequency dimensions of consumption (cf. Cheong et al., 2020) will inform more nuanced guidelines for lower-risk drinking patterns than are currently available.

Second, despite the emphasis placed by early behavior therapists on a broadly conceived functional analysis of drinking behavior, measures of functioning, well-being, and life circumstances relevant to characterizing AUD and recovery progress have not been widely incorporated into recovery research in a systematic way. As several chapters discussed, viable candidate measures exist and should receive wider adoption, so that a critical subset that reflects improved well-being and is important for recovery can be identified and used as best practices in research. This is in addition to the assessment of changes in the negative consequences of harmful alcohol use and those associated with reductions in alcohol use. There is also opportunity for improvement in the latter domain as well. Considerable evidence indicates that AUD is a heterogeneous disorder and that drinking problem severity is a multi-dimensional construct involving varying degrees of physiological dependence on alcohol and adverse psychosocial and health consequences (Litten et al., 2015; Witkiewitz et al., 2019b). Ideally, changes in domains reflecting negative effects of harmful drinking and benefits of drinking reductions should be assessed as routinely as changes in alcohol consumption, coupled with the routine assessment of functioning, well-being, and life circumstances.

Third, investigating the time course and dynamic changes involved in patterns of alcohol use, harmful use, remission, and relapse are essential to understanding how stable long-term recovery is achieved and merit greater research attention. Harmful drinking careers and their resolution are highly variable over time between and across individuals (Fillmore, 1988; Polich et al., 1980), and the causes of this variability remain poorly understood. As several chapters discussed, contextual factors such as life events, alcohol and alcohol-free reward availability, and family and social resources appear to be highly influential.

However, our ability to carefully measure and categorize relevant events in the environment lags far behind our ability to measure behavior and brain events, which has almost certainly contributed to their relative neglect in etiological accounts of AUD. This is an important area for future inquiry that is essential to support research guided by a broadened definition of recovery.

It is also vital to develop conceptual models and conduct research on how variables operating at different levels of analysis may interact with one another to promote or hinder recovery. For example, the efficacy, reach, and impact of a given treatment likely varies as a function of broader structural variables, such as economic and social factors and health care availability, access, and cost (Prado et al., 2013). However, such treatment by context interactions have rarely been investigated in the alcohol field and may be important to understanding and redressing health disparities affected by harmful drinking. The multi-level perspective on recovery presented in this volume offers a framework for exploring how variables established as influential within a given level of analysis influence or interact with influential variables at other levels.

Finally, knowledge about AUD recovery, particularly in light of the broadened definition, is at an early stage of development, and we cannot afford to take a view of evidence that is overly restrictive in focus or methodology. Using randomized controlled trial designs to evaluate treatment efficacy is a good fit between research and method, but, as discussed in several chapters, there are other questions relevant to understanding pathways to recovery that are not amenable to experimentation and are better addressed with non-experimental designs and methods, or a combination of the two approaches. For example, understanding what influences people with AUD to seek and engage in treatment and mutual-help groups and how these self-selection processes and contextual influences contribute to change are often better studied using observational research methods (Tucker & Roth, 2006). Rigorous observational studies that adhere to best research practices will continue to be essential to advancing understanding of recovery processes and outcomes that occur outside the context of formal treatment, including via AA or other mutual help group participation or in the absence of interventions. Mobile technology and sensing devices will likely be very useful for expanding understanding of the recovery process and the dynamic interactions between person, social networks, and contextual factors, which have been under-studied due to the limitations of traditional self-report assessments using longitudinal panel models that measure psychological variables across wide time frames (e.g., every three months).

In summary, we have learned a great deal in collating and editing this volume and hope that our readers have also expanded their horizons in considering future directions for research, prevention, treatment, and policy. We are hopeful that our field is at a turning point. It is time to acknowledge and carry forward all that we have learned about AUD recovery over the past 100 years, while leaving behind the rigid and fundamental belief that abstinence is the only path to recovery and the only meaningful change involved. There are many pathways to recovery, and it is best understood as a contextualized longitudinal process of change, as others have argued in the context of advancing intervention science (Hofmann & Hayes, 2019), including with respect to alcohol treatment (Moos et al., 1990). We encourage the field to embrace this heterogeneity and embark on new research, community action, and policy-making to support the many pathways to recovery.

References

Cheong, J., Lindstrom, K., Chandler, S. D., & Tucker, J. A. (2020). Utility of different dimensional properties of drinking practices to predict stable low-risk drinking outcomes of natural recovery attempts. *Addictive Behaviors, 106*, 106387 https://doi.org/10.1016/j.addbeh.2020.106387

Fillmore, K. M. (1988). *Alcohol use across the life course: A critical review of 70 years of international longitudinal research.* Addiction Research Foundation.

Grønbaek, M. (2009). The positive and negative health effects of alcohol – and the public health implications. *Journal of Internal Medicine, 265*, 407–420. https://doi.org/10.1111/j.1365-2796.2009.02082.x

Heather, N., Best, D., Kawalek, A., Field, M., Lewis, M., Rotgers, F., Wiers, R. W., & Heim, D. (2018). Challenging the brain disease model of addiction: European launch of the addiction theory network. *Addiction Research & Theory, 26*(4), 249–255. https://doi.org/10.1080/16066359.2017.1399659

Hoffman, S. G., & Hayes, S. C. (2019). The future of intervention science: Process-based therapy. *Clinical Psychological Science, 7*(1), 37–50. https://doi.org/10.1177/2167702618772296

Lambert, M. J. (2013). Outcome in psychotherapy: The past and important advances. *Psychotherapy, 50*(1), 42–51. http://dx.doi.org/10.1037/a0030682

Litten, R. Z., Ryan, M. L., Falk, D. E., Reilly, M., Fertig, J. B., & Koob, G. F. (2015). Heterogeneity of alcohol use disorder: Understanding mechanisms to advance personalized treatment. *Alcoholism: Clinical and Experimental Research, 39*(4), 579–584. https://doi.org/10.1111/acer.12669

Moos, R. H., Finney, J. W., & Cronkite, R. C. (1990). *Alcoholism treatment: Context, process, and outcome.* Oxford University Press.

Polich, J. M., Armor, D. J., & Braiker, H. B. (1980). *The course of alcoholism: Four years after treatment.* Rand Corporation (R-2433-NIAAA).

Prado, G., Lightfoot, M., & Brown C. H. (2013). Macro-level approaches to HIV prevention among ethnic minority youth: State of the science, opportunities, and challenges. *American Psychologist, 68*(4), 286–299. https://doi.org/10.1037/a0032917

Tucker, J. A., & Roth, D. L. (2006). Extending the evidence hierarchy to enhance evidence-based practice for substance use disorders. *Addiction, 101*(7), 918–932. https://doi.org/10.1111/j.1360-0443.2006.01396.x

Witkiewitz, K., Litten, R. Z., & Leggio, L. (2019b). Advances in the science and treatment of alcohol use disorder. *Science Advances, 5*(9), eaax4043. https://doi.org/10.1126/sciadv.aax4043

Witkiewitz, K., Stein, E. R., Votaw, V. R., Wilson, A. D., Roos, C. R., Gallegos, S. J., Clark, V. P., & Claus, E. D. (2019a). Mindfulness-based relapse prevention and transcranial direct current stimulation to reduce heavy drinking: A double-blind sham-controlled randomized trial. *Alcoholism: Clinical and Experimental Research, 43*(6), 1296–1307. https://doi.org/10.1111/acer.14053

Index

Printed in Dunstable, United Kingdom

76705167R00264